F

SURGICAL
CRITICAL
CARE

ESSENTIALS OF

SURGICAL CRITICAL CARE

EDITED BY

Jerome H. Abrams, M.D.

Assistant Professor of Surgery and Associate Director of Critical Care,
Department of Surgery, University of Minnesota; Staff Surgeon,
Minneapolis VA Medical Center,
Minneapolis, Minnesota

Frank B. Cerra, M.D.

Professor of Surgery, Department of Surgery, University of Minnesota;
Director of Surgical Critical Care and Director of Nutritional Support Services,
University of Minnesota Hospital and Clinic, Minneapolis, Minnesota,
and St. Paul–Ramsey Medical Center,
St. Paul, Minnesota

with 204 illustrations

QUALITY MEDICAL PUBLISHING, INC

ST. LOUIS, MISSOURI 1993

Copyright © 1993 by Quality Medical Publishing, Inc.

Printed in the United States of America.

PUBLISHER   Karen Berger

PROJECT MANAGER   Carlotta Seely

PRODUCTION   Judy Bamert

DESIGN   Diane M. Beasley

Quality Medical Publishing, Inc.
2086 Craigshire Drive
St. Louis, Missouri 63146

LIBRARY OF CONGRESS CATALOGING-IN-PUBLICATION DATA

Essentials of surgical critical care / edited by Jerome H. Abrams,
    Frank B. Cerra.
        p.   cm.
    Includes bibliographical references and index.
    ISBN 0-942219-31-7 (text)
    1. Surgical intensive care.   2.   Critical care medicine.
3. Therapeutics, Surgical.   I.   Abrams, Jerome H., 1949-
II.   Cerra, Frank B.
    [DNLM: 1.   Intensive Care—methods.   WX 218 E78]
RD51.5.E77   1993
617'.919—dc20
DNLM/DLC
for Library of Congress   92-49329
                                                              CIP

GW/M/M
5   4   3   2   1

CONTRIBUTORS

Jerome H. Abrams, M.D.
Assistant Professor of Surgery and
Associate Director of Critical Care,
Department of Surgery,
University of Minnesota;
Staff Surgeon,
Minneapolis VA Medical Center,
Minneapolis, Minnesota

David H. Ahrenholz, M.D.
Assistant Professor,
Department of Surgery,
University of Minnesota,
Minneapolis, Minnesota;
Associate Director, Burn Unit,
St. Paul–Ramsey Medical Center,
St. Paul, Minnesota

Roderick A. Barke, M.D.
Assistant Professor,
Department of Surgery,
University of Minnesota;
Director, Critical Care Units,
Minneapolis VA Medical Center,
Minneapolis, Minnesota

Richard G. Barton, M.D.
Assistant Professor of Surgery,
Department of Surgery,
University of Utah,
Salt Lake City, Utah

Jon F. Berlauk, M.D.
Assistant Professor of Anesthesiology,
Department of Anesthesiology, and
Assistant Director, SICU,
University of Minnesota,
Minneapolis, Minnesota

Joseph R. Bloomer, M.D.
Professor of Medicine,
Department of Gastroenterology, and
Director of Gastroenterology, Hepatology,
    and Nutrition,
University of Minnesota,
Minneapolis, Minnesota

Pamela K. Borchardt-Phelps, Pharm.D.
Clinical Assistant Professor,
College of Pharmacy, and
Clinical Supervisor,
Department of Pharmaceutical Services,
University of Minnesota Hospital and Clinic,
Minneapolis, Minnesota

John R. Border, M.D.
Professor of Surgery, Orthopaedics, and
    Biophysics,
Department of Surgery,
State University of New York at Buffalo,
Erie County Medical Center,
Buffalo, New York

Anthony Bottini, M.D.
Chief, Neurosurgery Service,
Department of Surgery,
Tripler Army Medical Center,
Honolulu, Hawaii

Philip G. Boysen, M.D.
Professor of Anesthesiology and Medicine,
University of Florida College of Medicine;
Chief, Anesthesia Services, and
Co-Director, Surgical Intensive Care,
VA Medical Center,
Gainesville, Florida

Timothy G. Buchman, M.D., Ph.D.
Associate Professor of Surgery,
Department of Surgery,
Johns Hopkins University School of
    Medicine,
Baltimore, Maryland

Richard W. Carlson, M.D., Ph.D.
Chairman and Professor of Medicine,
Department of Medicine,
University of Illinois College of Medicine,
Peoria, Illinois

Frank B. Cerra, M.D.
Professor of Surgery,
Department of Surgery,
University of Minnesota;
Director of Surgical Critical Care and
Director of Nutritional Support Services,
University of Minnesota Hospital and Clinic,
Minneapolis, Minnesota, and
St. Paul–Ramsey Medical Center,
St. Paul, Minnesota

Mark D. Cipolle, M.D., Ph.D.
Critical Care Fellow,
Department of Surgery,
University of Minnesota,
Minneapolis, Minnesota

Vivian L. Clark, M.D.
Clinical Instructor,
Department of Cardiology,
University of Michigan,
Ann Arbor, Michigan;
Senior Staff Cardiologist,
Henry Ford Hospital,
Detroit, Michigan

Ricardo Correa-Rotter, M.D.
Head, Department of Nephrology,
Instituto Nacional de la Nutrición/Salvador
    Zubiran,
Mexico City, Mexico

Alan J. Cropp, M.D.
Assistant Professor,
Northeastern Ohio Universities College of
    Medicine;
Assistant Director of Critical Care Medicine,
St. Elizabeth Hospital Medical Center,
Youngstown, Ohio

Robert E. Cunnion, M.D.
Senior Investigator and Chief,
Cardiovascular Section,
Department of Critical Care Medicine,
National Institutes of Health,
Bethesda, Maryland

Elizabeth A. Davis, M.D.
Assistant Professor,
Department of Physical Medicine and
    Rehabilitation,
University of Minnesota,
Minneapolis, Minnesota

James P. Davison, D.O.
Resident in Internal Medicine,
Department of Internal Medicine,
St. Elizabeth Hospital Medical Center,
Youngstown, Ohio

R. Phillip Dellinger, M.D., M.Sc.
Associate Professor and
Director of Critical Care,
Department of Medicine,
Baylor College of Medicine,
Houston, Texas

Paul Druck, M.D.
Clinical Instructor in Surgery,
Department of Surgery,
University of Minnesota,
Minneapolis, Minnesota

David L. Dunn, M.D., Ph.D.
Associate Professor of Surgery and
Head of Surgical Infectious Diseases,
Department of Surgery,
University of Minnesota,
Minneapolis, Minnesota

David C. Evans, M.D.
Chief Resident,
Department of Surgery,
McGill University,
Montreal, Quebec,
Canada

Steven D. Eyer, M.D.
Assistant Professor,
Department of Surgery,
University of Minnesota,
Minneapolis, Minnesota

Martha A. Fehr, M.D.
Staff Physician,
Department of Neurology,
University of Minnesota,
Minneapolis, Minnesota

Barry W. Feig, M.D.
Junior Faculty Associate,
Department of Surgery,
University of Texas M.D. Anderson Cancer
  Center,
Houston, Texas

Ian J. Gilmour, M.D.
Assistant Professor,
Department of Anesthesiology,
University of Minnesota,
Minneapolis, Minnesota

Paul Gustafson, R.N., C.R.T.T.
Cardiopulmonary Specialist,
Cardiopulmonary Services,
University of Minnesota Hospital and Clinic,
Minneapolis, Minnesota

Guillermo Gutierrez, M.D., Ph.D.
Professor,
Division of Pulmonary and Critical Care
  Medicine,
University of Texas Health Science Center
  Medical School,
Houston, Texas

James Hassett, M.D.
Associate Professor,
Department of Surgery,
State University of New York at Buffalo,
Buffalo, New York

Keith Henry, M.D.
Assistant Professor of Medicine,
Department of Medicine,
Section of Infectious Diseases,
University of Minnesota,
Minneapolis, Minnesota;
Director, HIV Programs,
St. Paul–Ramsey Medical Center,
St. Paul, Minnesota

Sharon Henry, M.D.
Assistant Professor,
Department of Surgery,
State University of New York
  Health Science Center,
Brooklyn, New York

Marshall I. Hertz, M.D.
Associate Professor,
Department of Internal Medicine,
University of Minnesota,
Minneapolis, Minnesota

Steven M. Hollenberg, M.D.
Senior Staff Fellow,
Department of Critical Care Medicine,
National Institutes of Health,
Bethesda, Maryland

John W. Hoyt, M.D.
Clinical Professor of Anesthesiology/Critical
  Care,
Department of Anesthesiology/Critical Care
  Medicine,
University of Pittsburgh,
Pittsburgh, Pennsylvania

David S. Knopman, M.D.
Associate Professor,
Department of Neurology,
University of Minnesota,
Minneapolis, Minnesota

James A. Kruse, M.D.
Associate Professor,
Division of Critical Care Medicine,
Wayne State University School of Medicine,
Detroit, Michigan

Becky Jo Lekander, R.N., M.S.N., C.C.R.N.,
C.S.
Clinical Nurse Specialist,
Department of Nursing Services,
University of Minnesota Hospital and Clinic,
Minneapolis, Minnesota

George M. Logan, M.D.
Assistant Professor of Medicine,
Section of Gastroenterology,
Department of Internal Medicine,
St. Paul–Ramsey Medical Center,
St. Paul, Minnesota

Bruce C. Lohr, Pharm.D.
Clinical Assistant Professor,
College of Pharmacy,
University of Minnesota;
Clinical Specialist,
Department of Pharmacy,
University of Minnesota Hospital and Clinic,
Minneapolis, Minnesota

Connie L. Manske, M.D.
Associate Professor,
Division of Nephrology,
Department of Medicine,
University of Minnesota,
Minneapolis, Minnesota

John E. Mazuski, M.D.
Assistant Professor of Surgery,
Department of Surgery,
St. Louis University School of Medicine,
St. Louis, Missouri

John W. McBride, M.D.
Assistant Professor of Medicine,
Division of Cardiology,
University of Minnesota,
Minneapolis, Minnesota;
Section of Cardiology,
St. Paul–Ramsey Medical Center,
St. Paul, Minnesota

Jonathan L. Meakins, M.D., D.Sc.
Professor and Chairman,
Department of Surgery,
McGill University,
Montreal, Quebec,
Canada

Larry Micon, M.D.
Medical Director,
Trauma Service,
Methodist Hospital of Indiana,
Indianapolis, Indiana

Beth M. Nelson, R.N., M.S.
Assistant Nurse Manager,
Department of Surgical Intensive Care,
University of Minnesota Hospital and Clinic,
Minneapolis, Minnesota

Michael D. Pasquale, M.D.
Critical Care Fellow,
Department of Surgery,
University of Minnesota,
Minneapolis, Minnesota

Elizabeth H. Perry, M.D.
Assistant Professor,
Department of Laboratory Medicine and
  Pathology,
University of Minnesota;
Assistant Medical Director,
Blood Bank,
University of Minnesota Hospital and Clinic,
Minneapolis, Minnesota

Michael R. Pinsky, M.D.
Professor and Director of Research,
Division of Critical Care Medicine,
Department of Anesthesiology and Critical
  Care Medicine,
University of Pittsburgh,
Pittsburgh, Pennsylvania

Mark E. Rosenberg, M.D.
Assistant Professor,
Division of Renal Diseases and
  Hypertension,
Department of Internal Medicine,
University of Minnesota,
Minneapolis, Minnesota

**Ori D. Rotstein, M.D., F.R.C.S.(C),
F.A.C.S.**
Associate Professor,
Department of Surgery,
University of Toronto,
Toronto, Ontario,
Canada

Richard L. Simmons, M.D.
George V. Foster Professor of Surgery;
Associate Dean for Clinical Affairs,
School of Medicine;
Associate Vice-President for Clinical Affairs,
University of Pittsburgh Medical Center,
Pittsburgh, Pennsylvania

Lynn D. Solem, M.D.
Assistant Professor,
Department of Surgery,
University of Minnesota;
Director, Burn Unit,
St. Paul–Ramsey Medical Center,
St. Paul, Minnesota

Oren K. Steinmetz, M.D.
Fellow,
Department of Surgery,
McGill University,
Montreal, Quebec,
Canada

David C. Templeman, M.D.
Assistant Professor of Orthopedic Surgery,
Department of Orthopedics,
University of Minnesota;
Staff Surgeon,
Hennepin County Medical Center,
Minneapolis, Minnesota

Fernando Torres, M.D.
Professor,
Department of Neurology,
University of Minnesota,
Minneapolis, Minnesota

Gregory M. Vercellotti, M.D.
Associate Professor,
Department of Internal Medicine,
University of Minnesota,
Minneapolis, Minnesota

Kathleen V. Watson, M.D.
Assistant Professor,
Department of Internal Medicine,
University of Minnesota,
Minneapolis, Minnesota

Larry A. Woods, D.O.
Assistant Professor of Internal Medicine,
Department of Internal Medicine,
Northeastern Ohio Universities
    College of Medicine;
Director, Critical Care Medicine,
St. Elizabeth Hospital Medical Center,
Youngstown, Ohio

Thomas Wozniak, M.D.
Senior Surgical Resident,
Department of Surgery,
Methodist Hospital of Indiana,
Indianapolis, Indiana

Carol H. Wysham, M.D.
Department of Internal Medicine,
Rockwood Clinic,
Spokane, Washington

Karl L. Yang, M.D.
Assistant Professor,
Division of Pulmonary and Critical Care
    Medicine,
University of Texas Health Science Center,
Houston, Texas

To the residents and fellows of the
UNIVERSITY OF MINNESOTA DEPARTMENT OF SURGERY

PREFACE

The rapid progress taking place in understanding of the pathophysiology and treatment of critically ill patients presents many challenges to the student of critical care. To place the new findings into a meaningful context requires a framework that includes global pathophysiology, specific organ dysfunction, systemic dysfunction, technical aspects of patient monitoring, and art of practice. This book is our effort to provide a framework for each of these components. It has been written for those individuals who are beginning their study of surgical critical care. Rooted in practical considerations, this book is meant for people who enjoy solving clinical problems.

Our goals have been to provide the foundation for understanding current ideas about the presentation and mechanism of the altered physiology and metabolism seen in the critically ill patient, to offer approaches to problems that are frequently encountered, and to suggest an approach when consensus about a clinical problem does not exist. Examples of the last consideration are found in "Strategies for Pulmonary Support When Conventional Ventilation Methods Fail" (Chapter 28). In the absence of clear agreement among all who treat the problems described in that chapter, we have offered our current practice, which has been useful in our experience. In addition, we have attempted to provide practical information for managing SICU patients and to present it in a concise format.

This book is neither an encyclopedia of critical care nor a brief outline. Our guiding principle has been to include the information that we wished someone had told us when we began to care for patients in the SICU. Since reading about principles of care and applying them to patients are not equal tasks, we have provided a companion volume of case studies that includes analysis of the cases by the chapter authors of this book. We hope that the reader, by comparing his or her thoughts with those of the authors, will have increased opportunity to learn.

We are indebted to the contributors to this volume for all their hard work. In addition, this book would have been impossible without the help of Joan M. Johnson. Her organizing strengths and literary skills kept the dark forces of chaos at bay. Working with everyone at Quality Medical Publishing, Inc., has been a great pleasure. We offer special thanks to Carlotta Seely, whose expert and comprehensive management kept this project on course and on time. We are especially indebted to Professor John S. Najarian for his continuing support, both of this book and of the surgical critical care program at the University of Minnesota.

We must bear responsibility for any errors that may remain in the text. Not only for that reason but also because of the rapidly occurring changes in critical care, we wish that this book could have been written in pencil.

Jerome H. Abrams
Frank B. Cerra

CONTENTS

PART THREE

PATHOPHYSIOLOGIC CONDITIONS

PART FOUR

SYSTEMIC DYSFUNCTION

PART FIVE

COMMON SICU PROCEDURES

PART SIX

MEASUREMENT AND INTERPRETATION OF DATA

PART SEVEN

THE ART OF PRACTICE

ESSENTIALS OF
SURGICAL
CRITICAL
CARE

PART ONE

ALTERED METABOLISM OF CRITICAL ILLNESS AND SHOCK

CHAPTER 1

Response to Injury and Multiple System Organ Failure

Jerome H. Abrams · Timothy G. Buchman · Frank B. Cerra

When the human response to stress is adaptive, it is a coordinated, integrated act of physiology and metabolism. As understanding of the stress response increases, the relations among genetic, cellular, tissue, organ, and physiologic reactions of the human increasingly become the focus of research and therapeutic trials. How do major injuries, such as multiple trauma, burns, sepsis, or pancreatitis, cause systemic cellular injury? How are subcellular and cellular events translated into macroscopic physiologic responses? The path to clinical organ failure illustrates current understanding of the relations between cellular responses and physiologic changes as well as the events that require further explanation. This chapter considers the features of the hypermetabolic response and the transition to the organ failure syndrome. A more comprehensive review of the metabolic response to injury, stress, and starvation has been done by Gann et al.[1]

The path to the multiple system organ failure (MSOF) syndrome begins with an indentifiable, and usually major, insult. Multiple trauma, sepsis, burns, severe pancreatitis, or a ruptured abdominal aortic aneurysm activate a carefully balanced stress response. In the absence of complications, the stress response is regulated and self-limited. If the result overwhelms the adaptive mechanisms, a continuing response occurs, the hypermetabolic response, and culminates in MSOF. The clinical consequences of injury are a result of the injury itself and, perhaps more significantly, the individual's own organ reserves and ability to maintain homeostasis.

MSOF, which has been recognized since the mid-1970s, is a process that evolves predominantly in those patients sustaining trauma, major surgery, and, especially, widespread infection. In the SICU 80% to 85% of deaths result from MSOF. Among patients who survive, the costs, including those of rehabilitation, are high, and the time for rehabilitation frequently exceeds twice the length of time spent in the SICU.[2]

CLINICAL FEATURES

MSOF syndrome does not involve isolated organ failure. Rather, it is the sequential and accumulated failure of all the major organ systems of the body that occurs until significant and concomitant dysfunction is seen in the lung, liver, kidneys, and nervous system. The stereotypic order of events is an inciting injury, adult respiratory distress syndrome, hypermetabolism, and, finally, MSOF syndrome. Several classes of injury have been associated with MSOF. These include microcirculatory failure (shock), ischemia/reperfusion, sepsis, significant soft tissue injury, necrotic tissue, and local inflammation with systemic effects, such as pancreatitis.[3]

Once the source of injury has been controlled, the patient seemingly responds to supportive measures such as IV fluids and ventilator therapy. After several days, low-grade fever, tachycardia, and dyspnea appear. The CXR reveals bilateral, diffuse, patchy infiltrates. The patient's mental status may be altered. Respiratory distress progresses, and intubation and mechanical ventilation may prove necessary. At this point when the patient demonstrates hemodynamic stability, as measured by heart rate and urine output, the characteristic features of hypermetabolism are already present. The cardiac index is elevated, often >4.5 L/min/m², the oxygen consumption is increased (>180 ml/min/m²), and the systemic vascular resistance is low. Another feature consistent with hypermetabolism is urinary nitrogen excretion of >15 g/day with no nutrient administration.

The clinical herald of MSOF is jaundice. After 7 to 10 days the bilirubin concentration exceeds 3 mg/dl. At the time jaundice appears, the biliary tree is dilated, cholestasis is present, and sludge is evident on ultrasound examination. These changes are mirrored by deterioration in other hepatic functions: hepatic protein synthesis of albumin, transferrin, prealbumin, and retinol-binding protein falls. Development of jaundice is temporally associated with measurable changes in other metabolic variables. Oxygen consumption rises and cardiac output increases, with a concomitant decrease in SVR. Wound healing deteriorates and pressure lesions of the skin are common. The patient becomes thrombocytopenic. As organ failure progresses, increased volume is needed to maintain preload and inotropes become necessary to maintain adequate cardiac output and oxygen delivery. In later organ failure, blood, urine, or sputum cultures often demonstrate the presence of *Candida* organisms and viruses. Between hospital days 14 and 21, renal failure worsens and dialysis may be necessary.

The transition to clinical MSOF is correlated with a change in mortality. Early MSOF has a mortality of 40% to 60%, whereas in late MSOF the mortality exceeds 90%. Clinically, the more pronounced liver failure and renal failure distinguishes early MSOF from late MSOF. In late MSOF, coma is profound, and the bilirubin concentration is >8 mg/dl. Indeed, the transition from hypermetabolism to MSOF is associated with clinically apparent liver failure. Persistent perfusion deficit, persistent systemic infection, recurrent episodes of hypotension, and pancreatitis all are implicated in the transition from hypermetabolism to MSOF. Evidence for hepatic failure includes progressive jaundice, decreasing amino acid clearance, reduction in hepatic protein synthesis, unrestricted ureagenesis in the absence of protein administration, and decreased triglyceride clearance. In late MSOF, the reduced redox potential of the liver is apparent in increased BOHB/AcAc, and terminally hypoglycemia occurs.

The primary overall response in MSOF is an increase in oxygen consumption. The patient must maintain adequate arterial oxygen saturation and increased cardiac output to provide the increased oxygen delivery necessary for survival. A pathologic condition of the lungs may interfere with arterial oxygen saturation. The lung may demonstrate a primary pathologic state in the form of pneumonitis. Secondary lung involvement, adult respiratory distress syndrome, can occur not only from a primary lung infection but also from hemorrhagic shock, systemic shock, pancreatitis, multiple trauma, and ischemia/reperfusion injury. One characteristic of acute lung injury is the increase in dead-space ventilation. The disease process and, perhaps, pulmonary therapy with increased airway pressure cause progressive mismatching between ventilation and blood flow, with increased numbers of nonperfused but ventilated alveoli. Patients with this condition must frequently develop an increased minute ventilation (15 to 25 L/min) to excrete carbon dioxide. In these patients the work of breathing demand, a result of the need for high minute ventilation, may exceed the patient's work of breathing reserve.[4]

Cardiac response may be limited by inadequate preload, previous cardiac disease, or acquired cardiac dysfunction. Inadequate resuscitation and redistribution of the body fluid compartments can lead to a decrease in preload. Preexisting cardiac valvular or coronary vascular disease may limit the patient's ability to respond with increased cardiac output. Acquired cardiac malfunction can arise from malnutrition or the presence of a soluble myocardial depressant factor. Experimental and clinical evidence demonstrates decreased ejection fraction in sepsis.[5,6]

Energy expenditure is increased during the hypermetabolic phase and the MSOF phase. Although both oxygen consumption and carbon dioxide production are elevated, the respiratory quotient (R/Q) usually is 0.8 to 0.9, a value consistent with a mixed fuel source. Carbohydrate, fat, and amino acids are used for high-energy phosphate production. Adequate metabolic support should include a mixture of carbohydrate, fat, and amino acids. Total body protein catabolism is increased and exceeds the protein synthetic rate. Lean body mass is lost in the phenomenon of autocannibalism, and urinary nitrogen excretion can exceed 20 g/day.[7] With protein loading, the uptake of amino acids by skeletal muscle is suppressed, but hepatic amino acid uptake is increased. The liver can synthesize increased amounts of acute-phase reactants, while albumin and transferrin synthesis is downregulated. The increased urea production and associated azotemia reflect the increased amino acid turnover. The lean body mass is redistributed to sites of active protein synthesis, to wounds for oxidation, and as necessary for conversion to other substrates.

Although the metabolic signals that cause catabolism are not suppressed by exogenous amino acid administration, the protein synthetic rate is increased with amino acid loading. When the synthetic rate equals the catabolic rate, nitrogen equilibrium is achieved. If metabolic support is absent or inadequate, hepatic protein synthesis fails, and the patient has a higher mortality risk.

In late organ failure, protein synthesis fails and catabolism is unabated. If the concentrations of plasma amino acids are examined, it is noted that all amino acids, including branched-chain amino acids, increase as total amino acid

clearance is reduced. Also, in later MSOF the endogenous R/Q exceeds 1, a value that suggests net lipogenesis. Further details of metabolic support are discussed in Chapter 3.

In a retrospective review of patients, the number of Gram-negative infections per patient was not significantly different in patients who survived compared to patients who died.[8] Discriminators of survival were arterial partial pressure of oxygen (Pao_2)/fraction of inspired oxygen (Fio_2) on day 1, serum lactate on day 2, serum bilirubin on day 6, and serum creatinine on day 12 (Table 1-1). Plasma transferrin concentration, serum glutamic-oxaloacetic transaminase (SGOT), and alkaline phosphatase were not discriminators. Patients who survived were younger, spent less time undergoing mechanical ventilation, and had shorter stays in the SICU. Total hospital days were not significantly different in both groups.

PATHOGENESIS

A description of the pathogenesis of MSOF must account for the time course of events, the persistence of hypermetabolism without continuing stimuli, and the increased susceptibility of patients to develop MSOF with multiple insults. Clinically, the path to MSOF proceeds through four phases: shock, resuscitation, stable hypermetabolism, and MSOF. Although current data do not explain on a cellular level the details of the time response, some comments can be made about the mechanism of MSOF. Gram-negative sepsis has been shown to be the most common antecedent of the MSOF syndrome. Gram-negative sepsis, and associated endotox-

TABLE 1-1 Discriminators of Survival (mean ± SEM)*

	SICU Day	No. of Patients Surviving	No. of Patients Expired
Pao_2/Fio_2	1	311 ± 25	233 ± 14
Lactate (mEq/L)	2	1.1 ± 0.2	3.4 ± 0.7
Bilirubin (m/dl)	6	2.2 ± 0.6	8.5 ± 2.2
Creatinine (m/dl)	12	1.9 ± 0.6	3.9 ± 0.3

* From Cerra FB, Negro F, Eyer S. Multiple organ failure syndrome: Patterns and effect of current therapy. Update Intensive Care Emerg Med 10:24, 1990.

emia, activate a cytokine-mediated mechanism that leads to MSOF. Other experimental data suggest that the same underlying mechanism is at work for ischemia/reperfusion injury. Current understanding assumes that the same type of mechanism applies to Gram-positive sepsis, pancreatitis, massive soft tissue injury, and necrotic tissue.

PROTOTYPE PATHWAY

The central hypothesis of the pathogenesis of MSOF states that circulating endotoxin lipopolysaccharide (LPS) stimulates the production of circulating tumor necrosis factor (TNF), which, in turn, produces circulating interleukin 1 (IL-1) (Fig. 1-1). This cascade produces MSOF and, in many patients, death. Endotoxin as a mediator of hypermetabolism was described in the 1960s by Porter et al.,[9] who linked endotoxin to a pathogenic role in severe infections. In their study, patients had evidence of circulating endotoxin at the time blood cultures demonstrated no bacteria. Although Porter et al. could not identify other mediators at the time, Michie et al.[10] administered *Escherichia coli* endotoxin to male volunteers. Circulating TNF was detectable and peaked at about 90 minutes after infusion of endotoxin. With the appearance of TNF, body temperature, pulse, adrenocorticotropic hormone (ACTH) secretion, and epinephrine secretion were increased. TNF then disappeared from the circulation. The systemic response could be blocked by administration of ibuprofen prior to administration of endotoxin.

Administration of TNF to rats produced hypotension, metabolic acidosis, dehydration, and death. TNF administered alone was a mediator of microcirculatory failure.[11] Anti-TNF monoclonal antibody produced increased survival in primates infused with a lethal dose of *E. coli*.[12] Endotoxin is not required for stimulating TNF production. In rat hepatic lobar ischemia, TNF was measurable after reperfusion. Further findings included pulmonary injury that occurred after reperfusion.[13]

Cell culture experiments demonstrated release of IL-1 by isolated endothelial cells after administration of TNF. IL-1 has been shown to produce shock in rabbits, and blocking of IL-1

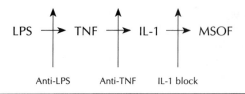

FIG. 1-1 Pathogenesis of multiple system organ failure. LPS, lipopolysaccharide; TNF, tumor necrosis factor; IL-1, interleukin-1.

can reduce mortality of endotoxin administration.[14,15] These data suggest a pathway from endotoxin to organ failure via the production of TNF and IL-1. Mortality is reduced by blocking agents at each level, namely, endotoxin, TNF, and IL-1.

Some of the systemic responses to stress are rapid, such as the response to glucagon and epinephrine. Through the second messengers, G-proteins, cyclic adenosine monophosphate (cAMP), and protein kinases, these hormones modify proteins that are preformed in the cell. The response occurs in minutes. In contrast, endotoxin, combined with its binding protein, stimulates TNF mRNA transcription from the TNF gene and stabilizes the otherwise highly unstable TNF mRNA. These signals are not preformed, and response has a characteristic time delay of minutes to hours. The cytokines TNF, IL-1, and IL-6 and other interleukins have local effects on nearby parenchymal cells and distinct systemic effects on endothelium. Locally, in the hepatocyte, for example, TNF and IL-1 lead to synthesis of acute-phase reactants.

Other stresses can produce alternate metabolic responses from cells. Increasing temperature, acid pH, and hypoxia/reperfusion produce expression of the stress genes. A hierarchy exists in the response of parenchymal cells to various stimuli. Response of the cell to glucagon and epinepherine is superseded by that of cytokines. The response to cytokines is superseded by the increase in temperature, decreased pH, and hypoxia/reoxygenation.[16-19] These responses, although hierarchical, might account for the early phase of hypermetabolism associated with resuscitation but do not explain persistent hypermetabolism. These responses are all reversible.

Sequestration of inflammatory cells in tissues may be responsible for persistence of the hypermetabolic response.[20,21] Persistent inflammatory response can produce findings of sepsis, even in the absence of bacteria. Zymosan injected intraperitoneally in rats, a nonbacterial model, produced findings similar to those of rat sepsis. Rats treated with zymosan showed aggregates of WBCs in capillaries of the lung and liver.[22] Could these effects be a consequence of the effects of mediators as they circulate?

Circulating WBCs, when treated with mediators such as TNF or endotoxin, produce proteins involved with adhesion of WBCs to the endothelium. Treatment with monoclonal antibody to adherence molecules improved survival in rabbits following shock and resuscitation.[23] Another WBC response to cytokines also has been shown. Exposure of endothelial cell lines to IL-1 and TNF produced increased neutrophil migration.[24] Reduced migration of WBCs and reduced symptoms were produced by anti-ICAM-1, an antibody to endothelial adhesion protein.[25] Mediators appear to have systemic effects by acting on endothelium to produce capillary injury directly and by increasing migration of neutrophils into the parenchyma. The stimulated neutrophils in the parenchyma may be a continuing source of organ injury.

Can mediators explain the increased susceptibility to organ failure in patients who receive multiple insults? Increased endothelial cell death under certain circumstances has been demonstrated. When cultured aortic endothelium was treated with endotoxin, cell viability was comparable to that of controls. When the endothelium was treated with a substance to produce heat shock, again, cell viability was not significantly different from that of controls. However, if the aortic endothelium was pretreated with endotoxin and then subjected to heat shock, cell death increased significantly. These findings suggest that priming of cells occurs with mediators and that additional injury enhances cell death and ultimately increases the chances of MSOF.[26,27]

IMPLICATIONS FOR TREATMENT

Current evidence suggests that a mediated pathway exists that links endotoxin to increased TNF production, increased IL-1 production, MSOF, and death. Mortality can be improved by blocking the pathway at the endotoxin level, the TNF level, or the IL-1 level. Additional effects of the mediators are the promotion of WBC adherence to endothelium and migration through endothelium. Ischemia/reperfusion also has been shown to increase TNF production. Although the mediators may have disappeared by the time of the clinical appearance of MSOF, they likely set in motion the parenchymal dysfunction and disseminated inflammation that culminates in MSOF.

Source control is of primary importance in reducing both short-term and long-term cell damage. Clearly, endotoxin challenge must be minimized. Abscesses must be drained, and infections must be treated as specifically as possible. Tissue hypoxia and repeated shock, both stimuli for TNF production, must be avoided. Necrotic tissue must be debrided. Hemorrhage must be controlled. The gut has been implicated as a possible source of continued endotoxin load. Loss of gut mucosal barrier function has been demonstrated after burns, 30 minutes of hemorrhagic shock, and endotoxin infusion.[28] Selective gut decontamination has been performed to control the possible endotoxin load from the gut. In the studies done to date, the incidence of organ failure and mortality has not been shown to be decreased.[29-32]

Along with source control, newer modes of therapy may help to reduce mortality. If endotoxemia occurs, antiendotoxin antibody may have a role. Anti-TNF antibody, the next cytokine stimulated, is another choice for therapy. Since TNF induces IL-1, IL-1 blockade also may be effective in improving outcome. Finally, agents that prevent WBC adhesion and migration, for example, anti-CD18 and anti-ICAM-1, may be of value. Several entry points into the TNF/IL-1 pathway exist. Optimum patient outcome requires management of multiple control points in the pathway.

New therapies for MSOF depend on accurate understanding of mechanisms of cell injury, organ dysfunction, cell death, and organ failure.

SUMMARY

- MSOF is sequential failure of all major organ systems of the body.
- Microcirculatory failure, ischemia/reperfusion, sepsis, soft tissue injury, tissue necrosis, and local inflammation with systemic effects (pancreatitis) are classes of injury associated with MSOF.
- Clinically apparent liver failure heralds the appearance of MSOF.
- Overall primary physiologic response is an increase in oxygen consumption.
- Energy expenditure is significantly increased in MSOF. Carbohydrate, fat, and amino acids are used for high-energy phosphate production.

- LPS → ↑ TNF → ↑ IL-1 → hypermetabolism → MSOF is the prototype mechanism for MSOF. Blockage of the pathway at LPS, TNF, or IL-1 or WBC adhesion decreases symptoms and reduces mortality in animal models.
- Source control is of primary importance to minimize endotoxin, TNF, and IL-1 challenge. It includes draining abscesses, treating infections, and controlling hemorrhage.
- Current therapy includes source control, restoration of oxygen transport, and metabolic support. Biologic therapy, with antibodies directed at specific mediators in the pathway, is promising for the future.

REFERENCES

1. Gann DS, Amaral JF, Caldwell MD. Metabolic response to injury, stress, and starvation. In Davis JH, ed. Clinical Surgery. St. Louis: CV Mosby, 1987, pp 337-376.
2. Cerra FB. Hypermetabolism, organ failure, and metabolic support. Surgery 101:1-14, 1987.
3. Barton R, Cerra FB. The hypermetabolism multiple organ failure syndrome. Chest 96:1153-1160, 1989.
4. Cerra FB. Multiple organ failure syndrome. In Bihari DS, Cerra FB, eds. New Horizons. Multiple Organ Failure. Fullerton, Calif.: Society of Critical Care Medicine, 1989, pp 1-24.
5. Parrillo JE, Burch C, Shelhamer JH, Parker MM, Natanson C, Schuette W. A circulating myocardial depressant substance in humans with septic shock. Septic shock patients with a reduced ejection fraction have a circulating factor that depresses in vitro myocardial cell performance. J Clin Invest 76:1539-1553, 1985.
6. Cunnion RE, Parrillo JE. Myocardial dysfunction in sepsis. Crit Care Clin 5:99-118, 1989.
7. Cerra FB, Siegel JH, Coleman B, Border JR, McMenamy RR. Septic autocannibalism. A failure of exogenous nutritional support. Ann Surg 192:570-580, 1980.
8. Cerra FB, Negro F, Eyer S. Multiple organ failure syndrome: Patterns and effect of current therapy. Update Intensive Care Emerg Med 10:22-31, 1990.

9. Porter PJ, Spievack AR, Kass EH. Endotoxin-like activity of serum from patients with severe localized infections. N Engl J Med 271:445-447, 1964.
10. Michie HR, Manogue KR, Spriggs DR. Detection of circulating tumor necrosis factor after endotoxin administration. N Engl J Med 318:1481-1486, 1988.
11. Tracey KJ, Bentler B, Lowry SE. Shock and tissue injury induced by recombinant human cachectin. Science 234:470-474, 1986.
12. Hinshaw LB, Tekamp-Olson P, Chang ACK. Survival of primates in LD100 septic shock following therapy with antibody to tumor necrosis factor (TNF$_\alpha$). Circ Shock 30:279-292, 1990.
13. Colletti LM, Remick DG, Burtch GD. Role of tumor necrosis factor-α in the pathophysiologic alterations after hepatic ischemia/reperfusion in the rat. J Clin Invst 85:1936-1943, 1990.
14. Dinarello CA, Cannon JG, Wolff SM. Tumor necrosis factor (cachectin) is an endogenous pyrogen and induces production of interleukin 1. J Exp Med 163:1433-1450, 1986.
15. Dinarello CA, Mier JW. Lymphokines. N Engl J Med 317:940-945, 1987.
16. DeMaio A, Buchman TG. Molecular biology of circulatory shock. Part IV. Translation and secretion of HEP G2 cell proteins are independently attenuated during heat shock. Circ Shock 34:329-335, 1991.
17. Cabin DE, Buchman TG. Molecular biology of circulatory shock. Part III. Human hepatoblas-

toma (HEP G2) cells demonstrate two patterns of shock-induced gene expression that are independent, exclusive, and prioritized. Surgery 108:902-912, 1990.

18. Buchman TG, Cabin DE, Vickers S. Molecular biology of circulatory shock. Part II. Expression of four groups of hepatic genes is enhanced after resuscitation from cardiogenic shock. Surgery 108:559-566, 1990.

19. Buchman TG, Cabin DE, Porter JM. Change in hepatic gene expression after shock/resuscitation. Surgery 106:283-291, 1989.

20. Fry DE, Pearlstein L, Fulton RL. Multiple system organ failure: The role of uncontrolled infection. Arch Surg 115:136-140, 1980.

21. Carrico CJ, Meakins JL, Marshall JC. Multiple-organ-failure-syndrome. Arch Surg 121:196-208, 1986.

22. Goris RIA, Boekholtz WKF, van Bebbler IPT. Multiple-organ failure and sepsis without bacteria. Arch Surg 121:897-901, 1986.

23. Vedder NB, Winn RK, Rice CL. A monoclonal antibody to the adherence-promoting leukocyte glycoprotein, CD18, reduces organ injury and improves survival from hemorrhagic shock and resuscitation in rabbits. J Clin Invest 81:939-944, 1988.

24. Moser R, Schleiffenbaum B, Groswerth P. Interleukin 1 and tumor necrosis factor stimulate human vascular endothelial cells to promote transendothelial neutrophil passage. J Clin Invest 83:444-455, 1989.

25. Wegner CD, Gundel RH, Reilly P. Intercellullar adhesion molecule-1 (ICAM-1) in the pathogenesis of asthma. Science 247:456-459, 1990.

26. Faist E, Baue AE, Dittmer H. Multiple organ failure in polytrauma patients. J Trauma 23:775-787, 1983.

27. Buchman TG. Cell-cell signals: Roles in the development and persistence of multiple organ system failure. Implications for therapy. Critical Care: Multisystem Failure, Postgraduate Course, New York: American College of Surgeons Spring Meeting, 1991.

28. Deitch EA. Bacterial translocation of the gut flora. J Trauma 30:S184-S189, 1990.

29. Blair P, Rowlands BJ, Lowry K, Webb H, Armstrong P, Smilie J. Selective decontamination of the digestive tract: A stratified, randomized, prospective study in a mixed intensive care unit. Surgery 110:303-310, 1991.

30. Stoutenbeck CP, VanSaene HKF, Miranda DR, Zandstra DF. The effect of selective decontamination of the digestive tract on colonisation and infection rate in multiple trauma patients. Intensive Care Med 10:185-192, 1984.

31. Ledingham I McA, Alcock SR, Eastaway AT, McDonald JC, McKay IC, Ramsay G. Triple regimen of selective decontamination of the digestive tract, systemic cefotaxime, and microbiological surveillance for prevention of acquired infection in intensive care. Lancet 1:785-790, 1988.

32. Kerver AJH, Rommes JH, Merissen-Verhage EAI. Prevention of colonisation and infection in critically ill patients: A prospective randomized study. Crit Care Med 16:1087-1093, 1988.

CHAPTER 2

Restoration of Oxygen Transport

Jerome H. Abrams · Frank B. Cerra

Restoration of oxygen transport is one of the three factors that form the foundation of modern critical care—source control, restoration of oxygen transport, and metabolic support. When combined, these factors can reduce mortality in the SICU. Once the airway has been safely maintained, source control becomes the hightest priority. Source control means that hemorrhage must be stopped. Abscesses must be drained since even small amounts of pus, if undrained, can produce grave systemic consequences, and other infections must be treated as specifically as possible. When adequate source control has been established, the next mandate is restoration of oxygen transport. After oxygen transport has been restored, appropriate metabolic support becomes the next goal. (See Chapter 3 for a detailed discussion of metabolic support.)

Restoration of oxygen transport requires supplying adequate oxygen to all tissues to satisfy the demand for oxygen. The critical care physician must be able to identify both the supply of oxygen to tissues and the demand for oxygen by tissues. The components of tissue oxygen supply and demand are shown in Table 2-1.

OXYGEN SUPPLY AND DEMAND

The clinical determinants of oxygen supply are well defined and may be measured routinely. The components of oxygen demand are less direct and reflect changes in oxygen use as a consequence of alterations in oxygen supply.

The fundamental assumption about oxygen transport is that increased use of oxygen with increased supply means that tissues are consuming oxygen in order to meet increased metabolic demands.

Hemoglobin is the physiologic carrier of oxygen. Providing sufficient hemoglobin to carry oxygen is an effective way of improving oxygen transport. Oxygen delivery (Do_2), is approximated by the relationship:

$$Do_2 = (1.36 \times Hb[g/dl] \times \% \text{ arterial saturation}) \times \text{cardiac output (L/min)} \times 10$$

Because of its small magnitude, the component $0.0034 Pao_2$ has been dropped. Providing sufficient oxygen carriers is one of the most important ways of improving oxygen delivery. Increasing hemoglobin concentration from 9 to 11.5 g/dl would increase Do_2 by nearly 30%, even if cardiac output remained constant. Changing the arterial oxygen partial pressure from 60 to 90 mm Hg would increase the arterial saturation from 88% to 95%. The increase in Do_2 would be only 7%. From this example, it can be seen that increasing the hemoglobin concentration is a very effective means of augmenting Do_2. The appropriate hemoglobin concentration depends on the clinical context. An elderly patient with coronary vascular disease who has intra-abdominal sepsis may require hemoglobin concentrations of approximately 12 g/dl. An increase of hemoglobin from 9 to 12 g/dl in such a patient could reduce

| TABLE 2-1 | Components of Tissue Oxygen Supply and Demand* |

Component	Clinical Variable
Oxygen supply	
Oxygen carrier	Hb concentration
Oxygen carrier saturation	Hb saturation
Oxygen carrier delivery	Do_2 = CO × Arterial oxygen content
	= $(1.36 × Hb × \%Sat + 0.0034 Pao_2) × CO × 10$
Oxygen demand	
Tissue oxygen demand	Flow-dependent oxygen consumption
	Delivery-dependent lactate production or acetate/pyruvate ratio
Oxygen consumption	$\dot{V}o_2$ = CO × DVo_2 × 10
	= $[CO × (1.36 × Hb (\% \text{ Arterial sat} − \% \text{ Venous sat})] × 10$
	$+ 0.0034 (Pao_2 − PVo_2)$

*From Abrams JH. Indications for hemodynamic monitoring. In Najarian JS, Delaney JP, eds. Progress in Trauma and Critical Care Surgery. St. Louis: Mosby–Year Book, 1992, p 278.
Do_2, oxygen delivery; Pao_2, partial pressure of arterial oxygen; $\dot{V}o_2$, oxygen consumption; PVo_2, partial pressure of venous oxygen; DVo_2, arteriovenous oxygen content difference.

| TABLE 2-2 | Determinants of Cardiac Output |

Component	Clinical Variable	Clinical Target
Preload	PCWP	12-15 mm Hg
Afterload	$SVR = \dfrac{MAP − CVP}{CO} × 80$	<1000 dynes/sec/cm^5
Contractility	Undefined	Undefined

PCWP, pulmonary capillary wedge pressure; SVR, systemic vascular resistance; MAP, mean arterial pressure; CVP, central venous pressure.

heart rate work, perhaps as much as 30%, and decrease myocardial oxygen consumption.

The target for saturation of hemoglobin is 90%. In an SICU, supplementary oxygen generally is required. For some patients oxygen administered by face mask may be sufficient. For other patients positive pressure ventilatory support may be necessary. Strategies for ensuring adequate oxygenation can be challenging. The various means of supporting gas exchange are discussed in Chapters 27 and 28.

OPTIMIZATION OF BLOOD FLOW

Once sufficient hemoglobin is available and saturated, the next issue is optimizing the flow of blood throughout tissues. Optimization of cardiac output (CO) in patients with multiple system organ failure is similar to that in other patients. Table 2-2 lists the determinants of CO.

Preload, afterload, and inotropic support are each evaluated in turn to minimize increases in myocardial oxygen consumption. A useful clinical target for preload is the pulmonary capillary wedge pressure (PCWP). In hypermetabolic states, oxygen needs are increased. To meet these needs, a CO greater than normal is generally necessary. Normal filling pressures may not be sufficient to produce increased cardiac flow. Rather, a PCWP of 12 to 15 mm Hg may be necessary. It is important to note that pressure measurements are not volume measurements. Fig. 2-1 shows the hysteresis involved in volume loading and volume unloading in the vascular system. Depending on whether the patient is volume loaded or volume unloaded, a given pressure may correspond to two left ventricular end-diastolic volumes. Nonetheless, the PCWP is a useful clinical guide.

Once preload is sufficient, afterload is addressed. A clinical target of systemic vascular resistance (SVR) <1000 dyne/sec/cm^5 is the usual clinical target. SVR is a proportionality constant that relates flow and pressure. From the means of calculation, SVR has the same role as resistance in Ohm's law (V = IR). When preload is adequate, a vasodilator may be added if the SVR is elevated and a need for increased CO exists. Nitroglycerin and nitroprusside are useful vasodilating agents. Frequently afterload reduction may cause a measurable decrease in PCWP, and additional volume may need to be infused.

If criteria addressed in the remaining discussion suggest that greater CO is necessary, and if preload and afterload are in the target range, inotropic support is considered. Cunnion and Parrillo have shown decreased ejection fraction in patients with sepsis and hypermetabolism in a model of synchronously beating cultured myocardial cells. Perfusion of these cells with the plasma of septic patients

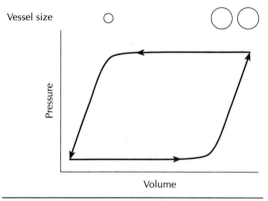

FIG. 2-1   Relationship between volume loading and volume unloading in vascular system. (From Cerra FB. Manual of Critical Care. St. Louis: CV Mosby, 1987, p 80.)

reduced the amplitude of contraction. Contraction returned to control values when cells were perfused with normal serum. The authors concluded that a soluble myocardial depressant factor was present in the serum of septic individuals. Patients may have a need for augmented contractility in such septic/hypermetabolic states. Dobutamine or amrinone both may be useful inotropes.

DETERMINATION OF RESTORATION OF OXYGEN TRANSPORT

How does the critical care physician decide when oxygen transport is restored? How can he/she decide if a patient requires greater CO? The following hypothetical cases may be considered:

Patient	Blood Pressure	Pulse	Urine Output (ml/hr)	Capillary Refill	Mental Status
A	60/0	160	0	⇊	⇊
B	105/65	110	35	⇈	↑
C	120/80	95	45	n1	↓

From the information supplied, is it possible to distinguish in which of these patients oxygen transport is restored? Could all of them be inadequately resuscitated at the time that these variables are measured? Are the variables presented sensitive for restoration of oxygen transport?

Variables that traditionally have been used to assess resuscitation (i.e., blood pressure, pulse, urine output, capillary refill, and mental status) do not provide sensitive and specific information about oxygen transport. If inadequate oxygen transport is defined as shock, most historical definitions of shock do not allow the critical care physician to easily develop an approach to restoring oxygen transport. Nearly all definitions emphasize a mismatch between existing blood volume and the volume of the vascular tree. As early as 1917, Archibald and McClain suggested: "While low blood pressure is one of the most consistent signs of shock, it is not the essential thing, let alone the cause of it."

What other information would help the physician to decide when oxygen transport is restored? Since this discussion relates to the general area of shock, the following definition of shock should be considered: Shock is a distribution of states in which tissue oxygen demand exceeds tissue oxygen supply for a single reason or a combination of reasons. This definition has three components. The first suggests that a given patient may be in a greater or lesser state of shock. The patient may be considered as resuscitated to a greater or lesser degree. The distribution of responses can be calculated from variables that reflect aerobic and anaerobic energy production to produce a response surface for SICU patients. The third part of the definition identifies the causes of shock as either single or multiple. For example, a patient with usually well-compensated congestive heart failure might be involved in a motor vehicle accident. The result might be hemorrhagic and cardiogenic shock. In a similar manner, a hypovolemic patient may acquire sepsis and demonstrate a combination of septic and hypovolemic shock.

The second component of the definition used here requires further discussion. How does one decide if tissue oxygen demand exceeds tissue oxygen supply? Clearly, a "tissue oxygen demandometer" would be valuable in determining whether tissue oxygen supply meets tissue oxygen demand. Since no such device exists, clinical variables must be found to identify this potential mismatch. Two criteria are used clinically: (1) the presence of flow-dependent oxygen consumption, and (2) flow-dependent lactate production (or its equivalent condition, an abnormal lactate/pyruvate ratio).

Flow-Dependent Oxygen Consumption

Flow-dependent oxygen consumption is a phenomenon that has been recognized for many years. Fig. 2-2 represents an idealization of this event. The steeply varying part of the curve is the flow-dependent area. The flat part of the curve is the flow-independent area. If a patient is in the flow-independent portion of the curve,

he/she is protected against sudden catastrophic decreases in oxygen consumption when oxygen delivery may be diminished. For example, if the patient were to develop hypovolemia and CO decreased, no significant changes in oxygen consumption would necessarily occur. Many studies support this concept of delivery-dependent oxygen consumption. Nonetheless, controversy exists about whether delivery-dependent oxygen consumption can be demonstrated in humans. Part of the controversy results from the way in which oxygen consumption and oxygen delivery are measured. In clinical practice, the Fick principle is used (oxygen consumption equals the cardiac index times the arteriovenous oxygen content difference):

$$\dot{V}O_2 = CI \times DVO_2$$

Oxygen delivery is the cardiac index times the arterial oxygen content:

$$DO_2 = CI \times CaO_2$$

Since cardiac index is a factor in both the dependent and the independent variables, some concern exists over whether a spurious correlation may result. This issue has been addressed by Archie and by Stratton and colleagues.

Flow-Dependent Lactate Production

The idea of flow-dependent oxygen consumption addresses the first criterion concerning

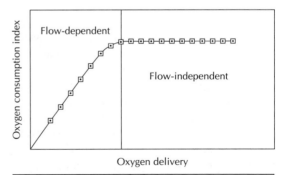

FIG. 2-2 Idealization of flow-dependent oxygen consumption. (From Abrams JH. Indications for hemodynamic monitoring. In Najarian JS, Delaney JP, eds. Progress in Trauma and Critical Care Surgery. St. Louis: Mosby–Year Book, 1992, p 275.)

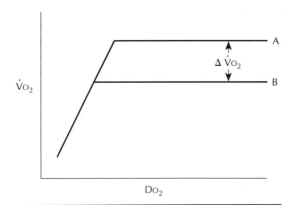

FIG. 2-3 Flow-dependent lactate production. (Modified from Abrams JH. Indications for hemodynamic monitoring. In Najarian JS, Delaney JP, eds. Progress in Trauma and Critical Care Surgery. St. Louis: Mosby–Year Book, 1992, p 276.)

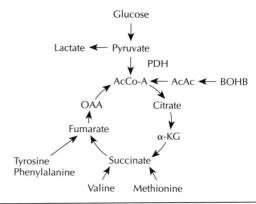

FIG. 2-4 Aerobic glycolysis. (From Abrams JH. Indications for hemodynamic monitoring. In Najarian JS, Delaney JP, eds. Progress in Trauma and Critical Care Surgery. St. Louis: Mosby–Year Book, 1992, p 277.)

whether oxygen transport is restored. Why is the second criterion necessary? The need for determining flow-dependent lactate production, or ratio of lactate to pyruvate, is equivalent to asking if one can imagine a situation in which flow-dependent oxygen consumption appears to be absent but the redox potential of the cell remains abnormal. Such a situation could occur if global extraction, as measured by the arteriovenous oxygen content difference (DVo_2), is limited in certain pathologic states. The clinician then would see a narrowed DVo_2, and the oxygen consumption would vary only with the change in CO. A common finding in septic shock, sepsis syndrome, adult respiratory distress syndrome, or liver failure is a narrowed, fixed DVo_2. In Fig. 2-3, a graphic equivalent of this question is demonstrated. Is it possible that the patient needs to be on curve A but has been able to achieve only the oxygen consumption of curve B? How could one ever tell? The use of lactate production (or the lactate/pyruvate ratio) is helpful in deciding whether a gap between the patient's oxygen consumption and tissue needs exists. If extraction of oxygen, as measured by DVo_2, is limited, the anaerobic metabolic pathways may be important. The use of serum lactate concentration is an aid in deciding whether additional delivery of oxygen, through increased hemoglobin concentration

or increased flow, might be of benefit. The use of the lactate/pyruvate ratio is also helpful. This ratio helps to identify the situation in which the concentration of lactate may be abnormally high, in the 2.5 to 3.4 mmol range, but the redox potential of the cell is normal. Such findings suggest the phenomenon of aerobic glycolysis, represented in Fig. 2-4. In hypermetabolism-mediated states, pyruvate dehydrogenase is down regulated. Entry of pyruvate into the tricarboxylic acid cycle is decreased, and increased lactate production occurs. Nonetheless, the lactate/pyruvate ratio remains normal. The redox potential of the cells stays normal because other carbon sources, fats, and amino acids (especially branched-chain amino acids) are used as sources of oxidative fuel. Therefore the lactate/pyruvate ratio is useful in identifying those patients with moderately elevated lactate concentrations, despite increased oxygen delivery, in whom aerobic metabolism is still an adequate source of energy production.

TREATMENT APPROACH

To accomplish restoration of oxygen transport with currently available technology, invasive hemodynamic monitoring must be used. A growing body of evidence indicates that survival is increased if patients are resuscitated by oxygen transport standards early in their clin-

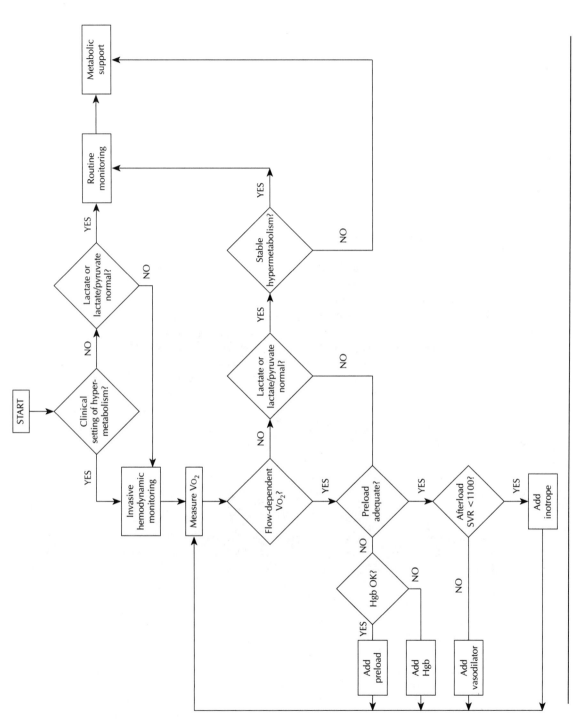

FIG. 2-5 Approach to restoration of oxygen transport.

ical course. The major indication for invasive hemodynamic monitoring, then, becomes restoration of oxygen transport. From the pulmonary artery catheter, PCWP, cardiac output/index, and mixed venous blood samples are obtained. Arterial blood is sampled to determine arterial oxygen content. With arterial oxygen content, Do_2 may be calculated, and, with the addition of mixed venous oxygen content, DVo_2 and the oxygen consumption index may be calculated. A serum lactate concentration should be considered a mandatory part of the data obtained. Other calculated hemodynamic quantities, such as SVR, then can be derived.

With the combined approach of source control, restoration of oxygen transport, and adequate metabolic support, a decrease in mortality can be demonstrated. In a prospective trial, Shoemaker and colleagues were able to demonstrate a significant decrease in mortality. In a retrospective review, Cerra and colleagues also were able to show a reduction in mortality by a factor of two.

Fig. 2-5 presents an approach to the problem of restoration of oxygen transport. The initial decision point addresses the presence or absence of hypermetabolism. Does the clinical setting suggest hypermetabolism? Does the patient have sepsis, pancreatitis, adult respiratory distress syndrome, or multiple trauma? If the answer is "yes," invasive hemodynamic monitoring with a pulmonary artery catheter is begun. What if the clinical setting does not suggest hypermetabolism? The clinician should determine whether serum lactate concentration is elevated. If the answer is "yes," very serious consideration should be given to increasing oxygen transport with the use of invasive he-

modynamic monitoring. The clinician should then measure CO, arterial and mixed venous blood gases, serum lactate, and serum pyruvate, if available. Oxygen consumption then may be calculated. If oxygen consumption is below expected values, or if lactate (or ratio of lactate to pyruvate) is elevated, oxygen delivery is increased and oxygen consumption and the metabolic variables, lactate (or the ratio of lactate to pyruvate) are again determined. Oxygen delivery is increased by providing sufficient hemoglobin at 90% oxygen saturation and increasing CO by optimizing preload, afterload, and contractility.

SUMMARY

- Shock is a distribution of states in which tissue oxygen demand exceeds tissue oxygen supply. Balance between demand and supply may be disturbed by one mechanism or by several mechanisms operating simultaneously.
- Shock is present when flow-dependent oxygen consumption and flow-dependent lactate production exist. An equivalent condition is a lactate/pyruvate ratio >20.
- Principles of management include source control, restoration of oxygen transport, and metabolic support.
- To restore oxygen transport, a sufficient number of hemoglobin molecules must be present, these molecules must be saturated, and CO must be optimized.
- CO is optimized in terms of preload, afterload, and inotropic support.

BIBLIOGRAPHY

Abrams JH, Barke RA, Cerra FB. Quantitative evaluation of clinical course in surgical ICU patients: The data conform to catastrophe theory. J Trauma 24:1028, 1984.

Archibald EW, McLean WS. Observations upon stroke, with particular reference to the condition as seen in war surgery. Ann Surg 66:280-286, 1917.

Archie JP. Mathematic compiling of data. Ann Surg 193:296, 1981.

Cerra FB. Hypermetabolism, organ failure, and metabolic support. Surgery 101:1, 1987.

Cerra FB. The multiple organ failure syndrome. Crit Care: State of Art 9:107, 1988.

Clowes GHA, Vucinic M, Weidner MG. Circulatory and metabolic alterations associated with survival and death in peritonitis. Ann Surg 163:861, 1966.

Cunnion RE, Parrillo JE. Myocardial dysfunction in sepsis. Crit Care Clin 5:99, 1989.

Danek SJ, Lynch JP, Weg JL, et al. The dependence of oxygen uptake in oxygen delivery in the adult respiratory distress syndrome. Am Rev Resp Dis 122:387, 1980.

Edwards JD, Brown GCS, Nightingale P, et al. Use of survivors' cardiorespiratory values in therapeutic goals in septic shock. Crit Care Med 17:1098, 1989.

Kaufman BS, Rackow EC, Falk JL. The relationship between oxygen delivery and consumption during fluid resuscitation of hypovolemic and septic shock. Chest 85:336, 1984.

Patel TB, Olson MS. Regulation of pyruvate dehydrogenase complex in ischemic rat heart. Am J Physiol 246:H858, 1984.

Schofield PS, McLees DJ, Kerbey AL, et al. Activities of cardiac and hepatic pyruvate dehydrogenase complex are decreased after surgical stress. Biochem Int 12:189, 1986.

Shoemaker WC. Cardiorespiratory patterns in complicated and uncomplicated septic shock. Ann Surg 174:119, 1971.

Shoemaker WC. Hemodynamic and oxygen transport patterns in septic shock. In Sibbald WJ, Sprung CL, eds. Perspectives in Sepsis and Septic Shock, New Horizons. Fullerton, Calif.: 1986, pp 203-234.

Shoemaker WC, Appel PL, Bland R. Use of physiologic monitoring to predict outcome and to assist in clinical decisions in critically ill postoperative patients. Am J Surg 146:43, 1983.

Shoemaker WC, Appel PL, Bland R, et al. Clinical trial of an algorithm for outcome prediction in acute circulatory failure. Crit Care Med 10:390, 1982.

Shoemaker WC, Montgomery ES, Kaplan E, et al. Physiologic patterns in surviving and nonsurviving shock patients. Arch Surg 106:630, 1973.

Stratton HH, Feustel PJ, Newell JC. Regression of calculated variables in the presence of shared measurement error. J Appl Physiol 62:2083, 1987.

Waxman K, Nolan LS, Shoemaker WC. Sequential peri-operative lactate determination. Crit Care Med 10:96, 1982.

Weil MH, Abdelmonen AD. Experimental and clinical studies in lactate and pyruvate as indicators of the severity of acute circulatory failure (shock). Circulation 41:989, 1970.

CHAPTER 3

Nutritional and Metabolic Support

Frank B. Cerra · Jerome H. Abrams

Metabolic support is the third major foundation of modern surgical critical care. With source control and resuscitation by oxygen transport standards, metabolic support is the next priority for the critically ill patient. Improved patient outcome depends on early recognition of malnutrition, an estimate of patient stress, and a strategy for support matched to the patient's clinical state. A definition of malnutrition is necessary for early recognition. Malnutrition is altered body composition that includes a reduction in lean body mass or visceral protein mass inappropriate for the age, sex, height, weight, and activity status of the patient. When malnutrition is severe enough, compromise of major organ function may prevent recovery. Malnutrition is an acquired condition that results from a generalized lack of nutrient supply (starvation) or from a disease process, or both. Trauma, burns, infection with a systemic response, major surgical procedures, perfusion shock, inadequate resuscitation, and thyrotoxicosis can induce alterations in body composition characteristic of malnutrition, despite administration of an adequate nutrient supply.

Current nutritional support is designed to eliminate that component of malnutrition that is due to starvation. Modern nutrition support is effective in preventing starvation, a generalized lack of nutrient supply. In the presence of disease states, which affect body composition, the principles of nutritional support developed for starvation alone produce ineffective support and increased major complications. Increased

benefit at decreased risk requires the clinician to avoid calorie, glucose, and fat overload; to provide adequate doses of amino acids or protein; to administer multivitamins; and to provide trace elements and minerals in accord with the patient's renal function (see box). The reduction in morbidity and mortality of metabolic

---

Guidelines for Nutritional Support in SICU Patients

1. Avoid calorie and glucose overload:
   Total kcal, 25-30/kg/day
   Glucose, 3-5 g/kg/day
2. Avoid fat overload:
   No more than 1.5 g/kg/day of current long-chain fatty acid formulations as continuous infusion
3. Provide adequate doses of amino acids or protein:
   1.5-2 g/kg/day
   Modified formulations are more efficient— less ureagenesis, better nitrogen retention, and more support of protein synthesis
4. Provide multivitamins:
   Balanced formula
   IV formulations require added vitamin K
5. Provide trace elements daily*
6. Provide minerals*
   Magnesium, 15-20 mEq/day
   Zinc, 15-20 mg/day

*Glomerular filtration >20 ml/min is assumed.

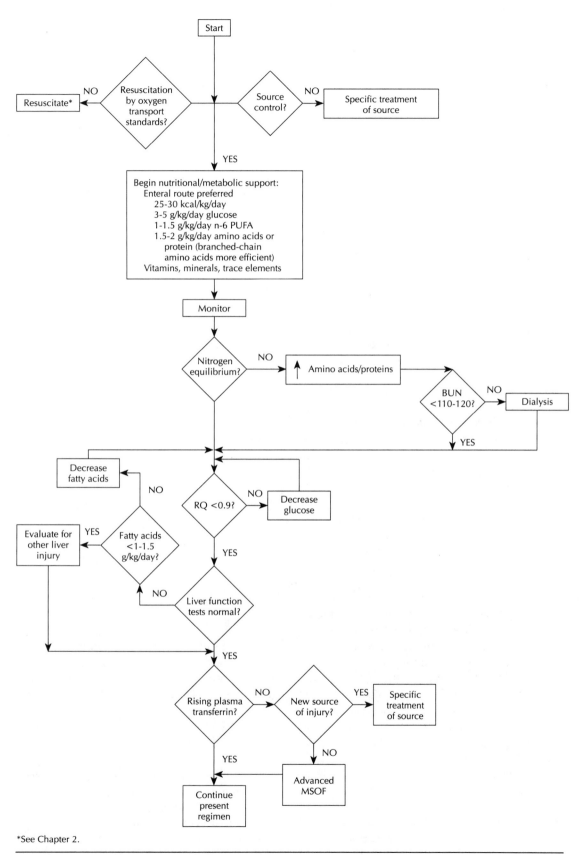

*See Chapter 2.

FIG. 3-1 General approach to nutritional and metabolic support for SICU patient.

support does not depend on the route of administration. Both the enteral and the parenteral routes allow adequate nutritional replacement. In a general way metabolic support is beneficial because it prevents both specific and generalized nutrient deficiencies from contributing to the disease process. New forms of nutritional support are designed to alter these disease processes. Nutrients are administered not only to provide replacement but also to alter disease-induced metabolic effects. The use of specific nutrients to alter disease processes and improve morbidity and mortality is defined as metabolic support.

Nutritional and metabolic support begin after resuscitation. During shock states, nutritional and metabolic support are not well studied and are associated with adverse outcome in experimental conditions. The general goals of nutritional and metabolic support are:

1. Do no harm.
2. Prevent starvation from either specific or generalized nutrient deficiency from contributing to morbidity and mortality.
3. Support organ structure and function.
4. Favorably alter metabolism associated with the systemic inflammatory response.
5. Improve patient outcome.

Fig. 3-1 summarizes the general approach to nutritional and metabolic support. Benefits are best achieved after resuscitation has been completed and source control is well under way.

ADVERSE EFFECTS OF STARVATION

Starvation, viewed as inadequate nutrient supply, results in reduced lean body mass, reduced visceral protein mass, and associated tissue/organ dysfunction. These clinical effects can result from a specific or a generalized nutrient deficiency. Table 3-1 summarizes the effects of specific nutrient deficiencies. Generalized nutrient deficiencies, for example, inadequate amino acids or calories, can result in major organ system dysfunction, such as the altered cardiac function that occurs with semistarvation. In experimental semistarvation, atrial muscle is lost, ventricular muscle is lost, global cardiac function is depressed, and cardiac output is decreased. For the starved patient, cardiac function is adequate because energy demands are reduced. In clinical settings of trauma and sep-

TABLE 3-1 Effects of Specific Nutrient Deficiencies

Nutrient Deficiency	Effect
Branched chains, lysine, methionine	Increased bacterial infections
Arginine	Decreased T-cell and macrophage function
↓ Methionine	Decreased complement levels (C3)
↓ Phenylalanine, tyrosine	Decreased phagocytic function
Vitamins	
C	Reduced chemotaxis and random migration
A	Lymphoid atrophy; decreased T- and B-cell function; decreased phagocytosis
E	Antioxidant; high doses— suppressant; low doses— stimulant to immune function
Trace elements	
Iron	Decreased phagocytic and bactericidal activity
Zinc	Lymphoid atrophy; T- and B-cell dysfunction; impaired phagocytosis
Selenium	Impaired antibody production; cardiomyopathy

sis, where demand on circulation is increased, these physiologic alterations significantly impair the ability of the heart to respond adequately. Loss of contractility increases the likelihood of ventricular failure. Reduced myocardial compliance more easily produces pulmonary edema in response to fluid administration.

A second example comes from the research on the gut response to injury in the absence of enteral nutrition. A major portion of colonocyte nutrition and a significant component of enterocyte nutrition depends on the presence of food substances in the gut lumen. The lack of such nutrients results in gut atrophy, bacterial overgrowth, and altered gut immunity. Perfusion deficit has important effects on the gut. It responds to decreased perfusion with increased permeability, a transient increase in bacterial translocation, and altered immunologic function. If started very early postinjury, enteral nutrition attenuates these problems.

In general, appropriate nutritional support does not allow starvation to become a major comorbidity or comortality factor in the SICU. The effects of starvation on body composition and organ function are accelerated after injuries such as hemorrhage or sepsis and after major surgery. For this reason, after immediate source control and resuscitation have been established, nutritional support is initiated, especially when a prolonged SICU stay is likely. Clinical studies indicate that this approach prevents the damaging effects of a specific or generalized nutrient deficiency.

EFFECTS OF TISSUE INJURY ON NUTRITIONAL THERAPY

Following trauma, infection, or surgical intervention requiring SICU care, patients typically manifest four stages of response to the injury: shock, resuscitation, stable hypermetabolism, and organ failure. Not all patients exhibit all four stages. If source control and resuscitation are effective, or if the injury is uncomplicated, the hypermetabolic response peaks on day 3 to 5 postinjury and abates by day 7 to 10. For a very severe injury, the response can be a rapid death. If the response persists after 3 to 5 days, a complication is frequently present. Prompt recognition and treatment of the complication can result in complete patient recovery. Sometimes the hypermetabolic response continues unabated, even though the causes have been removed or treated. The patient then enters the phase of multiple organ dysfunction or multiple system organ failure. Mortality at this point is high (Fig. 3-2).

The patterns of response to injury were originally described following multiple trauma. The same pattern has since been observed after severe infections, septic shock, hypovolemia, hypovolemic shock, inadequate resuscitation, and severe inflammation, such as pancreatitis. Different etiologies, and in the case of infection

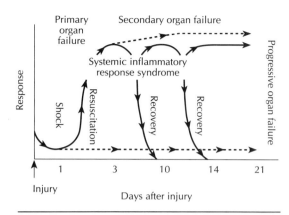

FIG. 3-2 Commonly observed clinical responses to injury. Which response occurs depends on type and severity of injury, delay in effective treatment, type of treatment received, and chronic disease status of patient.

different microorganisms, do not produce distinguishable alterations in vital signs, physiology, or metabolism. The concept of the systemic inflammatory response syndrome (SIRS) has evolved, and the term "sepsis" is reserved for SIRS with evidence of infection.

Most of the investigations of nutritional support have been performed after resuscitation and during the systemic inflammatory response. The physiology and metabolism of this phase of response is markedly different from that of starvation (see box, p. 22). The clinical manifestations reflect the modulation of the physiology and metabolism by the neuroendocrine and cell-cell communication systems. The responses, therefore, are regulated by the intensity and duration of the inflammatory mediator signals (Tables 3-2 and 3-3).

When the systemic inflammatory response is present, total calories or glucose calories in excess of demand can result in adverse effects, including fatty infiltration of the liver with hepatic dysfunction, hyperosmolar states, excess carbon dioxide production, increased oxygen consumption, stimulation of catecholamine release, and increased lactate production. Excess enteral feedings will, in addition, produce increased intestinal gas and bowel distention. Excess calories fail to suppress gluconeogenesis and to alter catabolic or synthetic rates. Limiting caloric and glucose load to the usable total ca-

Characteristics of Systemic Inflammatory Response

Clinical observations

Persistent inflammatory response—fever, leukocytosis, hypermetabolism, activated macrophage

Nosocomial infection

Wound failure

Malnutrition—altered body composition, specific or generalized nutrient deficiencies

Organ failure—lung, liver, kidney, gut

Immune dysfunction—anergy, decreased B-cell function, decreased T-cell function

Physiologic observations

Increased oxygen consumption demand

Increased cardiac output and oxygen delivery

Increased demand for ventilation

Decreased systemic vascular resistence

Peripheral oxygen extraction abnormality

Metabolic observations

Increased gluconeogenesis and lipolysis

Relative nonresponsiveness of gluconeogenesis and lipolysis to down regulation by exogenous glucose

Energy production by process of aerobic glycolysis

Utilization of mixed carbon source for energy production—glucose, fatty acids of all chain length, and amino acids

Increased catabolic rate that exceeds that of anabolism; anabolic rate responsive to exogenous amino acids while catabolic rate is poorly responsive

Change in body composition characterized by rapid reduction in lean body mass that is poorly responsive to exogenous amino acids and anabolic hormone administration

Redistribution of body nitrogen to areas of active protein synthesis such as viscera, wounds, and white cell mass

TABLE 3-2   Correlation Between Metabolic Parameters and Degree of Stress Response

Stress Level*	Clinical Prototype	Urinary Nitrogen (g/day)	Oxygen Consumed (ml/M²)	Blood Glucose (mg/dl)	Plasma Lactate (mM/L)	Glucagon Insulin Ratio
0	Starvation	<5	90 ± 10	100 ± 20	100 ± 50	2 ± 0.5
1	Elective surgery	5-10	130 ± 10	150 ± 25	1200 ± 200	2.5 ± 0.8
2	Trauma	10-15	150 ± 20	150 ± 25	1200 ± 200	3 ± 0.7
3	Sepsis	>15	180 ± 20	250 ± 50	2500 ± 500	8 ± 1.5

*Levels represent a continuum within which ranges of values or patterns of use can be identified. Likewise, an individual patient may not coincide with the clinical prototype (e.g., all septic patients do not exhibit level 3 metabolism).

TABLE 3-3   Examples of Metabolic Support

Stress Level	Total Calories (g/kg)	Nonprotein Calories (g/kg)	Amino Acids (g/kg)	Nonprotein Calorie/ Nitrogen Ratio	Basal Energy Expenditure Multiple
0	25	20	1	150/1	1
1	30	25	1.5	100/1	1
2	35	30	2	100/1	1.5
3	35	30	2	100/1	2

loric and glucose requirement (25 to 30 kcal/kg/day and 3 to 5 kcal/kg/day, respectively) and substituting fat calories for glucose calories can minimize these adverse effects. The glucose load should be adjusted to maintain a blood sugar concentration <225 mg/dl. A serum concentration of glucose >225 mg/dl alters white cell function. In the absence of diabetes mellitus, insulin does not appear to increase the oxidation rate of glucose and may contribute to the adverse hepatic effects of excess glucose.

Current fat emulsions primarily contain n-6 polyunsaturated long-chain fatty acids and were designed to treat or prevent essential fatty acid deficiency. These emulsions have been used as a caloric source, particularly when glucose administration is restricted. High doses of n-6 fatty acid–based emulsion (>1.5 g/kg/day), given when they are used as a caloric source, can produce increased turnover and release of eicosanoids, hepatic steatosis, bile duct proliferation, periportal inflammation, and clinical cholestatic jaundice. Other adverse effects include decreased pulmonary diffusion capacity, decreased particulate and bacterial clearance, decreased cell-mediated immunity, decreased phagocytosis, and decreased bactericidal function. In the presence of excess n-6 fatty acids, decreased lymphoproliferation in response to an antigenic stimulus occurs. Further, increased release of macrophage-derived dienoic series prostaglandins and cytokines, such as interleukin 1 and 6 and tumor necrosis factor, has been observed. Adverse clinical outcomes also have been documented. During a 4- to 6-week SICU course, no added benefit arises from achieving caloric equilibrium. Nitrogen equilibrium, rather than caloric equilibrium, produces survival advantage. Many of the commonly employed enteral formulas contain high percentages of n-6 fatty acids and are associated with the same problems. For these reasons, current recommendations call for no more than 1.5 g/kg/day of these fats, administered either enterally or parenterally.

Clearance of these fat emulsions occurs by both enzymatic and particulate mechanisms and needs to be monitored. As the hypermetabolism progresses, lipoprotein lipase function decreases in skeletal muscle, and fat and the hepatic output of very low density lipoprotein triglyceride increases. With reduced triglyceride clearance, continuous infusion of fat over a 24-hour period may improve the patient's tolerance.

In hypermetabolic-mediated states, the skeletal muscle mass is rapidly mobilized. Some of the amino acids are oxidized for energy production in skeletal muscle; others are transported to the liver for gluconeogenesis or protein synthesis. A fraction of the amino acid pool is taken up by the mononuclear cell mass and active wounds for protein synthesis. Clinically, skeletal muscle mass rapidly disappears. Exogenous amino acid administration does not significantly reduce the catabolic rate. However, the total body synthetic rate is sensitive to amino acid infusion. As the load of exogenous amino acids is increased, the synthetic rate is increased. This process can occur until the synthetic rate equals the catabolic rate, at which point nitrogen equilibrium is achieved. Achieving nitrogen equilibrium results in less total nitrogen loss over the course of the illness and better support of visceral protein synthesis. Plasma concentrations of visceral proteins and measurements of synthetic rates increase. The visceral protein concentrations, however, do not return to normal values until the inflammatory process has subsided, a consequence of acute-phase protein gene activation and the effects of cytokine mediators on hepatic protein synthesis.

The measurement of nitrogen balance in the stressed patient should probably be done by total urine nitrogen rather than by urine urea nitrogen. In stressed patients, the urinary urea nitrogen can vary between 40% and 90% of the total nitrogen. Current formulas do not accurately compensate for this discrepancy between urea nitrogen and total nitrogen. The objective measure most strongly correlated with improved outcomes is nitrogen balance. Approaching nitrogen equilibrium in the clinical setting of hypermetabolism is of major importance.

The different effects of exogenous amino acids on synthetic and catabolic rates account for the observed dose-dependent nitrogen retention and the need for 1.5 to 2 g/kg/day to achieve nitrogen equilibrium. Because of these nitrogen kinetics, a search for a more efficient amino acid profile was undertaken. In a number of randomized, prospective clinical trials, modified amino acids were demonstrated to be significantly more efficient "protein" sources. None of the studies, however, was designed to evaluate improved patient outcomes, and the question awaits clinical testing.

METABOLIC SUPPORT
Route of Administration

Most practitioners would use the gut whenever possible. Early enteral feeding is safe and nutritionally efficacious. The GI tract is more functional than initially thought. Most of the ileus is related to the stomach and colon. Intubation beyond the ligament of Treitz facilitates enteral nutrition and minimizes morbidity. Enteral feeding of 0.6/kg/day nitrogen appears to maintain gut integrity and immune function, and enteral feeding of essential fatty acids can control bacterial translocation in experimental models. Early postinjury feeding via the GI tract may blunt the hypermetabolic response, preserve GI immune competence, and decrease translocation of luminal bacteria. However, translocation as a pathogenic mechanism in this setting remains to be demonstrated. In the burn patient, early enteral feeding diminishes hypermetabolism and preserves gut integrity. Once hypermetabolism has been established (2 to 3 days postinjury), the enteral route does not appear to confer special advantage in reducing the hypermetabolic response.

Enterocyte Nutrient Effects

Enterocytes appear to have some special requirements that necessitate nutrients within the intestinal lumen. When total parenteral nutrition (TPN) is used as the sole form of nutritional support, these requirements may not be met. Glutamine is one of these nutrients. The lack of glutamine may be partially responsible for the breakdown in the gut mucosal barrier when enteral nutrition is not employed. Once formulation problems have been solved, glutamine can be added to TPN formulas. Whether its addition will improve patient outcome, however, remains to be demonstrated. In a similar way, little clinical evidence exists that adding glutamine to enteral formulas improves patient outcome. Most enteral formulas contain glutamine that is biologically available. A number of other components of enteral formulas, including ketone bodies, short- and long-chain fatty acids, and branched-chain amino acids, also appear to have the same enterocyte-supporting effects.

Short-chain fatty acids are a preferred fuel source for the colonocyte. The combination of bowel rest and TPN results in colonic mucosal atrophy in experimental animals. Providing beta-hydroxybutyric acid in TPN can reduce the TPN-associated colonic mucosal involution. Experimental data demonstrate that short-chain fatty acids, either added directly to enteral formulas or as fiber to be metabolized, can improve the healing of colonic anastomoses.

Polyunsaturated Fatty Acids

The administration of lipid can alter the membranes of cells and produce a fatty acid composition similar to that of the administered lipid. This altered membrane phospholipid composition also changes many of the basic membrane functions: fluidity, peroxidation, signal transduction, and the type of prostanoid/leukotriene released in response to a stimulus. Lipid emulsions currently in use are predominantly omega-6 (n-6) polyunsaturated fatty acids (PUFAs) the precursors of the dienoic series of arachidonic acid metabolites. Omega-3 (n-3) PUFA promotes the formation of the trienoic series of prostaglandins and leukotrienes, reduces thrombogenesis, and blunts inflammation. Reducing the n-6/n-3 PUFA ratio of the macrophage membrane can reduce the stimulated release of dienoic prostaglandins and leukotrienes and decrease the release of interleukin 1 and tumor necrosis factor in response to a lipopolysaccharide (LPS) stimulus.

Medium-chain triglyceride fatty acids, with 8 to 10 carbon atoms, have a number of potential benefits, including rapid clearance with less interference in the reticuloendothelial system pathways, carnitine-independent uptake by the mitochondria, and protein-sparing effects at least equal to long-chain triglycerides. Short-chain triglycerides also offer an alternate, readily oxidizable source of energy. Demonstration of clinical efficacy for short-chain triglycerides awaits clinical trials.

Growth Factors

Human growth hormone (GH) can improve nitrogen balance in highly catabolic burn patients. GH enhances the ability of the stressed individual to utilize endogenous fat stores as a fuel source. In septic patients with systemic inflammation, GH has no improved nutritional or overall patient outcome. In contrast, low-stressed, routine postoperative patients derive a clear nutritional benefit from administered GH. Altered carbohydrate metabolism in sepsis produces hyperglycemia and insulin resistance. The increased incidence of hepatic steatosis and the inability to increase glucose oxidation, despite lowering serum glucose concentrations, do not support the aggressive use of exogenous insulin.

Immune System Modulation

Despite aggressive nutritional support, immune dysfunction persists in the critically ill patient. This continued dysfunction reflects abnormalities in at least two portions of the specific antigen response system: (1) antigen processing by macrophages, and (2) a reduced ability of T cells to proliferate in response to antigen stimulation. An excess of suppressive substances such as prostaglandin E_2, appears to be a major contributing factor. Specific nutrients, arginine, uracil, and n-3 PUFA, are now being used to reverse these effects. This form of metabolic support is referred to as nutrient pharmacology.

Dietary nucleotides, specifically uracil, can restore skin test response, enhance in vitro T-cell proliferation to IL-2 stimulation, correct T-helper cell maturation arrest, and enhance induction of adenosine deaminase and purine nucleoside phosphorylase activities. Both adenosine deaminase and purine nucleoside phosphorylase are important in T-cell maturation. In animals fed nucleotide-free diets, these activities are reduced. Arginine has multiple effects on the immune response. It acts as a secretagogue for GH, improves wound healing, and improves T-cell proliferative responses.

These three agents, along with standard nutrients, have been formulated into an enteral product. When this product was used in patients with sepsis, in vitro tests showed restoration of immune function after 7 days of therapy. A multicenter trial has now demonstrated a significant reduction in the length of SICU stay.

ASSESSMENT AND MONITORING

The assessment of body composition and the response to nutritional therapy in the SICU patient is difficult. Bedside methods of quantifying body composition are limited. Of those available, impedance plethysmography is probably the most useful type, but its use is limited in the presence of increased total body water, a finding common in SICU patients. In addition, alterations in body composition reflect the disease process, such as systemic inflammation. Recovery of lean body mass does not occur until the inflammatory process has abated. A similar situation is present for the visceral proteins. The redistribution of body protein to the visceral compartment, particularly in the presence of nutritional support, is modulated by the mediator systems. Mediator systems favor acute phase-protein synthesis over nonacute-phase proteins. Thus low albumin and transferrin concentrations may reflect inadequate nutrient supply or an active inflammatory process. With optimum metabolic support, the concentrations of such proteins as plasma transferrin should rise in response to amino acid/protein loading, particularly with modified amino acid formulations enriched with branched chains. Failure of transferrin concentration to rise, despite amino acid loading, suggests advanced organ failure.

Assessment of nutritional status, then, relies heavily on the physical examination and the clinical setting. Measurement of nitrogen excretion and oxygen consumption are useful in judging the degree of hypermetabolism that is present. Predicting energy and caloric needs from the many formulas is difficult. The kilogram guidelines presented in the box on p. 18 have been useful for management of stressed patients. Direct measurement of the respiratory quotient can be done to assess the adequacy of mix and the amount of metabolic fuels. How-

Metabolic Complications of Nutritional Support

Substrate intolerance as origin:
  Hyperglycemia
  Hypoglycemia
  Excess carbon dioxide production
  Hyperlipidemia
  Abnormal liver function tests (e.g., cholestasis, steatosis)
Fluid/electrolyte intolerance as origin:
  Hypovolemia/hypervolemia
  Hyponatremia/hypernatremia
  Hypokalemia/hyperkalemia
  Hypophosphatemia/Hyperphosphatemia
  Hypomagnesemia/hypermagnesemia
  Hypocalcemia/hypercalcemia
  Metabolic acidosis/alkalosis

ever, measurement of the respiratory quotient does not have utility on a routine basis.

Monitoring is essential to maximize benefit and to minimize complications. In general, if the protocol of Fig. 3-1 is followed, metabolic complications should be rare events (see box). Monitoring of daily weights is essential. SICU patients will not gain weight from nutritional support in most cases. Weight gain or absence of weight loss of up to 0.5 kg/day usually indicates water retention. Electrolytes need to be monitored on a daily basis until stability of the patient's condition is achieved. Zinc and magnesium need to be provided in doses that maintain reasonable blood concentrations to promote wound healing and minimize cardiac dysrhythmias, respectively. Other intracellular ions, such as phosphate and potassium, need to be kept in the high normal range to facilitate appropriate metabolism of the nutrients provided. Adequate doses of vitamins and trace elements need to be given on a daily basis when the glomerular filtration rate is adequate, and a number of commercial preparations are available for this purpose. Medication incompatibilities are a major potential problem with nutritional support, both enteral and parenteral. The list is long and increasing. It is strongly recommended that a clinical pharmacist be involved in the nutritional and metabolic management of SICU patients.

BUN usually will increase with nutritional support. Most of this increase is from the hypermetabolism itself. The remainder is a result of the amino acids/protein provided. A wide variety of utilization efficiency for amino acids/protein is present, varying from low in regular food to high for the modified amino acids. The higher utilization efficiency, the less urea is generated per gram of administered protein. In general, BUN is not a cause for major concern when the concentration is <110 mg/dl. In some cases, however, altered mental status and platelet dysfunction can occur. Renal injury from amino acid loading to achieve nitrogen retention has not been observed over the course of the SICU stay in such patients. The single best index of adequacy of nutritional support remains nitrogen retention as measured by nitrogen balance.

Line care is essential. When appropriate line care is provided, complications should be <1% for placement and <3% per patient for infection. The central line should be used for TPN administration only. In practice, however, exclusive use of the TPN line for TPN only is seldom possible. Nonetheless, with appropriate line care and attention, infection rates can still be maintained in the 3% range per patient.

The major enteral feeding complication is aspiration. Since gastric atony usually is present, aspiration generally occurs during gastric feeding. When feeding is administered distal to the pylorus, this complication becomes rare. Placing the feeding tube in this position can be done at surgery, under fluoroscopy, or by endoscopy. Contraindications to enteral nutrition include bowel obstruction, ileus with thick-walled small bowel, and fresh anastamoses. A relative contraindication is large-volume diarrhea induced by a drug, disease, or microbe. More than 95% of patients can be fed via the enteral route. Diarrhea is a common occurrence in SICU patients in the absence of enteral feeding and is mainly related to the administration of antibiotics. Diarrhea can occur with enteral feeding, but it is not usually related to formula osmolality and normally does not preclude successful enteral feeding. Most patients will tolerate full feeding volume within 36 to 48 hours by using continuous administration with an enteral tube feeding pump.

SPECIAL CLINICAL PROBLEMS

With both enteral and parenteral nutrition, several special clinical problems arise that necessitate modification of the basic approach. Such cases include patients requiring volume restriction, those with advanced pulmonary insufficiency, and those with cirrhosis of the liver or liver failure.

Volume Restriction

The volume of nutritional support administration is sometimes restricted by renal insufficiency, requirements for blood and blood products, pulmonary edema, and a need for diuresis of total body water. In general, the nutritional requirements do not change, but the administration volume may change. In progressive renal insufficiency, restriction of such components as magnesium, zinc, trace elements, and phosphate may be necessary, especially when the creatinine clearance is <20 ml/min. It also may be necessary to reduce the amount of nitrogen administered in order to allow the BUN to remain <110 mg/dl. In the latter situation, however, if restriction is under 1 g/kg/day, some form of dialysis or hemofiltration should be started to allow administration of adequate nutrition. The use of amino acid formulas marketed for renal failure is neither necessary nor beneficial. The renal insufficiency is usually not an isolated organ dysfunction. Standard or branched-chain-enriched formulas produce the same results as special renal formulas.

Volume restriction can be accomplished by concentrating the formula. Current technology for mixing TPN permits a broad range of formulations. Cost can be controlled with the use of a single bag for administration of glucose and amino acids. High-density enteral formulations are also available and well tolerated. In unusual cases enteral modular technology offers almost the same flexibility as custom mixing for TPN. For such special situations a knowledgeable clinical pharmacist or dietitian can be of great help.

Advanced Pulmonary Insufficiency

Advanced intrinsic lung disease, restrictive or obstructive, can require specialized formulations to minimize carbon dioxide production.

In general, carbohydrate administration increases carbon dioxide production, amino acid/protein consumption, and oxygen consumption. Excess glucose calories can increase energy expenditure and carbon dioxide production to a level that is clinically important in the management of a patient with pulmonary insufficiency.

To prevent increased carbon dioxide production, the glucose load is reduced and the fat load is increased. Amino acid/protein necessary to achieve nitrogen equilibrium is administered. Note that the fat load still should not exceed 1 to 1.5 g/kg/day of n-6 PUFA triglyceride. Medium-chain fats should be used for additional calories, if necessary. Patients receiving such supplementation may require expired gas monitoring to maintain a respiratory quotient under 0.9.

Cirrhosis With Liver Failure

Patients with end-stage liver disease may enter the SICU with overt liver failure resulting from trauma or a surgical procedure or as a complication of cirrhosis (e.g., variceal bleeding). For these patients, the major change in nutritional formulation involves the amino acids. Amino acids should not be restricted in the presence of encephalopathy. Rather, administration of amino acid formulations designed for this problem can improve the encephalopathy status and survival.

Intravenous and enteral formulations (e.g., Hepatamine, Hepatic Aid, or Travesorb Hepatic) contain amino acid formulations designed for liver cirrhosis with encephalopathy. The patient's mental status can be used as an aid in guiding the use of such formulations. In the presence of cirrhosis, standard amino acid formulations can be used effectively as long as encephalopathy is not present. When encephalopathy occurs, the special formulations should be used in doses that will result in nitrogen retention, until encephalopathy has subsided and is not likely to recur. These amino acid formulations should *not* be used in the absence of cirrhosis with encephalopathy, including patients with the systemic inflammatory response who have hepatic dysfunction. The branched-chain-enriched formulas are more appropriate in the latter situation.

SUMMARY

- Metabolic support is one of the major foundations of modern critical care.
- Begin metabolic support after source control and restoration of oxygen transport have been achieved.
- Malnutrition is altered body composition that includes a reduction in lean body mass or visceral protein mass inappropriate for the patient's age, sex, height, weight, or activity status.
- Malnutrition is an acquired condition that results from either a specific nutrient deficiency, a general nutrient deficiency, or both.
- Modern metabolic support can prevent specific and generalized nutrient deficiencies.
- Benefits of metabolic support do not depend on route of administration. Enteral and parenteral routes are both effective.

- Systemic inflammatory response is regulated by inflammatory mediators. Principles of nutritional support developed for starvation do not apply.
- Kilogram rules (see box, p. 18) are useful guidelines for management of hypermetabolic patients.
- Enteral feeding may support the gut mucosal barrier.
- Altering composition of fatty acid infusions may change the systemic response.
- Monitoring is essential for maximizing benefits and minimizing complications of nutritional support (see Fig. 3-1).
- Placement of feeding tubes distal to pylorus minimizes aspiration.
- Advanced pulmonary insufficiency, liver failure, and requirements for volume restriction mandate alterations in metabolic support.

BIBLIOGRAPHY

Abraham E, Chang Y-H. The effects of hemorrhage on mitogen-induced lymphocyte proliferation. Circ Shock 15(2):141-149, 1985.

ACCP - SCCM Consensus Conference: Definitions for sepsis and organ failure and guidelines for the use of innovative therapies in sepsis. Chest 101:1644-1655, 1992.

Barbul A, Sisto DA, Wasserkrug HL, et al. Metabolic and immune effects of arginine in post-injury hyperalimentation. J Trauma 21:970-974, 1981.

Barton R, Cerra FB. The hypermetabolism multiple system organ failure. Chest 96:1153-1160, 1989.

Cerra FB, Hirsch J, Mullen K, Blackburn G, Luther W. The effect of stress level, amino acid formula, and nitrogen dose on nitrogen retention in traumatic and septic stress. Ann Surg 205:282-287, 1987.

Cerra FB, Lehman S, Konstantinides N, Konstantinides F, Shronts EP, Holman R. Effect of enteral nutrient on in vitro tests of immune function in ICU patients: A preliminary report. Nutrition 6:84-87, 1990.

Cerra FB, McPherson J, Konstantinides FN, Konstantinides NN, Teasley KM. Enteral nutrition does not prevent multiple organ failure syndrome after sepsis. Surgery 104(4):727-733, 1988.

Cerra FB, Siegal JH, Coleman B, Border JR, McMenamy RH. Septic autocannibalism: A failure of exogenous nutritional support. Ann Surg 192:570-580, 1980.

Cuthbertson D, Tilstone W. Metabolism during the post-injury period. Adv Clin Chem 12:1-55, 1977.

Dinarello CA. Interleukin-1 and the pathogenesis of the acute-phase response. N Engl J Med 311:341-344, 1984.

Elwyn D, Kinney JM, Juvanandum M. Influence of increasing carbohydrate intake of glucose kinetics in injured patients. Ann Surg 190:117-127, 1979.

Feuerstein G, Hallenbeck JM. Prostaglandins, leukotrienes, and platelet-activating factor in shock. Ann Rev Pharmacol Toxicol 27:301-313, 1987.

Kinsella JE, Lokesh B, Broughton S, Whelan J. Dietary polyunsaturated fatty acids and eicosanoids: Potential effects on the modulation of inflammatory and immune cells—An overview. Nutrition 6(1):24-44, 1990.

Kulkarni AD, Fanslow WC, Rudolph FB, Van Buren CT. Effect of dietary nucleotides on response to bacterial infections. J Parenter Enter Nutr 10:169-171, 1986.

McCord JM. The superoxide free radical: Its biochemistry and pathophysiology. Surgery 94:412-414, 1983.

Moore EE, Dunn EL, Jones TN: Immediate jejunostomy feeding. Its use after major abdominal trauma. Arch Surg 116:681-684, 1981.

Saito H, Trocki O, Wang S, et al. Metabolic and immune effects of dietary arginine supplementation after burn. Arch Surg 122:784-789, 1987.

Siegel JH, Cerra FB, Coleman B, Giovannini I, Shetye M, Border JR, McMenamy RH. Physiological and metabolic correlation in human sepsis. Surgery 806:163-193, 1979.

Vilcek LEJ. Biology of disease TNF and IL-1: Cytokines with multiple overlapping biological activities. Lab Invest 56:234-248, 1987.

Wilmore DW, Aulick LH. Systemic responses to injury and the healing wound. J Parenter Enter Nutr 4(2):147-151, 1980.

Wolfe R. Allsop J. Burke J. Glucose metabolism in man: Responses to intravenous glucose infusion. Metabolism 28:210-220, 1979.

CHAPTER 4

Lactic Acidosis

Paul Druck

The term "lactic acidosis" embodies two separate pathologic processes: *hyperlactatemia* and *metabolic acidosis*. The accumulation of excess lactate itself (a weak base) does not cause acidemia. However, inadequate tissue oxygen delivery or utilization, the most common cause of hyperlactatemia, may simultaneously cause acidemia; hence the common use of the combined term "lactic acidosis." Although lactic acidosis generally indicates a severe metabolic derangement, there are many causes of hyperlactatemia, some of lesser clinical significance.

PATHOGENESIS
Hyperlactatemia

Lactate, a metabolic "dead end," is derived exclusively from pyruvate (rare exceptions will be noted later) and must be converted back to pyruvate to be utilized.[1] Lactate and pyruvate exist in a cytosolic equilibrium catalyzed by lactate dehydrogenase (LDH) and regulated by concentrations of hydrogen ion (H+) and the NAD$^+$/NADH (nicotinamide adenine dinucleotide [oxidized form/reduced form]) ratio:

$$\text{Pyruvate + NADA + H}^+ \xrightleftharpoons{\text{LDH}} \text{Lactate + NAD}^+$$

The cellular NAD$^+$/NADH ratio in turn depends on O$_2$ availability and intact mitochondrial function. Lactate concentrations are thus a reflection of pyruvate metabolism (production vs. utilization) and cellular oxidative capacity. Hyperlactatemia thus may be contributed to by a shift in the lactate/pyruvate equilibrium toward lactate, decreased pyruvate utilization, or increased pyruvate production (Fig. 4-1).

The most important cause of a shift in the lactate/pyruvate ratio toward lactate is decreased mitochondrial oxidative capacity, which may result from cellular hypoxia or toxins. Lactate production consumes NADH; oxidation back to pyruvate requires NAD$^+$. NAD$^+$ is regenerated from NADH indirectly via mitochondrial oxidative phosphorylation and cytosolic/mitochondrial shuttles. During cellular hypoxia this mechanism is depressed, and as the NAD$^+$/NADH ratio falls, lactate accumulates. Reduction of pyruvate to lactate during cellular hypoxia actually may be useful because it produces NAD$^+$, which is necessary for glycolysis.

The usual metabolic fate of pyruvate is oxidation in the tricarboxylic acid (TCA) cycle. The rate-limiting step is oxidation to acetyl-CoA by the pyruvate dehydrogenase complex (PDH). Acetyl-CoA also may be utilized for the biosynthesis of fatty acids, cholesterol, and other substances. Sepsis specifically inhibits PDH, thereby interfering with cellular energy production and pyruvate utilization.[2] The principal disposal route for pyruvate under this circumstance is gluconeogenesis via the Cori cycle, which occurs in the liver and kidney only. When inhibition of oxidative pathways directs accumulating pyruvate to gluconeogenesis, glycolysis eventually returns the three carbon moieties back to the expanding pyruvate pool (futile cycling) for eventual repeated gluconeogenesis and further lactate buildup.

Normally, the liver clears up to 70% of a lactate load, and the kidneys clear 20% to 30%.

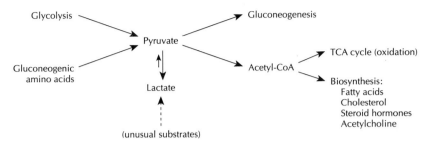

FIG. 4-1   Overview of lactate and pyruvate metabolism.

Other tissues, such as skeletal muscle and heart, also can extract lactate. Hepatic extraction follows saturable, second-order kinetics with a V_{max} equal to 5.72 mmol/kg$^{0.75}$/hr (approximately 3300 mmol/day @ 70 kg), as determined in lactate-loading studies of animals. Acidosis, hepatic ischemia or hypoxia, or hepatic parenchymal disease can markedly impair extraction, under which circumstance renal extraction increases significantly. Renal utilization involves gluconeogenesis and oxidation; excretion is minimal with a tubular transport maximum of 6 to 10 mmol/L. Basal lactate production averages 20 mmol/kg/day (1400 mmol/day @ 70 kg).[1] Normal plasma lactate concentrations are 1 to 2 mmol/L.

Pyruvate overproduction is probably a minor contributor to hyperlactatemia. The principal sources of pyruvate are glycolysis and transamination of gluconeogenic amino acids (especially alanine). Glycolysis may be accelerated by hypoxia since a falling ATP/(ADP, AMP) ratio stimulates phosphofructokinase (Pasteur's effect). Hypoxia rapidly activates glycogen phosphorylase, providing increased substrate for glycolysis. Alkalosis also stimulates glycolysis at the phosphofructokinase level, but its effect on lactate levels may be partially offset by a shift in the lactate/pyruvate equilibrium away from lactate. Sepsis and hypermetabolism drive protein catabolism, with mobilization of large quantities of gluconeogenic amino acids, which contribute to the pyruvate pool.

Associated Acidemia

Hyperlactatemia associated with acidemia is usually caused by mitochondrial dysfunction resulting from inadequate oxygen delivery or by toxic interference with oxidative phosphorylation. An important endogenous source of H^+ is ATP hydrolysis:

$$ATP^{-4} + H_2O \rightarrow ADP^{-3} + Pi + H^+$$

Normally the H^+ thus produced is consumed (indirectly) at the final step of mitochondrial electron transport:

$$2H^+ + 2e^- + \frac{1}{2}O_2 \rightarrow H_2O$$

Inadequate oxygen delivery or electron transport function interferes with this pathway. Thus ATP utilization proceeds without clearance of H^+, and acidemia results.

ETIOLOGY

The traditional classification scheme of Cohen and Woods[3] subdivides lactic acidosis into type A (low-flow, hypoperfusion, or inadequate tissue oxygen delivery) and type B (sepsis, toxins, or metabolic derangements) (see box, p. 32). Combined processes are common, particularly sepsis complicated by hypoperfusion or diabetic decompensation complicated by hypovolemia.

Anemia itself rarely causes lactic acidosis, unless the anemia is life-threatening. More commonly, anemia exacerbates perfusion deficits by further impairing oxygen delivery. Similarly, vitamin deficiencies usually are complicating factors in stressed patients with other causes of hyperlactatemia. Thiamine is a necessary cofactor for PDH; biotin is necessary for pyruvate carboxylase (which catalyzes the first step in gluconeogenesis from pyruvate).

Hepatic insufficiency does not usually cause elevated lactate concentrations in unstressed

| Etiology of Lactic Acidosis

Type A—inadequate tissue oxygen delivery

Shock (cardiogenic, septic, hypovolemic)
Regional ischemia (limb, splanchnic)
Severe hypoxemia
Severe anemia
Relative hypoperfusion (generalized seizure, intense anaerobic skeletal muscle activity)

Type B—sepsis, toxins, metabolic derangements

Sepsis
Diabetes mellitus
Liver insufficiency
Neoplasms (especially lymphomas, metastatic oat cell carcinoma)
Vitamin deficiencies (thiamin, biotin)
Inborn errors of metabolism:
  Glucose-6-phosphatase deficiency
  Fructose 1,6-diphosphatase deficiency
  Pyruvate carboxylase deficiency
  Pyruvate dehydrogenase deficiency
  Mitochondrial oxidative defects
Toxins:
  Acetaminophen
  Biguanides (phenformin)
  Cyanide
  Ethanol
  Ethylene glycol
  Fructose
  Isoniazid
  Methyl isocyanate
  Nitroglycerin
  Nitroprusside
  Propylene glycol
  Salicylates
  Sorbitol
  Streptozotocin
  Xylitol
Other: D-lactatic acidosis in intestinal bypass

patients. However, it will prolong the half-life of a lactate load produced during a metabolic insult, particularly if accompanied by hypoxemia, acidosis, or splanchnic hypoperfusion. In general, lactic acidosis in a patient with liver disease has the same clinical significance as in a patient with normal liver function.[4]

The various short-chain alcohols may consume intermediates necessary for pyruvate utilization (PO_4^{-3}, NAD^+) or may be converted directly to lactate without pyruvate intermediates (ethylene glycol, propylene glycol). Propylene glycol is a vehicle for certain water-insoluble drugs. If administered in sufficiently high doses, particularly in the patient with preexisting liver disease, it can cause hyperlactatemia.

Hyperlactatemia also may be seen in some solid and hematologic malignancies, especially metastatic oat cell carcinoma. Hepatic replacement by tumor may play a role in this condition.[5]

CLINICAL CORRELATES

Lactic acidosis has been associated with weakness, malaise, anorexia, vomiting, changes in mental status, hyperventilation, tachycardia, hemodynamic instability, mild hypochloremia, hyperphosphatemia, and hyperuricemia (competition for renal excretion). In general, the manifestations of lactic acidosis are integral parts of, or are overshadowed by, the underlying disorder.[1]

A crude correlation exists between the magnitude of lactic acidosis and the prognosis.[6-8] The rate and magnitude of response to therapy and the etiology of the lactic acidosis are probably better indicators of prognosis and adequacy of treatment (see treatment of sepsis and shock in Chapters 1 and 2, respectively).

If pyruvate determinations are available, the lactate/pyruvate ratio may be indicative of the predominant class of derangement. A normal ratio (<20) is associated with sepsis and some intoxications. An elevated ratio (>20) is consistent with hypoperfusion, hypoxemia, or interference with mitochondrial oxidation.[9]

TREATMENT

Once hyperlactatemia, with or without metabolic acidemia, has been identified, the underlying cause(s) should be sought and corrected. Although some data support an independent deleterious effect of lactate (e.g., as a negative inotrope),[10-12] the basic metabolic derangement greatly overshadows this effect. Specific therapy and general supportive care will be dictated by the patient's diagnosis and his/her general condition.

Inadequate tissue oxygen delivery should be corrected by improving cardiac performance, oxygen content, and regional perfusion (see Chapter 2). Compartmental ischemia (extremity or splanchnic) may require restoration of arterial or venous patency or resection.

If sepsis is suspected, it should be treated by elimination of the infectious source, administration of antibiotics, and restoration of microcirculatory perfusion. The presence of toxins should be considered and excluded. Preexisting metabolic disorders, such as diabetes mellitus or thiamine deficiency, should be addressed.

Signs of resolving hyperlactatemia and acidemia indicate metabolic improvement, but occult hypoperfusion can exist in the face of a normal or near-normal lactate concentration. Acidemia in particular is a *late* consequence of tissue hypoxia. The principles of establishment of flow-independent oxygen consumption should be considered (see Chapter 2).

The management of severe metabolic acidemia is controversial. The basic strategy always should be correction of the underlying derangement and restoration of adequate perfusion. A growing body of evidence suggests that alkali therapy (bicarbonate) is deleterious since it causes intracellular acidosis with paradoxical worsening of hyperlactatemia, a shift in the oxyhemoglobin dissociation curve to the left with impairment of tissue oxygenation, increased susceptibility to cardiac dysrhythmias, and, in patients with congestive heart failure, sodium and fluid overload. Bicarbonate should be withheld for all but the most severe cases of acidemia (pH <7.2). If administered, only enough bicarbonate to raise the pH from dangerously low levels should be used. Attempts to titrate the pH to near-normal before perfusion is restored will result in dangerous "overshoot alkalemia." Equimolar sodium carbonate/bicarbonate prevents some of these deleterious side effects; however, this agent is not widely available.[13,14]

Hemodialysis or peritoneal dialysis may be useful in severe lactic acidosis associated with renal insufficiency or congestive heart failure.[1]

Dichloroacetic acid (DCA), which specifically reverses the septic inhibition of PDH, can lower blood lactate concentration and has been used successfully in humans. Responders have a better prognosis, but the response to DCA may be a mere marker of better underlying prognosis. The lack of adequate randomized prospective data makes it difficult to draw firm conclusions about the role of DCA.[15]

SUMMARY

- Hyperlactatemia and metabolic acidemia, two separate pathologic processes, contribute to lactic acidosis.
- Accumulation of excess lactate does not cause acidemia. Associated inadequate tissue oxygen delivery or use usually produces acidemia.
- Lactate concentrations reflect pyruvate metabolism and cellular oxidative capacity.
- A shift in equilibrium toward lactate production is usually caused by decreased cellular oxidative capacity, resulting from hypoxia or toxins.
- Sepsis inhibits PDH, the rate-limiting step in pyruvate oxidation.

- The liver clears up to 70% of a lactate load, and the kidneys clear 20% to 30%.
- In patients with liver disease, lactic acidosis has the same clinical significance as in patients with normal liver function.
- In the presence of mild hyperlactatemia, a lactate/pyruvate ratio >20 is associated with hypoperfusion, hypoxemia, or impaired mitochondrial function.
- Presence of hyperlactatemia should result in prompt recognition and therapy of the underlying disorder.

REFERENCES

1. Madias NE. Lactic acidosis. Kidney Int 29:752-774, 1986.
2. Vary TC, Seigel JH, Nakatani T, et al. Effect of sepsis on activity of pyruvate dehydrogenase complex in skeletal muscle and liver. Am J Physiol 250:E634-E640, 1986.
3. Cohen RD, Woods HF. Clinical and Biochemical Aspects of Lactic Acidosis. Boston: Blackwell Scientific, 1976.
4. Kruse JA, Zaidi SAJ, Carlson R, et al. Significance of blood lactate levels in critically ill patients with liver disease. Am J Med 83:77-82, 1987.
5. Spechler SJ, Esposito AL, Raymond S, et al. Lactic acidosis in oat cell carcinoma with extensive hepatic metastases. Arch Int Med 138:1663-1664, 1978.
6. Weil MH, Afifi AA. Experimental and clinical studies on lactate and pyruvate as indicators of the severity of acute circulatory failure (shock). Circulation 41:989-1001, 1970.
7. Vitek V, Cowley RA. Blood lactate in the prognosis of various forms of shock. Ann Surg 173:308-313, 1971.
8. Peretz DI, Scott HM, Duff J, et al. The significance of lactic acidemia in the shock syndrome. Ann N Y Acad Sci 119:1133-1141, 1965.
9. Seigel JH, Cerra FB, Coleman B, et al. Physiological and metabolic correlations in human sepsis. Surgery 86:163-193, 1979.
10. Yatani A, Funini T, Kinoshita K, et al. Excess lactate modulates ionic currents and tension components in frog atrial muscle. J Mol Cell Cardiol 13:147-161, 1981.
11. Jurkowitz M, Scott KM, Altschuld RA, et al. Ion transport by heart mitochondria: Retention and loss of energy coupling in aged heart mitochondria. Arch Biochem Biophys 165:98-113, 1974.
12. Mochizuki S, Kobayashi K, Neely JR, et al. Effect of L-lactate on glyceraldehyde 3-phosphate dehydrogenase in heart muscle. Recent Adv Stud Cardiol Struct Metab 12:175-182, 1976.
13. Narins RG, Jones ER, Dornfeld LP, et al. Alkali therapy of the organic acidoses: A critical assessment of the data and the case for the judicious use of sodium bicarbonate. In Narins RG, ed. Controversies in Nephrology and Hypertension. London: Churchill Livingstone, 1984, pp 359-376.
14. Bersin RM, Arieff AI. Improved hemodynamic function during hypoxia with carbicarb, a new agent for the management of acidosis. Circulation 77:227-233, 1988.
15. Stacpoole PW, Lorenz AC, Thomas RG, et al. Dichloroacetate in the treatment of lactic acidosis. Ann Int Med 108:58-63, 1988.

PART TWO

CARE OF THE CRITICALLY ILL PATIENT

CHAPTER 5

Initial Approach to the Injured Patient

Richard G. Barton

INITIAL MANAGEMENT AND STABILIZATION

As in any immediately life-threatening situation, management of the trauma patient begins with the establishment or maintenance of the *A*irway, the insurance of adequate *B*reathing or ventilation, and restoration of the *C*irculation. As part of this initial resuscitation effort, a brief survey of the patient should be performed to identify and immediately treat life-threatening injuries such as tension pneumothorax, hemothorax, or brisk external hemorrhage. In addition, the patient must be managed in such a way as to prevent permanent *D*isability. Such management simultaneously involves protection and immobilization of the cervical, thoracic, and lumbar spines. Finally, a comprehensive *E*valuation of the patient's injuries should be accomplished with a detailed physical examination, laboratory tests, and appropriate x-ray and diagnostic procedures.

Although the basic treatment approach for the initial management of trauma is a simple one, the key to successful trauma management is continuous reassessment and reorganization of priorities as the clinical condition of the patient changes.

Airway

Initial airway management will vary depending on the presence or absence of shock, respiratory compromise, maxillofacial injuries, the mental status of the patient, and the potential for neurologic or cervical spine injury. A patient who is alert, talking, breathing comfortably, and hemodynamically stable may require only mask or nasal cannula oxygen. In the multiple trauma patient, however, there is frequently a need to establish an airway, protect an existing airway (with depressed mental status, oropharyngeal blood or vomitus, extensive facial fractures, expanding neck hematoma, facial or other large burns), or provide ventilatory support in the setting of existing or impending respiratory failure (Fig. 5-1).

Clinical signs of respiratory failure include tachypnea; shallow, labored breathing; use of accessory muscles; stridor; paradoxical chest wall movement, as in flail chest; cyanosis; confusion; or abnormal ABGs (partial pressure of oxygen [Po_2] <60 or partial pressure of carbon dioxide [Pco_2] >50, particularly with a pH <7.3). Apnea or cardiopulmonary arrest mandates immediate intubation, and intubation should be considered for the patient with on-

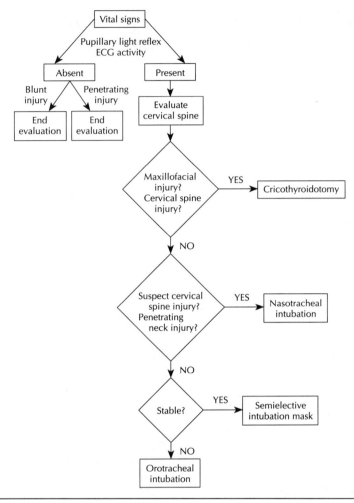

FIG. 5-1   Decision-making related to establishing an airway in the injured patient.

going hemorrhage and hemodynamic instability, particularly when surgery is anticipated. If tracheal intubation can be performed semielectively, a cross-table lateral cervical spine x-ray should be taken first to identify obvious cervical spine fractures. An adequate airway must take precedence over all other potential problems, and intubation should be performed immediately, if necessary.

Standard orotracheal intubation is the most reliable method of intubation. It is the method of choice in the setting of apnea or cardiopulmonary arrest, but such intubation usually requires manipulation of the head and neck. Orotracheal intubation should be avoided in the patient with known or suspected cervical spine injury.

Blind nasotracheal intubation requires minimal head and neck manipulation and is perhaps the tracheal intubation method of choice in the spontaneously breathing patient with known or suspected cervical spine injury. In experienced hands, nasotracheal intubation can be performed successfully in 90% of cases.[1] Nasotracheal intubation should be avoided when midfacial fractures or basilar skull fractures are suspected. This type of intubation is not possible in the apneic patient.

Cricothyroidotomy has replaced tracheostomy as the surgical procedure of choice for emergency airway access in all but a few cases, such as laryngeal fracture or complete tracheal disruption. Cricothyroidotomy is particularly

TABLE 5-1 Airway Management in the Trauma Patient

	Advantages	Disadvantages
Orotracheal intubation	Reliable Usually easy Method of choice in cardiopulmonary arrest	Requires manipulation of head and neck Relatively contraindicated with known or suspected cervical spine fracture
Blind nasotracheal intubation	Does not require neck manipulation Can be done in the awake patient	Requires considerable experience Requires that patient is breathing (air flow or vapor in tube) Contraindicated with midfacial or basilar skull fracture Sinusitis with long-term use
Cricothyroidotomy	Method of choice when cervical spine and facial fractures are present Technically easier than tracheostomy	Requires surgical procedure
Tracheostomy	Good long-term airway access (ventilator weaning, secretion control) More comfortable than cricothyroidotomy Appropriate in laryngeal fracture, laceration	Technically demanding, particularly in emergency situations (bleeding, poor lighting, etc.)

appropriate in patients with obvious maxillofacial injuries and suspected cervical spine injury. In an adult patient, a size 6 tracheostomy tube, a size 6 endotracheal tube, or even a 12-gauge angiocatheter usually can be placed through the cricothyroid membrane. If appropriate connectors are not available, a 5 ml plastic syringe barrel can be cut in half and the Luer tip inserted into the angiocatheter hub. The ventilator tubing is then connected to the cut end of the syringe barrel.

Airway management is summarized in Table 5-1 and discussed in more detail in Chapter 11.

Breathing and Ventilation

Bag/mask ventilation should be continued until airway access has been achieved. Even after intubation, bagged ventilation by hand may be appropriate until the cardiopulmonary status of the patient has been stabilized. Ventilatory support to obtain Pco_2 and pH in the normal range and oxygen saturation >90% are the usual goals

of mechanical ventilation, although in the head-injured patient, hyperventilation to obtain a Pco_2 of 25 to 30 mm Hg is appropriate.

Circulation

After the airway has been secured and ventilation has been ensured, the next priority is restoration or support of the circulation. In the seriously injured patient, at least two large-bore (14-gauge) peripheral IV cannulae should be placed, preferably in an uninjured upper extremity, usually in the antecubital veins. When IV access cannot be established percutaneously, cutdown catheterization is appropriate; it is usually performed in the saphenous vein at the ankle or in the cephalic vein at the antecubital fossa. Central venous lines, whether internal jugular, subclavian, or femoral, are generally not recommended in the acute setting because difficulties in placement arise in the hypovolemic patient. However, many physicians are now more comfortable with the placement of central lines than with cutdown IV access, and central lines are used with increasing frequency in the initial management of trauma. If central lines are placed for rapid fluid administration, the relatively short, large-bore introducers (e.g., Cordis or Arrow) should be placed with a dilator via the Seldinger technique. These large-bore introducers also can be placed into large peripheral veins by "rewiring" previously placed IV catheters. Procedures for central venous access are discussed in Chapter 50.

External hemorrhage should be controlled with direct, manual pressure. In general, tourniquets should be avoided.

Fluid resuscitation is initiated with crystalloid (lactated Ringer's solution) at a rate that is commensurate with the degree of shock but one that may exceed several liters per hour. Colloid solutions (plasmanate or 5% albumin) can be used safely as an adjunct to crystalloid and are more efficient for the expansion of intravascular volume. The disadvantages of colloid solutions include expense, viscosity (flow slowly through IV tubing), and the fact that most are packaged in glass bottles, preventing the use of pressure bags or powered infusion systems for rapid infusion.

Indications for blood transfusion include massive or ongoing hemorrhage and persistent hypotension or shock after crystalloid infusion exceeding 2 to 4 L (50 ml/kg). If cross-matched blood is not yet available, type-specific or O-negative blood may be appropriate, particularly with ongoing hemorrhage or hemodynamic instability. In the more stable patient, the decision to transfuse blood should be made carefully. The expense, availability, and risk of transfusion-associated viral infections need to be considered. A young, healthy patient in whom hemorrhage has been controlled generally will tolerate a hematocrit concentration of 20% to 25%, whereas the older patient with underlying cardiopulmonary disease should generally be transfused to maintain a hematocrit of 30% to 35%. Transfusions are discussed in more detail in Chapter 45.

When ongoing hemorrhage is present, the decision to transfuse platelets or clotting factors (fresh-frozen plasma, cryoprecipitate) generally should be based on the results of standard clotting tests and platelet counts. "Automatic" replacement of clotting factors and platelets is probably not indicated, except perhaps with "massive" transfusions, exceeding 8 to 10 units of packed RBCs. Disorders of coagulation are discussed in more detail in Chapter 44.

Vasopressors have little, if any, place in the management of shock in the trauma patient. Use of vasopressors may produce adverse effects on peripheral tissue perfusion.

CPR is appropriate for the trauma patient in cardiopulmonary arrest, although the prognosis for the trauma patient who requires chest compressions is usually grim. Persistent hypotension or cardiac arrest in the trauma patient is usually a consequence of exsanguinating hemorrhage, but it may result from one of several treatable causes.

The most common cause of intractable shock in the trauma patient is ongoing hemorrhage, and patients with massive hemorrhage (brisk external bleeding, expanding abdomen) should be assigned to the operating room within minutes of arrival in the emergency room. Less obvious but equally lethal sources of ongoing hemorrhage are extremity and pelvic fractures. The hematoma from a femur fracture may contain 2 to 4 units of blood, and pelvic fractures may be responsible for 6 to 20 units of blood, depending on the severity of the injury.

Other treatable causes of intractable shock include flail chest, tension pneumothorax, hemothorax, or pericardial tamponade. Flail chest, caused by four or more ribs fractured in two places in a single hemithorax or by a similar number of ribs fractured anterolaterally in both hemithoraces, presents as discordant chest wall movement and is usually treated with intubation and positive pressure ventilation.

Tension pneumothorax presents as diminished breath sounds and hyperresonance to percussion in the affected hemithorax, with deviation of the trachea to the opposite side. The neck veins may be distended. CXR, which should be taken early in the management course of the trauma patient, will confirm the diagnosis, but treatment should not be delayed in the deteriorating patient if the diagnosis is suspected. If tension pneumothorax is suspected, a 16- to 18-gauge angiocatheter or needle can be inserted into the pleural space anteriorly through the second intercostal space at the midclavicular line as a temporary lifesaving measure. The definitive treatment is placement of a chest tube.

Tension hemothorax presents in a similar fashion, except that there will be dullness to percussion in the affected hemithorax. Treatment includes placement of a large (36 to 40 Fr) chest tube directed from the midaxillary line into the posterior or dependent portions of the pleural space. Continued bleeding from a tube thoracostomy may warrant surgical exploration and repair of the injured lung or blood vessels.

Pericardial tamponade is suspected in the presence of persistent hypotension and dilated neck veins, particularly in the presence of a penetrating injury to the chest. Muffled heart sounds and pulsus paradoxus are classic signs of pericardial tamponade, but they may be difficult to appreciate in a noisy emergency department. Definitive treatment of pericardial tamponade requires thoracotomy or median sternotomy to drain the blood-filled pericardium and to repair the source of pericardial hemorrhage. Needle pericardiocentesis via a subxyphoid approach can be lifesaving, but it must be considered a temporary measure in the trauma patient. Significant hemodynamic improvement should be noted after 50 to 75 ml of blood (usually nonclotting) has been withdrawn from the pericardium, if pericardial tamponade is the cause of unexplained hypotension.

Disability

Simultaneously addressed with the initial management of airway, breathing, and circulation is the prevention of long-term or permanent neurologic disability. The spine, in particular the cervical spine, must be carefully protected and stabilized until adequate diagnostic maneuvers have been completed. In the awake, cooperative, neurologically intact patient, the lack of neck pain, tenderness, or neurologic deficit may be sufficient evidence to forego x-ray evaluation. However, cervical spine x-ray films are mandatory in the patient who complains of neck, shoulder, or back pain; in the patient with cervical spine tenderness or neurologic deficit; in any patient with penetrating neck trauma; and in any blunt trauma patient unable to cooperate with the examination, such as the head-injured or intoxicated patient. A mechanism of injury associated with an increased risk of cervical spine injury, such as a high-speed motor vehicle accident, also must be considered an indication for cervical spine x-ray examination. A cross-table lateral cervical spine x-ray film, demonstrating all seven cervical vertebrae adequately, will allow identification of the majority of unstable cervical spine fractures, but the cervical spine should not be considered to be uninjured until anteroposterior, odontoid, and oblique views have been obtained. Although the cross-table lateral film does provide some assurance of cervical spine stability, particularly when airway management and diagnostic or surgical procedures are top priorities, the neck should be maintained in a hard cervical collar until the full cervical spine x-ray series has been completed.

Criteria for x-ray evaluation of the thoracic and lumbar spines are similar to those for cervical spine x-ray but are of secondary priority. Taking the time to obtain all the x-ray films in the radiology department during this acute phase is frequently associated with complications. The patient at risk should be placed supine on a firm surface and "log-rolled" as needed until appropriate anteroposterior and lateral x-ray views have been obtained.

Evaluation and Initial Treatment

Once the airway has been secured, breathing or ventilation has been established, and resuscitation of the circulation is under way, a thorough and comprehensive evaluation of the patient's injuries is initiated. Such an evaluation is precluded only when the patient requires immediate assignment to the operating room for hemodynamic instability or for emergency neurosurgical intervention.

Early in the emergency department phase of a patient's care, blood samples should be sent for appropriate laboratory tests, including type and cross-match, CBC, electrolytes, BUN, creatinine, amylase, coagulation studies, and ABGs.

A urinalysis should be obtained for any penetrating wound to the trunk and for all cases of significant blunt trauma.

A nasogastric tube should be placed in the patient with chest or abdominal trauma, in the intubated patient, or in the patient with a depressed mental status. If extensive midfacial or basilar skull fracture is suspected, then an orogastric tube is appropriate.

In the seriously injured patient, a Foley catheter should be placed, both to obtain urine for diagnostic purposes and to assess the adequacy of resuscitation. Blood at the urethral meatus or a "high-riding prostate" noted on rectal examination suggests urethral injury. In this situation a urethrogram should be obtained before Foley catheter placement is attempted.

In the multiply injured patient, anteroposterior chest and lateral cervical spine radiographs should be obtained early in the course of the evaluation since processing of these films will take several minutes. Other radiographs and diagnostic procedures are obtained as dictated by the history and physical examination.

PHYSICAL EXAMINATION

If relative hemodynamic stability is presumed, the patient should be disrobed to undergo a thorough physical examination. As much as possible, a complete medical history should be obtained simultaneously with the examination of the patient, with particular attention given to the mechanism of injury and to medication or drug abuse.

Head and Neck

In addition to the usual eye, ear, nose, and throat examination, the head and neck examination should include careful palpation of the cranium and facial bones for tenderness or deformity suggestive of fractures. Dental occlusion should be assessed. Hemotympanum, otorrhea, rhinorrhea, or "raccoon's eyes" are suggestive of basilar skull fracture. A thorough cranial nerve examination, including pupillary light responses and funduscopic examinations, should be performed. In the alert, cooperative patient, the posterior cervical spine should be palpated carefully to assess tenderness or bony deformity. In penetrating neck trauma, a pulse deficit or expanding hematoma should be sought as evidence of a major vascular injury. Crepitus in the neck suggests esophageal or laryngeal injury. Hoarseness, unilateral hypoventilation, or upper extremity neurologic deficit are all suggestive of significant skeletal or nerve injury.

Early in the course of the evaluation, the Glasgow Coma Scale score and its three individual subscores (see Chapter 18) should be obtained and recorded, both for communication with other health care professionals and as a baseline for comparison in the patient with a changing neurologic status.

Chest

Examination of the chest should include inspection of the chest wall for penetrating injuries or contusions and palpation of bony prominences for evidence of fracture. Tenderness to anteroposterior or lateral compression suggests sternal or rib fractures. Any abnormalities in the heart and lung examination (e.g., murmurs, rubs, gallops, dysrhythmias) or signs of congestive heart failure should be noted. Pneumothorax and hemothorax should be identified and treated as previously described. An upper extremity or carotid artery bruit or pulse deficit may suggest an unsuspected great vessel injury.

Abdomen

Inspection may reveal abdominal wall hematoma or contusion, which can suggest possible injury to underlying solid organs. Tenderness, particularly in the upper abdomen, may suggest liver or spleen injury, whereas signs of peritoneal irritation suggest hemoperitoneum or hollow viscus injury. The back and flanks should be inspected, which may require logrolling of the patient. An expanding abdomen may be a sign of exsanguinating intra-abdominal hemorrhage. In the patient in cardiopulmonary arrest, an expanding, tympanitic abdomen suggests esophageal placement of the endotracheal tube. The pelvis should be examined for stability and tenderness to anteroposterior and lateral compression. Rectal and vaginal examinations are performed in any patient with injuries to the abdomen, pelvis, or perineum and in any patient with significant blunt trauma. Pelvic fractures often are associated with vaginal and rectal tears and injuries to the male urethra are suggested by a "high-riding" or hematoma-surrounded prostate.

Extremities

The extremities should be inspected for obvious deformities, contusions, and hematomas and palpated for bony tenderness or deformity. A detailed neurovascular examination should be performed in all cases, particularly with extremity injuries or suspected spinal cord injury. If major skeletal injuries are not suspected, passive and active range of motion should be tested and joint ligamentous integrity assessed. Joint dislocation, particularly with a distal pulse deficit, requires emergency relocation and vascular evaluation to minimize further compromise of perfusion distal to the joint.

EVALUATION AND TREATMENT OF SPECIFIC INJURIES

A detailed discussion of all potential injuries, diagnostic procedures, and therapeutic interventions is beyond the scope of this chapter. Although the initial steps in the management of trauma, as described here, are relatively standard, the treatment of specific problems is much more controversial. As a result, even the diagnostic approach for the evaluation of specific injuries may be controversial. Some commonly encountered problems are discussed here.

Head Injury

Patients requiring immediate neurosurgical evaluation and treatment are those with evidence of brainstem dysfunction from transtentorial (uncal) herniation. Usually an expanding intracranial mass lesion causes the herniation. Transtentorial herniation is suggested by the triad of abnormal pupillary light reflex, depression of consciousness, and asymmetric motor signs. Pupillary dilation, the most reliable localizing sign, is ipsilateral to the lesion in 95% of patients. CT scan is the diagnostic procedure of choice in the head-injured patient and should be performed urgently to localize surgically correctable lesions. Emergency bur-hole explo-

---

Indications for Head CT Scan in the Trauma Patient
Decreased or decreasing level of arousal
Change in mental status
Unilateral dilation of a pupil
Cranial nerve VI palsy
Hemiparesis
Seizures
Suspected depressed or open skull fracture
Penetrating head injury
Glasgow coma score ≤ 10
History of prolonged loss of consciousness

ration is still performed by some neurosurgeons, particularly when CT scan is unavailable.[2] In the absence of signs of brainstem compression, head CT scan usually can be delayed until chest and abdominal injuries have been evaluated. General indications for head CT scan in the trauma patient are included in the box.

Although plain skull radiographs may be appropriate for trauma patients in the pediatric population (up to approximately 2 years of age), they are of little value in the adult population, especially if head CT scanning is available. The identification of a skull fracture, even though such a fracture is associated with an increased risk of intracerebral injury, does not establish the diagnosis of intracerebral injury; nor does the lack of a skull fracture rule out the presence of an intracerebral injury. Even when a depressed skull fracture is noted (a diagnosis that usually requires surgical intervention and can be made with skull radiographs), the patient probably still should undergo CT scanning to evaluate the brain for associated injuries.

Initial therapy in the head-injured patient is directed at control or prevention of secondary injury from compression of, or swelling within, the normal brain tissue. Urgent neurosurgical intervention may be required to control bleeding, drain mass lesions, establish intracranial pressure monitoring, or perform ventriculostomy for monitoring and treatment of cerebral edema. If increasing intracranial pressure is suspected on the basis of clinical or CT scan criteria (compressed ventricles, midline shift, loss of sulci and gyri), initial management should include elevation of the head of the bed, hyperventilation to a PCO_2 of 25 to 30 mm Hg, control of systemic hypertension, and intravenous administration of mannitol with an initial dose of 0.5 to 1.5 g/kg. Although the use of steroids in the management of severe head injuries is controversial, most evidence suggests that steroids are of no benefit in reducing intracranial pressure or increasing meaningful survival. Therefore the use of steroids is not routinely recommended in the management of the head-injured patient.[3-9] Phenytoin and benzodiazapines are appropriate for control of seizures. A more detailed discussion of the management of head injuries is included in Chapter 18.

Neck Injury

Suspected cervical spine injury is managed with the use of a hard cervical collar and immobilization of the head and torso. Evaluation requires full cervical spine x-rays, including lateral, odontoid, anteroposterior, and, in some cases, oblique views. All seven cervical vertebrae need to be visualized. If necessary, a "swimmer's view" is obtained. In the absence of identifiable fracture, neck pain or tenderness warrants flexion-extension views. After neurosurgical consultation, a CT scan with coronal or sagittal reconstructions may further demonstrate the extent of fractures. The hard cervical collar must be left in place until fractures or ligamentous injury have been excluded or until other therapy (e.g., traction or operative stabilization) is undertaken. Spinal cord injury is discussed further in Chapter 19.

The evaluation and management of penetrating neck injuries is controversial.[10] The controversy relates to the concept of mandatory vs. elective exploration of penetrating (through the platysma) neck injuries.

If a policy of mandatory exploration is followed, all patients with penetrating injuries undergo exploratory surgery in the operating room immediately. The only diagnostic study obtained preoperatively is a cervical spine x-ray.

If a policy of selective exploration is observed, the patient undergoes exploration early for signs of significant injury (e.g., airway compromise, expanding hematoma, pulse deficit suggesting a major vascular injury, air in the soft tissues suggesting an esophageal, laryngeal, or tracheal injury) or for evidence of nerve injury. Patients who do not meet the criteria for immediate exploration are admitted to the hospital and observed. Controversy exists regarding the need for further diagnostic evaluation in patients selected for observation. Suspected esophageal injury is best evaluated with a water-soluble contrast esophagram. Esophagoscopy may not detect small perforations. Angiography can be used to rule out major vascular injury and is particularly helpful in determining penetrating injuries above the angle of the mandible and at the thoracic inlet. Fiberoptic laryngoscopy or bronchoscopy is appropriate for identification of tracheal and laryngeal injuries.

Chest Injury

High-velocity penetrating wounds to the heart or great vessels are usually lethal and consequently rarely require evaluation. On the other hand, patients who sustain stab wounds or other low-velocity penetrating injuries often survive to be evaluated in the emergency department. CXR is the primary diagnostic study required. Pneumothorax or hemothorax from suspected injury to the lung or intercostal vessels often can be managed by tube thoracostomy as the only mode of treatment. The "sucking chest wound" is managed by covering the wound with a sterile, occlusive dressing and placing a chest tube through a separate incision. Surgical intervention is generally indicated for an initial chest tube output exceeding 1000 ml, continuing bleeding exceeding 200 to 300 ml/hr, or a total chest tube output exceeding 1500 to 2000 ml of blood in the adult patient. Suspected penetrating injury to the heart or great vessels requires surgical intervention.

Serious chest injuries after blunt trauma include pulmonary or myocardial contusion and injuries to the aorta and great vessels. Laceration or free rupture of the great vessels usually is associated with death at the scene of the accident. Contained ruptures or leaks of the aorta

---

CXR Findings Consistent With Injury of Aorta and Great Vessels

Mediastinal widening (>8 cm)
Deviation of trachea or nasogastric tube to right
Left pleural cap
Left pleural effusion
Depression of left main bronchus
Indistinct aortic knob
Obscuration of aortopulmonary window
First and second rib fractures*
Fractured scapula*

---

*Suggests deceleration injury of sufficient magnitude to result in aortic injury.

---

should be suspected from characteristic CXR findings, some of which are listed in the box. Similar x-ray findings, a carotid or upper extremity pulse deficit, or a bruit often are present with great vessel injury. The diagnostic procedure of choice is arch aortogram with great vessel run-off. In the stable patient, angiography should be performed before the patient goes to the operating room for treatment of other injuries. In the unstable patient, immediately life-threatening injuries should be addressed first. Free rupture of an aortic arch injury is rapidly (almost instantaneously) fatal. Gradually decreasing blood pressure is usually the result of other injuries, such as intra-abdominal hemorrhage.

Pulmonary contusion is diagnosed through CXR. Cardiac contusion can be diagnosed with serial cardiac enzymes (CPK-MB) and ECG (any new abnormalities). In most cases treatment involves cardiac monitoring and management of dysrhythmias. Cardiogenic shock may occur if the injury is severe enough. Echocardiography is usually reserved for signs of cardiac dysfunction. Cardiac contusion should not preclude necessary surgical intervention for other injuries.[11]

Emergency department thoracotomy

Penetrating injury to the chest in a rapidly deteriorating or moribund patient is the primary indication for emergency department thoracotomy. When the left chest has been opened

via an anterolateral thoracotomy, pericardial tamponade can be relieved by opening the pericardium, and cardiac bleeding can be controlled by direct digital pressure until suture repair can be performed. Massive bleeding from the lung can be controlled by cross-clamping the pulmonary hilum after division of the inferior pulmonary ligament. Injuries of the great vessels are controlled with finger pressure until suture repair can be accomplished.

In collected reviews, meaningful survival after emergency department thoracotomy has been noted as approximately 8%. In one large series, survival after emergency department thoracotomy was 19.8% for stab wounds isolated to the chest, 3.4% for gunshot wounds, and 3.8% for blunt trauma. Emergency thoracotomy should not be performed if ECG activity or pupillary light reflexes are absent. Emergency department thoracotomy generally is not recommended for blunt chest or abdominal trauma and should be performed only if the patient's vital signs are noted in the emergency department.[12]

Abdominal Injury

The management of penetrating abdominal injuries, like that of penetrating neck injuries, is somewhat controversial. General agreement exists that gunshot wounds require surgical exploration. Stab wounds have been managed by exploration or observation, with or without peritoneal lavage. In general, I favor surgical exploration for any stab wound suspected of penetrating the peritoneal cavity.

Diagnostic procedures for the evaluation of blunt abdominal trauma include peritoneal lavage, either by percutaneous or open technique, or abdominal CT scan. Plain abdominal radiographs have little value with blunt abdominal trauma. The percutaneous peritoneal lavage procedure is reported to have a complication rate of 0% to 5%, whereas the complication rate of the open technique is reported to be half that of the percutaneous technique.[13-15] Peritoneal lavage by either technique should identify 95% to 98% of intra-abdominal surgical pathology. The incidence of a false positive lavage (leading to negative laparotomy) is <6%.[13-15] Generally accepted criteria for a pos-

---

Criteria for "Positive" Peritoneal Lavage

1. Immediate aspiration of gross intraperitoneal blood
2. Lavage fluid containing:
   RBC $\geq$ 100,000/mm^3
   WBC $\geq$ 500/mm^3
   Any bile
   Any bacteria
   Meat fibers or food particles

Special considerations

Retroperitoneal hematoma from pelvic fractures may confound results. Consider supraumbilical lavage.

Place nasogastric tube and Foley catheter *prior* to lavage.

Abdominal surgical scars are relative contraindication to diagnostic peritoneal lavage.

Must retrieve 600 to 700 ml of 1000 ml lavage fluid.

---

itive peritoneal lavage in the setting of blunt trauma are listed in the box. Prior to peritoneal lavage, a nasogastric tube and Foley catheter should be placed to decompress the stomach and bladder and to minimize the risk of puncturing these organs. Extreme care should be used when peritoneal lavage is being considered in the patient with previous abdominal surgery. Abdominal CT scan has been suggested as a replacement for peritoneal lavage in selected patients and is used effectively at many institutions.[16,17] Advantages of CT scan include the ability to assess the severity of solid organ injuries and to evaluate retroperitoneal structures including the duodenum, pancreas, and kidneys. Disadvantages of the CT scan are that it is time-consuming and it does require interpretation by surgeons or radiologists with extensive experience in reading CT scans in trauma patients. Ideally, scans should be performed with both oral and intravenous contrast media. CT scan is probably the diagnostic procedure of choice for blunt abdominal trauma in children.

Peritoneal lavage or CT scanning is appropriate in any patient in whom physical examination is unreliable, including the patient with head injury or spinal cord injury and the intoxicated patient. In patients with unexplained hemodynamic instability or a falling hematocrit concentration, the possibility of abdominal injury must be evaluated. I favor the use of peritoneal lavage in the unstable patient. In the stable patient, CT scanning may provide more information, particularly when urinary tract or retroperitoneal injuries are suspected. The only absolute contraindication to either diagnostic procedure is a surgical (acute) abdomen, which mandates exploratory laparotomy.

Genitourinary Injury

Intravenous pyelogram (IVP) and cystogram are appropriate for penetrating injuries to the back or flanks and for hematuria, regardless of the mechanism of injury. Angiography is appropriate when a kidney cannot be visualized on IVP, but it must be done rapidly if a devascularized kidney is to be salvaged. The limit to warm ischemia time with renal artery injury is 30 to 60 minutes. CT scan with intravenous contrast provides excellent visualization of the kidneys and collecting system; it is particularly appropriate if a CT scan is to be performed for evaluation of other abdominal injuries. A single-shot IVP provides limited but very important information in the patient with hematoma, who must be explored urgently to control intra-abdominal hemorrhage. Specifically, the single-shot IVP demonstrates the number of functioning kidneys within the abdomen, an observation that may be important for intraoperative decisions regarding renal exploration, renal repair, or nephrectomy. Suspected urethral trauma requires a retrograde urethrogram and a voiding cystourethrogram for evaluation. When a urethral injury is suspected, a retrograde urethrogram should be obtained before Foley catheterization is done. Signs of urethral injury include blood at the urethral meatus or a high-riding prostate noted on digital rectal examination.

Musculoskeletal Injury

Suspected fractures require appropriate plain x-ray evaluation when time and the patient's condition permit. The patient with suspected fractures is immobilized with appropriate

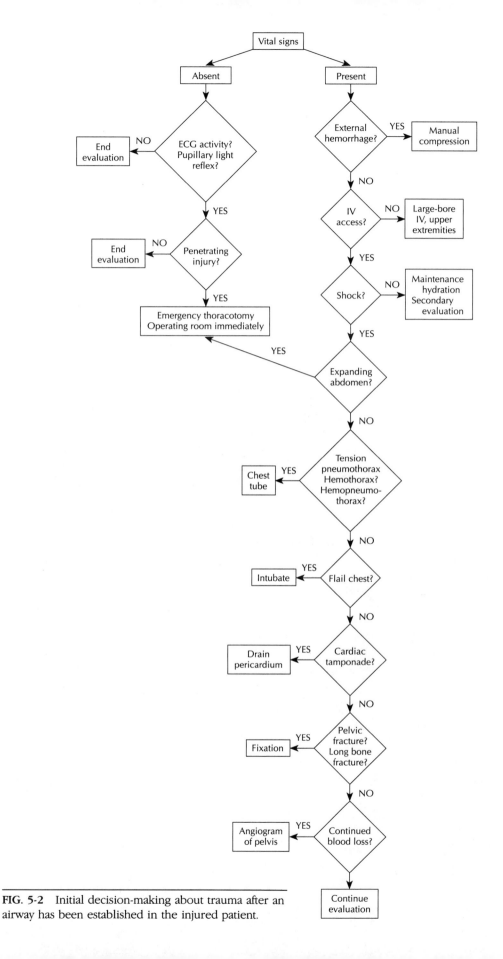

FIG. 5-2 Initial decision-making about trauma after an airway has been established in the injured patient.

splints until definitive therapy can be undertaken. Open fractures require operative irrigation and debridement, and plain films of open fractures or joint injuries should be obtained to identify any foreign body or unsuspected fractures. Bones proximal and distal to a joint injury should be evaluated radiographically.

Angiography is appropriate when a pulse deficit or neurovascular compromise is associated with blunt extremity trauma. The place of angiography in the management of penetrating extremity trauma with suspected vascular injury is less clear. When the diagnosis and location of vascular injury are obvious, many surgeons explore the wound immediately. Others favor angiography in the stable patient. The diagnosis must be made early, and treatment must be initiated rapidly since a devascularized extremity will tolerate only 4 to 6 hours of ischemia before irreversible injury occurs. Angiography is generally favored when extensive or multiple extremity wounds are present, such as a gunshot wound.

Angiography may be particularly useful for extensive pelvic fractures with major hemorrhage, both as a diagnostic and a therapeutic procedure. Angiographic embolization of bleeding sites within the pelvis is usually favored over surgical repair of such injuries.[18-21] External fixation[22-24] or military antishock trousers (MAST)[25,26] also have been used effectively in the setting of exsanguinating hemorrhage from pelvic fractures. The management of extremity injuries is covered in more detail in Chapters 36 and 37.

SUMMARY

- Initial management of trauma includes establishing an adequate airway, providing oxygen and ventilation, controlling hemorrhage, and replacing lost blood volume.
- An initial survey is done to identify and treat immediately life-threatening injuries: tension pneumothorax, tension hemothorax, flail chest, pericardial tamponade, and brisk external bleeding.
- After hemodynamic stability has been achieved, a thorough physical examination and diagnostic evaluation are done. For the unresuscitatable patient, thoracotomy or laparotomy may be necessary to control hemorrhage.
- During trauma evaluation and treatment, the patient must be protected from further neurologic injury.
- Successful management of trauma demands that life-threatening or limb-threatening injuries receive highest priority.
- The patient must be reevaluated continuously and priorities must be changed to match the patient's changing clinical needs.

REFERENCES

1. Moore FA, Moore EE. Trauma Resuscitation. In Wilmore DW, Brennan MF, Harken AH, Holcroft JW, Meakins JL, eds. Care of the Surgical Patient. New York: Scientific American, 1989, pp 1-15.
2. Pitts LH, Martin N. Head injuries. Surg Clin North Am 62:47-60, 1982.
3. Braakman R, Schouten HJA, Dishoeck MB, et al. Megadose steroids in severe head injury: Results of a prospective double blind trial. J Neurosurg 58:326-330, 1983.
4. Cooper PR, Moody SS, Clark WK, et al. Dexamethasone and severe head injury: A prospective double blind study. J Neurosurg 51:307-316, 1979.
5. Dearden NM. Management of raised intracranial pressure after severe head injury. Br J Hosp Med 36:94-103, 1986.
6. Gudemen SK, Miller JD, Becker DP. Failure of high-dose steroid therapy to influence intracranial pressure in patients with severe head injury. J Neurosurg 51:301-306, 1979.
7. Faupel G, Ruelen HJ, Muller D, et al. Double blind study on the effects of steroids on severe closed head injury. In Pappius HM, Feindel W, eds. Dynamics of Brain Edema. Berlin: Springer-Verlag, 1976, pp 337-343.
8. Becker DP, Gudeman SK. Textbook of Head Injury. Philadelphia: WB Saunders, 1989.
9. Pitts LH, Wagner FC. Craniospinal Trauma. New York: Thieme Medical, 1990.
10. Carducci B, Lowe RA, Dalsey W. Penetrating neck trauma: Consensus and controversies. Ann Emerg Med 15:208-215, 1986.
11. Feliciano DV, Bitondo CG, Cruse PA, Mattox KL, Burch JM, Beall AC, Jordan GL. Liberal use of emergency center thoracotomy. Am J Surg 152:654-660, 1986.
12. Flancbaum L, Wright J, Siegel JH. Emergency surgery in patients with post-traumatic myocardial contusion. J Trauma 26:795-803, 1986.
13. Pachter HL, Hofstetter SR. Open and percutaneous paracentesis and lavage for abdominal trauma. Arch Surg 116:318, 1981.
14. Lazarus HM, Nelson JA. A technique for peritoneal lavage without risk or complication. Surg Gynecol Obstet 149:889, 1979.
15. Fischer RP, Bryce CB, Engrav LH, Benjamin CI, Perry JF Jr. Diagnostic peritoneal lavage: Fourteen years and 2,586 patients later. Am J Surg 136:701-704, 1978.
16. Peitzman AB, Makaroun MS, Slasky S, Ritter P. Prospective study of computed tomography in initial management of blunt abdominal trauma. J Trauma 26:585-592, 1986.
17. Fabian TC, Mangiante EC, White TJ, Patterson CR, Boldreghini S, Britt LG. A prospective study of 91 patients undergoing both computed tomography and peritoneal lavage following blunt abdominal trauma. J Trauma 26:602-608, 1986.
18. Gilliland MG, Ward RE, Flynn TC. Peritoneal lavage and angiography in the management of patients with pelvic fractures. Am J Surg 144:744-747, 1985.
19. Matalon TS, Athanasoulis CA, Margolies MN, et al. Hemorrhage with pelvic fractures: Efficacy of transcatheter embolization. Am J Roentgenol 133:859-864, 1979.
20. Yellin AE, Lundell CJ, Finck EJ. Diagnosis and control of posttraumatic pelvic hemorrhage. Arch Surg 118:1378-1383, 1983.
21. Panetta T, Sclafani SJA, Goldstein AS, et al. Percutaneous transcatheter embolization for massive bleeding from pelvic fractures. J Trauma 25:1021-1029, 1985.
22. Gylling SF, Ward RE, Holcroft JW. Immediate external fixation of unstable pelvic fractures. Am J Surg 150:721-724, 1985.
23. Mears DC, Fu FH. Modern concept of external fixation of the pelvis. Clin Orthop 151:65-72, 1980.
24. Peltier LF. Complications associated with fractures of the pelvis. J Bone Joint Surg 47A:1060-1069, 1965.
25. Batalden DJ, Wickstrom PH, Ruiz E, et al. Value of the G suit in patients with severe pelvic fracture. Arch Surg 109:326-328, 1974.
26. Flint LM, Brown A, Richardson JD. Definitive control of bleeding from severe pelvic fractures. Ann Surg 189:709-716, 1979.

CHAPTER 6

Cardiovascular Risk: Assessment and Reduction

Jon F. Berlauk

Heart disease, especially coronary artery disease (CAD), is the primary health care problem in the United States. Nearly one out of every two deaths in this country can be attributed to cardiovascular disease. Therefore it is not surprising that CAD is also the major cause of morbidity (myocardial infarction, unstable angina, congestive heart failure, or serious dysrhythmia) and mortality after surgery. Unfortunately, the outlook does not improve with time. In 1988, 25 million patients in all age groups underwent noncardiac surgical procedures. One millon of these patients had diagnosed CAD, and another 2 to 3 million were estimated to be at risk for the disease. Many of these patients were elderly, who now constitute the fastest growing segment of our population. In 1988, 25 million people (10%) were over 65 years old. This figure is projected to grow to 66 million by the year 2055. In 1988, elderly patients comprised 25% (6 million) of the noncardiac surgery group, and this figure is expected to grow to 35% (12 million) within 30 years.[1] The implied magnitude of the problem of CAD is enormous. In the aging surgical population, how can the preoperative patient who is at high risk for perioperative cardiac morbidity (PCM) be identified? Can the patient's risk be reduced? For the past 35 years, clinical studies have focused primarily on the factors involved in cardiac risk assessment, but in recent years more emphasis has been devoted to risk reduction. This chapter provides a framework for assessing and reducing the risk of PCM in the surgical patient.

RISK FACTORS

Over several decades, investigators have studied thousands of surgical patients in order to determine which preoperative risk factors can be used to predict perioperative morbidity and mortality.* Several historical risk factors have been identified and are supported by the majority of studies (see box). As might be expected because of the number of studies involved, few of these risk factors are undisputed. Nevertheless, two factors consistently have been found to predict poor outcome following surgery, recent myocardial infarction (MI) and current congestive heart failure (CHF).

---

*For an excellent comprehensive review of this subject, see reference 1.

Historical Predictors of Surgical Risk*
Age
Recent myocardial infarction (<6 mo)
Old myocardial infarction (>6 mo)
Angina
Congestive heart failure
Hypertension
Diabetes mellitus
Dysrhythmia
Peripheral vascular disease
Valvular heart disease
Previous coronary artery bypass graft surgery

*Modified from Mangano DT. Perioperative cardiac morbidity. Anesthesiology 72:153, 1990.

In 1964 Topkins and Artusio[2] reported the first comprehensive, large-scale study describing the risk of previous MI in relation to subsequent noncardiac surgery. They found that the incidence of postoperative MI in patients without a previous MI was 0.66%, as compared with 6.5% in patients who had a known preoperative MI. The mortality rate following this postoperative MI was high (26.5%) in the patients without a previous MI but even worse (72%) in the patients who had a prior MI. In addition, these authors found that the rate of reinfarction was 54.5% in patients who had had an MI less than 6 months before surgery, compared to only 4.5% if the prior MI occurred more than 6 months before surgery (Table 6-1). It was clear that, depending on the timing, a prior MI placed a surgical patient at extraordinary risk for reinfarction and death. Such findings did not change appreciably over the next 20 years despite dramatic advances in surgery and anesthesia. Even today the reinfarction rate within the first 3 months of a prior MI is generally estimated to be 30%; between 3 to 6 months it is approximately 15%, and after 6 months it is about 5%. Overall risk of postoperative reinfarction is 6% to 8%, with associated mortality exceeding 50% (see Table 6-1).

In 1983 Rao et al.[12] confirmed these reinfarction rates in a group of 364 patients who were studied retrospectively. More important, in a second group of 733 prospectively studied patients, a significant decrease in reinfarction rates was demonstrated for each time period following the prior MI. This decrease was achieved by implementing invasive hemodynamic monitoring and aggressively treating cardiovascular variables that deviated from normal. These authors found that reinfarction occurred in only 1.9% of all patients with a previous MI (see Table 6-1) if these patients had arterial and pulmonary artery catheters placed intraoperatively followed by extended postoperative SICU care. Based on these findings, some have inferred that preoperative optimization of the patient's status, aggressive monitoring and therapy, plus an extended SICU stay may reduce the risk of reinfarction. I would agree with this approach in selected patients. However, further confirmation of the findings of Rao et al.[12] are necessary in order to substantiate the clinical and financial implications of this approach for all patients with a previous MI.

TABLE 6-1   Studies of Perioperative Myocardial Infarction

	Year	No. of Patients	Previous MI	Reinfarction (%)			Patients With Reinfarction (%)	Reinfarction Mortality (%)
				0-3 Mo	3-6 Mo	>6 Mo		
Knapp et al.[3]	1962	8,984	427	100	100	4.5	6.1	58
Thompson et al.[4]	1962	*	192	*	*	*	5.7	63
Topkins and Artusio[2]	1964	12,712	658	← 54.5 →		4.5	6.5	72
Arkins et al.[5]	1964	1,005	267	11	← 7.5 →		7.9	81
Tarhan et al.[6]	1972	32,877	422	37	16	3	6.6	54
Steen et al.[7]	1978	73,321	587	27	11	5.4	6.1	69
Goldman et al.[8]	1978	1,001	101	← 4.5 →		2.5	3	33
Eerola et al.[9]	1980	2,063	89	*	*	*	6.7	50
von Knorring[10]	1981	12,654	157	← 25 →		12	15.9	28
Schoeppel et al.[11]	1983	981	53	0	0	4.5	3.8	50
Rao et al.[12]	1983	*	364	36	26	5	7.7	57
Rao et al.[12]	1983	*	733	5.8	2.3	0.8	1.9	36

*Data not provided.

CHF is also a reliable predictor of perioperative risk. In 1988, 2.3 million people in the United States were found to have CHF. Its incidence doubles in each decade of life after age 45, and CHF is now the leading diagnosis related group in hospitalized patients older than 65 years.[1] After 40 years of clinical studies, only one study[13] has not found CHF to be a major risk factor for PCM. Is there a problem? Only if we try to objectively define CHF. There is more controversy about the predictive value of specific markers of heart failure than there is about the condition itself. Since CHF is a constellation of clinical symptoms rather than a specific disease, such controversy is understandable. Goldman et al.[14] assigned an S_3 gallop or jugular venous distention the highest point weight in their cardiac risk index (CRI). Cardiomegaly was not a significant variable in their study, but Charlson et al.[15] disagree. Detsky et al.[16] used "alveolar pulmonary edema" in their modification of the CRI. Using multivariant analysis, Foster et al.[17] found that only dyspnea on exertion and left ventricular wall motion abnormality (during angiography) were predictors of PCM. Less qualitative measures of left ventricular performance have fared no better. Left ventricular ejection fraction (LVEF) by angiography has been shown to be the best prognostic indicator of survival in nonsurgical patients with CAD.[18] Several studies have validated LVEF that is <50% of normal to be a predictor of poor outcome in patients undergoing noncardiac surgery[19,20]; however, Kopecky et al.[21] and Franco et al.[22] have not confirmed the predictive value of resting or exercise LVEF. In summary, although controversy exists about how to best identify the condition, CHF is a reliable predictor of PCM.

Although MI and CHF are good predictors of PCM, they are by no means the only variables that determine outcome. In 1977 Goldman et al.[14] used multivariate analysis of 39 clinical variables in 1001 surgical patients to select nine variables that were predictors of PCM. A point score was given to each variable to reflect its statistical weight in the analysis, and the cardiac risk index was formulated (Table 6-2). Detsky et al.[16] later modified this index to include severe and unstable angina. More recently Shah et al.[13] used stepwise logistic regression to analyze 24 preoperative variables in 688 patients with cardiac disease. They found that eight risk factors could be used to predict outcome. Only two of these factors, chronic stable angina and ischemia on ECG, do not have a counterpart in the CRI, which underscores the validity of this index. Currently the CRI is the most widely used and best validated risk assessment index. It was derived from an unselected patient group undergoing noncardiac surgery. Therefore if the CRI is not used to predict risk in a highly selected patient group with either unusual med-

TABLE 6-2 Computation of Cardiac Risk Index*

Criteria	Points
History	
Age >70 yr	5
MI in previous 6 mo	10
Physical examination	
S_3 gallop or jugular venous distention	11
Important valvular aortic stenosis	3
Electrocardiogram	
Rhythm other than sinus or PACs on last preoperative ECG	7
>5 PVCs/min documented at any time before operation	7
General status	
Po_2 <60 or Pco_2 >50 mm Hg, K <3 or HCO_3 <20 mEq/L, BUN >50 or Cr >3 mg/dl, abnormal SGOT, signs of chronic liver disease, or patient bedridden from noncardiac causes	3
Operation	
Intraperitoneal, intrathoracic, or aortic operation	3
Emergency operation	4
TOTAL POSSIBLE	53

*From Miller RD, ed. Anesthesia, 3rd ed. New York: Churchill Livingstone, 1990, p 829.

Note: To calculate a patient's score, the number of points from all factors he/she possesses are summed.

Patients are further segregated into class I (0-5 points), with a risk of 1-7% of major complications; class II (6-12 points), risk 7-11%; class III (13-25 points), risk 14-38%; and class IV (≥26 points), risk 30-100%.

PAC, premature atrial contraction; PVC, premature ventricular contraction.

ical conditions or high baseline risk, it appears to be useful to stratify, if not accurately predict, risk.[23]

SCREENING

Clearly, surgical patients who have either clinically overt or occult ischemic heart disease with or without left ventricular dysfunction are at greatest risk for perioperative complications. Who should be screened for these conditions? Which tests should be used? Is the expense justified? Many of these questions remain unanswered. Eagle and Boucher[24] estimate that adverse "event rates above 10 to 15 percent (but probably not below 5 percent) are likely to be high enough to justify screening all patients in the category by further laboratory testing." One approach to screening the noncardiac surgical patient (Fig. 6-1) involves laboratory testing of selected patients to subject only high-risk patients to costly and invasive procedures.

The assessment begins with a complete history and physical examination along with baseline blood chemistries, CXR, and ECG. Such a traditional approach to risk assessment may seem antiquated in view of our high-technology medical orientation. Nevertheless, a thorough clinical history may be the best indicator of CAD. The sensitivity and specificity of history alone to detect the presence of CAD ranges from 80% to 91% in several studies.[25] The physical examination will reveal signs of CHF, cardiac dysrhythmia, valvular heart disease, and general medical status, all important variables in popular cardiac risk indexes. In fact, history and physical examination account for 20 of 53 points in Goldman's CRI.[14] Hypokalemia appears to be an independent risk predictor.[13,14] Cardiomegaly on CXR also has been found to predict PCM. Finally, 40% to 70% of patients with CAD who are undergoing noncardiac surgery have an abnormal ECG.[1]

Although an abnormal ECG may be diagnostic of underlying CAD, a normal resting ECG is not necessarily reassuring. Only 25% to 50% of old MIs can be detected by ECG. Tomatis et al.[26] found that 38% of patients with a normal ECG and a negative history of CAD still had 50% stenosis of one or more coronary vessels. Hertzer et al.[27] found that 37% of similar patients had 70% stenosis of one or more coronary arteries. Benchimol et al.[28] found three-vessel CAD in 15% of patients with a normal ECG. Unlike the other factors, a normal ECG does not preclude significant disease.

At this point in the evaluation, select patients will require further testing. Given a surgical patient with suspected or proven CAD, it would seem prudent to test his/her ability to tolerate myocardial stress under controlled conditions. The increased respiratory, metabolic, and cardiovascular work demanded in the postoperative period will surely provide uncontrolled stress. Therefore, for those patients who are physically able, exercise ECG stress testing is inexpensive, noninvasive, and reasonably predictive for PCM. Several investigators have shown that patients who cannot exercise to low cardiac workloads or those who develop a positive ischemic response to exercise are at high risk for postoperative cardiac events.[1] Gerson et al.[29] found that the inability to exercise was 80% sensitive and 53% specific for PCM. For patients who are unable or unwilling to exercise, the dipyridamole-thallium scan provides an alternative stress test. However, this test should be done after Holter monitoring, which is less expensive and noninvasive. In addition, the 24-hour Holter monitor has been shown to provide a 99% negative predictive value for PCM.[30] When this sequence is used, only those patients at risk would receive the dipyridamole-thallium scan. Thallium-201 is taken up by myocardial cells in proportion to their blood flow. Intravenous dipyridamole dilates coronary vessels, which increases the blood flow to myocardium supplied by nonstenotic vessels. However, myocardium supplied by stenotic vessels shows poor uptake (+ defect) on early scintigraphic scan. Later this defect will "fill in" (+ redistribution) if viable myocardium is available. An old MI will appear as a persistent defect on thallium scan. In several uncontrolled studies, the dipyridamole-thallium scan appeared to be very sensitive (89% to 100%), reasonably specific (53% to 80%), and had a negative predictive value of 78% for PCM.[1] The positive predictive value of dipyridamole-thallium scan was found to be low because of the many false positives that were noted. Combining 24-hour Holter monitoring with this type of scanning may improve discrimination.

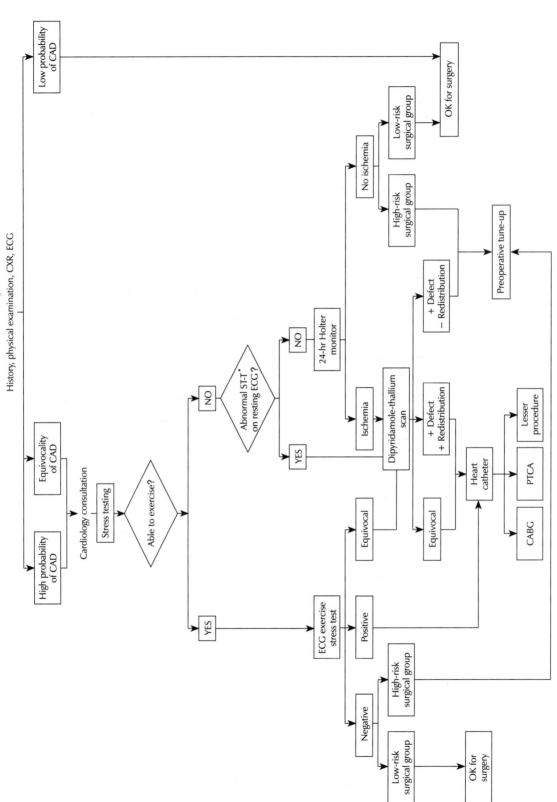

*Caused by left bundle branch block, left ventricular hypertrophy with strain, digoxin.

FIG. 6-1 Preoperative screening tests for the noncardiac surgical patient. CAD, coronary artery disease; CABG, coronary artery bypass graft; PTCA, percutaneous transluminal coronary angioplasty.

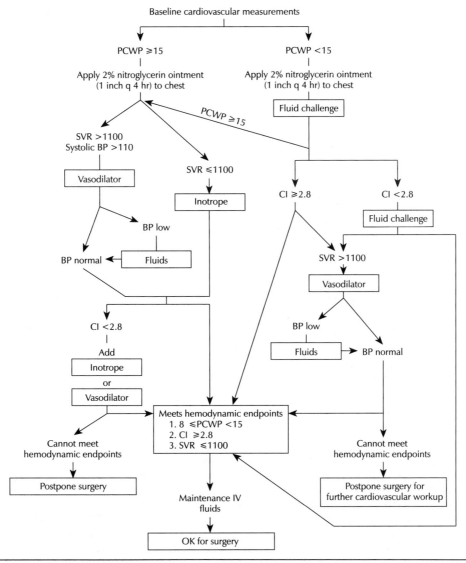

FIG. 6-2 Preoperative cardiovascular "tune-up." Cardiovascular measurements were repeated after each intervention. Inotropes: dobutamine or dopamine. Vasodilators: nitroglycerin or nitroprusside. PCWP, pulmonary capillary wedge pressure; SVR, systemic vascular resistance; CI, cardiac index. Measurement units are mm Hg for pressure, dyne · sec · cm^{-5} for resistance, and L · min^{-1} · m^{-2} for cardiac index. (From Berlauk JF, Abrams JH, Gilmour IJ, et al. Preoperative optimization of cardiovascular hemodynamics improves outcome in peripheral vascular surgery: A prospective randomized clinical trial. Ann Surg 214:289, 1991.)

General considerations

1. A complete history and physical examination of the patient are required.
2. Recent laboratory data, including CXR, ECG, and blood chemistries, should be available. If not available, these baseline studies are obtained.
3. All special screening or diagnostic testing should be completed before the tune-up.
4. The use of antihypertensive medication, except for beta-blocker agents and clonidine, is discontinued during the tune-up.
5. Serum electrolyte abnormalities are corrected. The serum potassium concentration is maintained in the 4 to 5 mEq/L range; serum magnesium, in the 2 to 2.5 mEq/L range.

Invasive catheter placement

1. Both arterial and pulmonary artery catheters are generally required. Insertion of invasive catheters should be done under appropriate supervision.
2. Arterial catheter sites in order of preference are (1) radial, (2) dorsalis pedis, (3) femoral, and (4) axillary. Brachial artery catheters should not be used routinely. Patients with arthritis, diabetes mellitus, arteriovenous shunts, peripheral vascular disease, or a renal or pancreatic transplant are at high risk for complications from injudiciously placed arterial catheters. An automated sphygmomanometer may be preferable in these patients.
3. The pulmonary catheter is usually placed via the internal jugular vein or via the subclavian vein (with the Seldinger technique used).

General principles

The pulmonary artery catheter is used to assess a patient's baseline cardiovascular status and his/her response to an intravenous fluid challenge. If cardiovascular derangements are detected, the aim of the tune-up is to improve myocardial performance without significantly increasing the myocardial workload in order to assess a patient's ability to meet the increased tissue oxygen demands of the postoperative period. This goal is accomplished by infusing appropriate fluids, vasodilators, and inotropes to obtain a target cardiac output (see Fig. 6-2). Target cardiac output does NOT mean *maximal* cardiac output. Although certain surgical procedures do impose different levels of stress and hence create risk, the tune-up should not push the patient's limits of myocardial performance.

1. After baseline measurements of cardiovascular parameters have been taken, all patients are given low-dose nitroglycerin, usually as an ointment. Nitroglycerin is used for its salutary effects on coronary arteries rather than the mild systemic venous and arterial vasodilation it produces.
2. Patients are classified according to their initial pulmonary capillary wedge pressure (PCWP) measurement. In preoperative patients, the optimal PCWP is probably 12 to 15 mm Hg, based on the few available studies.

a. *PCWP >15 mm Hg*

In general, these patients have left ventricular dysfunction. Many will require the intravenous administration of either a vasodilator agent (nitroglycerin or sodium nitroprusside) or an inotropic agent (dopamine or dobutamine*) to optimize left ventricular function. In patients with serious myocardial dysfunction, both vasodilator and inotropic agents may be necessary to achieve the desired hemodynamic endpoints. Such patients have been found to be at highest risk for postoperative complications by some investigators. Therefore modification or postponement of the anticipated surgical procedure may be judicious in these patients.

Diuretic therapy is conspicuously absent from this treatment approach. Since relative hypovolemia is a common problem in preoperative patients, improvement of myocardial function is attempted while optimal intravascular volume is maintained. Diuretics should be given only to patients in frank congestive heart failure.

b. *PCWP ≤15 mm Hg*

These patients have inadequate intravascular volume because of chronic hypertension or dehydration. Generally they have good left ventricular function and respond well to minimal pharmacologic intervention. Fortunately, the majority of unselected, high-risk surgical patients fall into this category. Those patients with poor left ventricular function but a "normal" baseline PCWP (i.e., chronic compensated congestive heart failure) will be identified after a fluid challenge. They will demonstrate an inability to redistribute an acute volume load to the left ventricle.

Appropriate colloids (albumin, hetastarch, or RBCs) rather than crystalloid are used for the fluid challenge in order to increase circulating blood volume most efficiently. The majority of patients will meet hemodynamic endpoint criteria with the use of fluids alone.

---

*See Chapter 15 for a discussion of the pharmacologic aspects of these agents.

PREOPERATIVE TUNE-UP

All the screening tests, except perhaps exercise ECG stress testing, focus exclusively on the detection of ischemic heart disease. Such a focus, however, leaves a significant population of surgical patients with left ventricular dysfunction who will not be identified as "at risk." In fact, there are no reliable screening tests to identify these patients. Precordial echocardiography has never been shown to predict outcome in preoperative patients, and LVEF as measured by angiography is controversial, as previously discussed. Yet a patient's ability to sustain a hyperdynamic stress response postoperatively has been clearly linked to survival.[31,32] Therefore several investigators have used the pulmonary artery (PA) catheter to identify and correct physiologic hemodynamic abnormalities before operation.[33-35] My associates and I also have used the PA catheter preoperatively to study a group of patients with severe peripheral vascular disease who were undergoing limb salvage procedures. Such patients are recognized to be at high risk for PCM.[26] In a randomized prospective study,[36] we found that optimizing left ventricular function (LVF) and oxygen transport before operation significantly reduced postoper-

ative cardiac complications. We refer to this preoperative hemodynamic assessment and optimization as the preoperative "tune-up" (see box on p. 56 and Fig. 6-2). We use the tune-up to evaluate and optimize cardiac performance in all patients believed to be at high risk for perioperative cardiac complications.

Several studies have confirmed that about 35% of patients undergoing the tune-up will meet hemodynamic endpoints on initial evaluation. An additional 25% will require only fluids, and about 40% will require pharmacologic intervention.[36,37] If the magnitude of myocardial dysfunction can be estimated by the level of pharmacologic intervention necessary to meet hemodynamic endpoints and if the degree of ventricular dysfunction predicts postoperative risk, then the response to the tune-up should predict risk. This theory remains controversial. In our study[36] we could not correlate pharmacologic intervention and outcome. However, as noted throughout this chapter, risk is multifactorial. We need to further identify the risk factors that are essential and refine our approach to the cardiac patient in order to reduce the patient's perioperative morbidity and mortality.

SUMMARY

- Predictors of perioperative cardiac morbidity include (1) reliable predictors (MI within previous 6 months, current CHF), (2) less consistent predictors (aortic stenosis, diabetes mellitus), and (3) controversial predictors (old MI, angina, previous episodes of CHF, hypertension, age).
- Specialized testing for cardiovascular problems includes exercise stress test, dipyridamole-thallium scanning, and radionuclide ejection fraction. All these methods are considered controversial.
- Current diagnostic approaches focus on evaluation of ischemia. No screening test is currently available for assessing left ventricular function.

REFERENCES

1. Mangano DT. Perioperative cardiac morbidity. Anesthesiology 72:153, 1990.
2. Topkins MJ, Artusio JF. Myocardial infarction and surgery: A five-year study. Anesth Analg 43:716, 1964.
3. Knapp RB, Topkins MJ, Artusio JF Jr. The cerebrovascular accident and coronary occlusion in anesthesia. JAMA 182:332, 1962.
4. Thompson GJ, Kelalis PP, Connolly DC. Transurethral prostatic resection after myocardial infarction. JAMA 182:908, 1962.
5. Arkins R, Smessaert AA, Hicks RG. Mortality and morbidity in surgical patients with coronary artery disease. JAMA 190:485, 1964.
6. Tarhan S, Moffitt E, Taylor WF, et al. Myocardial infarction after general anesthesia. JAMA 220:1451, 1972.
7. Steen PA, Tinker JH, Tarhan S. Myocardial reinfarction after anesthesia and surgery. JAMA 239:2566, 1978.
8. Goldman L, Caldera DL, Southwick FS, et al. Cardiac risk factors and complications in noncardiac surgery. Medicine 57:357, 1978.
9. Eerola M, Eerola R, Kaukinen S, et al. Risk factors in surgical patients with verified preoperative myocardial infarction. Acta Anaesthesiol Scand 24:219, 1980.
10. von Knorring J. Postoperative myocardial infarction: A prospective study in a risk group of surgical patients. Surgery 90:55, 1981.
11. Schoeppel LS, Wilkinson C, Waters J, et al. Effects of myocardial infarction on perioperative cardiac complications. Anesth Analg 62:493, 1983.
12. Rao TLK, Jacobs KH, El-Etr AA. Reinfarction following anesthesia in patients with myocardial infarction. Anesthesiology 59:499, 1983.
13. Shah KB, Kleinman BS, Rao TLK, et al. Angina and other risk factors in patients with cardiac diseases undergoing noncardiac operations. Anesth Analg 70:240, 1990.
14. Goldman L, Caldera DL, Nussbaum SR, et al. Multifactorial index of cardiac risk in noncardiac surgical procedures. N Engl J Med 297:845, 1977.
15. Charlson ME, MacKenzie CR, Gold JP, et al. The preoperative and intraoperative hemodynamic predictors of postoperative myocardial infarction or ischemia in patients undergoing noncardiac surgery. Ann Surg 210:637, 1989.
16. Detsky AS, Abrahms HB, McLaughlin JR, et al. Predicting cardiac complications in patients undergoing non-cardiac surgery. J Gen Intern Med 1:211, 1986.
17. Foster ED, Davis KB, Carpenter JA, et al. Risk of noncardiac operation in patients with defined coronary disease: The Coronary Artery Surgery Study (CASS) Registry Experience. Ann Thorac Surg 41:42, 1986.
18. Mock MB, Ringquist I, Fisher LD, et al. Survival of medically treated patients in the Coronary Artery Surgery Study (CASS) Registry. Circulation 66:562, 1982.
19. Pasternack PF, Imparato AM, Bear G, et al. The value of radionuclide angiography as a predictor of perioperative myocardial infarction in patients undergoing abdominal aortic aneurysm resection. J Vasc Surg 1:320, 1984.
20. Pasternack PF, Imparato AM, Riles TS, et al. The value of the radionuclide angiogram in the prediction of perioperative myocardial infarction in patients undergoing lower extremity revascularization procedures. Circulation 2 (Suppl II): II-13, 1985.
21. Kopecky SL, Gibbons RJ, Hollier LH. Preoperative supine exercise radionuclide angiogram predicts perioperative cardiovascular events in vascular surgery [abstract]. J Am Coll Cardiol 7 (Suppl A): 226A, 1986.
22. Franco CD, Goldsmith J, Veith FJ, et al. Resting gated pool ejection fraction: A poor predictor of perioperative myocardial infarction in patients undergoing vascular surgery for infrainguinal bypass grafting. J Vasc Surg 10:656, 1989.
23. Goldman L. Multifactorial index of cardiac risk in noncardiac surgery: Status report. Cardiothorac Vasc Anesth Update 1:1, 1990.
24. Eagle KA, Boucher CA. Cardiac risk of noncardiac surgery [editorial]. N Engl J Med 321:1330, 1989.
25. Roizen MF. Anesthetic implications of concurrent diseases. In Miller RD, ed. Anesthesia, 3rd ed. New York: Churchill Livingstone, 825, 1990.
26. Tomatis LA, Fierens EE, Verbrugge GP. Evaluation of surgical risk in peripheral vascular disease by coronary angiography: A series of 100 cases. Surgery 71:429, 1972.
27. Hertzer NR, Beven EG, Young JR, et al. Coronary artery disease in peripheral vascular patients. A classification of 1000 angiograms and results of surgical management. Ann Surg 199:223, 1984.
28. Benchimol A, Harris CL, Desser KB, et al. Resting electrocardiogram in major coronary artery disease. JAMA 224:1489, 1973.
29. Gerson MC, Hurst JM, Hertzberg VS, et al. Cardiac prognosis in noncardiac geriatric surgery. Ann Intern Med 103:832, 1985.
30. Raby KE, Goldman L, Creager MA, et al. Correlation between preoperative ischemia and major

cardiac events after peripheral vascular surgery. N Engl J Med 321:1296, 1989.

31. Clowes GHA Jr, Del Guercio LR, Barwinsky J. The cardiac output in response to surgical trauma. A comparison between patients who survived and those who died. Arch Surg 81:212, 1960.

32. Bland RD, Shoemaker WC, Abraham E, et al. Hemodynamic and oxygen transport patterns in surviving and non-surviving postoperative patients. Crit Care Med 13:85, 1985.

33. Whittemore AD, Clowes AW, Hechtman HB, et al. Aortic aneurysm repair. Reduced operative mortality associated with maintenance of optimal cardiac performance. Ann Surg 192:414, 1980.

34. Schultz RJ, Whitfield GF, LaMura JJ. Role of physiologic monitoring in patients with hip fractures. J Trauma 25:309, 1985.

35. Del Guercio LRM, Savino JA, Morgan JC. Physiologic assessment of surgical diagnosis-related groups. Ann Surg 202:519, 1985.

36. Berlauk JF, Abrams JH, Gilmour IJ, et al. Preoperative optimization of cardiovascular hemodynamics improves outcome in peripheral vascular surgery: A prospective randomized clinical trial. Ann Surg 214:289, 1991.

37. Babu SC, Pathanjali Sharma PV, Raciti A, et al. Monitor-guided responses. Arch Surg 115:1384, 1980.

CHAPTER 7

Life Support and Management of Cardiac Arrest

Michael D. Pasquale

OVERVIEW

Cardiorespiratory arrest is defined as loss of pulse, blood pressure, and spontaneous respiration. This state results in cardiac output that is inadequate to sustain life. The brain and the kidneys are the organs most susceptible to irreversible ischemic damage after successful but prolonged resuscitation. With time, dialysis, and careful medical management, the kidney often may be salvaged. However, no such time-proven protocol exists for salvage of brain function, and therefore the brain is usually regarded as the barometer of success or failure of resuscitation.

Although the means of reversing death has occupied the thoughts and efforts of man since antiquity, the technique of modern CPR (i.e., effective ventilation, closed-chest cardiac massage, and external defibrillation) has evolved over only the past 30 years. The four basic principles of modern CPR are to (1) ensure airway patency, (2) ensure ventilation, (3) provide artificial circulation, and (4) restart the arrested heart.[1]

AIRWAY MANAGEMENT

Management of the patient's airway is the first priority of resuscitation. It begins with ensuring airway patency and relief of airway obstruction. The most common cause of airway obstruction in the unconscious human is the tongue, which falls backward against the posterior pharynx.

Jaw-thrust or chin-lift maneuvers should be attempted before any airway adjuncts are used. In the patient with blunt trauma, the chin lift is preferred since it is less likely to produce injury to the spinal cord in a patient with a cervical spine fracture.[2] Obstructing foreign bodies always should be suspected, and blood, teeth, vomitus, secretions, or other debris, if present, should be evacuated from the airway. Abdominal thrusts may be useful in a patient with an airway that is totally obstructed by a foreign body. Once optimal positioning and removal of any foreign body have been achieved, the patient should be checked for return of spontaneous ventilation.

The presence of inspiratory stridor, gurgling, choking, hoarseness, increased respiratory effort, or difficulty with speech may be associated with partial airway obstruction, and optimization of airway patency should be pursued. A variety of airway adjuncts may be used. The oropharyngeal airway is a means of improving airway patency in unconscious patients since it prevents the tongue from falling back onto the posterior pharynx.[2] This type of airway should not be used in the conscious patient because it may stimulate the gag reflex and induce vomiting and subsequent aspiration.[2,3] The patient with an intact gag reflex will better tolerate a rubber nasopharyngeal airway even though it provides a less effective route than the oropharyngeal device does.[2]

Endotracheal intubation (ETI) is the definitive procedure for establishing an airway and optimizing ventilation in the patient with cardiac arrest. It also provides a conduit to evacuate secretions and administer drugs for resuscitation. The trachea can be intubated by the

60

oral, nasal, or transcricoid route. In noninjured patients without airway obstruction, the oral route is preferred. Nasotracheal intubation (NTI) can be used if the patient is breathing spontaneously.[4] In the patient with trauma, if there is no need for an immediate airway, a cervical spine x-ray film can be obtained first. If this film reveals no evidence of fracture, orotracheal intubation (OTI) may be done safely.[5] If there is evidence of fracture or if an immediate airway is needed, NTI is preferred in the spontaneously breathing patient. If the patient is apneic, OTI with in-line manual cervical immobilization should be used.[4,5] In the patient with severe maxillofacial injury or one in whom orotracheal and nasotracheal techniques have been unsuccessful, a surgical airway must be established.[6-8] In adults, surgical cricothyroidotomy is preferred. In children under the age of 12 years, needle cricothyroidotomy and subsequent tracheostomy should be done. Formal cricothyroidotomy should be avoided in children because the cricoid cartilage of children provides the only circumferential support to the upper trachea and therefore should not be damaged.[6,8] A very useful procedure in ETI is the application of firm pressure over the cricoid cartilage to occlude the upper end of the esophagus (Sellick's maneuver).[9] This maneuver reduces the incidence of aspiration of gastric contents during intubation.

VENTILATION

Once airway control has been established, adequate oxygenation and ventilation should be ensured. Mouth-to-mouth or mouth-to-mask ventilation should be initiated immediately. The fractional concentration of oxygen (FiO_2) in a rescuer's exhaled air is approximately 0.16, which is sufficient to meet a victim's needs. Conversion to bag/valve/mask ventilation, when available, is done with 100% FiO_2 and flow rates of 10 to 15 L/min. In this way an inspired oxygen concentration of approximately 75% can be delivered.[3,7] Potential problems with this technique include air leak, inadequate lung inflation, atelectasis, arteriovenous shunting, and hypoxemia. Also, gastric inflation secondary to high peak inspiratory pressures and decreased lung compliance during CPR increase the risk

of pulmonary aspiration. Optimal oxygenation and ventilation is achieved with ETI and subsequent bag/valve/tube respiration with 100% oxygen.[3,7]

CIRCULATION

In the absence of a pulse, chest compressions are necessary. In adults, standard two-person CPR involves 100 compressions per minute with a ventilation delivered every fifth compression.[3,10,11] The generation of a forward cardiac output as a result of chest compression is a subject of controversy. Kouwenhoven[12] popularized the cardiac pump theory, which suggests that during CPR the heart is squeezed like a pump between the sternum and the spine. Antegrade flow is ensured because of the cardiac valves.[13] The relaxation phase also mimics the natural circulation with a fall in intracardiac pressures and flow of blood into the heart as the sternum returns to its normal position. Ventilation and compression are alternated so that inflation does not impede flow during compression.[13,14] Interestingly, no data confirmed this assumption; however, an associated rise in venous pressure was noted during compression.[15] It was speculated that the thorax was acting as the pump (thoracic pump).[15,16] This theory suggests that with sternal compression there is an abrupt increase in intrathoracic pressure that propels blood into the arterial tree.[17,18] If this theory is true, then maneuvers to increase intrathoracic pressure may prove useful in resuscitation.[16] Unidirectional flow is ensured via one-way valves in the superior vena cava and venous collapse while arteries remain open.[17,18] The heart is considered simply a passive conduit, and flow depends on an arteriovenous pressure gradient outside the chest.

The relative contributions of the cardiac and thoracic pumps are still unsettled. Each mechanism probably contributes to perfusion, depending on the configuration and stiffness of the chest wall, the presence of cardiac enlargement, and the method of CPR.[19,20]

The blood flow established during CPR is barely life-sustaining since cardiac output is only about 25% of normal. Although systolic pressures of 90 mm Hg may be attainable, diastolic pressures are usually low (<20 mm Hg).[7] The cerebral cortex and the myocardium are inadequately perfused. The use of epinephrine in conjunction with CPR improves pressure, but perfusion remains suboptimal. New techniques and adjuncts to external compression (i.e., simultaneous ventilation and compression CPR [SVC-CPR], abdominal binders, volume loading during CPR, interposed abdominal counter pressure during CPR) intended to harness the thoracic pump have been tried, but there has been no conclusive evidence to suggest that they enhance vital organ perfusion or resuscitability.[16] Efforts to recruit the cardiac pump (i.e., high-frequency, high-impulse CPR) have demonstrated increases in cardiac output, aortic diastolic blood pressure, and coronary perfusion pressure.[21] It seems that squeezing the cardiac pump is essential to generating a coronary perfusion gradient, neurologic recovery, and increasing survival. Currently, the American Heart Association recommends compressions of moderate force and short duration to be delivered at a rate of 100 to 120/min.[21]

Open cardiac massage has been shown to provide a two- to threefold increase in cardiac output along with generation of higher arterial pressures and lower venous pressures.[22] These changes would suggest enhanced neurologic recovery and survival, but prospective randomized clinical trials are lacking. Possible indications for open cardiac massage are failure of conventional CPR, refractory ventricular fibrillation, hypothermia-associated arrest, cardiac tamponade, massive pulmonary embolism, abdominal aortic aneurysm, hemothorax, hemoperitoneum, air embolism, flail chest, third trimester of pregnancy, postoperative state, arrest in young patients, and thoracic deformities.[22]

THE ARRESTED HEART: A PHARMACOLOGIC APPROACH*
Epinephrine

Epinephrine is an endogenous catecholamine with both alpha- and beta-receptor–stimulating actions. It is the drug of choice for primary cardiac arrest. In addition, epinephrine is rec-

ommended for patients with ventricular fibrillation and pulseless tachycardia who are unresponsive to initial defibrillation attempts and electromechanical dissociation with asystole. The mechanism of action of epinephrine is related to its alpha vasopressor effects; cardiovascular responses include increases in heart rate, myocardial contractile force, systemic vascular resistance, arterial blood pressure, myocardial oxygen consumption, and automaticity. Clinically, epinephrine increases perfusion pressure, improves the contractile state, stimulates spontaneous contraction, and increases the vigor of ventricular fibrillation. Current evidence suggests epinephrine provides higher cardiac blood flow, higher cerebral blood flow, and more favorable oxygen delivery/consumption balance than other alpha agonists (e.g., phenylephrine, methoxamine). The recommended dose of epinephrine is 0.5 to 1 mg intravenously.[3] This dose may be repeated at 5-minute intervals because of the drug's short duration of action. Epinephrine also may be given transbronchially or by direct injection into the heart.

Atropine

Atropine sulfate is a parasympatholytic drug that accelerates the rate of discharge of the sinus node and may improve atrioventricular conduction. It is currently recommended for bradycardic dysrhythmias with hypotension, high-degree atrioventricular block at the nodal level, and ventricular asystole. The recommended dosage is 0.5 mg IV, repeated at 5-minute intervals until the desired rate is achieved (not to exceed 2 mg).[3] Atropine should not be given for atrioventricular block related to overdosage of beta-blockers or calcium channel blockers, which are treated with glucagon and calcium, respectively.

Isoproterenol

Isoproterenol hydrochloride is a sympathomimetic amine that is structurally related to epinephrine but acts almost exclusively on beta-receptors. Because it increases myocardial oxygen consumption, decreases coronary perfusion, and predisposes to ventricular dysrhythmia, isoproterenol is not recommended as a first-line agent for cardiac arrest. It is useful as a secondary drug in patients with sinus brady-

---

*For complete treatment approaches to the various conditions associated with the arrested heart, see Figs. 7-1 through 7-3 at the end of this chapter.

cardia and atrioventricular blocks associated with hypotension who do not respond to atropine.[3] Isoproterenol is generally given as a continuous intravenous infusion of 2 to 20 μg/min.

Dopamine

Dopamine has strong beta-$_1$ inotropic and alpha-adrenergic vasoconstrictor effects. It is the drug of choice for hypotension in the patient who has been successfully resuscitated from cardiac arrest that was caused by myocardial ischemia.[3] Dopamine is usually given as a continuous intravenous infusion of 2 to 20 μg/kg/min. Transition from a primarily renal dopaminergic effect to a primarily inotropic effect occurs at 2 to 5 μg/kg/min. At doses >25 μg/kg/min, the actions of dopamine are similar to those of norepinephrine.

Norepinephrine

Norepinephrine is a naturally occurring catecholamine that acts as a potent alpha- and beta-receptor stimulus to increase vasoconstriction and inotropy. Significant hypotension or cardiogenic shock are the principal indications for its use; however, there may be substantial increases in myocardial oxygen consumption due to increased left ventricular wall tension. Norepinephrine also has the disadvantage of causing renal and mesenteric vasoconstriction. The initial response of the coronary circulation to norepinephrine is vasoconstriction; however, this response is transient and vasodilation usually ensues because of increased myocardial metabolic activity and increased perfusion pressures. Norepinephrine is given by continuous intravenous infusion starting at 2 to 4 μg/min with titration done for desired blood pressure.

Sodium Bicarbonate

Acidemia during prolonged CPR is caused by alveolar hypoventilation and anaerobic metabolism.[23] The acidosis produced exerts detrimental effects on circulation; that is, increased pulmonary vasoconstriction, decreased systemic vascular resistance, arteriolar dilation, venous constriction, and capillary stasis. The acidosis also decreases the vascular and cardiac responses to adrenergic amines, while enhancing the effects of vagal stimulation. Overall, there is decreased chronotropy, inotropy, and

vascular tone. With a decrease in pH, the patient is also predisposed to ventricular dysrhythmias. Primary treatment of acidemia is adequate ventilation, which removes carbon dioxide. Correction of respiratory acidosis is more critical since partial pressure of carbon dioxide ($Paco_2$) more closely reflects intracellular pH because of the rapid diffusibility of carbon dioxide.[24,25] Recently, considerable controversy has been generated regarding the routine use of intravenous sodium bicarbonate during arrest.[26] The reason for this controversy is that it has been shown that above a pH of 7.2 there is no direct correlation between pH and success of defibrillation or resuscitation. Also, when given intravenously, sodium bicarbonate will produce carbon dioxide as it dissociates. This additional carbon dioxide passes into cells more quickly than does sodium bicarbonate and thus decreases intracellular pH.[25,27,28] Current recommendations regarding administration of sodium bicarbonate are a pH <7.2, prolonged (>10 minutes) interval prior to CPR, and failure of standard drug therapy. Iatrogenic alkalosis may lead to dysrhythmias, lactate production, and cerebral and peripheral vasoconstriction. Sodium bicarbonate should be given as an intravenous bolus of 1 mg/kg.[3]

Calcium

Calcium is no longer recommended as first-line therapy in cardiac arrest (excepting arrest due to hypokalemia) since it has not been shown to be effective.[3,26,29] Injection of calcium is also associated with detrimental effects, such as sinus node arrest, ventricular ectopy, and increased calcium levels in cytosol leading to mitochondrial damage (particularly in the brain and heart).[26,29,30]

Lidocaine

Lidocaine has been found to be most useful in the suppression of ventricular dysrhythmias. It decreases automaticity by slowing phase 4 depolarization. In infarcted tissue lidocaine has been shown to reduce conduction velocity and prolong the effective refractory period. Lidocaine also has been demonstrated as further depressing cells that form part of a reentrant pathway in ischemic zones while producing little or no effect on normal or moderately depressed cells. This effect prevents emergence of a wavefront from ischemic zones and thus terminates reentrant ventricular dysrhythmias. Lidocaine also reduces the disparity in action potential duration between ischemic and normal zones and prolongs conduction and refractoriness in ischemic zones. Last, lidocaine has been shown to increase the fibrillation threshold. Dosage should be a 1 mg/kg intravenous bolus followed by an infusion of 2 to 4 mg/min. An additional bolus of 0.5 mg/kg may be given 10 minutes after the initial bolus was administered if ventricular ectopy is still present. Excessive doses of lidocaine are capable of producing myocardial and circulatory depression, and clinical indications of lidocaine toxicity primarily include CNS effects. Since lidocaine is metabolized in the liver, dosages should be reduced in patients with hepatic impairment.

Procainamide

Procainamide suppresses phase 4 diastolic depolarization and thus slows the rate of ectopic pacemaker discharge. It also decreases the rate of rise of phase 0 of the action potential and terminates reentrant pathways by slowing conduction in already depressed areas. Procainamide is useful in suppressing premature ventricular complexes and recurrent ventricular tachycardia, which cannot be controlled with lidocaine. It also can be used in persistent ventricular fibrillation. The dosage for premature ventricular contractions and ventricular tachycardia is 100 mg every 5 minutes at a rate of approximately 20 mg/min until dysrhythmia is suppressed, hypotension ensues, the QRS complex is widened by 50%, or a total of 1 g has been injected. The maintenance infusion rate is 1 to 4 mg/min. Alternatively, a loading dose of 17 mg/kg can be given as an infusion over 1 hour followed by a maintenance infusion of 2.8 mg/min. Since procainamide is cleared by the kidney, in patients with renal impairment, the maintenance dose is reduced to 1.4 mg/kg/hr. In the presence of cardiac impairment, the recommended loading dose should be reduced to 12 mg/kg followed by a maintenance infusion of 1.4 mg/kg/hr. Side effects of procainamide administration include a hypotensive response, widening of the QRS complex, length-ening of the PR and QT intervals, and atrioventricular conduction disturbances.

Bretylium

Bretylium tosylate is a quaternary ammonium compound with postganglionic adrenergic-blocking properties, antidysrhythmic effects, and a positive inotropic action. It has been shown to elevate the ventricular fibrillation threshold and to increase the action potential duration and effective refractory period in normal ventricular muscle and Purkinje's fibers without lengthening the effective refractory period relative to action potential duration. Bretylium produces little increase in action potential duration in infarcted tissue; thus there is an overall reduction in disparity between normal and infarcted tissue. This drug has been shown to be useful in treating ventricular fibrillation and ventricular tachycardia refractory to other therapy. In ventricular fibrillation, 5 mg/kg is given intravenously at a rapid rate. If fibrillation persists despite administration of this dose and the use of countershock, the dose can be increased to 10 mg/kg and repeated as necessary. In refractory or recurrent ventricular tachycardia, 5 to 10 mg/kg can be injected over 8 to 10 minutes. If ventricular tachycardia persists, a second dose can be given 1 to 2 hours later and repeated every 6 to 8 hours. Alternatively, the drug can be given as a continuous infusion of 2 mg/min. On injection, postural hypotension is the most common adverse reaction.

EXPECTATIONS FOR RESUSCITATION

It is generally thought that the efforts of an organized health care team effectively increases the patient's long-term survival following unexpected cardiac arrest. Despite this impression, only 10% to 20% of those patients who sustain a cardiac arrest survive to be discharged home.[7] Considering the time, money, and effort allocated to resuscitation efforts, prearrest and arrest parameters must be recognized for their prognostic implications in predicting outcome of cardiac arrest in the hospital.

Prearrest Factors
Age

Although Stephenson[30a] noted that resuscitation was less successful in both the extremely old and the very young, most authors have not found age to significantly affect outcome.[31-33] Rozenbaum and Shenkman[34] noted that patients over 65 years old had a 20% survival, compared to a 16% survival in those under 65.

Sex

No significant differences in survival have been noted based solely on the sex of the patient undergoing arrest.[31,32,35]

Associated disease

In patients with significant associated illness, most notably cancer, sepsis, pneumonia, renal failure, left ventricular dysfunction, and cerebrovascular accident with residual defect, the outcome is generally poor.[31,32,35,36] In patients with one or more of these associated illnesses, Bedell et al.[32] noted 95% to 100% mortality after cardiac arrest. Also, a homebound life-style was associated with a 95% mortality.

Arrest Factors
Duration of resuscitation

Most authors concur that there is an inverse correlation between duration of resuscitation and survival. In general, if resuscitation is accomplished in less than 15 minutes, survival is more likely.[31,32,34-37] In contrast, efforts lasting longer than 30 minutes are almost always associated with death.

Initial cardiac rhythm

Patients found to be asystolic or having electromechanical dissociation are less likely to survive than those having ventricular fibrillation or ventricular tachycardia. Castagna et al.[31] noted that there were no survivors in patients whose initial rhythm was asystolic. Stiles et al.[37a] noted a 6% survival for patients in asystole, compared to a 30% survival for those in ventricular fibrillation.

Recurrent arrest

The likelihood of survival after a second or third cardiac arrest is remote, particularly in those patients with progressive metabolic or multisystem organ failure.[36] DeBard[35] has noted no survival in patients having more than three cardiac arrests.

Care setting

Rozenbaum and Shenkman,[34] Bedell et al.,[32] Castagna et al.,[31] DeBard,[35] and Sanders[19] have shown no significant differences in survival in relation to location of care administered for cardiac arrest.[31,32,34,35] Peatfield et al.[38] and Hershey and Fisher[39] however, have shown that survival after cardiac arrest on the ward ranges from 2% to 3%. One explanation may be that more resuscitative attempts are performed in this setting despite the presence of multiple associated disease.

Arterial blood gases

Most studies are not conclusive regarding the use of ABGs or oxygen saturations as determinants of survival. This uncertainty results from the fact that ABGs are not always obtained during the arrest phase. When ABGs are obtained, they are taken at different times during the resuscitation effort and do not take into account whether or not the patient has been intubated.[32,40] Sanders et al.[41] noted no significant differences in pH or $Paco_2$ in survivors vs. nonsurvivors, but they did find that survivors tended to have a higher initial Pao_2.

Other factors

No differences in outcome have been noted regarding time of cardiac arrest, presence of senior vs. junior members of the staff, and presence or absence of an anesthesiologist.

Patient Outcome

Of patients surviving cardiac arrest and subsequently being discharged, there is an annual death rate of approximately 10% for the first 5 years. Thereafter the death rate approaches that of the general population.[7,32,42] The brain is especially vulnerable to the ischemic and anoxic insults associated with cardiac arrest. Indeed, many patients who die after cardiac arrest have ischemic brain damage as a secondary cause.[43] Also, neurologic dysfunction has been noted in 2% of the long-term survivors.[43] Ischemic brain injury probably results from anoxia, which leads to a shift from aerobic to anaerobic metabolism. The ensuing lactic acidosis, besides being directly cytotoxic, leads to failure of critical membrane-bound ion pumps, most notably calcium pumps. Calcium rapidly enters the neurons and leads to mitochondrial dysfunction and uncoupling of oxidative phosphorylation. Calcium also activates phospholipase and leads to generation of free fatty acids, particularly arachidonic acid. Metabolism of arachidonic acid then leads to production of oxygen free radicals, which cause further necrosis.[44] It is important to note that approximately 90% of patients who are comatose after resuscitation will either regain consciousness or die within 36 hours, whereas the remaining 10% will remain in a vegetative state.[43-45]

Experimentally, there is evidence of a beneficial effect of calcium channel blockers in preventing neurologic dysfunction.[46,47] Clinically, however, no beneficial effects have been demonstrated.[48]

DO-NOT-RESUSCITATE ORDERS

In addition to moral and ethical considerations, the decision to perform CPR should be based on medical considerations, including an assessment of the expected outcome.

Recently, the Council of Ethical and Judicial Affairs[49] updated its resuscitation guidelines as follows:

1. Efforts should be made to resuscitate patients who suffer cardiac or respiratory arrest except when circumstances indicate that administration of CPR would be futile or not in accord with the desires or best interests of the patient.
2. Physicians should discuss with appropriate patients the possibility of cardiopulmonary arrest. Patients who are at risk of cardiac or respiratory failure should be encouraged to express, in advance, their preferences regarding the use of CPR. These discussions should include a description of the procedures encompassed by CPR and, when possible, should occur in an outpatient setting when general treatment preferences are discussed, or as early as possible during hospitalization, when the patient is likely to be mentally alert. Early discussions that occur on a nonemergency basis help to ensure the patient's active participation in the decision-making process. In addition, subsequent discussions are desirable, on a periodic basis, to allow for changes in the patient's circumstances or in available treatment alternatives that may alter the patient's preferences.
3. If a patient is incapable of rendering a decision regarding the use of CPR, a decision may be made by a surrogate decision maker, based on the previously expressed preferences of the patient or, if such preferences are unknown, in accordance with the patient's best interests.
4. The physician has an ethical obligation to honor the resuscitation preferences expressed by the patient or the patient's surrogate. Physicians should not permit their personal value judgments about quality of life to obstruct the implementation of a patient's or surrogate's preferences regarding the use of CPR. However, if, in the judgment of the treating physician, CPR would be futile, the treating physician may enter a do-not-resuscitate (DNR) order into the patient's record. When there is adequate time to do so, the physician must first inform the patient, or the incompetent patient's surrogate, of the content of the DNR order, as well as the basis for its implementation. The physician also should be prepared to discuss appropriate alternatives, such as obtaining a second opinion or arranging for transfer of care to another physician.
5. Resuscitative efforts should be considered futile if they cannot be expected either to restore cardiac or respiratory function to the patient or to achieve the expressed goals of the informed patient.
6. DNR orders, as well as the basis for their implementation, should be entered by the attending physician in the patient's medical record.
7. DNR orders only preclude resuscitative efforts in the event of cardiopulmonary arrest and should not influence other therapeutic interventions that may be appropriate for the patient.
8. Hospital medical staffs should periodically review their experience with DNR orders, revise their DNR policies as appropriate, and educate physicians regarding their proper role in the decision-making process for DNR orders.

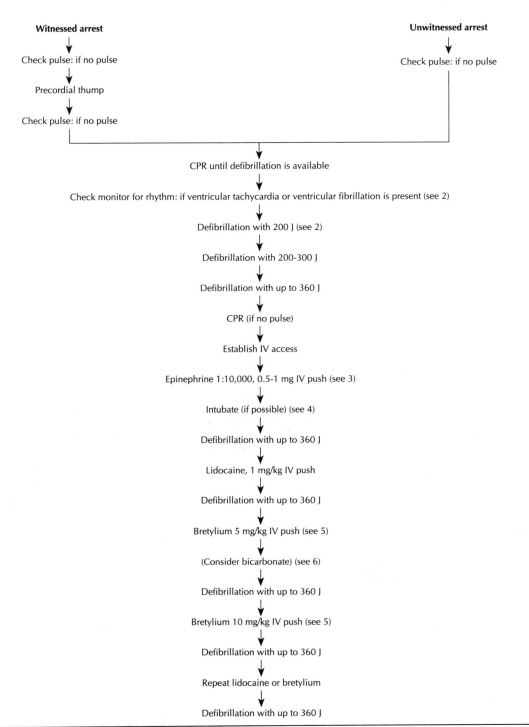

FIG. 7-1 Treatment approach for ventricular fibrillation or pulseless ventricular tachycardia. (1) Flow chart presumes that dysrhythmia is continuing. (2) Check pulse and rhythm after every shock. If ventricular fibrillation recurs after transiently converting, use whatever energy level had previously been successful. (3) Epinephrine should be repeated every 5 minutes. (4) Intubation is preferable, the sooner the better; however defibrillation and epinephrine are more important initially if patient can be ventilated without intubation. (5) May prefer repeated doses of lidocaine given in 0.5 mg/kg boluses every 8 minutes to total of 3 mg/kg. (6) Initial dose of sodium bicarbonate is 1 mEq/kg; one half of this dose may be repeated every 10 minutes, if necessary. (Data from Standards and guidelines for cardiopulmonary resuscitation and emergency cardiac care. JAMA 255:2841, 1986.)

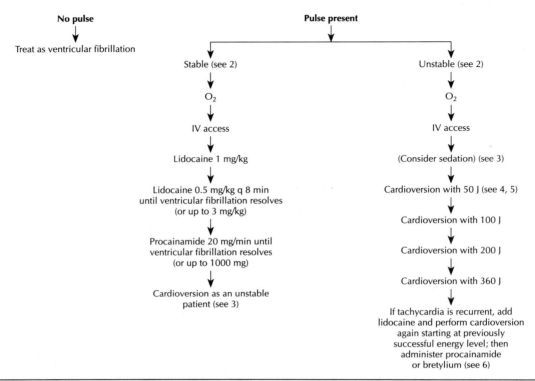

FIG. 7-2 Treatment approach for sustained ventricular tachycardia. (1) Flow chart presumes that ventricular tachycardia is continuing. (2) If patient becomes unstable (chest pain, dyspnea, hypotension, congestive heart failure, ischemia, infarction) at any time, move the "unstable" arm of flow chart. (3) Sedation should be considered for all patients except those who are hemodynamically unstable or unconscious. (4) If hypotension, pulmonary edema, or unconsciousness is present, unsynchronized cardioversion should be done to avoid delay associated with synchronization. (5) In absence of hypotension, pulmonary edema, or unconsciousness, a precordial thump may be employed prior to cardioversion. (6) Once ventricular tachycardia has resolved, begin intravenous infusion of antiarrhythmic agent that has aided resolution of ventricular tachycardia. (Data from Standards and guidelines for cardiopulmonary resuscitation and emergency cardiac care. JAMA 255:2841, 1986.)

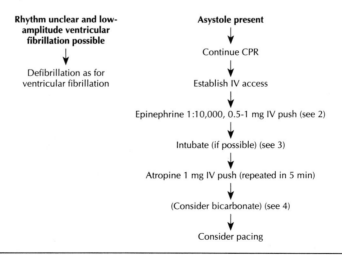

FIG. 7-3 Treatment approach for asystole (cardiac standstill). (1) Flow chart presumes asystole is continuing. (2) Epinephrine should be repeated every 5 minutes. (3) Intubation is preferable, the earlier the better; however, CPR and use of epinephrine are more important initially if patient can be ventilated. (4) Sodium bicarbonate should be given in a dose of 1 mEq/kg; one half of original dose may be repeated every 10 minutes (if used). (Data from Standards and guidelines for cardiopulmonary resuscitation and emergency cardiac care. JAMA 255:2841, 1986.)

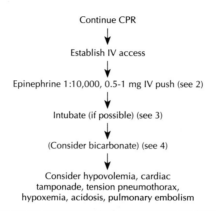

Continue CPR

↓

Establish IV access

↓

Epinephrine 1:10,000, 0.5-1 mg IV push (see 2)

↓

Intubate (if possible) (see 3)

↓

(Consider bicarbonate) (see 4)

↓

Consider hypovolemia, cardiac
tamponade, tension pneumothorax,
hypoxemia, acidosis, pulmonary embolism

FIG. 7-4   Treatment approach for electromechanical dissociation. (1) Flow chart presumes that electrome-chanical dissociation is continuing. (2) Epinephrine should be repeated every 5 minutes. (3) Intubation is preferable, the earlier the better; however, CPR and epinephrine are more important initially if patient can be ventilated. (4) Sodium bicarbonate (if used) should be given in a dose of 1 mEq/kg; one half of original dose may be repeated every 10 minutes, if necessary. (Data from Standards and guidelines for cardiopulmonary resuscitation and emergency cardiac care. JAMA 255:2841, 1986.)

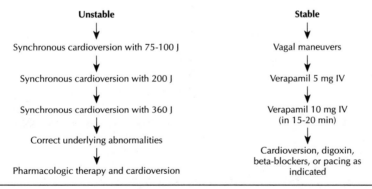

Unstable	**Stable**
↓	↓
Synchronous cardioversion with 75-100 J	Vagal maneuvers
↓	↓
Synchronous cardioversion with 200 J	Verapamil 5 mg IV
↓	↓
Synchronous cardioversion with 360 J	Verapamil 10 mg IV (in 15-20 min)
↓	↓
Correct underlying abnormalities	Cardioversion, digoxin, beta-blockers, or pacing as indicated
↓	
Pharmacologic therapy and cardioversion	

FIG. 7-5   Treatment approach for paroxysmal supraventricular tachycardia. Flow chart presumes that tachycardia is continuing. (Data from Standards and guidelines for cardiopulmonary resuscitation and emergency cardiac care. JAMA 255:2841, 1986.)

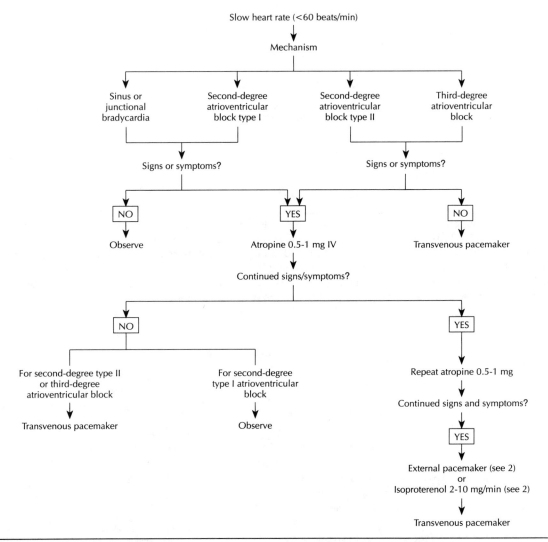

FIG. 7-6   Treatment approach for bradycardia. (1) Flow chart presumes continuing bradycardia. (2) Temporizing therapy. (Data from Standards and guidelines for cardiopulmonary resuscitation and emergency cardiac care. JAMA 255:2841, 1986.)

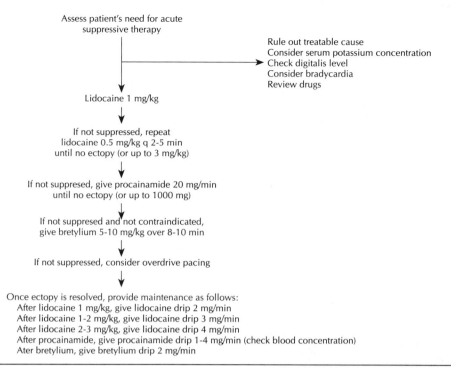

Assess patient's need for acute
suppressive therapy

Rule out treatable cause
Consider serum potassium concentration
Check digitalis level
Consider bradycardia
Review drugs

Lidocaine 1 mg/kg

If not suppressed, repeat
lidocaine 0.5 mg/kg q 2-5 min
until no ectopy (or up to 3 mg/kg)

If not suppresed, give procainamide 20 mg/min
until no ectopy (or up to 1000 mg)

If not suppresed and not contraindicated,
give bretylium 5-10 mg/kg over 8-10 min

If not suppressed, consider overdrive pacing

Once ectopy is resolved, provide maintenance as follows:
    After lidocaine 1 mg/kg, give lidocaine drip 2 mg/min
    After lidocaine 1-2 mg/kg, give lidocaine drip 3 mg/min
    After lidocaine 2-3 mg/kg, give lidocaine drip 4 mg/min
    After procainamide, give procainamide drip 1-4 mg/min (check blood concentration)
    Ater bretylium, give bretylium drip 2 mg/min

FIG. 7-7 Treatment approach for ventricular ectopy in acute suppressive therapy. Flow chart presumes continuing ventricular ectopy. (Data from Standards and guidelines for cardiopulmonary resuscitation and emergency cardiac care. JAMA 255:2841, 1986.)

SUMMARY

- Basic principles of management of the patient with cardiac arrest are to (1) establish a secure, patent airway; (2) ventilate the patient; (3) provide artificial circulation; (4) restart the arrested heart.
- Use jaw-thrust or chin-lift maneuvers to establish patent airway. ETI is definitive procedure. In emergencies, use oral, nasal, or transcricoid approach. Avoid surgical cricothyroidotomy in children.
- After airway has been established, use mouth-to-mouth resuscitation immediately, when necessary. Convert to bag/valve/mask as soon as possible.
- Begin chest compression in absence of a pulse. Use compressions of moderate force and short duration at rate of 90 to 100/min.
- Pharmacologic guidelines:

Use:

Epenephrine for patients with ventricular fibrillation and pulseless tachycardia when unresponsive to defibrillation attempts

Atropine for bradycardia with hypotension, nodal atrioventricular block, and ventricular asystole

Isoproterenol only as a secondary drug for bradycardia and atrioventricular block treated unsuccessfully with atropine

Dopamine in the successfully resuscitated patient with persistent hypotension

Norepinephrine for profound hypotension and cardiogenic shock

Sodium bicarbonate for pH <7.2, >10-minute interval prior to CPR, and failure of standard drug therapy

Lidocaine for suppression of ventricular dysrhythmias

Procainamide for suppression of PVCs and ventricular tachycardia not controlled with lidocaine

Bretylium in refractory ventricular tachycardia and ventricular fibrillation

Do not use:

Calcium as initial therapy except with hypocalcemia or hyperkalemia

REFERENCES

1. Hermreck AS. The history of cardiopulmonary resuscitation. Am J Surg 156:430, 1988.
2. Guildner CW. Resuscitation-opening the airway. A comparative study of techniques for opening an airway obstructed by the tongue. J Am Coll Emerg Physicians 5:588, 1976.
3. Standards and guidelines for cardiopulmonary resuscitation and emergency cardiac care. JAMA 255:2841, 1986.
4. Iserson KV. Blind nasotracheal intubation. Ann Emerg Med 10:468, 1981.
5. Majernick TG, Bierrick R, Houston JB. Cervical spine movement during orotracheal intubation. Ann Emerg Med 15:417, 1986.
6. Attia RR, Battit GE, Murphy JD. Transtracheal ventilation. JAMA 234:1152, 1975.
7. Dellinger RP, Mattox KL. Emergency resuscitation: What the books do not tell you. In Civetta JM, Taylor RW, Kirby RR, eds. Critical Care. Philadelphia: JB Lippincott, 1988.
8. Kress TD. Cricothyroidotomy. Ann Emerg Med 11:197, 1982.
9. Sellick BA. Cricoid pressure to control regurgitation of stomach contents during induction of anesthesia. Lancet 2:404, 1961.
10. Shipman KH, McCrady W, Bradford HA. Closed chest cardiac resuscitation. Am J Cardiol 10:551, 1962.
11. Sykes MK, Orr DS. Cardiopulmonary resuscitation. Anaesthesia 21:363, 1966.
12. Kouwenhoven WB, Jude JR, Knickerbocker GG. Closed chest massage. JAMA 173:1064, 1960.
13. Deshmukh NG, Weil MH, Gudapati CV, et al. Mechanisms of blood flow generated by precordial compression during CPR. I. Studies of closed chest precordial compression. Chest 95:1092, 1989.
14. Halperin HR, Tsitlik JE, Guerci AD, et al. Determinants of blood flow to vital organs during cardiopulmonary resuscitation in dogs. Circulation 73:539, 1986.
15. Kaplin BM, Knott AP. Closed-chest cardiac massage for circulatory arrest. Arch Intern Med 114:5, 1964.
16. Ewy GA. Alternative approaches to external chest compression. Circulation 74 (Suppl IV):98, 1986.
17. Luce JM, Ross BK, O'Quinn RJ, et al. Regional blood flow during cardiopulmonary resuscitation in dogs using simultaneous and nonsimultaneous compression and ventilation. Circulation 67:258, 1983.
18. Martin GB, Carden DL, Nowak RM, et al. Aortic and right atrial pressures during standard and simultaneous compression and ventilation CPR in human beings. Ann Emerg Med 15:125, 1986.
19. Sanders AB, Meislin NW, Ewy GA. The physiology of cardiopulmonary resuscitation: An update. JAMA 252:3283, 1984.
20. Swenson RD, Weaver WD, Hiskaner RA, et al. Hemodynamics in humans during conventional and experimental methods of cardiopulmonary resuscitation. Circulation 19:1220, 1988.
21. Maier GW, Newton JR Jr, Wolfe JA, et al. The influence of manual compression rate on hemodynamic support during cardiopulmonary resuscitation. Circulation 74(Suppl IV):51, 1986.
22. Rosenthal RE, Turbiak TW. Open-chest cardiopulmonary resuscitation. Am J Emerg Med 4:248, 1986.
23. Stacpoole PW. Lactic acidosis: The case against bicarbonate therapy. Ann Intern Med 105:276, 1986.
24. Grundler W, Weil MH, Rackow EC, et al. Selective acidosis in venous blood during human cardiopulmonary resuscitation: A preliminary report. Crit Care Med 13:886, 1985.
25. Weil MH, Rackow EC, Trevino R, et al. Difference in acid-base state between venous and arterial blood during cardiopulmonary resuscitation. N Engl J Med 315:153, 1986.
26. Schleien CL, Berkowitz ID, Traystman R, et al. Controversial issues in cardiopulmonary resuscitation. Anesthesiology 71:133, 1989.
27. Weil MH, Ruiz CE, Michaels S, et al. Acid-base determinants of survival after cardiopulmonary resuscitation. Crit Care Med 13:888, 1985.
28. Weil MH, Trevino RP, Rackow EC. Sodium bicarbonate during CPR: Does it help or hinder? Chest 88:487, 1985.
29. Hughes WG, Ruedy JR. Should calcium be used in cardiac arrest? Am J Med 81:285, 1986.
30. Fiskum G. Mitochondrial damage during cerebral ischemia. Ann Emerg Med 14:810, 1985.
30a. Stephenson NE. Cardiac Arrest and Resuscitation. St. Louis: CV Mosby, 1958.
31. Castagna J, Weil MH, Shubin H. Factors determining survival in patients with cardiac arrest. Chest 65:527, 1974.
32. Bedell SE, Delbanco TL, Cook EF, Epstein FH. Survival after cardiopulmonary resuscitation in the hospital. N Engl J Med 309:569, 1983.
33. Gulati RS, Bhan GL, Horan MA. Cardiopulmonary resuscitation of old people. Lancet 2:267, 1983.
34. Rozenbaum EA, Shenkman L. Predicting outcome of inhospital cardiopulmonary resuscitation. Crit Care Med 16:583, 1988.

35. DeBard ML. Cardiopulmonary resuscitation: Analysis of six years' experience and review of literature. Ann Emerg Med 10:408, 1981.

36. Peterson MW, Geist LJ, Schwartz DA, et al. Outcome after cardiopulmonary resuscitation in a medical intensive care unit. Chest 100:168, 1991.

37. Scott RPF. Cardiopulmonary resuscitation in a teaching hospital: A survey of cardiac arrests outside intensive care units and emergency rooms. Anaesthesia 36:526, 1981.

37a. Stiles QR, Tucker BL, Meyer BW, et al. Cardiopulmonary arrest—Evaluation of an active resuscitation program. Am J Surg 122:282, 1971.

38. Peatfield RC, Taylor D, Sillett RW, et al. Survival after cardiac arrest in hospital. Lancet 2:1223, 1977.

39. Hershey CO, Fisher L. Why outcome of cardiopulmonary resuscitation in general wards is poor. Lancet 1:31, 1982.

40. Snyder AB, Salloum LJ, Barone JE, et al. Predicting short-term outcome of cardiopulmonary resuscitation using central venous oxygen tension measurements. Crit Care Med 19:111, 1991.

41. Sanders AB, Kern KB, Otto CW, et al. End-tidal carbon dioxide monitoring during cardiopulmonary resuscitation: A prognostic indication for survival. JAMA 262:1347, 1989.

42. Messert B, Quaglieri CE. Cardiopulmonary resuscitation: Perspectives and problems. Lancet 2:410, 1976.

43. Safar P. Cerebral resuscitation after cardiac arrest: A review. Circulation 74(Suppl IV):138, 153, 1986.

44. Seisjo BK. Mechanisms of ischemic brain damage. Crit Care Med 16:954, 1988.

45. Henneman EA. Brain resuscitation. Heart Lung 15:3, 1986.

46. Vaagenes P, Cantadore R. Safar P, et al. Amelioration of brain damage by lidoflazine after prolonged ventricular fibrillation cardiac arrest in dogs. Crit Care Med 12:846, 1984.

47. Winegar CP, Henderson O, White BC, et al. Early amelioration of neurologic deficit by lidoflazine after fifteen minutes of cardiopulmonary arrest in dogs. Ann Emerg Med 12:471, 1983.

48. Brain Resuscitation Clinical Trial 2 Study Group: A randomized clinical study of a calcium-entry blocker (lidoflazine) in the treatment of comatose survivors of cardiac arrest. N Engl J Med 324:1225, 1991.

49. Council on Ethical and Judicial Affairs, American Medical Association. Guidelines for the appropriate use of Do-Not-Resuscitate orders. JAMA 265:1868, 1991.

CHAPTER 8

Evaluation of Hepatic Function

George M. Logan · Joseph R. Bloomer

The liver is involved in a wide variety of metabolic processes. Its roles include synthesis, biotransformation, and detoxification. Derangements in any of these functions can occur in the postoperative period as a result of the stress of surgery, the effects of anesthesia, or the unmasking of underlying liver disease. Patients with preexisting liver disease are at increased risk for hepatic decompensation after surgery. The lack of controlled studies makes the precise prediction of the risk of surgery in patients with liver disease difficult. This chapter considers the evaluation of hepatic function to aid in the understanding and prediction of surgical risk.

EFFECTS OF ANESTHESIA AND SURGERY

Surgery, independently of the type of anesthesia administered, may produce transient increased concentrations in the tests used to evaluate liver status. Transaminase concentrations show modest increases, usually in the range of doubling to tripling.[1] These increases occur in 20% of surgical procedures. Rates as high as 61% are found in patients undergoing biliary tract surgery. Increased concentrations of alkaline phosphatase and bilirubin have been documented in 25% to 75% of patients after administration of most types of anesthetics.[2] These findings are rarely of clinical significance.

The anesthetic agents used today for biliary tract surgery are not direct hepatotoxins, but they do reduce hepatic blood flow. Despite hepatic blood flow reduction, liver hypoxia has not been demonstrated in studies of normal volunteers undergoing general anesthesia.[3] Additional intraoperative factors leading to liver dysfunction may be positive pressure ventilation, hypovolemia, and the use of vasoactive drugs. Patients with liver disease, especially those with portal hypertension, are more likely to have a decrease in hepatic blood flow during surgery. They also may have impaired metabolism of anesthetic agents and other drugs. Doses of sedatives, especially benzodiazepines and narcotics, should be reduced. In patients with decompensated liver disease, if the disease is severe, the use of sedatives should be eliminated. The metabolism of other agents also is affected. For example, the half-life of lidocaine is increased by 300% in liver disease.

RISK FACTORS FOR SURGERY

Liver dysfunction can be broadly divided into *acute* and *chronic* liver disease. *Cirrhosis* is the advanced and irreversible stage of liver disease. Any of these three conditions are risk factors for hepatic surgery.

Acute Hepatitis

Acute hepatitis is associated with increases in the transaminase concentrations of aspartate aminotransferase (AST) and alanine aminotransferase (ALT), which rise more than three times normal. Frequently, acute hepatitis is associated with increases of 10 to 20 times normal. Often the cause is viral, especially in hepatitis types A, B, or C. Currently, viral hepatitis can be diagnosed serologically. However, serologic tests were not available at the time of the series reported in this discussion, which was done before 1970.

A 12-year series of more than 18,000 operations for hepatobiliary disorders at the Mayo Clinic included 42 patients with presumed viral hepatitis.[4] Of these 42 patients, 10% died postoperatively and an additional 12% had major morbidity.

In 1967 a retrospective study from the Massachusetts General Hospital that reported on 46,923 patients undergoing surgery revealed 73 patients with postoperative hepatic dysfunction.[5] Of these 73 patients, 12 had unsuspected preoperative hepatic dysfunction and 11 of the 12 patients died. In this study no distinction was made between acute and chronic liver disease. Finally, Turner and Sherlock[6] reported 42% mortality and 33% hepatic decompensation in patients with acute hepatitis.

In contrast, Hardy and Hughes[7] reported on a series of 14 patients with acute viral hepatitis who underwent laparotomy and suffered no morbidity or mortality.

These observations support the delay of elective surgery in acute viral hepatitis until the patient recovers clinically and biochemically.

Chronic Hepatitis

Chronic hepatitis is defined by an increase in serum transaminase concentrations that persists for 6 months or more. A wide variety of hepatic disorders, including alcoholic liver disease, chronic viral hepatitis, drug-induced hepatitis, autoimmune hepatitis, and primary biliary cirrhosis, are causes of chronic hepatitis. Although this population has not been studied for surgical risk, the risk of surgery, in general, would be expected to correlate with the level of impairment in hepatic synthetic function.

Cirrhosis

Cirrhosis is the irreversible stage of chronic liver disease characterized by fibrosis that disrupts the normal hepatic lobular architecture. The most common cause of cirrhosis in the United States is chronic alcoholism, but chronic hepatitis B infection is the most common cause worldwide. Less common causes include viral hepatitis C, viral hepatitis D, chronic active hepatitis of autoimmune origin, primary biliary cirrhosis, and secondary biliary cirrhosis. Secondary biliary cirrhosis is usually a result of chronic extrahepatic biliary obstructions. The inherited disorders, hemochromatosis, alpha-1-antitrypsin deficiency, and Wilson's disease, also may cause cirrhosis. In addition, cirrhosis may arise from chronic right heart failure. Those cases in which no cause is determined are called cryptogenic cirrhosis.

Patients with chronic liver disease and cirrhosis who are undergoing surgery have been the focus of several studies. A review of 429 patients undergoing cholecystectomy during a period of 8 years at the Hines VA hospital in Illinois revealed that 12.8% of patients had cirrhosis.[8] The operative mortality among those patients free of liver disease was 1.1%. Among those with cirrhosis, prothrombin times (PTs) within 2.5 seconds of control were found in 78%. In this group operative mortality was elevated (9.3%). Operative mortality rose to 83% among those patients with prothrombin times prolonged >2.5 seconds above control.

The Child's classification for cirrhosis and the Pugh modification of this classification provide a method of predicting surgical risk in patients with cirrhosis (Table 8-1). Garrison et al.[9] have retrospectively studied various predictors of surgical risk in a series of 100 cirrhotic patients undergoing abdominal operations other than portasystemic shunts. Predictors of surgical mortality were prolonged PT, prolonged partial thromboplastin time (PTT), preexisting infection, depressed serum albumin, and Child's classification (Table 8-2). Similar findings were reported by Doberneck et al.[10] In their series of 102 patients, an increased mortality was demonstrated for a wide variety of operative procedures. The operative mortality for intraperitoneal procedures was 35%, and the overall mortality was 20%. The major risk factors identified in this study were jaundice and prolonged PT.

A series of 51 patients with alcoholic cirrhosis undergoing abdominal surgery reported on by Aranha and Greenlee[11] in 1986 had an overall mortality of 67%. The risk factors associated with increased mortality were PTs >2.5 seconds

TABLE 8-1	Methods of Predicting Surgical Risk in Patients With Cirrhosis

*Child's classification**

Factor	A (minimal)	B (moderate)	C (advanced)
Serum bilirubin (mg/dl)	<2	2-3	>3
Serum albumin (mg/dl)	>3.5	3-3.5	<3
Ascites	None	Controlled	Refractory
Encephalopathy	None	Minimal	Advanced, "coma"
Nutrition	Excellent	Good	Poor, "wasting"

Pugh modification†

Clinical/Biochemical Measurements	Points for Increasing Abnormality		
	1	2	3
Encephalopathy	None	Minimal	Advanced
Ascites	Absent	Slight	Moderate
Bilirubin (mg/dl)	1-2	2-3	>3
Albumin (g/dl)	>3.5	2.8-3.5	<2.8
Prothrombin time (seconds prolonged)	1-4	4-6	>6
For primary biliary cirrhosis, bilirubin (mg/dl)	1-4	4-10	>10
Child's-Pugh class	A	B	C
SCORING (points)	5-6	7-9	10-15

*Modified from Child CG III, Turcotte J. In Child CG III, ed. The Liver and Portal Hypertension. Philadelphia: WB Saunders, 1965.
†Modified from Pugh RNH, Murray-Lyon IM, Dawson JL, et al. Transection of the esophagus for bleeding esophageal varices. Br J Surg 60:646-649, 1973.

TABLE 8-2	Predictors of Surgical Mortality in Patients With Cirrhosis

Variable	Mortality (%)
Child's class:	
A	10
B	31
C	76
Ascites	58
Infection	64
Prothrombin time >1.5 sec >control	63
Albumin <3 mg/dl	58

above control, emergency surgery, and ascites.

The importance of hepatic reserve is shown in a series that assessed hepatic function via the aminopyrine breath test.[12] In this study, 30 of 31 patients with a normal preoperative test survived abdominal surgery, whereas 6 of 7 patients with depressed values died. Despite its small size, this study showed statistically significant differences in survival.

INDICATIONS FOR PREOPERATIVE METABOLIC SUPPORT

Patients with liver disease are at risk for nutritional deficits. In a group of 284 patients with alcoholic liver disease, Mendenhall et al.[13] showed that all of the patients showed some evidence of malnutrition. Although malnutrition increases surgical risk, patients with liver disease are often intolerant to oral repletion. Their associated malabsorption and anorexia limit oral diet. Parenteral nutrition may cause an increase in ascites and also may promote hepatic encephalopathy. However, modification of total parenteral nutrition formulas to provide branched-chain amino acids has been shown to improve hepatic encephalopathy. Fisher et al.[14-15] used an amino acid mixture that was enriched in branched-chain amino acids and deficient in aromatic amino acids and methionine, along with hypertonic glucose. This approach was based on the knowledge that increased serum concentrations of aromatic amino acids occur in patients with cirrhosis. The aromatic amino acids usually are catabolized in the liver. This function is diminished in liver disease as a result of decreased functional capacity and, in patients with cirrhosis, shunting of portal blood around the liver. The branched-chain-enriched amino acids stimulate protein synthesis, which results in a decrease in the circulating concentration of the aromatic amino acids. Further, the branched-chain amino acids compete with aromatic amino acids for transfer across the blood-brain barrier. This competition reduces the level of aromatic amino acids in the brain and cerebral spinal fluid and improves the aminergic neurotransmitter profile. Prospective randomized controlled trials on protein-intolerant patients with liver disease who were resistant to standard treatments for hepatic encephalopathy have shown that infusions of branched-chain-enriched amino acids produce faster and more complete recovery of patients and greater improvement in encephalopathy.[16] These solutions permitted nutritional support in this group of patients, who would be otherwise intolerant of such supplementation. Patients with encephalopathy that cannot be controlled by the usual measures of lactulose and/or neomycin administration should have metabolic support to clear the encephalopathy in the preoperative period.

ASSESSMENT OF THE PREOPERATIVE PATIENT

The history and physical examination of the preoperative patient is the most important part of the evaluation. When the history is taken, attention should be given to inclusion of hepatitis, icteric episodes, exposure to hepatotoxins, and transfusion of blood products. Because many drugs produce deleterious hepatic effects, the use of current and recent medications (including over-the-counter agents) should be documented. Any family history of liver disease should be noted. Past and present alcohol use should be documented. Direct inquiries about DWI arrests and prior chemical dependency treatment should be made. Systemic symptoms of chronic liver disease, such as easy fatigue and lassitude, should be documented.

On physical examination, signs of liver disease should be sought. These signs include spider nevi, palmar erythema, gynecomastia, hepatosplenomegaly, and caput medusae. When signs of portal hypertension are present, the Child's classification should be determined. This classification includes an examination for ascites, hepatic encephalopathy, and nutritional status.

Laboratory evaluation should be undertaken for patients with a history of hepatitis. Testing of these individuals should include screening for hepatitis C antibody, hepatitis A antibody, fraction, hepatitis A antibody IgG fraction, hepatitis B surface antigen, AST, ALT, total and direct bilirubin, alkaline phosphatase, gamma-glutamyl transpeptidase (GGT), albumin, PT, and complete blood count. If these values are normal, the patient is probably not at increased risk for surgery. If the findings suggest acute hepatitis, elective surgery should be deferred until resolution of the condition is complete. In the case of significant laboratory abnormalities, a thorough evaluation for the cause should be undertaken before all but urgent surgery is done.

Patients with evidence of chronic hepatitis may require liver biopsy to determine the cause and extent of liver damage. Those with cholestasis, evidenced by increased alkaline phosphatase and confirmed by increased GGT or 5'-nucleotidase, require imaging of the biliary tree. Usually the use of ultrasonography is satisfactory, but sometimes endoscopic retrograde cholangiopancreatography is necessary to evaluate the possibility of extrahepatic ductal disease. Patients with evidence of cirrhosis should have careful evaluation of coagulation function. Many of these patients have poor nutrition and are deficient in vitamin K. If PTs are elevated, testing should be repeated 12 to 24 hours after administration of a subcutaneous dose of vitamin K_1, which may be repeated if no improvement in the PT is observed. PTs that remain elevated >3 seconds beyond the control values after administration of vitamin K may respond to infusion of fresh frozen plasma. Unfortunately, large volumes of plasma often are required and the response is transient. The splenomegaly of portal hypertension may cause thrombocytopenia. In cirrhotic patients with chronic alcohol use, direct toxic effects on the bone marrow also may reduce the platelet count.

Patients with cirrhosis should be evaluated for ascites. If present, the ascitic fluid should be tested for evidence of infection. A total white blood cell count of >500 cells/mm³ or a polymorphonuclear cell count of >250 cells/mm³ provides the best evidence of presumptive bacterial infection. Ascitic fluid and blood cultures should be obtained. Ascitic fluid should be sterile and controlled with diuretics to whatever extent is possible before abdominal surgery. Treatment should include salt restriction to 1 g of sodium chloride per day and a potassium-sparing diuretic. Careful monitoring of serum electrolytes, weight, girth, urine sodium, and

renal function all are important in the preoperative management of these patients. If the patient's volume status is uncertain, central venous pressure monitoring is helpful.

Patients with decompensated hepatic function are at risk for renal impairment. Care should be taken to avoid the use of potentially nephrotoxic drugs. Patients who are in this group appear to be at particular risk for renal toxicity from NSAIDs and aminoglycoside antibiotics.

The patient also should be evaluated for the presence of hepatic encephalopathy. At one extreme, the diagnosis is apparent. Clinical findings include confusion, asterixis, and increased serum ammonia concentration. However, mild encephalopathy can be detected by the more subtle findings of day-night reversal and psychometric testing. Hepatic encephalopathy should be treated medically prior to surgery, if possible. Therapy includes the use of oral lactulose, neomycin, or both. Lactulose acts as a laxative and creates an acidic colonic lumen in which the conversion of absorbable ammonia (NH_3) to nonabsorbable ammonium (NH_4^+) is favored. If these measures do not control the hepatic encephalopathy, or if the patient is malnourished and requires protein supplementation (which worsens the hepatic encephalopathy), nutritional support with solutions enriched in branched-chain amino acids should be administered.

SUMMARY

- Patients with liver disease have increased surgical risk.
- Surgical risk is proportional to severity of liver disease. Risk correlates with Child's-Pugh classification.
- Delay all surgery, except emergency surgery, in Child's-Pugh classification C cirrhosis, acute viral hepatitis, or acute alcoholic hepatitis.
- Correct reversible features of liver disease, in-

cluding malnutrition, hepatic encephalopathy, coagulopathy, renal insufficiency, and ascites, before surgery.
- Evaluate ascitic fluid preoperatively for possibility of bacterial infection.
- Carefully evaluate and treat malnutrition, hepatic encephalopathy, coagulopathy, renal insufficiency, and ascites in postoperative period for improved patient outcome.

REFERENCES

1. Ayres PR, Williard TB. Serum glutamic oxalacetic transaminase levels in 266 surgical patients. Ann Intern Med 52:1279-1288, 1960.
2. LaMont JT. Postoperative jaundice. Surg Clin North Am 54:637-645, 1974.
3. Price HL, Deutsch S, Davidson IA, et al. Can general anesthetics produce splanchnic visceral hypoxia by reducing regional blood flow? Anesthesiology 27:24-32, 1966.
4. Harville DD, Summerskill WHJ. Surgery in acute hepatitis: Causes and effects. JAMA 184:257-261, 1963.
5. Dykes MHM, Walzer SG. Preoperative and postoperative hepatic dysfunction. Surg Gynecol Obstet 124:747-751, 1967.
6. Turner MD, Sherlock S. In Smith R, Sherlock S, eds. Surgery of the Gallbladder and Bile Ducts. London: Butterworth, 1964.
7. Hardy KJ, Hughes ESR. Laparotomy in viral hepatitis. Med J Aust 1:710, 1968.
8. Aranha GV, Sontag SJ, Greenlee HB. Cholecystectomy in cirrhotic patients: A formidable operation. Am J Surg 143:55-59, 1982.
9. Garrison RN, Cryer HM, Howard DA, Polk HC. Clarification of risk factors for abdominal operations in patients with hepatic cirrhosis. Ann Surg 199:648-655, 1984.
10. Doberneck RC, Sterling WA Jr, Allison DC. Morbidity and mortality after operation in nonbleeding cirrhotic patients. Am J Surg 146:306, 1983.
11. Aranha GV, Greenlee HB. Intra-abdominal surgery in patients with advanced cirrhosis. Arch Surg 121:275, 1986.
12. Gill RA, Goodman MW, Golfus GR, et al. Aminopyrine breath test predicts surgical risk for patients with liver disease. Ann Surg 198:701-704, 1983.
13. Mendenhall CL, Anderson S, Weesner RE, et al. Protein-calorie malnutrition associated with alcoholic hepatitis. Am J Med 76:211-222, 1984.
14. Fisher JE, Funovics JM, Aguirre A, et al. The role of plasma amino acids in hepatic encephalopathy. Surgery 78:276-290, 1975.
15. Fisher JE, Rosen HM, Ebeid AM, et al. The effect of normalization of plasma amino acids on hepatic encephalopathy in man. Surgery 80:77-91, 1976.
16. Cerra FB, Cheung NK, Fisher JE, et al. Disease-specific amino acid infusion (F080) in hepatic encephalopathy: A prospective, randomized, double-blind, controlled trial. J Parenter Enter Nutr 9:288-295, 1985.

CHAPTER 9

The Surgical Patient and Renal Failure

Ricardo Correa-Rotter · Mark E. Rosenberg

ACUTE RENAL FAILURE

Acute renal failure (ARF) constitutes a highly lethal condition when associated with surgery or trauma (45% to 70% mortality) despite significant improvement in dialytic treatment in the last decade. Prevention of this complication relies on early identification of predisposing risk factors and careful preoperative evaluation of the patient's renal function. Since a variety of conditions may be responsible for the development of ARF in the surgical patient, it is imperative to determine the cause in order to provide adequate therapy. The classification of ARF into prerenal, renal, or postrenal causes is presented in Chapter 30. Acute tubular necrosis (ATN), a term often used interchangeably with ARF, is the most common form of ARF observed after trauma or surgery.

This chapter first focuses on predisposing risk factors and measures for preventing the development of ARF, with particular emphasis given to the basic principles for preoperative assessment of renal function. Next, special problems often encountered in association with the development of ARF are discussed. Finally, guidelines for the preoperative evaluation and management of the patient with known chronic renal failure (CRF) are presented.

Risk Factors and Precipitating Conditions

Common risk factors and precipitating conditions that favor the development of ARF are listed in the accompanying box. When two or more of these conditions are present in a given patient, there is an additive effect, which increases the risk for the development of ARF. In addition to the factors shown in the box, conditions that may favor the development of ARF are the severity of the disease that leads the patient to the surgical intervention, the nature of the surgery (emergency or elective), and the presence and severity of underlying medical conditions, particularly heart failure, diabetes mellitus, and liver disease. The presence of severe Gram-negative sepsis accompanied by diminished effective circulating volume (septic shock) constitutes a common cause of ARF in the surgical patient and often may constitute

---

Factors Associated With Development of ARF in Surgical Patients

Age over 50 years
Volume depletion
Diabetes mellitus
Nephrotoxic agents
   Aminoglycosides
   Radiocontrast agents
   Others
Underlying intrinsic renal disease
Underlying vascular disease
Hypertension
Sepsis
Major cardiovascular intervention
Intravascular hemolysis
   Transfusion reactions
Abdominal aortic aneurysm surgery
Cardiopulmonary bypass
Long-standing obstructive uropathy

part of a syndrome of sequential organ system failure. In this condition prompt diagnosis and early aggressive treatment should be undertaken because Gram-negative sepsis is associated with extremely high mortality.

Preoperative Evaluation of Renal Function

An adequate assessment of the patient's renal function and fluid and electrolyte balance provides vital information for recognizing those who are prone to develop ARF in the postoperative period. A complete history and thorough physical examination provide valuable data regarding previous and current pathologic conditions, drug intake history, and estimation of extracellular volume status. Laboratory determination of glomerular filtration rate (GFR), plasma creatinine (PCr), serum electrolytes, and urinalysis complement the preoperative evaluation.

Assessment of volume status

Maintenance of adequate extracellular volume is mandatory since volume depletion is a major risk factor for the development of ARF. Some of the clinical and laboratory variables useful in estimating volume status are listed in the accompanying box. The history of intake/output and weight can prove to be of great value in conjunction with the physical examination. If apparent volume depletion is noted (with or without overt oliguria), urinary sodium determination, urinalysis, and urinary indexes, in conjunction with GFR estimation, can aid in distinguishing prerenal azotemia from established ATN (see Chapter 30). In some patients, particularly those with sepsis and hepatic or cardiac failure, estimation of volume status may be difficult. If the volume status is in doubt, central venous pressure (CVP) or pulmonary capillary wedge pressure (PCWP) measurements are warranted.

Assessment of renal function

Determination of GFR is the best way to estimate the degree of preoperative renal function. Clinical measurement of GFR can be performed by calculating plasma clearance of exogenously administered substances, such as inulin or ra-

diolabeled iothalamate, or by determining endogenous creatinine clearance (CrCl). Although plasma clearance determination of exogenous compounds (inulin or ^{125}iothalamate) is more accurate than CrCl, the latter is the most widely used method to estimate GFR since urinary and plasma measurements of creatinine are readily available in most laboratories. CrCl is determined by the following formula:

$$CrCl \ (ml/min) = \frac{Urinary\ creatinine\ (mg/dl)\ \times\ Urinary\ volume\ (ml/min)}{PCr\ (mg/dl)}$$

Urinary creatinine and volume are usually measured in a 24-hour collection since shorter collections may give unreliable results. A complete urine collection is essential to ensure accuracy

Estimation of Extracellular Volume Status

History

Fluid input and output history
    Decreased intake
    Gastrointestinal loss (vomiting, diarrhea, hemorrhage, bowel obstruction)
    Renal loss (diuretics, glycosuria, adrenal insufficiency)
    Internal loss or redistribution of extracellular fluid (pancreatitis, peritonitis, severe hypoalbuminemia)

Physical examination

Skin turgor
Moisture of mucous membranes (oral, vaginal, anal)
Postural blood pressure changes
Jugular venous distention
Chest examination for evidence of compromised cardiopulmonary function (pulmonary edema, arrhythmias, S_3 gallops, pericardial rub)
Abdominal examination (ascites, hepatomegaly)
Peripheral edema or anasarca
CVP or PCWP

Laboratory values

Urinary sodium
Urinary indexes (see Chapter 30)
BUN/PCr
Serum electrolytes

of CrCl. To determine if a urine collection corresponds to a 24-hour period, total creatinine excretion in mg/kg/day is used because normal urinary creatinine excretion remains constant. Normal values for creatinine excretion are shown in Table 9-1.

Creatinine, derived from skeletal muscle creatine metabolism, is produced, released to the circulation, and excreted by the kidney at a relatively constant rate. In the patient who is in steady state, PCr varies inversely with the GFR. This reciprocal relation between PCr and GFR is demonstrated in Fig. 9-1. Athough PCr may be useful as a diagnostic test for the estimation of renal function in an individual in steady state, it loses its clinical applicability when acute changes in GFR are occurring. For instance, a rapid fall in GFR will be followed by a delayed creatinine increase since it takes some time for creatinine to accumulate in plasma. It is also important to note the nonlinear relation between these two parameters; an apparently small increase in PCr (from 1 to 2 mg/dl) can represent a loss of almost 50% of the GFR (see Fig. 9-1). The interpretation of PCr measurements is also subject to potential errors since PCr may be elevated in the absence of GFR changes (see box).

CrCl can be estimated from the Cockroft and Gault formula. This formula provides a rough estimation of CrCl and allows the clinician to determine GFR both to establish the level of renal function and for dose correction of drugs excreted by the kidney:

$$CrCl = \frac{(140 - age) \times Lean\ body\ weight}{PCr \times 72}$$

For females, multiply above by 0.85.

Determination of the levels of serum electrolytes (Na, Cl, K, HCO_3), BUN, PCr, serum Ca, P, and Mg should be part of the preoperative assessment of renal function. Identification of potentially hazardous electrolyte abnormalities, such as hyperkalemia in the patient with volume depletion or established renal insufficiency, is critical. In addition, serum electrolyte levels give important information in patients suspected of having acid-base disorders, as often happens in the setting of an acute surgical emergency. If an acid-base disorder is suspected, an analysis of arterial blood gases should be done.

TABLE 9-1 Normal Values for Urinary Creatinine Excretion

	Male (mg/kg*)	Female (mg/kg*)
Adult, age <60	20-25	15-20
Adult, age >60	10-20	8-15

*Lean body weight.

PCr Increase Without Change in GFR

Substances measured as noncreatinine chromagens with alkaline picrate method
  Acetoacetate and acetone
  Ascorbic acid
  Cephalosporins
Massive increase in creatinine production
  Rhabdomyolysis
Decrease in creatinine excretion (PCr increase of <0.5 mg/dl)
  Trimethoprim
  Cimetidine

Specific Problems
Radiocontrast medium–induced ARF

Although noninvasive body imaging procedures, such as ultrasonography, are in widespread use, CT and MRI, radiographic procedures requiring infusion of a contrast medium, are often required for diagnostic purposes in the surgical patient. ARF develops in a significant number of patients who receive radiocontrast material. Although ARF has been reported after exposure to a contrast medium given by various routes (oral, intravenous, intra-arterial), its incidence following intra-arterial administration seems to be greater.

In the general population, the incidence of radiocontrast medium–induced ARF is very low (0% to 5%), but it is significantly higher (10% to 50%) in some high-risk subpopulations.

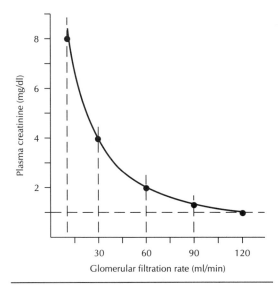

FIG. 9-1 Reciprocal relation between glomerular filtration rate (GFR) and plasma creatinine (PCr) concentration. Hyperbolic nature of this relationship is illustrated: in a patient with normal renal function, an apparently small increase in PCr (from 1 to 2 mg/dl) reflects a major fall in GFR (from 120 to 60 ml/min), whereas in a patient with established renal failure, an increase in PCr from 4 to 8 mg/dl represents a relatively small reduction in GFR (from 28 to 14 ml/min).

Identification of risk factors associated with radiocontrast medium–induced ARF plays a key role in preventing the development of this complication. These risk factors include the following:

Established factors:
Preexisting renal failure
Diabetes mellitus
Severe cardiovascular disease with diminished renal blood flow
Large dose of contrast material
Repeated doses of contrast material

Probable factors:
Dehydration
Advanced age
Multiple myeloma
Peripheral vascular disease

The principal predisposing factor for contrast nephropathy is the presence and severity of underlying renal insufficiency. Diabetic patients with normal renal function do not have increased risk for development of contrast nephropathy, yet those with moderate or severe renal impairment appear to be at significantly greater risk than those with similar degrees of renal dysfunction from other causes. Exposure to large amounts or repeated doses of radiocontrast material also may increase the risk and severity of contrast nephropathy. Administration of nonionic radiocontrast material, as compared to a traditional ionic contrast agent, does not reduce nephrotoxicity.

Once the risk factors have been identified, the following strategies aimed at preventing the development of contrast nephropathy should be followed:

1. Use of noninvasive imaging studies whenever possible
2. Administration of smallest possible dose of contrast medium
3. Hydration and maintenance of high urine flow rate
   a. Target urine output: 150 to 200 ml/hr
   b. Example of hydration protocol:
      ▪ IV administration of 1 L 5% dextrose in 0.45% normal saline with 25 g mannitol at 150 ml/hr, beginning 2 hours prior to procedure
      ▪ Continue hydration up to 24 hours after procedure
4. Close monitoring of urine output
   a. Adjust fluid intake/urine output in congestive heart failure and/or severe renal failure
   b. Mannitol may be contraindicated in these conditions (low cardiac output)
   c. Loop diuretics (20 to 40 mg IV bolus of furosemide) could enhance urine output

Whenever a noninvasive imaging procedure can provide adequate diagnostic information, it should be performed rather than the invasive radiocontrast study. Using the smallest possible dose of contrast medium also may prevent the development of, or reduce the severity of, renal dysfunction.

Multiple studies have shown that adequate hydration accompanied by high urine flow rates can play a key role in preventing the development of ARF. Several different hydration schemes have been used, some of which are based solely on the administration of intravenous solutions. Others have added the infusion of an osmotic agent (e.g., mannitol) or a loop diuretic (e.g., furosemide) to achieve optimal hydration and high urine output. The outline on p. 83 includes a proposed regimen for adequate hydration to be administered before and during performance of a radiocontrast study.

Drug-induced ARF

Treatment of intercurrent medical problems (e.g., infection, analgesia) requires the use of drugs, most of which undergo renal excretion. In the patient with established renal failure, accumulation of these drugs and their metabolites will reach toxic levels unless adequate dosage adjustments are made. On the other hand, the administration of a nephrotoxic drug to a surgical patient constitutes a risk factor for the development of ARF (see box, p. 80). The addition of a nephrotoxic agent in the presence of other concomitant risk factors may have an additive effect for the induction of renal dysfunction. The best way to prevent drug nephrotoxicity is to avoid using nephrotoxic drugs in the surgical patient, particularly if other risk factors are also present. Yet this approach is often not possible. Therefore it is important to keep in mind the possibility of inducing renal dysfunction in order to detect it early and adjust drug dosages. Newer, less nephrotoxic drugs, such as the third-generation cephalosporins and fluoroquinolones, should be used when appropriate instead of more nephrotoxic drugs, such as the aminoglycosides. A list of the most common nephrotoxic drugs encountered in clinical practice follows:

Antibiotics
    Aminoglycosides
    Cephalosporins
    Sulfonamides
    Vancomycin
    Pentamidine
    Amphotericin B
NSAIDs
Cyclosporine A
Chemotherapeutic agents
    Cisplatin

It is important to emphasize that this is not a comprehensive list of all drugs reported to induce renal dysfunction.

The degree of renal dysfunction directly influences the extent of drug accumulation. For proper adjustment of drug doses, the level of renal function must be determined. Endogenous CrCl or its estimation from serum creatinine (see equation on p. 81) can be used to establish the patient's renal function and provide guidelines for adjusting drug doses. If renal function is already decreasing rapidly, as happens in ARF, PCr will overestimate renal function; therefore drug doses should be administered as for a patient with severe renal failure (CrCl <10 ml/min). Dosage adjustment in these patients can be performed according to clinical course, continued monitoring of CrCl, and serum drug levels, if available. Tables are available that provide information regarding dose reduction and degree of removal by dialysis for most drugs (see Bibliography).

Cardiovascular surgery and ARF

ARF occurs in a high percentage of patients who undergo open heart surgery (5% to 25%). During cardiopulmonary bypass, the kidneys are underperfused. The duration of bypass usually correlates with the severity of renal failure. Although renal circulatory compromise is the major determinant of renal dysfunction after open heart surgery, other factors participate in its pathogenesis. For example, trauma to the blood from extracorporeal circulation induces hemolysis and can activate the complement system. Other contributing factors for the development of ARF are the common occurrence of postoperative cardiac dysfunction leading to continued renal circulatory compromise and the use of postoperative artificial ventilation, which may alter inferior vena cava hemodynamics by impairing venous return to the thorax. The increased intrathoracic pressure generated by positive pressure ventilation may lead to pooling of blood in the inferior vena cava and to an increase in renal venous pressure.

Adequate blood flow and perfusion pressure should be ensured during the period of extracorporeal circulation to reduce the incidence of ARF. Careful monitoring of blood pressure, maintenance of a cardiac index exceeding 2.5 L min^{-1}m^{-2}, and cautious use of vasodilators are recommended in the postoperative period in order to avoid significant reductions in renal flow below the kidney's autoregulatory range. Also, the period of mechanical artificial ventilation should be as short as possible to avoid hemodynamically mediated impairment of renal function.

Aortic surgery (e.g., grafting of an aortic aneurysm) poses a very high risk for the development of ARF. Suprarenal aortic clamping, a procedure sometimes necessary to perform the grafting, is responsible for temporary interruption of blood flow to the kidneys. The incidence of ARF and the degree of renal dysfunction seem to be closely related to the length of the surgical procedure. If a lengthy interruption of renal artery blood flow is expected, consideration should be given to a shunt to the distal renal artery in order to maintain renal perfusion.

CHRONIC RENAL FAILURE

During the past two decades a significant improvement has occurred in the prognosis of patients with renal disease who are subjected to elective or emergency surgery. Better dialytic procedures are probably the major element in this improved outcome since more intensive dialysis ensures better fluid and electrolyte balance and may improve impaired clotting mechanisms, immune function, and wound healing. In addition to the routine preoperative evaluation, the renal patient will require special assessment of factors that may favor the development of perioperative complications.

Dialysis

The patient already under dialytic treatment must undergo preoperative dialysis to correct hyperkalemia and acidosis, improve volume status, and reduce the level of uremic toxins that may be involved in the platelet dysfunction of CRF. Since heparin is usually required for hemodialysis, having the patient undergo dialysis the day prior to surgery will allow sufficient time for the metabolism of the remaining heparin. If patients are having peritoneal dialysis and are not undergoing abdominal surgery,

then dialysis can be performed according to the patient's usual schedule in the preoperative period and as needed in the postoperative period. Often switching to an automated peritoneal dialysis cycler will be necessary postoperatively. Abdominal surgery in the peritoneal dialysis patient will necessitate a temporary change to hemodialysis.

Patients with moderate renal insufficiency who are not yet having long-term dialysis and require surgery may undergo the surgical procedure safely with adequate conservative management of their fluid and electrolyte and metabolic abnormalities. This subset of patients must be monitored very closely because dialysis may need to be initiated in the event of renal function deterioration, in order to prevent the appearance of uremic complications that would further complicate the patient's course. The presence of uremic manifestations as well as volume and electrolyte abnormalities unresponsive to conservative treatment are indications for immediate dialytic therapy (see Chapter 30).

Anesthesia

When the choice of general anesthetic agent to be used in a patient with CRF is being considered, the drug's metabolism and elimination route need to be taken into consideration. Metabolic acidosis may potentiate the effect of some neuromuscular blocking agents. In addition, some of these drugs (neuromuscular blockers) can favor the development of acute hyperkalemia. In general, common gas anesthetics, such as halothane and methoxyflurane, are well tolerated by the patient with CRF, although the latter should be avoided in patients with residual renal function since it is potentially nephrotoxic.

Bleeding Disorders

Bleeding disorders are common in CRF. Platelet dysfunction and abnormal platelet-vessel interactions are the most significant clotting defects seen in uremia, and they are adversely influenced by anemia. The following therapeutic measures are aimed at minimizing bleeding in the patient with CRF: (1) avoidance of anticoagulants, aspirin, and NSAIDs; (2) aggressive dialysis; and (3) use of DDAVP (desmopressin) and estrogens.

In most instances platelet dysfunction will not cause excessive operative bleeding, if the patient has undergone proper dialysis and is not under the influence of chronic antiplatelet treatment sometimes prescribed to maintain patency of arteriovenous fistulas. If a bleeding tendency is present, administration of 8-D-arginine vasopressin (DDAVP or desmopressin) (0.3 μg/kg IV or 3 μg/kg intranasally) will aid hemostasis within 1 hour of administration and its effect will last up to 8 hours. The effects of DDAVP are attenuated with repeated dosing. Conjugated estrogens also have been shown to reduce bleeding tendency when given at a dose of 0.6 mg/kg/day, starting 6 to 12 hours before the surgery and for a period of up to 5 days. It is critical to discontinue those drugs that interfere with platelet function such as NSAIDs or aspirin.

Anemia

Anemia is an almost universal complication of CRF. The hematocrit level starts to decrease when the GFR falls below 50 ml/min. The primary mechanism of the anemia is erythropoietin deficiency, but other factors, such as decreased RBC lifespan, iron deficiency, and blood loss, may contribute to the anemia. Recombinant erythropoietin is available to treat the anemia of renal failure in both predialysis and dialysis patients. Therapy with erythropoietin results in a dose-dependent increase in hematocrit level, obviating the need for transfusion therapy. The target hematocrit level is 30% to 35%, which is easily achieved in most patients by administration of erythropoietin three times a week, either subcutaneously (predialysis and peritoneal dialysis patients) or intravenously (hemodialysis patients). In anticipation of elective surgery in patients with CRF, the hematocrit level can be optimized by initiating or adjusting the erythropoietin dose. The usual dose range is 4000 to 10,000 U administered three times per week.

Calcium, Phosphorus, Magnesium

As renal function deteriorates, abnormalities in calcium, phosphorus, and magnesium homeostasis occur. (For a review of the pathophysi-ologic aspects of these changes, see the Bibliography.) Lowering serum phosphorus is a major goal of therapy in patients with renal insufficiency both to prevent the development of secondary hyperparathyroidism and to keep the calcium-phosphorus product below 70 to avoid metastatic calcification. Aluminum-containing antacids have been used as phosphate binders and are still the agents of choice when the calcium-phosphorus produce is elevated. Problems with aluminum accumulation leading to a form of osteodystrophy have led to a search for alternative long-term phosphate binders. At present, calcium carbonate is the best alternative. If time permits, serum calcium and phosphorus levels should be normalized prior to surgery and monitored closely during the postoperative period. Since magnesium balance is normally maintained by the kidney, hypermagnesemia can occur as a complication of renal failure. Magnesium levels should be followed closely; as a general rule, excessive magnesium intake should be avoided in patients with end-stage renal disease. This restriction includes avoiding magnesium-containing antacids and enemas, which are rich sources of magnesium.

In the postoperative period, in addition to the usual care measures, the renal patient needs to be monitored very closely for abnormalities in intravascular volume, electrolytes, and acid-base balance since the normal homeostatic mechanisms provided by the kidney are lacking (see Chapter 30). Increased catabolism of sepsis may favor a faster accumulation of nitrogenous compounds, and dialysis requirements need to be evaluated on a continuing basis as the patient is recovering from the surgical procedure.

■ ■ ■

Editor's note: This chapter summarizes a number of issues related to renal failure in the surgical patient. One of the points relates to the relationship among serum creatinine, GFR, and lean body mass. In SICU patients who have sustained prolonged hypermetabolism for several weeks, the lean body mass becomes considerably reduced, even in the presence of nutritional support. Thus the serum creatinine may be low, implying a much higher GFR than is actually present. As the authors point out, periodic creatinine clearance measurements need to be performed to validate the relationship between the serum creatinine and the GFR.

SUMMARY

Acute Renal Failure

- Early identification of risk factors for ARF (see box, p. 80) can help prevent complications.
- Preoperative evaluation of renal function:
  Assess volume status by history, body weight, urinary electrolytes, or invasive hemodynamic monitoring, when necessary.
  Assess renal function by clinical measurement of GFR or creatinine clearance. Plasma creatinine concentration loses sensitivity when rapid changes in GFR occur.
  Measure concentrations of serum Na, Cl, K, HCO_3, BUN, PCr, Ca, P, and Mg.
  If question of acid-base disorder exists, obtain analysis of ABGs. Underlying renal insufficiency is important risk factor for radiocontrast-induced ARF. Hydrate these patients prior to x-ray study and monitor urine output closely. Administration of nephrotic drug to a surgical patient is a risk factor for development of ARF. Avoid nephrotoxic agents, if possible. Adjust doses of nephrotoxic drugs to CrCl.

Chronic Renal Failure

- For patients with CRF managed with dialysis, have dialysis done on day prior to elective surgery.
- Metabolic acidosis may potentiate neuromuscular blocking agents.
- Avoid anticoagulants, aspirin, and NSAIDs.
- Institute or increase erythropoietin dose in anticipation of surgery.
- Normalize serum calcium and phosphorus levels whenever possible.

BIBLIOGRAPHY

Bennett WM, Aronoff GR, Morrison G, Golper TA, Pulliam J, Wolfson M, Singer I. Drug prescribing in renal failure: Dosing guidelines for adults. Am J Kid Dis 3:155, 1983.

Brezis M, Rosen S, Epstein FH. Acute renal failure. In Brenner BM, Rector FC. The Kidney. Philadelphia: WB Saunders, 1991, p 993.

Lazarus JM. Prophylaxis of acute renal failure in the intensive care unit. In Bihari D, Neild G. Acute renal failure in the intensive therapy unit. London: Springer-Verlag, 1990, p 279.

Lazarus JM, Morgan AP, Tilney NL. Patients with chronic renal failure: General management and acute surgical illness. Philadelphia: WB Saunders, 1982, p 1.

Manske CL, Sprafka JM, Strony JT, Wang Y. Contrast nephropathy in azotemic diabetic patients undergoing coronary angiography. Am J Med 89:615, 1990.

Mehler PS, Schrier RW, Anderson RJ. Clinical presentation, complications and prognosis of acute renal failure. In Jacobson HR, Striker GE, Klahr S. The principles and practice of nephrology. Philadelphia: BC Decker, 1991, p 660.

Paganini EP, Bosworth CR. Acute renal failure after open heart surgery: Newer concepts and current therapy. Semin Thorac Cardiovasc Surg 3:63, 1991.

Rose BD. Clinical assessment of renal function: Pathophysiology of renal disease. New York: McGraw-Hill, 1987, p 1.

Schwab SJ, Hlatky MA, Pieper KS, Davidson CJ, Morris KG, Skelton TN, Bashore TM. Contrast nephrotoxicity: A randomized controlled trial of a nonionic and an ionic radiographic contrast agent. N Engl J Med 320:149, 1989.

Tilney NL, Morgan AP, Lazarus JM. Acute renal failure in surgical patients. In Tilney NL, Lazarus JM. Surgical care of the patient with renal failure. Philadelphia: WB Saunders, 1982, p 30.

Wish JB, Moritz CE. Preventing radiocontrast-induced acute renal failure. J Crit Illn 5:16, 1990.

CHAPTER 10

Perioperative Pulmonary Evaluation

Philip G. Boysen

The measurement of preoperative pulmonary function, when combined with the history and the physical examination, can alert the clinician to the need for interventional therapy that will improve outcome. In addition, the site and nature of the surgical procedure may alter pulmonary function and pose increased perioperative and postoperative risk to an individual patient. In the assessment of the pulmonary component of surgical risk, the part of the preoperative evaluation that provides the most information at minimum cost is the combination of spirometric testing and arterial blood gas analysis. More sophisticated and more expensive types of testing, such as the measurement and compartmentalization of lung volumes and the measurement of diffusing capacity, generally corroborate information obtained through spirometry and blood gas measurements. In the patient being considered for thoracotomy, lung compartment volumes and lung diffusing capacity may better quantify the risk of lung resection.

PULMONARY FUNCTION TESTING

A major advantage of spirometric testing is that it can be performed simply and rapidly. A potential limitation is that it requires patient cooperation. The test is performed by having the patient inspire to total lung capacity, then exhale forceably into a measurement device while lung volume decreases to residual volume. The normal spirogram, which is a measurement of volume vs. time, is easily recorded on a revolving drum or a similar device (Fig. 10-1). To achieve the best results, three separate spirometric determinations are made and their reproducibility is examined. Following the initial measurement, the patient receives a nebulized bronchodilator and three additional measurements are taken. With this procedure, the recorded data represent a maximum envelope for pre- and postbronchodilator efforts in a given patient (Fig. 10-2).

These data provide the total volume delivered into the device (i.e., forced vital capacity [FVC]) and specific volumes related to time during the forced expiration. The forced expiratory volume at one second (FEV_1) is an index of airflow obstruction. The ratio of FEV_1 to FVC for a given patient is reduced when obstructive ventilatory defects are present. In patients with ob-

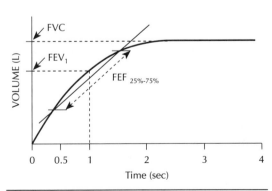

FIG. 10-1 Normal spirogram and derived data. (From Boysen PG. Preoperative assessment of the patient undergoing noncardiac thoracic surgery. In Mangano DT, ed. Preoperative Cardiac Assessment. Philadelphia: JB Lippincott, 1990, p 127.)

structive diseases, the FVC is well preserved until late in the course of the disease. In contrast, the FVC may be dramatically reduced in patients who have a restrictive ventilatory defect. A further evaluation of airflow obstruction is obtained by recording and analyzing midflows during the vital capacity maneuver. The forced expiratory flow between 25% and 75% of the vital capacity ($FEF_{25\%-75\%}$) is most useful in assessing midflows during the FVC maneuver. This range of flow is particularly important for the surgical patient since the ability to improve midflow after bronchodilation has been correlated with improved postoperative outcome.

For many years these two elements, restrictive ventilatory defects (RVDs) and obstructive ventilatory defects (OVDs), have been the physiologic linchpins in presurgical assessment. Investigators have tried to plot the FEV_1/FVC vs. the FVC and to define a line of marginal reserve. Strict limitations in function have not correlated well with postoperative complications, but the more severely compromised patient tends to have a stormier postoperative course.

Recently, the FVC maneuver has been used to record flow vs. volume instead of volume vs. time (Figs. 10-3 and 10-4). This flow volume loop can be combined with an inspiratory effort at the end of the FVC maneuver to return to total lung capacity. The flow volume loop provides similar spirometric data but offers important additional data describing upper airway function. Partial or fixed obstruction of the upper airway will manifest itself by changes in the loop. Intrathoracic airway obstruction is most evident during expiration, whereas extrathoracic upper airway obstruction is most evident during inspiration (Fig. 10-5). In the preoperative period, measurement of flow volume loop, both with and without a bronchodilator, is often useful in assessment (see Fig. 10-2).

POSTOPERATIVE CHANGES IN LUNG FUNCTION

Specific changes in lung function have been well delineated in the postoperative patient. Such changes occur most commonly if the surgical procedure is done at or near the diaphragm. These postoperative changes have all the elements of a superimposed RVD. Since changes in RVD are expected postoperatively, the goal of preoperative assessment is to demonstrate preexisting RVD or OVD. In the postoperative patient who has undergone a thoracic

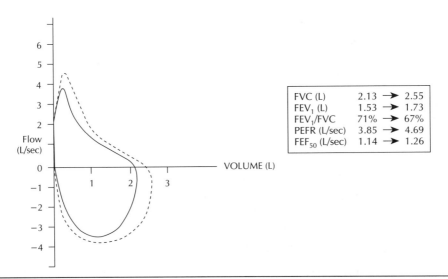

FVC (L)	2.13	2.55
FEV_1 (L)	1.53	1.73
FEV_1/FVC	71%	67%
PEFR (L/sec)	3.85	4.69
FEF_{50} (L/sec)	1.14	1.26

FIG. 10-2 Comparison of flow volume loops before (solid line) and after (dotted line) administration of nebulized bronchodilator. Note marked increase in both FEV_1 and FVC, with little change in FEV_1/FVC ratio. Both peak expiratory flow rate (PEFR) and forced expiratory midflow (FEF_{50}) also show dramatic increases. (Modified from Boysen PG. Evaluation of pulmonary function tests and arterial blood gases. In Kaplan JA, ed. Thoracic Anesthesia. New York: Churchill Livingstone, 1991, p 9.)

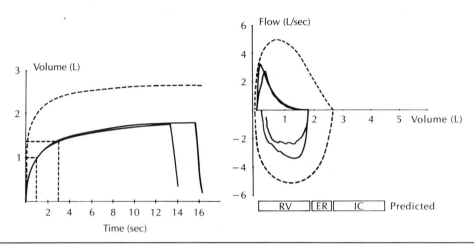

FIG. 10-3 Preoperative vital capacity maneuver (solid lines) represented as both spirogram and flow volume loop showing combined obstructive and restrictive ventilatory defect. Predicted normal values for this patient are represented by dotted lines. Normal predicted values for lung volumes depicted along abscissa of flow volume loop indicate hyperinflation and gas trapping. RV, residual volume; ER, expiratory reserve volume; IC, inspiratory capacity.

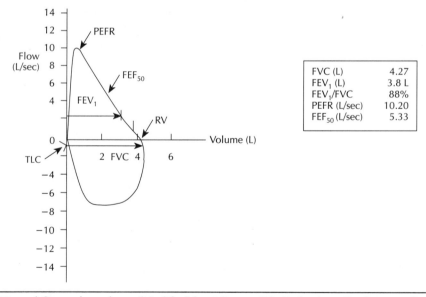

FIG. 10-4 Normal flow volume loop. (Modified from Boysen PG. Evaluation of pulmonary function tests and arterial blood gases. In Kaplan JA, ed. Thoracic Anesthesia. New York: Churchill Livingstone, 1991, p 4.)

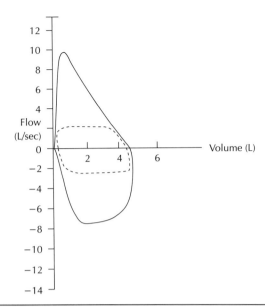

FIG. 10-5   Changes in flow volume loop with upper airway obstruction. Fixed obstruction throughout respiratory cycle results in "square" loop. Peak inspiratory flow and expiratory flow are fixed. (From Boysen PG. Evaluation of pulmonary function tests and arterial blood gases. In Kaplan JA, ed. Thoracic Anesthesia. New York: Churchill Livingstone, 1991, p 4.)

or an abdominal procedure, a dramatic decrease in lung volume can occur postoperatively. The functional residual capacity (FRC) and the total lung capacity (TLC) are both reduced, even when changes on the x-ray film consistent with a loss in lung volume are absent (Fig. 10-6). This observation has led to the term "microatelectasis" to describe the known volume loss in the absence of an anatomic radiographic correlate. Associated with the changes in lung volume is increased intrapulmonary shunt and consequent widened alveolar-to-arterial gradient for oxygen. The loss of lung volume is associated with a change in lung/thorax compliance, and affected patients will demonstrate a decreased tidal volume and an increased respiratory rate. For these reasons patients generally have mild respiratory alkalosis with a normal or slightly lowered arterial carbon dioxide tension postoperatively. Breathing patterns change because the yawn or the sigh, present in the normal pattern of breathing, may

be altered. The patient may not be able to use the normal physiologic mechanisms to reinflate a lung that has already begun to lose volume.

The postoperative pulmonary complications that result are most often directly related to the change in lung volume. The loss of lung volume and the stasis associated with segmental or lobar atelectasis may produce infection, especially tracheobronchitis or pneumonia. Other postoperative pulmonary complications include bronchospasm, pulmonary edema, pulmonary embolism, and complications of prolonged endotracheal intubation. The latter complications are not specifically related to measurement of preoperative function.

Postoperative pain can affect postoperative ventilation by both altering breathing patterns and eliminating the tendency to breathe deeply. The duration of the anesthestic state or the surgical procedure also has been correlated with postoperative complications. Alterations in diaphragmatic function, the incision site, abdom-

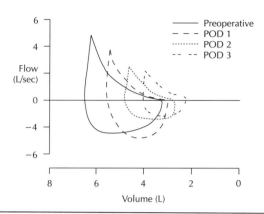

FIG. 10-6   Preoperative flow volume loop (solid line) and flow volume loops on postoperative days 1 through 3 show superimposed restricted ventilatory defect and recovery of function.

inal distention, patient position, restrictive bandages, or obesity are other factors that may adversely affect postoperative pulmonary function. The administration of narcotics may alleviate pain but may present other problems. Narcotics alter central respiratory drive, breathing patterns, and function of the upper airway. The presence of normal pulmonary function preoperatively does not protect the patient from postoperative pulmonary complications. Many studies have shown that such complications occur in 6% to 10% of normal patients. In upper abdominal procedures the incidence of postoperative complications is doubled. Factors such as smoking or established chronic obstructive pulmonary disease (COPD) may triple the complications normally encountered.

DEFINITION OF PULMONARY RISK

Specific tests of pulmonary function have not been shown consistently to correlate with postoperative pulmonary complications. Nonetheless, some guidelines are useful in assessing which patients may be at increased risk. Those individuals at high risk have pulmonary function criteria as shown in the top box on p. 93. For these patients, thoracotomy, with resection of only small amounts of lung tissue, is not possible. If the patient requires an upper abdominal surgical procedure, these limitations

of pulmonary function are likely to necessitate the use of postoperative mechanical ventilation. Those individuals deemed to be at moderate risk exceed the pulmonary performance presented in the top box on p. 93 but have pulmonary function studies as shown in the middle box on p. 93. For these individuals, if thoracotomy is being contemplated, some assessment of right lung vs. left lung function must be done preoperatively. For patients undergoing abdominal procedures, attention to maximizing perioperative function (bottom box, p. 93) has been of major benefit. The regimen shown in the box improves lung function for the patient with COPD through maximal bronchodilation, elimination of secretions, and treatment of underlying colonization or infection. Patients with restrictive disease generally have a pathologic process that is not likely to be improved by any therapeutic maneuver.

For the patient undergoing thoracotomy, in whom separate right lung and left lung function studies are desired, several procedures are available. The most direct technique, bronchospirometry, involves endotracheal intubation with a double-lumen endotracheal tube that allows isolation of the right and the left lung. An FVC maneuver done with each lumen connected to a bronchospirometer will enable the clinician to determine how much volume comes from each lung and to assess the re-

Pulmonary Function Criteria Indicating High Risk	
Factor	*Value*
FVC	<15 cc/kg
FEV_1	<1 L
FEV_1/FVC	<35%
$FEF_{25\%-75\%}$	<14 min

Pulmonary Function Criteria Indicating Moderate Risk	
Factor	*Value*
FVC	<50% predicted
FEV_1	<2 L
RV/TLC	>50%
D_{LCO}	<50% predicted
$FEV_{1/FVC}$	<70%
MVV	<50% predicted or <50 L/min

RV, respiratory volume; D_{LCO}, diffusion capacity; MVV, maximal volume ventilation.

Pharmacologic Approach to Maximizing Perioperative Pulmonary Function
Sympathomimetics: beta-2 agonists Parasympatholysis: atropine and atropine analogs Catecholamines (e.g., epinephrine) Cromolyn sodium Corticosteroids (if indicated) Antibiotics (if indicated)

maining lung function if a pneumonectomy should be performed. To evaluate the effects of interruption of blood flow, the clinician can pass a balloon into the pulmonary artery of the lung to be resected and occlude blood flow to that side. By using this technique, the clinician can determine whether an unacceptable ele-vation of pulmonary artery pressure or arterial oxygen desaturation occurs. Such studies are valuable preoperatively because, in patients who do not survive lung resection, the immediate postoperative course is generally one of hemodynamic decompensation, hypoxemia, and cor pulmonale.

Similar information has been obtained non-invasively with the combination of ventilation perfusion lung scans and pulmonary function studies. To determine the probable effect of lung resection on postoperative pulmonary function, either the ventilation or the perfusion study, whichever is limiting, is used. With these studies the percentage of blood flow or ventilation that goes to each lung can be assessed. In the case of lung volume, the remaining function can be estimated by multiplying this percentage and the FEV_1 and substracting this product from the total FEV_1. In general, the predicted postoperative FEV_1 calculated in this fashion must be between 800 and 1000 cc to ensure immediate postoperative survival. When selective pulmonary artery occlusion is done, the arterial oxygen tension should not fall below 45 mm Hg and the mean pulmonary artery pressure should not rise above 35 mm Hg.

POSTOPERATIVE MANEUVERS

The general postoperative approach has been to reverse the compromised physiology described here. The therapeutic goal is to increase or improve lung volume, decrease intrapulmonary shunt, and improve arterial oxygen tension and saturation. The postoperative maneuvers that have been used to achieve these goals are listed in the box on p. 94. Postoperatively, encouraging a cough or offering a blow-bottle or a bottle-glove is useful. Successful patient participation implies that prior to each effort a deep inspiration is accomplished. Since many patients attempt to cough at very low volumes, they may experience exacerbation of airway collapse. To be successful, postoperative pulmonary care requires careful attention and supervision. Carbon dioxide–induced hyperventilation also can be problematic in patients who have altered respiratory drive caused by

---

Postoperative Maneuvers to Improve Lung Inflation

Deep inspiration
Forced expiration (blow-bottles)
Hyperventilation
Intermittent positive pressure breathing (IPPB)
Continuous positive airway pressure (CPAP)
Sustained maximal inspiration (incentive spirometry)
Upright position

---

underlying disease, administration of sedatives or narcotics, or use of volatile anesthetic agents. Intermittent positive pressure breathing (IPPB) as a means of passive lung inflation may be of use in certain patients who cannot cooperate with voluntary deep breathing and coughing. In general, the use of voluntary maximal inhalation is the most physiologic means of restoring lung volume because this type of inhalation produces a coincident drop in intrapleural pressure that is necessary to achieve deep inspiration and sustains a subatmospheric pleural pressure during full lung inflation.

To assist patients with voluntary maximal inhalation, the incentive spirometer has been developed. It is a volumetric device that enhances the spontaneous breath that the patient is encouraged to take. A biofeedback mechanism associated with the device makes the patient aware of the vital capacity he/she has inspired and the number of maximal inspirations accomplished per hour. With appropriate coaching of the patient, the incentive spirometer results in improvement in lung volumes and oxygenation and also produces a decrease in postoperative pulmonary complications (e.g., infection, atelectasis). In addition to good results with IPPB, several authors have described improvement in lung volumes in postoperative patients using low levels of continuous positive airway pressure (CPAP). CPAP can be administered by face mask at a level of 5 to 7 cm of water; it can be used for 20-minute periods four to six times per day.

In summary, an improvement in pulmonary physiology will enhance outcome in the postoperative patient. The observed postoperative decrease in lung volumes and the hypoxemia that result are complicated by postoperative pain. Because the maneuvers are painful, patients are unwilling to take deep breaths, cough, or clear secretions. With attention given to adequate pain control, a periodic sustained maximal inspiration will reverse the pattern of alveolar collapse, improve lung volume, augment oxygenation, and result in a return to normal ventilatory patterns.

PAIN MANAGEMENT

For the postoperative surgical patient, intermittent administration of a bolus dose of narcotic presents problems. With intermittent doses, pain control is either inadequate or the patient alternates between periods of subtherapeutic blood levels of narcotic and toxic concentrations. Newer procedures have not only improved pain management but often have resulted in lower blood concentrations of narcotic, which avoid the deleterious side effects on central respiratory drive and breathing patterns.

Patient controlled analgesia (PCA) allows the patient to interact with his/her own pain management system. A control device delivers a programmed dose of narcotic when it is activated by the patient. A lanyard extending from the device to the patient allows the patient to administer a specific number of small doses per hour. Since the delay in pain perception to receipt of dose is eliminated, the use of a PCA results in a lower total dose of narcotic.

The second pain management system of importance is epidural analgesia. Whether or not epidural anesthesia is used for the surgical procedure, the postoperative placement of an epidural catheter allows continuous infusion or intermittent administration of narcotic into the epidural space. Since pain often is mediated at the level of the spinal cord, this approach interrupts nociception and results in a low or minimal dose of narcotic in the patient's plasma. Complications of epidural analgesia include urinary retention, pruritus, and alterations in respiratory drive. The last response tends to be biphasic for agents such as morphine. Initially, respiratory depression occurs within several hours and is followed by a lesser degree of respiratory depression at about 8 to 10 hours. The delayed and reduced degree of respiratory depression is thought to result from rostral spread of the narcotic after epidural administration.

Both PCA and epidural analgesia have been shown to improve postoperative lung function and to decrease postoperative complications in certain patients. Pleural installation of local anesthetics also has been used to lessen pain that follows upper abdominal surgery. This therapy has been particularly successful after cholecystectomy. An epidural catheter is introduced into the pleural space with a Tuohy needle, and a local anesthetic is infused into the pleural space. The mechanism of mediation of pain is unknown, but some patients are completely pain-free postoperatively and do not require the concomitant administration of intravenous or intramuscular narcotics.

SUMMARY

- Spirometric testing combined with arterial blood gas analysis provides cost-effective information about pulmonary function.
- FEV, FVC, FEV/FVC, and $FEF_{25\%-75\%}$ may be obtained from spirometry.
- FVC may be approximately normal in a patient with COPD but is significantly reduced in patients with restrictive lung disease.
- The pulmonary flow volume loop provides information comparable to that of the standard spirogram but offers additional information about upper airway obstruction.
- Postoperative pulmonary changes have the characteristics of superimposed restrictive ventilatory disease. Postoperative complications are most often related to loss of lung volume.
- FRC may be reduced in the postoperative patient despite the absence of radiographic evidence of lung volume loss.

- Postoperative pain can potentiate complications by altering breathing patterns and compromising deep breathing. Both PCAs and epidural analgesia are effective treatments for postoperative pain that also reduce plasma narcotic concentrations.
- Characteristics of patients at high risk for pulmonary complications are listed in the top box on p. 93.
- Characteristics of patients at moderate risk for pulmonary complications are listed in the middle box on p. 93.
- For moderate-risk patients, individual lung function tests may be necessary to determine whether pulmonary resection can be tolerated.
- Postoperative therapy attempts to improve lung volume, reduce shunting, and improve oxygenation. Deep breathing and coughing, incentive spirometry, and, if necessary, IPPB and CPAP are useful therapies.

BIBLIOGRAPHY

Amesbury SR, Humphrey HJ. Preoperative evaluation of pulmonary function. Hosp Pract (Off) 27(5A):40-41, 51-54, 1992.

Boysen PG. Pulmonary disease. In Brown D, ed. Risk and Outcome in Anesthesia. Philadelphia: JB Lippincott, 1992, pp 77-102.

Boysen PG, Clark CA, Block AJ. Graded exercise testing and postthoracotomy complications. J Cardiothorac Anesth 4:68-72, 1990.

Cottrell JJ, Ferson PF. Preoperative assessment of the thoracic surgical patient. Clin Chest Med 13:47-53, 1992.

Gerson MC, Hurst JM, Hertzberg VS, Baughman R, Rouan GW, Ellis K. Prediction of cardiac and pulmonary complications related to elective abdominal and noncardiac thoracic surgery in geriatric patients. Am J Med 88:101-107, 1990.

Melendex JA, Alagesan R, Reinsel R, Weissman C, Burt M. Postthoracotomy respiratory muscle mechanics during incentive spirometry using respiratory inductance plethysmography. Chest 101:432-436, 1992.

Nunn JF. Effects of anesthesia on respiration. Br J Anaesth 65:54-62, 1990.

Shapira N, Zabatino SM, Ahmed S, Murphy DM, Sullivan D, Lemole GM. Determinants of pulmonary function in patients undergoing coronary bypass operations. Ann Thorac Surg 50:268-273, 1990.

Wahba RW. Perioperative functional residual capacity. Can J Anaesth 38:384-400, 1991.

Weissman C. Flow-volume relationships during spontaneous breathing through endotracheal tubes. Crit Care Med 20:615-620, 1992.

Zibrak JD, O'Donnell CR, Marton KI. Indications for pulmonary function testing. Ann Intern Med 112:763-771, 1990.

Zibrak JD, O'Donnell CR, Marton KI. Preoperative pulmonary function testing. Ann Intern Med 112:793-794, 1990.

CHAPTER 11

Airway Management

Ian J. Gilmour

Airway management decisions should not be based solely on the patient's need for mechanical ventilatory support. Consideration also must be given to the patient's ability to maintain his/her airway. Mental status, associated musculoskeletal disorders, and the amount of pulmonary toilet required all enter into the decision-making process. Approaches to airway support other than endotracheal tubes (ETTs) or tracheostomy tubes (TTs) include nasopharyngeal (Fig. 11-1) and oropharyngeal (Fig. 11-2) airways and continuous positive airway pressure (CPAP) masks (Fig. 11-3). The intensivist must be familiar with these commonly used airway adjuncts. The Brain laryngeal mask is receiving attention in Europe, particularly for emergency airway management, but it is not currently available in the United States.[1]

INDICATIONS FOR ENDOTRACHEAL INTUBATION

Indications for endotracheal intubation (ETI) include (1) continuing threat to airway patency (trauma, edema, hemorrhage); (2) risk for aspiration of gastric contents or other substances (blood, foreign objects); (3) removal of substances (sputum, blood); (4) diagnostic procedures (bronchoscopy); (5) general anesthesia requiring muscle relaxation; and (6) mechanical ventilation.

ROUTE OF INTUBATION AND SELECTION OF TUBE

Translaryngeal intubation may be attempted through either the nares (nasotracheal intuba-

tion [NTI]) or the mouth (orotracheal intubation [OTI]). The advantages and disadvantages of each route are listed in Table 11-1.

Several observations deserve emphasis. In an emergency, OTI is faster than NTI. If use of the ETT will be required for longer than 48 to 72 hours, the potential for sinus and middle ear infections is increased with NTI and therefore OTI may be preferable. If the patient is hypovolemic, the judicious use of sedatives and muscle relaxants is mandatory. Establishment of the airway must take precedence over patient comfort. NTI is not suitable for the patient at risk for regurgitation and aspiration of gastric contents or the patient with facial trauma, bleeding diathesis, sinusitis, or retropharyngeal abscess. Because any manipulation of the airway can increase intracranial pressure markedly in patients with reduced intracranial compliance, intubation in these patients should follow adequate resuscitation and aggressive measures to obtund reflex responses. After three or four failed attempts, laryngoscopy may cause sufficient soft tissue trauma and edema that the physician may be unable to ventilate the patient. An alternative route should be considered if three or four efforts with laryngoscopy have been unsuccessful. Additional complications of intubations are listed in the boxes shown on pp. 99 and 100.

STANDARD APPROACHES TO INTUBATION

Standard approaches to intubating patients include blind nasal or oral intubation, direct lar-

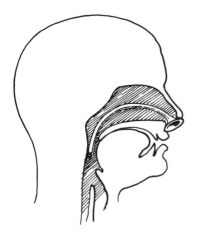

FIG. 11-1 Nasopharyngeal airway in place. Airway passes through the nose and ends at a point just above the epiglottis. (Redrawn from Dorsch JA, Dorsch SE. Understanding Anesthetic Equipment, 2nd ed. Baltimore: Williams & Wilkins, 1984, pp 326-337.)

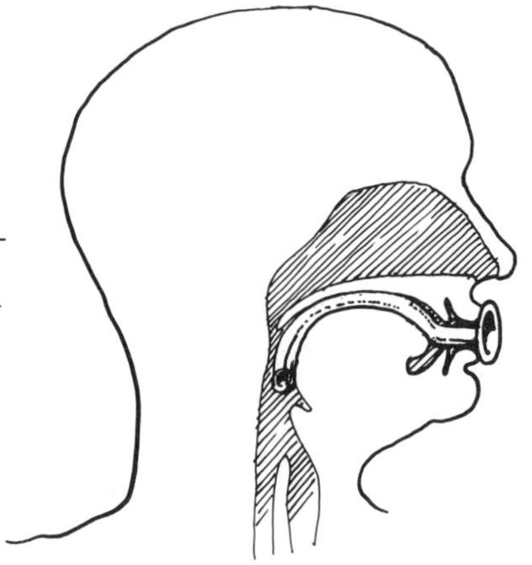

FIG. 11-2 Oropharyngeal airway in place. Airway follows curvature of the tongue, pulling it and the epiglottis away from the posterior pharyngeal wall and providing a channel for air passage. (Redrawn from Dorsch JA, Dorsch SE. Understanding Anesthetic Equipment, 2nd ed. Baltimore: Williams & Wilkins, 1984, pp 326-337.)

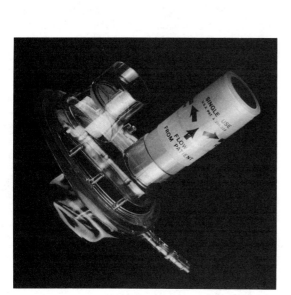

FIG. 11-3 CPAP mask. (Courtesy Vital Signs Inc., Totowa, N.J.)

TABLE 11-1 Comparison of Nasotracheal and Orotracheal Intubation

	Nasotracheal	Orotracheal
Specifications	Smaller diameter	Larger diameter
	Longer length	Shorter length
	Increased resistance	Decreased resistance
Instrumentation	May be done blind	Requires instrumentation
Usefulness	More useful in difficult airway	More easily used with adjuncts (i.e., bronchoscope)
Endobroncheal intubation	Decreased possibility	Increased possibility
Stability	More stable	Less stable
Possibility of sinus infection	Risk of sinusitus	Low risk
Risk of hemorrhage	Increased risk	Lesser risk
Cuff damage	Increased potential*	Less potential*
Trauma	To retropharynx, conchae, larynx	To tongue, teeth, larynx
Patient comfort	More comfortable	Less comfortable

*Inversely related to tube diameter.

Complications of Endotracheal Intubation*

During intubation

Laryngospasm
Laceration, bruising of lips, tongue, and pharynx
Fracture, chipping, dislodgment of teeth or dental appliances
Perforation of trachea or esophagus
Retropharyngeal dissection
Fracture or dislocation of cervical spine
Trauma to eyes
Hemorrhage
Aspiration of gastric contents or foreign bodies
Endobronchial or esophageal intubation
Dislocation of arytenoid cartilages or mandible
Hypoxemia, hypercarbia
Bradycardia, tachycardia
Hypertension
Increased intracranial or intraocular pressure

With tube in situ

Accidental extubation
Endobronchial intubation
Obstruction or kinking

Bronchospasm
Ignition of tube by laser device
Aspiration
Excoriation of nose or mouth

Evident after extubation

Laryngospasm
Aspiration of secretions, gastric contents, blood, or foreign bodies
Glottic, subglottic, or uvular edema
Dysphonia, aphonia
Paralysis of vocal cords or hypoglossal, lingual nerves
Sore throat
Noncardiogenic pulmonary edema
Laryngeal incompetence
Sore, dislocated jaw
Tracheal collapse
Sinusitis
Glottic, subglottic, or tracheal stenosis
Vocal cord granulomata or synechiae

*From Stehling LC. Management of the airway. In Barash PG, Cullen FB, Stoelting RK, eds. Clinical Anesthesia. Philadelphia: JB Lippincott, 1989, pp 543-561.

Complications of Nasotracheal Intubation*
Epistaxis
Turbinectomy
Sinusitis
Nasal infection
Ulceration of ala nasi or septum
Otitis media
Nasal pain
Nasal adhesion
Bacteremia
Submucosal dissection
Pharyngeal perforation
Eustachian tube damage

*Modified from Berlauk JF. Intubation in the ICU: A review from a different perspective. Perspect Crit Care 3(2):95, 1990.

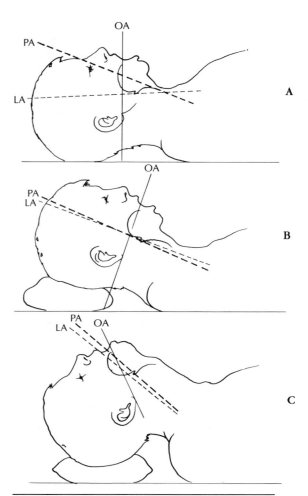

FIG. 11-4   Demonstration of head position for endotracheal intubation. **A,** Successful direct laryngoscopy for exposure of glottic opening requires alignment of oral *(OA),* pharyngeal *(PA),* and laryngeal *(LA)* axes. **B,** Elevation of head approximately 10 cm with pads underneath to occiput and shoulders remaining on table aligns laryngeal and pharyngeal axes. **C,** Subsequent head extension at atlanto-occipital joint serves to create shortest distance and straightest line possible from incisor teeth to glottic opening. (Redrawn from Stone DJ, Gal TJ. Airway management. In Miller RD. Anesthesia, 3rd ed. New York: Churchill Livingstone, 1990, pp 1265-1292.)

yngoscopy, and fiberoptic bronchoscopy. With blind nasal or oral intubation, instrumentation of the oropharynx is not done and patient comfort is improved. The procedure is useful in patients who have reduced movement of the mandible or the neck. However, it requires considerable practice. These methods should not be used in children or in patients with pathologic conditions of the upper airway or neck.

Direct laryngoscopy is the most familiar approach. Although easier to learn and less influenced by blood and secretions than other methods, this procedure is affected by the patient's anatomy. The instrumentation necessary produces a high level of patient discomfort.

Fiberoptic bronchoscopy/laryngoscopy is being used more frequently. This approach is useful when direct laryngoscopy is difficult or dangerous, and it permits visual confirmation of ETT tip location. The procedure produces less patient discomfort than does direct laryngoscopy. Fiberoptic approaches are more difficult to learn, are difficult to perform in the unconscious or sedated patient, and may be more difficult to perform in the presence of large volumes of blood or mucus.

THE DIFFICULT AIRWAY

The goal of laryngoscopy is to position the head and neck so that the axes of mouth, pharynx and larynx are aligned (Fig. 11-4). Syndromes and clinical conditions that may make endotracheal intubation difficult are listed in the box on p. 101 and Tables 11-2 and 11-3. Occasionally, even in the absence of predisposing factors, laryngoscopy will be difficult. However, by having the patient open his/her mouth, one can

Conditions in Which Intubation Is Potentially Dangerous*

Conditions associated with atlantoaxial subluxation

Congenital
  Down's syndrome
  Odontoid anomalies
  Mucopolysaccharidoses
Acquired
  Rheumatoid arthritis
  Still's disease
  Ankylosing spondylitis
  Psoriatic arthritis
  Enteropathic arthritis
    Crohn's disease
    Ulcerative colitis
    Reiter's syndrome

Trauma
  Odontoid fracture
  Ligamentous disruption

Syndromes associated with odontoid hypoplasia

Morquio's syndrome
Klippel-Feil syndrome
Down's syndrome
Spondyloepiphyseal dysplasia
Dysproportionate dwarfism
Congenital scoliosis
Osteogenesis imperfecta
Neurofibromatosis

*From Crosby ET, Lui A. The adult spine: Implications for airway management. Can J Anaesth 37:77-93, 1990.

TABLE 11-2 Selected Congenital Syndromes Associated With Difficult Endotracheal Intubation*

Syndrome	Difficulty
Down's	Large tongue, small mouth make laryngoscopy difficult; small subglottic diameter possible
	Laryngospasm frequent
Goldenhar's (oculoauriculovertebral anomalies)	Mandibular hypoplasia and cervical spine abnormality make laryngoscopy difficult
Klippel-Feil	Neck rigidity because of cervical vertebral fusion
Pierre Robin	Small mouth, large tongue, mandibular anomaly; awake intubation essential in neonate
Treacher Collins' (mandibulofacial dysostosis)	Laryngoscopy difficult
Turner's	High likelihood of difficult intubation

*From Stone DJ, Gal TJ. Airway management. In Miller RD. Anesthesia, 3rd ed. New York: Churchill Livingstone, 1990, pp 1265-1292.

| TABLE 11-3   Selected Pathologic States That Influence Airway Management* |

Infectious

Epiglottitis	Laryngoscopy may worsen obstruction
Abscess (submandibular, retropharyngeal, Ludwig's angina)	Distortion of airway renders mask ventilation or intubation extremely difficult
Croup, bronchitis, pneumonia (current or recent)	Airway irritability with tendency for cough, laryngospasm, bronchospasm
Papillomatosis	Airway obstruction
Tetanus	Trismus renders oral intubation impossible

Traumatic

Foreign body	Airway obstruction
Cervical spine injury	Neck manipulation may traumatize spinal cord
Basilar skull fracture	Nasal intubation attempts may result in intracranial tube placement
Maxillary/mandibular injury	Airway obstruction, difficult mask ventilation, and intubation; cricothyroidotomy may be necessary with combined injuries
Laryngeal fracture	Airway obstruction may worsen during instrumentation
	Endotracheal tube may be misplaced outside larynx and worsen injury
Laryngeal edema (post intubation)	Irritable airway, narrowed laryngeal inlet
Soft tissue, neck injury (edema, bleeding, emphysema)	Anatomic distortion of airway
	Airway obstruction

Neoplastic

Upper airway tumors (pharynx, larynx)	Inspiratory obstruction with spontaneous ventilation
Lower airway tumors (trachea, bronchi, mediastinum)	Airway obstruction may not be relieved by tracheal intubation
	Lower airway distorted
Radiation therapy	Fibrosis may distort airway or make manipulations difficult

Inflammatory

Rheumatoid arthritis	Mandibular hypoplasia, temporomandibular joint arthritis, immobile cervical spine, laryngeal rotation, cricoarytenoid arthritis all make intubation difficult and hazardous
Ankylosing spondylitis	Fusion of cervical spine may render direct laryngoscopy impossible
Temporomandibular joint syndrome 　True ankylosis 　"False" ankylosis (burn, trauma, radiation, temporal craniotomy)	Severe impairment of mouth opening
Scleroderma	Tight skin and temporomandibular joint involvement make mouth opening difficult
Sarcoidosis	Airway obstruction (lymphoid tissue)
Angioedema	Obstructive swelling renders ventilation and intubation difficult

*From Stone DJ, Gal TJ. Airway management. In Miller RD. Anesthesia, 3rd ed. New York: Churchill Livingstone, 1990, pp 1265-1292.

TABLE 11-3 Selected Pathologic States That Influence Airway Management—cont'd	
Endocrine/metabolic	
Acromegaly	Large tongue, bony overgrowths
Diabetes mellitus	May have reduced mobility of atlanto-occipital joint
Hypothyroidism	Large tongue, abnormal soft tissue (myxedema) make ventilation and intubation difficult
Thyromegaly	Goiter may produce extrinsic airway compression or deviation
Obesity	Upper airway obstruction with loss of consciousness
	Tissue mass make successful mask ventilation difficult.

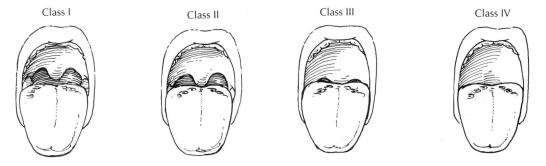

FIG. 11-5 Classification of pharyngeal structures as seen during conduction of tests. *Note:* Class III, soft palate visible; class IV, soft palate not visible. (Redrawn from Samsoon GLT, Young JRB. Difficult tracheal intubation: A retrospective study. Anaesthesia 42:487-490, 1987.)

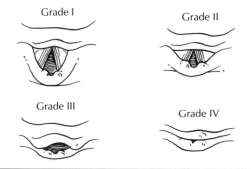

FIG. 11-6 Classification of laryngoscopic views obtained by modifying drawings used by Cormack and Leane in their original classification. (Redrawn from Samsoon GLT, Young JRB. Difficult tracheal intubation: A retrospective study. Anaesthesia 42:487-490, 1987.)

often predict the ease of laryngoscopy by which pharyngeal structures are visible (Figs. 11-5 and 11-6). If a class III or IV anatomic configuration is seen (see Fig. 11-5), referral of the patient's intubation to an expert should be considered.

The most appropriate method of intubation depends on the circumstances. A variety of laryngoscope blades have been designed to be used in difficult airways. Intubating stylets, some with lights, allow easier manipulation of ETTs. Blind ETI should not be used in a patient with marked airway distortion (i.e., epiglottitis, soft tissue tumors). In skilled hands, fiberoptic laryngoscopy may have a significant advantage when difficult airway access is expected. Intubation over a wire passed retrograde through the cricothyroid membrane and out through the mouth is also an option. For alternative approaches in the patient with an unstable cervical spine, see Table 11-4.

When the skill and experience necessary for the above methods are lacking, esophageal obturator airways are a practical alternative. For the difficult airway, the consultation of an anesthesiologist or otorhinolaryngologist may be lifesaving. Because the inability either to intubate or to ventilate is life-threatening, everyone in the SICU should be familiar with the necessary additional steps in airway management. The keys to successful emergency airway management in the SICU include:

1. Having immediately available: oxygen, functioning bag/valve/mask, a selection of oral/nasal pharyngeal airways, a selection of ETTs, a functioning laryngoscope, preferably with several different blades and suctions.
2. Adequate evaluation of the patient and his/her airway
3. Knowledgeable assistance
4. Immediate, accurate confirmation of tube placement
5. Appropriate alternatives being immediately available
6. Recognition of limitations of the physician

CONFIRMATION OF SUCCESSFUL INTUBATION

Confirmation of correct placement must be undertaken immediately after intubation. Standard methods of confirming tube placement are shown in Table 11-5. Any of these methods depends on the skill and experience of the operator (fiberoptic bronchoscopy/laryngoscopy,

TABLE 11-4   Methods of Intubation for Unstable Cervical Spine*

Patient State	Technique
Awake	Blind nasotracheal
	Fiberoptic orotracheal/ nasotracheal
	Retrograde catheter
	Cricothyrotomy
Anesthetized; no relaxants	Blind nasotracheal
	Fiberoptic orotracheal/ nasotracheal
Anesthetized; rapid sequence, muscle relaxants	Orotracheal laryngoscopic

*Modified from Crosby ET, Lui A. The adult spine: Implications for airway management. Can J Anaesth 37:77-93, 1990.

TABLE 11-5   Methods of Confirmation of Endotracheal Tube Placement

Method	Esophageal	Endobronchial	Too High
Auscultation	Not reliable	Decreased reliability in children	Good
Chest x-ray examination	Not reliable, very delayed	Very delayed	Very delayed
Observation of chest movement	Not reliable	Not reliable	Poor
Condensation in tube	Not reliable	N/A	N/A
Palpation of cuff	N/A for uncuffed tubes, not reliable for cuffed	Good	Good
Persistent expired CO_2 (capnometry)	Good	Not reliable	Not reliable
Pulse oximetry	Delayed	Very delayed	Not reliable
Direct visual confirmation			
Rigid	Good in experienced hands	N/A	Good in experienced hands
Fiberoptic	Good, delayed	Good, delayed	Good, delayed

auscultation), and his/her knowledge of the inherent limitations of the technique (cuff palpation, capnometry, pulse oximetry). Capnometry is the best technique available, but it is not wholly reliable.[2]

Incorrect placement of an ETT means either that the tube is in the esophagus or has been advanced too far or not far enough in the airway (Table 11-6).

Neck flexion and extension can cause significant movement of the ETT. Furthermore, fixation of the external portion of the tube does not guarantee that, as the ETT becomes softer

and more malleable with time and body heat, it will not migrate with coughing and tongue movements. Accordingly, tube position should be established by x-ray examination daily. Approximate distances for ETT insertion can be found in Table 11-7.

CHANGING OF OROTRACHEAL TUBE

If for some reason the exchange of one orotracheal tube (OTT) for another becomes necessary, consideration should be given to the use of an intubating stylet. Limitations of the intubating stylet procedure include laryngeal

TABLE 11-6 Consequences of Misplaced Endotracheal Tubes

Placement	Consequence
Esophageal intubation	No alveolar ventilation
	Rapid development of hypoxia, hypercapnea
Endobronchial intubation	May be continuous or intermittent
	May cause hypoxia, barotrauma
High endotracheal tube	May be continuous or intermittent
	May cause inadequate alveolar ventilation
	May allow loss of positive end-expiratory pressure, causing hypoxia
	Promotes accidental extubation
	May increase potential for aspiration

TABLE 11-7 Endotracheal Tube Size and Position Based on Patient Age*

Age	Internal Diameter (mm)	External Diameter (mm)†	French Unit	Distance Inserted from Lips (cm)‡
Premature	2.5	3.3	10	10
Full-term newborn	3.0	4.0-4.2	12	11
1-6 mo	3.5	4.7-4.8	14	11
6-12 mo	4.0	5.3-5.6	16	12
2 yr	4.5	6.0-6.3	18	13
4 yr	5.0	6.7-7.0	20	14
6 yr	5.5	7.3-7.6	22	15-16
8 yr	6.0	8.0-8.2	24	16-17
10 yr	6.5	8.7-9.3	26	17-18
12 yr	7.0	9.3-10	28-30	18-20
14 yr and older	7.0 (women)	9.3-10	28-30	20-24
	8.0 (men)	10.7-11.3	32-34	

*From Stehling LC. Management of the airway. In Barash PG, Cullen FB, Stoelting RK, eds. Clinical Anesthesia. Philadelphia: JB Lippincott, 1989, pp 543-561.
†Approximate, varying among manufacturers.
‡For tip placement in midtrachea. *Note:* Add 2 to 3 cm for nasal tubes.

edema, which makes passage of the tube difficult; laryngospasm/coughing; and lack of patient cooperation (biting). The technique is not useful for NTT because of the narrowness of the airway and the large number of twists and turns encountered with NTI.

EXTUBATION

Extubation should not be equated with weaning. The indications for and the methods of weaning are described in Chapter 27. Extubation should be considered only when weaning goals have been reached *and* the patient is expected to have an unobstructed airway that he/she will be capable of protecting after extubation. Uncertainty regarding either of these conditions should lead to postponement of extubation and consideration of tracheostomy.

TRACHEOSTOMY

A tracheostomy is indicated in the following situations:
1. Prolonged necessity for mechanical ventilation/artificial airway
2. Airway obstruction/lack of access to airway at or above the larynx
3. Inadequate pulmonary toilet, particularly if reintubation is necessary
4. Inability to wean the patient from mechanical ventilatory support

For many years, routine tracheostomy was undertaken whenever ETI was required for more than 24 to 48 hours because the high-pressure, low-volume cuffs on older ETTs caused tracheal stenosis at the cuff site. With the advent of low-pressure, high-volume cuffs, long-term translaryngeal intubation has become common.[3] Additional benefits, such as lower incidence of aspiration past the cuff with the ETT vs. the TT, have supported the trend to delaying tracheostomy until the third or fourth week of intubation.[4] Associated with this trend has been an increase in damage to the vocal cords and the larynx.[3] However, it is not certain that subsequent tracheostomy decreases laryngeal complications caused by prolonged translaryngeal intubation.[5,6] For this reason most authors recommend an anticipatory approach. Some suggest regular fiberoptic examination of the upper airway, with creation of a tracheostomy only when significant laryngeal

injury becomes apparent. Other complications of tracheostomy are listed in the box.

"Inadequate pulmonary toilet" or "inability to wean" are judgments often made in debilitated patients with severe chronic obstructive pulmonary disease in whom repeated attempts to extubate are foiled by the patient's failure to clear secretions or to wean past a low intermittent mandatory ventilation rate. Such patients may benefit from tracheostomy because of the improved toilet and/or small decrease in airway resistance and dead space.

Tube Selection
Cuffed vs. noncuffed

In adults, noncuffed tubes can be considered for patients who are capable of spontaneous ventilation and airway protection.

Inner cannula

For long-term tracheostomy, particularly when the patient is no longer in the hospital, an inner cannula that can be removed and cleaned can be very helpful. However, an inner cannula de-

---

Complications of Tracheostomy*
First 48-72 hours
Bleeding (usually vein or thyroid vessel)
Pneumothorax
Pneumomediastinum
Accidental decannulation
After 72 hours
Infection at stomal site
Mucous plug obstruction
Innominate artery fistula
Sinusitis
Otitis media
Tracheobronchitis
Pneumonia (nosocomial)
Late
Dilation of trachea at cuff site
Granulation tissue at stoma
Tracheoesophageal (T-E) fistula
Delayed
Difficulty decannulating
Persistent tracheocutaneous fistula
Tracheal stenosis at stoma or cuff site

*From Adams GL. Complications of tracheostomy. Perspect Crit Care 3(2):117, 1990.

creases the internal diameter, thereby augmenting resistance. Also, a TT with a rigid inner cannula often has a larger outer diameter for a given inner diameter, which may increase the risk of stenosis at the stomal site following decannulation.

Shape and Construction of Tube

The length of the extratracheal portion of the TT is important when the distance between the incision and the tracheal stoma is longer than normal (obesity, edema, induration, subcutaneous emphysema). A tracheostomy appliance that is too short greatly increases the risk of accidential decannulation. By adapting to the shape of the patient's airway, malleable TTs have fewer pressure points and thus reduce tracheal damage.

Special Considerations With Recent Tracheostomy

Accidental decannulation of a recent tracheostomy may be life-threatening. Just as for failed intubation, each SICU should have a procedure for avoiding accidental decannulation. Taking preventive measures is clearly superior to managing such a difficult problem. Attention to several features of tracheostomy placement are helpful:

1. All tracheostomies should have "stay" sutures inserted into the third or fourth tracheal rings.[7] These sutures should ex-

trude from the stoma to facilitate emergency recannulation.

2. The selected TT should be of appropriate size, length, and shape (Fig. 11-7).

3. Tracheal ties should be snug and secure so that the wings of the tube rest against the skin. As swelling dissipates, the ties may need to be tightened.

4. Manipulation of the airway should be avoided for at least 72 hours. Ventilator hoses/oxygen tubing should be disconnected when the patient is being moved. When the mouth is wired shut, wire cutters must be kept at the bedside.

5. Emergency airway materials including a tracheostomy/cricothyrotomy tray with tracheostomy hooks, laryngoscope, and ETTs, and a bag/valve/mask setup must be immediately available.

If the patient should be decannulated, the following steps must be taken:

1. Call for experienced airway assistance and emergency airway materials.

2. While help and equipment are arriving:

   a. If the patient is moving air, increase F_{IO_2} at the nose and mouth or the tracheostomy site (if the stoma in the trachea is visible) and request indirect monitors (pulse oximetry, capnometry).

   b. If the patient is making respiratory efforts but not moving air, look for easily

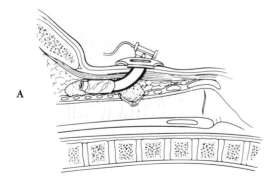
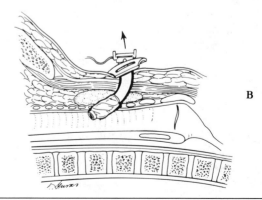

FIG. 11-7 Accidental decannulation is one of the most common complications of tracheostomy. Proper size and length of tracheostomy tube and incision are important in preventing this complication. **A,** Fenstra can be lost during changing of a tracheostomy tube. **B,** A tube that is too short can decannulate. (From Adams GL. Complications of tracheostomy. Perspect Crit Care 3(1):117, 1990.)

remediable problems, such as a blood clot in the tracheal stoma.

   c. If the patient is not making respiratory efforts and the upper airway is potentially available, attempt bag/valve/mask ventilation with oxygen. Blind passes with a suction catheter may cannulate the distal trachea. The catheter then can be used as a stylet to reintroduce the TT or an ETT.

3. Once equipment and personnel arrive, proceed as follows:

   a. If the patient is ventilating/being ventilated and if stay sutures were placed, use gentle traction on the sutures and suction to attempt recannulation. Adequate light is mandatory to adequately visualize the tracheal stoma.

   b. If the patient is not being ventilated and the upper airway is potentially open (i.e., the patient has not had a laryngectomy), proceed with OTI.

   c. If (a) and (b) are not successful, use the emergency tracheostomy equipment.

   d. Although its use is difficult when blood and secretions are present, a fiberoptic laryngoscope occasionally may be used to replace the TT.

4. Do not attempt to ventilate the patient through the newly reestablished airway unless (1) correct position has been determined by fiberoptic laryngoscopy, (2) a suction catheter can be passed freely through the tube, or (3) the patient is ventilating spontaneously through the cannula. Capnometry will confirm appropriate placement. Subcutaneous/mediastinal/submucosal emphysema due to positive pressure ventilation (PPV) through a misplaced tube can make subsequent intubation/ventilation impossible.

Changing of Tracheostomy Tube
Indications for tube change in recent tracheostomies (<72 hours after tracheostomy)

1. Obstructed tube
2. Inappropriate tube size or shape
3. Mechanical problems—leaky cuff, leaky inner cannula
4. Change in patient status—necessity for PPV, cuffed vs. uncuffed tube

Procedure (Fig. 11-8)

1. Ensure that all ancillary equipment is available (intubation, tracheostomy, bag/valve/mask, replacement TT).
2. Procure a stylet about 12 inches long, malleable but not floppy.
3. Preoxygenate the patient; consider sedation/analgesia.
4. Loosen the tracheostomy ties and lubricate the replacement tube.
5. Consider application of a local anesthetic. Injection may cause bleeding.
6. Pass the stylet through the TT, deflate the cuff, and remove the old tube. Thread the replacement tube over the stylet into the trachea.
7. Establish correct placement as above.
8. Tie or suture the tube into place.

Fiberoptic laryngoscopes may be used for this procedure, but their use necessitates losing the airway momentarily after the old TT has been removed. Tracheostomy instruments also may be used, but their use requires some knowledge and experience.

PULMONARY HEMORRHAGE/MASSIVE HEMOPTYSIS

Minor hemoptysis occurs frequently in the SICU. Typically it is associated with a mucosal ulcer in the trachea and a concomitant mild bleeding diathesis (i.e., platelet dysfunction, renal failure). Although such bleeding occasionally warrants intervention, most commonly correction of the bleeding disorder is sufficient. Bleeding in excess of 200 cc per 24 hours is defined as massive hemoptysis. By this definition, massive hemoptysis is rare, occurring in only 1.5% of cases.

The most common causes of massive hemoptysis are tuberculosis, bronchiectasis (including cystic fibrosis), and lung cancer (see box, p. 110). The mortality rate may be as high as 78%; patients usually die of suffocation from airway obstruction.[8] Underlying pulmonary

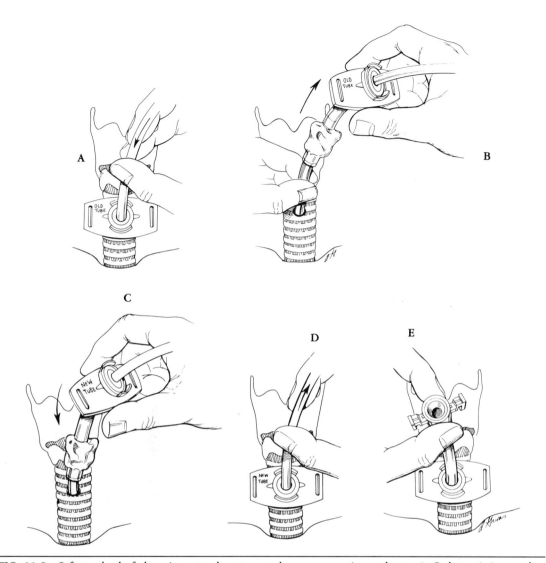

FIG. 11-8 Safe method of changing a tracheostomy tube over a suction catheter. **A**, Catheter is inserted. **B**, Old tracheostomy tube is removed over catheter. **C**, New tracheostomy tube is placed over catheter. **D**, Catheter is removed. **E**, Inner cannula is inserted into new tube. (From Adams GL. Complications of tracheostomy. Perspect Crit Care 3(1):117, 1990.)

dysfunction may make even minor hemoptysis life-threatening.

Approaches to the treatment of hemoptysis include ongoing life support and resuscitation, brochoscopy, balloon tamponade, angiography/ embolization, radio nuclear scanning, and surgery.

All cases. All patients in need of airway management require ongoing life support and resuscitation, including oxygen, mechanical ventilation (if required), correction of coagu-

lopathies, and consideration of the use of double-lumen ETTs or broncheal blockers if the bleeding site is known or suspected.

Bronchoscopy. Rigid bronchoscopy is the treatment of choice because it allows concomitant ventilation, suctioning, and application of local treatments (vasoactive agents, iced saline lavage). This approach is particularly useful in massive bleeding. The disadvantages are the need for general anesthesia and transport to the operating room. When the source of bleed-

Common Causes of Massive Hemoptysis*

Infectious
    Tuberculosis
    Lung abscess
    Bronchopneumonia
    Fungus ball
    Parasitic infestations
Neoplastic
    Bronchogenic carcinoma
    Bronchial adenoma
    Lymphoma
    Metastatic disease
    Carcinoma of contiguous structures
Cardiovascular
    Mitral stenosis
    Arteriovenous malformation
    Thoracic aortic aneurysm
    Vasculitis
    Pulmonary hypertension

Immunologic
    Goodpasture's syndrome
    Collagen-vascular diseases
Congenital
    Cystic fibrosis
    Bronchiectasis associated with Kartagener's syndrome
Other
    Bronchiectasis
    Retained foreign body
    Broncholithiasis
    Idiopathic pulmonary hemosiderosis
    Iatrogenic
    Trauma
    Idiopathic

*From Rudzinski JT, del Castillo J. Massive hemoptysis. Ann Emerg Med 16:561-564, 1987.

ing is not in the large airways, rigid bronchoscopy allows localization of the bleeding.

Fiberoptic bronchoscopy is available in most SICUs. It allows for visualization of the smaller branches of the tracheobronchial tree, and some forms of localized treatment (Fogarty catheters, epinephrine, gel foam) can be applied. Fiberoptic bronchoscopy is less useful in the presence of massive or diffuse bleeding. The efficacy of either type of bronchoscopy is reduced when the patient is not actively bleeding.

Balloon tamponade. Balloon tamponade is usually used in conjunction with bronchoscopy. Along with tamponade, balloon catheters allow distal irrigation with vasoactive substances or iced saline. Balloon tamponade is most useful when the site of bleeding has been localized. Although inflating the balloon blindly in a larger bronchus can be effective, it frequently leaves the patient with insufficient residual pulmonary function. When the bleeding source is thought to be pulmonary artery rupture associated with the use of a Swan-Ganz catheter, leaving the catheter in position and inflating the balloon may be lifesaving.[9]

Angiography/embolization. Massive hemoptysis usually results from systemic (bronchial) artery bleeding. Unfortunately, the anatomy of the bronchial arteries is highly variable, and with chronic disease there are widespread anastomoses. Since the anterior spinal artery may arise close to the bronchial arteries, there is potential for embolic material to cause neurologic dysfunction. Although useful only in the presence of active bleeding, angiography with embolization can be highly effective and is associated with only a small recurrence rate. This approach has the added advantage of being minimally invasive, but it does require the patient to be moved to the radiology suite.

Radionuclear scanning. Radionuclear scanning is noninvasive and relatively benign but can be used only with heavy, active bleeding (>60 ml/hr).[10] This approach is diagnostic rather than therapeutic.

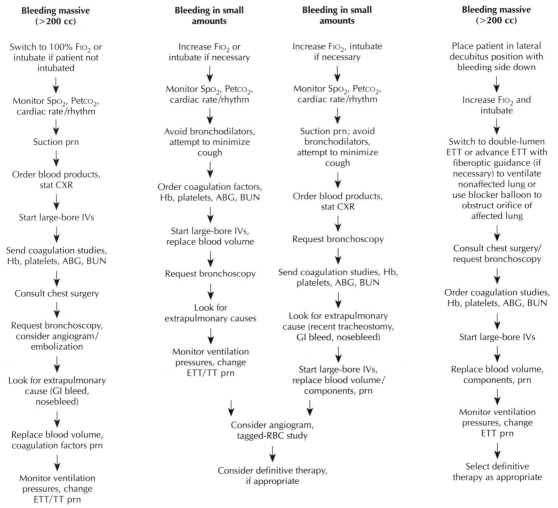

SITE UNKNOWN

**Bleeding massive
(>200 cc)**

Switch to 100% F_{IO_2} or
intubate if patient not
intubated
↓
Monitor Sp_{O_2}, Pet_{CO_2},
cardiac rate/rhythm
↓
Suction prn
↓
Order blood products,
stat CXR
↓
Start large-bore IVs
↓
Send coagulation studies,
Hb, platelets, ABG, BUN
↓
Consult chest surgery
↓
Request bronchoscopy,
consider angiogram/
embolization
↓
Look for extrapulmonary
cause (GI bleed,
nosebleed)
↓
Replace blood volume,
coagulation factors prn
↓
Monitor ventilation
pressures, change
ETT/TT prn

**Bleeding in small
amounts**

Increase F_{IO_2} or
intubate if necessary
↓
Monitor Sp_{O_2}, Pet_{CO_2},
cardiac rate/rhythm
↓
Avoid bronchodilators,
attempt to minimize
cough
↓
Order coagulation factors,
Hb, platelets, ABG, BUN
↓
Start large-bore IVs,
replace blood volume
↓
Request bronchoscopy
↓
Look for
extrapulmonary causes
↓
Monitor ventilation
pressures, change
ETT/TT prn

SITE KNOWN/SUSPECTED*

**Bleeding in small
amounts**

Increase F_{IO_2}, intubate
if necessary
↓
Monitor Sp_{O_2}, Pet_{CO_2},
cardiac rate/rhythm
↓
Suction prn; avoid
bronchodilators,
attempt to minimize
cough
↓
Order blood products,
stat CXR
↓
Request bronchoscopy
↓
Send coagulation studies, Hb,
platelets, ABG, BUN
↓
Look for extrapulmonary
cause (recent tracheostomy,
GI bleed, nosebleed)
↓
Start large-bore IVs,
replace blood volume/
components, prn

Consider angiogram,
tagged-RBC study
↓
Consider definitive therapy,
if appropriate

**Bleeding massive
(>200 cc)**

Place patient in lateral
decubitus position with
bleeding side down
↓
Increase F_{IO_2} and
intubate
↓
Switch to double-lumen
ETT or advance ETT with
fiberoptic guidance (if
necessary) to ventilate
nonaffected lung or
use blocker balloon to
obstruct orifice of
affected lung
↓
Consult chest surgery/
request bronchoscopy
↓
Order coagulation studies,
Hb, platelets, ABG, BUN
↓
Start large-bore IVs
↓
Replace blood volume,
components, prn
↓
Monitor ventilation
pressures, change
ETT prn
↓
Select definitive
therapy as appropriate

*Swan-Ganz catheter balloon rupture.

FIG. 11-9   Treatment approach to pulmonary hemorrhage/massive hemoptysis.

Surgery. Surgery is the treatment of last resort for massive hemoptysis primarily because many patients with this disease have insufficient pulmonary reserve to allow resection of adequate amounts of lung tissue. For surgery to be effective, the site of the bleeding must be known and the patient must be adequately resuscitated. Furthermore, surgery requires transport to the operating room, general anesthesia, and additional blood loss. In selected patients, however, surgery can be highly effective, with some studies showing a greater than 50% decrease in mortality.

For a presentation of the treatment of pulmonary hemorrhage/massive hemoptysis, see Fig. 11-9.

SUMMARY

- Use ETT for (1) trauma, edema, or hemorrhage that threatens airway patency; (2) significant risk of aspiration; (3) suctioning of airway repeatedly and frequently; (4) diagnostic procedures; (5) general anesthesia requiring muscle relaxation; and (6) mechanical ventilation.
- Standard intubating approaches include blind nasal or oral intubation, direct laryngoscopy, and fiberoptic bronchoscopy/laryngoscopy.
- Emergency airway management requires extensive preparation, evaluation of patient, skilled assistance, immediate and accurate determination of tube location, necessary equipment for managing difficult airway.
- Indications for tracheostomy include prolonged mechanical ventilation, airway obstruction at or above larynx, and chronic suctioning for pulmonary toilet.
- Accidental decannulation of recent tracheostomy:
  Minimize chance of decannulation by using tracheostomy appliance of appropriate size, length, and shape; securing tracheal ties; adjusting tracheal ties as edema resolves; and avoiding airway manipulation for at least 12 hours.

Take precautions to avoid accidental decannulation. Have immediately available tracheostomy tray with tracheostomy hooks, laryngoscope, ETTs, bag/valve/mask, and wire cutter (if patient's mouth is wired shut).
If accidental decannulation occurs:
  1. Call for help. Increase F_{IO_2} at nose, mouth, or stoma (if visible). Look for blood clot in stoma. If upper airway is patent, attempt bag/valve/mask ventilation.
  2. If unable to ventilate patient, attempt oral intubation.
  3. Confirm correct position of newly established airway.
- Massive hemoptysis:
  Establish a secure, patent airway.
  Resuscitate with volume oxygen and mechanical ventilation.
  Correct coagulopathies (if present).
  Rigid bronchoscopy is preferred with massive bleeding.
  Balloon tamponade may be used to stop bleeding when bleeding site is known.
  Angiography with embolization may be effective.

REFERENCES

1. Maltby JR, Loken RG, Watson NC. The laryngeal mask airway: Clinical appraisal in 250 patients. Can J Anaesth 37:509-513, 1990.
2. Dunn SM, Mushlin PS, Lind CJ, Raemer D. Tracheal intubation is not invariably confirmed by capnography. Anesthesiology 73:1285-1287, 1990.
3. Berlauk JF. Intubation in the ICU: A review from a different perspective. Perspect Crit Care 3(2):89-107, 1990.
4. Stauffer JL, Olson DE, Petty TL. Complications and consequences of endotracheal intubation and tracheostomy: A prospective study of 150 critically ill patients. Am J Med 70:65-76, 1981.
5. Bishop MJ. Mechanisms of laryngotracheal injury following prolonged tracheal intubation. Chest 96:185-186, 1989.
6. Sasaki CT, Horiuchi M, Koss N. Tracheostomy related subglottic stenosis: Bacteriologic pathogenesis. Laryngoscope 139:857-877, 1979.
7. Adams GL. Complications of tracheostomy. Perspect Crit Care 3(2):105-123, 1990.
8. Jones DK, Davies RJ. Massive hemoptysis. Br Med J 300:889-890, 1990.
9. Thomas R, Siproudhis L, Laurent JF, et al. Massive hemoptysis from iatrogenic balloon catheter rupture of pulmonary artery: Successful early management by balloon tamponade. Crit Care Med 15:772-773, 1987.
10. Haponik EF, Rothfeld B, Britt ES, Bleecker ER. Radionuclide localization of massive pulmonary hemorrhage. Chest 86:208-212, 1984.

SUGGESTED READINGS

Airway management

Stone DJ, Gal TJ. Airway management. In Miller RD. Anesthesia, 3rd ed. New York: Churchill Livingstone, 1990, pp 1265-1292.

Wilson RS. Upper airway problems. Resp Care 37:533-550, 1992.

Difficult intubation

Crosby ET, Lui A. The adult spine: Implications for airway management. Can J Anaesth 37:77-93, 1990.

Davies JM, Weeks S, Crone LA, Pavlin EG. Difficult intubation in the parturient. Can J Anaesth 36:668-674, 1989.

King TA, Adams AP. Failed tracheal intubation. Br J Anaesth 65:400-414, 1990.

Mallampati SR, Gatt SP, Gugino LD, et al. A clinical sign to predict difficult tracheal intubation: A prospective study. Can Anaesth Soc J 32:429-434, 1985.

Samsoon GLT, Young JRB. Difficult tracheal intubation: A retrospective study. Anaesthesiology 42:487-490, 1987.

Tracheostomy

Adams GL. Complications of tracheostomy. Perspect Crit Care 3(2):105-123, 1990.

Berlauk JF. Intubation in the ICU: A review from a different perspective. Perspect Crit Care 3(2):89-107, 1990.

Hemoptysis

Metzdorff MT, Vogelzang RL, LoCicero J, et al. Transcatheter broncheal artery embolization in the multimodality management of massive hemoptysis. Chest 97:1494-1496, 1990.

Wedzicka JA, Pearson MC. Management of massive hemoptysis. Resp Med 84:9-12, 1990.

CHAPTER 12

Pulmonary Embolism

Mark D. Cipolle

Historically, the diagnosis and treatment of pulmonary embolism (PE) have presented a challenge for clinicians,[1] and this challenge remains today. In the SICU the diagnosis of PE is often complicated by superimposed lung injury, and treatment decisions are affected by relative or absolute contraindications to anticoagulation or thrombolytic therapy. In fact, most critically ill patients manifest some findings consistent with PE (i.e., dyspnea, chest pain, ventilation-perfusion [V/Q] mismatch, or elevated central venous pressure) at some point during their disease course. Therefore an approach to patients that optimizes the use of diagnostic tests and therapy is necessary.

INCIDENCE

PE remains the most common preventable cause of inhospital mortality. Fatal PE is found in 4% to 7% of emergency hip surgery patients, 0.34% to 1.7% of elective hip surgery patients, and 0.1% to 0.8% of general surgery patients.[2-4] PE occurs in approximately 35% to 50% of patients with documented proximal deep venous thrombosis (DVT).[5,6] These figures include both silent and clinically suspected PE.

It is estimated that the incidence of PE in the United States is approximately 600,000 cases per year and that the annual mortality exceeds 200,000. PE is the third leading cause of death in the United States. Ten percent of PE victims die within 1 hour of the event. Of the remaining 90%, only one third will have the diagnosis of PE made; of these patients in whom therapy is instituted, 8% will die. In the larger group with undiagnosed PE, there is a 30% mortality.[4] Therefore when the diagnosis of PE has been established, the mortality is decreased by three- to fourfold. Fig. 12-1 outlines the scope of the problem of PE.

RISK FACTORS

Several well-documented risk factors for the development of venous thromboembolism are shown in the accompanying box. The incidence of DVT can be as high as 30% and 70% in major abdominal surgery and orthopedic surgery, respectively. The incidence of fatal PE is 1% to 2% in major abdominal surgery and 2% to 5% in orthopedic procedures. The contribution of a surgical procedure to the risk of venous thromboembolism is not easily separable from

---

Risk Factors for Venous Thromboembolism

Heart disease
Advanced age
Shock
Trauma
Obesity
Estrogen therapy, pregnancy
Malignancy
Surgery
Immobility, paralysis
Previous PE or DVT
Antithrombin III deficiency
Other hypercoagulable disorders

the risk associated with underlying disease, age, and preoperative immobility. Of patients over the age of 40 who undergo major surgery, 15% to 50% develop DVT.[4] Not all detectable deep venous thrombi carry the same risk of embolism: only venous thrombi located in or above the popliteal vein have been associated with a high risk of PE.[7]

The estimated prevalence of fatal PE in trauma patients, in whom the incidence of PE is 2%, is about 1%. DVT has a greater probability of occurrence in adult trauma patients. In patients with head and chest trauma, the incidence is 40%; and in those with femur fracture, the incidence approaches 80%. In lower extremity fractures, venous thrombi are often found bilaterally. All patients with trauma, regardless of the site of injury or the patient's age, have increased risk of PE.[4] A cumulative risk may be present when more than one risk factor is identified; therefore the surgical intensivist must maintain a high index of suspicion for venous thromboembolism in all patients admitted to the SICU or trauma unit. All such patients should have adequate thromboembolism prophylaxis. If PE occurs, the diagnosis and treatment of venous thromboembolism must be made rapidly and efficiently.

CLINICAL MANIFESTATIONS

Clinical findings are notoriously unreliable in the diagnosis of PE. The classic clinical triad of PE—dyspnea, pleuritic chest pain, and hemoptysis—occurs in only 20% of patients with major PE.[8] The nonspecificity of the clinical diagnosis of PE was well demonstrated in the Urokinase Pulmonary Embolism Trial (UPET).[9] In this study over 60% of more than 2500 patients who entered with clinically suspected PE had the diagnosis excluded by a negative perfusion scan.

The signs and symptoms of PE are listed in Table 12-1. In SICU patients concomitant cardiopulmonary disease or lung injury make the clinical signs and symptoms less sensitive and less specific. Therefore clinical and laboratory data are sufficient to indicate only those patients who need further evaluation. Adding to the diagnostic difficulties is the fact that the presentation may be either abrupt and catastrophic or quite subtle.

The SICU physician should always include

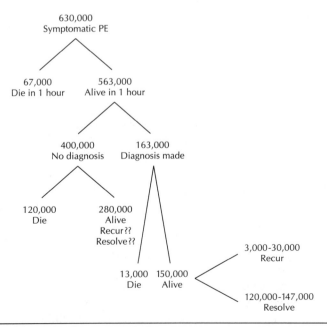

FIG. 12-1 Scope of problem of pulmonary embolism.

TABLE 12-1 Clinical Manifestations of Pulmonary Embolism

Sign/Symptom	% Seen
Tachypnea	85
Pleuritic chest pain	73
Rales (localized)	60
Increased S_2	60
Apprehension	60
Cough	60
Tachycardia	40
Fever	45
Thrombophlebitis	40
Hemoptysis	34
Supraventricular tachycardia	15
Proximal DVT	70-90 (majority "silent")

PE in the differential diagnosis of shock and look for subtle manifestations of PE, such as (1) worsening hypoxemia and respiratory alkalosis in a ventilated patient; (2) dyspnea that is unresponsive to bronchodilators in a patient with chronic obstructive pulmonary disease; (3) unexplained fever, atelectasis, or peripheral infiltrate on CXR; and (4) sudden pulmonary hypertension or elevated CVP.[10,11]

ECG, CXR, and the pulmonary artery catheter may be of some benefit in making the diagnosis of PE. Acute myocardial infarction must often be distinguished from PE in the differential diagnosis. When shock is caused by myocardial infarction, ECG findings are consistent with ischemia. The right heart strain pattern of PE, namely $S_1Q_3T_3$, is generally evident only with massive PE and in itself is not specific for PE. The CXR generally shows interstitial or pulmonary edema with myocardial infarction; only occasionally are asymmetric hyperlucent areas found in PE. Rarely will pulmonary infarct resulting from a PE present itself on initial CXR. Occasionally, the pulmonary artery catheter will be helpful in distinguishing PE from acute myocardial infarction or cardiac tamponade. Elevated right atrial and right ventricular diastolic pressures with a normal or low pulmonary artery wedge pressure favor the diagnosis of PE.

In contrast, patients with cardiogenic shock from myocardial infarction generally have no, or only slight, elevations in right atrial or right ventricular pressures and a markedly increased pulmonary artery wedge pressure. In shock resulting from cardiac tamponade, the right heart pressure and wedge pressure are elevated and equal. The finding of pulsus paradoxicus also may occur in cardiac tamponade[10] (Table 12-2).

"Massive" PE has been defined by the National Heart, Lung, and Blood Institute as a significant filling defect in two or more pulmonary lobar arteries noted on pulmonary angiogram. This finding implies occlusion of at least 40% of the pulmonary arterial tree.[12] Angiographic studies suggest that between 30% and 60% of pulmonary emboli are anatomically massive.[13] The clinician must remember that the consequences of a pulmonary embolus are a function not only of size but also of underlying cardiopulmonary disease and the neuroendocrine response to the emboli. In autopsy series only half of fatal emboli met the anatomic definition of "massive."[14] The mortality in patients without shock is 5% to 8%. It rises to 22% to 33% in PE patients who present with hemodynamic compromise.[15]

DIAGNOSIS

Making the diagnosis of PE and instituting appropriate therapy decreases the mortality from approximately 30% to 8% (see Fig. 12-1). Since none of the signs or symptoms of PE are sensitive or specific, the success of making a correct antemortem diagnosis of PE is difficult. This difficulty is emphasized by Goldhaber and Hennekens.[16] Of 54 patients with *massive* PE, only 16 had the diagnosis made before death. Furthermore, patients older than 70 years or patients with pneumonia had the correct antemortem diagnosis of PE made only 10% and 21% of the time, respectively.

Important research has been conducted on the diagnostic approach to patients suspected of having venous thromboembolism. Some studies have focused on the correlation between V/Q scanning and pulmonary angiography. Other studies have investigated the relationship between DVT and PE.

TABLE 12-2 Pulmonary Artery Catheter Pressure Reading in Differential Diagnosis of Pulmonary Embolism

Diagnosis	PA Catheter Pressure			
	RA	RV	PAP	PCWP
Acute myocardial infarction with shock	Normal or ↑	Normal or ↑	Normal or ↑	↑ ↑
Massive PE	↑	↑	↑	Normal or ↓
Cardiac tamponade	↑	↑ *	↑	↑
Right ventricular infarction	↑	↑ (diastolic)	Normal*	↓

RA, right atrial; RV, right ventricular; PAP, pulmonary artery pressure; PCWP, pulmonary capillary wedge pressure; ↑, increased pressure; ↓, decreased pressure.
*Narrow pulse pressure.

Pulmonary Angiography

Pulmonary angiography is the accepted diagnostic reference standard for establishing the presence or absence of PE.[17,18] Selective techniques and magnification have made this tool even more powerful in the last few years.

A diagnosis of PE is made when the angiogram demonstrates a constant intraluminal filling defect on multiple films or when a sharp cutoff, consistent in multiple views, is seen in a vessel >2.5 mm. Abnormalities such as oligemia, vessel pruning, and loss of filling of vessels are nonspecific and may be the result of pneumonia, atelectasis, adult respiratory distress syndrome, pulmonary hypertension, chronic obstructive pulmonary disease, or carcinoma.

Morbidity and mortality associated with pulmonary angiography is not trivial. Clinically significant complications, including tachycardia, myocardial injury, cardiac perforation, cardiac arrest, and hypersensitivity due to contrast material, occur in 3% to 4% of patients. Hull et al.[5] established that approximately 20% of patients with clinically suspected PE and abnormal perfusion lung scans could not undergo pulmonary angiography because of the severity of their primary illness. The mortality associated with pulmonary angiography varies from 0.2% to 0.5%. The only absolute contraindications to its use are allergy to contrast material and severe pulmonary hypertension.[10] Because of these issues and the unavailability of angiography at smaller centers, radionuclide scanning has become an increasingly important diagnostic tool.

Ventilation/Perfusion Scanning

Perfusion lung scanning occupies a pivotal role in the diagnostic workup of PE. Injection of technetium-99m–labeled macroaggregated human albumin particles, 10 to 30 μm in diameter, temporarily occludes <0.5% of pulmonary capillary beds. Ventilation scanning has been added to perfusion scanning in an attempt to differentiate embolic occlusions from other causes of perfusion defects resulting from a primary disturbance in ventilation, such as pneumonia or atelectasis. Ventilation scanning is usually performed with ^{133}Xe.[10]

Several prospective studies have been done to determine the probability of PE based on detection of defects through various scanning techniques vs. pulmonary angiography.[5,19-22] Diagnostic problems with V/Q scanning arise from this method's lack of specificity. Only a normal scan, which occurs 5% to 10% of the time, or a high-probability scan in a patient with a high index of suspicion is useful as a diagnostic endpoint. The overwhelming majority of patients suspected of having PE will have V/Q scans that fall in the categories of low, intermediate, or indeterminant probability of having PE. Unfortunately, the criteria used for classifying V/Q scans is not uniform, and the most variability occurs in the intermediate probability category.[23] In general, the probability of PE increases with the size of the perfusion defect and the amount of V/Q mismatch.

To date, the best prospective studies for determining the accuracy of V/Q scanning are those of Hull and colleagues[5,22] and the Prospective Investigation of Pulmonary Embolism Diagnosis (PIOPED).[21] Hull and his group found that patients with segmental, or greater, perfusion defects with V/Q mismatch (high probability) had an 86% probability of having a PE on pulmonary angiogram. Twenty-five to 40% of patients with a low-probability scan had PE demonstrated by angiography. Hull and colleagues recommended not withholding anticoagulation therapy solely on the basis of the results of a low-probability V/Q scan.[5]

PIOPED was a multicenter trial that included 931 patients with clinically suspected PE. Eighty-eight percent of patients with a high-probability scan had PE shown by angiogram (102 of 116 patients). However, only 41% of patients with PE (102 of 251 patients) had a high-probability V/Q scan. Of 322 patients with intermediate-probability scans, 105 (33%) had PE. The researchers found a 12% frequency of PE in patients classified as "low probability" on the V/Q scan. Overall, the sensitivity of the V/Q scan was determined to be 98%. However, the overall specificity was only 10% according to PIOPED. Although the specificity could be increased by making the criteria for PE more stringent, then sensitivity was lost.[21]

Several studies have shown that noninvasive lower extremity studies are acceptable screening tools for ruling out proximal DVT. Wheeler and Anderson[24] showed that impedance plethysmography (IPG) had a 93% sensitivity and a 94% specificity for diagnosis of proximal DVT. They used contrast venography as the standard. Their figures were obtained by analyzing 16 studies, which included over 2000 patients. Venous duplex ultrasonography seems to be even better for diagnosing above-knee DVT. Recent reports of this method show a sensitivity of 95% to 100% and a specificity of 99% in diagnosing above-knee DVT.[25-27]

Hull and colleagues[5,22,28] performed three studies to outline the role of noninvasive DVT testing in the diagnosis of PE. Several important observations were made in these studies. The frequency of proximal DVT differed depending on a wide spectrum of V/Q defects, ranging from <1% in patients with normal lung scans to 49% in patients with large perfusion defects and V/Q mismatch. Patients with low- and intermediate-probability V/Q scans had a 15% to 27% rate of proximal DVT.[22] These findings were interpreted to show that patients with clinically suspected PE and abnormal V/Q scans have a substantial frequency of proximal DVT. Also, failure to treat proximal DVT is associated with a high rate of recurrent venous thromboembolism. In these studies 30% of patients with angiographically proven PE had a negative venogram for proximal DVT.[5] It follows that a patient with a low- or intermediate-probability V/Q scan and a positive IPG should be treated for venous thromboembolism.

Should a patient with a non–high-probability V/Q scan and a negative noninvasive examination be treated for DVT? Hull et al.[28] recently conducted a study addressing this issue. They showed that 371 patients with low- or intermediate-probability V/Q scans and normal serial IPGs (six times over a 2-week period) had a <3% chance of having DVT or PE during a 3-month follow-up. Also, no patient died of venous thromboembolism during this 3-month period. This study was limited to patients with "good" cardiopulmonary reserve. The authors concluded that withholding anticoagulation therapy is an acceptable strategy for managing patients with adequate cardiopulmonary reserve, nondiagnostic lung scan results, and negative serial IPGs.

Fig. 12-2 presents an approach to the diagnosis of PE. Portable duplex scanning is a valuable diagnostic tool for ruling out lower extremity DVT in SICU patients.

PROPHYLAXIS

The key to reducing morbidity and mortality from venous thromboembolism is prophylaxis. Although anticoagulant therapy is very effective in preventing death from this condition, the vast majority of patients die of PE either within the first hour of the event or without a diagnosis. Prophylaxis is more effective for prevention of death and morbidity from PE than for treatment of an established embolus. Routine use of effective prophylaxis in patients undergoing elective general surgery could prevent 4000 to 8000 postoperative deaths yearly in the United States.[29] Studies proving the efficacy of venous thromboembolism prophylaxis, particularly in surgical patients, have been well-summarized.[29-31] Subcutaneous low-dose heparin, adjusted-dose heparin, pneumatic compression devices, graduated compression stockings, and dextran have been the most carefully studied forms of prophylaxis. Table 12-3 outlines the risk stratification of venous thromboembolism for surgical patients.

Low-Dose Heparin

Low-dose heparin is generally given as a dose of 5000 U sc 2 hours preoperatively and every 8 to 12 hours postoperatively. Much lower doses of heparin are required to inhibit the initiation of blood coagulation than are needed for the treatment of established DVT or PE.[30]

A large multicenter international trial involving over 4000 patients[31] and an analysis of 70 randomized trials that included over 16,000 patients[30] have established the efficacy of low-dose heparin as a prophylactic agent against postoperative venous thromboembolism.

Collins et al.[30] performed an exhaustive overview of 70 studies involving 16,000 patients in general, orthopedic, and urologic surgery. They demonstrated a reduction in DVT from 22% to

TABLE 12-3 Classification of Risk of Postoperative Venous Thromboembolism*

Risk Category	Risk (%) Related to:		
	Calf Vein Thrombosis	Proximal Vein Thrombosis	Fatal Pulmonary Embolism
High risk	40-80	10-20	1-5
General surgery in patients >40 years with recent history of DVT or PE			
Extensive pelvic or abdominal surgery for malignant disease			
Major orthopedic surgery of lower limbs			
Moderate risk	10-40	2-10	0.1-0.7
General surgery in patients >40 years lasting 30 minutes or more			
Low risk	<10	<1	<0.01
Uncomplicated surgery in patients >40 years with no additional risk factor			
Minor surgery (<30 minutes) in patients >40 years with no additional risk factors			

*From Hull RD, Raskob GE, Hirsch J. Prophylaxis of venous thromboembolism: An overview. Chest (Suppl) 89:374S, 1986.

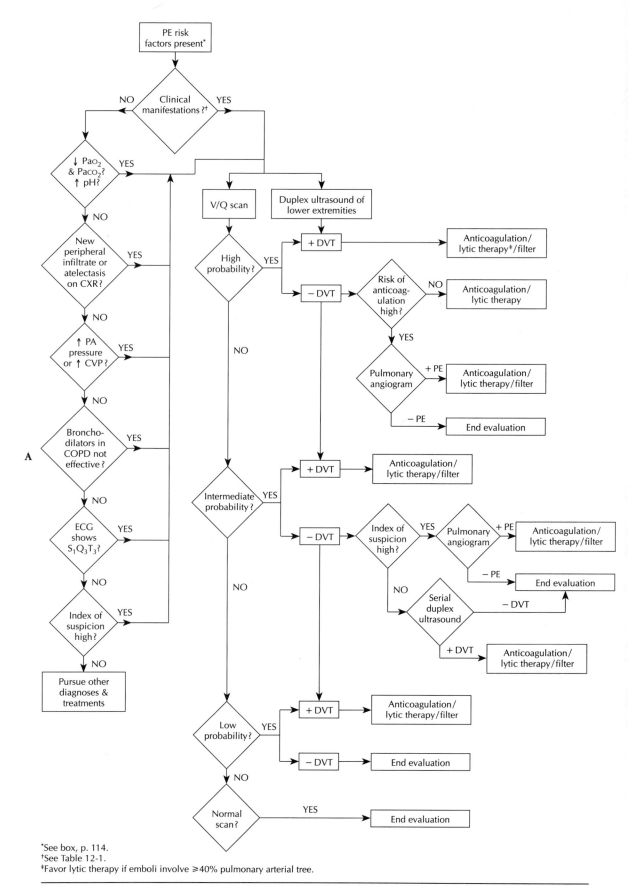

A

*See box, p. 114.
†See Table 12-1.
‡Favor lytic therapy if emboli involve ≥40% pulmonary arterial tree.

FIG. 12-2 A, Approach to diagnosis and treatment of pulmonary embolism in a stable patient.

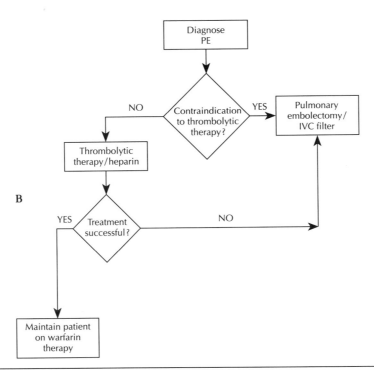

B

FIG. 12-2, cont'd **B,** Approach to diagnosis and treatment of pulmonary embolism in an unstable patient.

9% with the use of subcutaneous heparin and found a significant reduction in fatal PE in the patients treated with low-dose heparin. Low-dose heparin caused no apparent increase in deaths. Collins et al. estimated that using low-dose subcutaneous heparin decreased the odds of having proximal DVT by about two thirds and of having postoperative PE by one half.

In major orthopedic surgery, the administration of low-dose heparin reduced DVT by approximately two thirds in elective surgery and trauma. In hip fracture patients, the use of low-dose heparin may be limited. Kakkar et al.[32] reported that 22 of 50 hip fracture patients still sustained a postoperative DVT despite receiving low-dose heparin therapy.

Data on increased bleeding associated with the use of low-dose heparin in postoperative patients have been incomplete and inadequate in many trials. In their overview of the randomized trials, Collins et al.[30] demonstrated that the absolute excess of bleeding attributable to low-dose heparin was approximately 2%. Although the multicenter trial showed a slight increase in bleeding morbidity in the low-dose-heparin

group (117 wound hematomas in control patients vs. 158 in heparin-treated patients), there was no difference between groups in deaths due to hemorrhage.[31]

Adjusted-Dose Heparin

Because of the limited efficacy of low-dose heparin in high-risk patients (hip surgery), a moderate adjusted dose of subcutaneous heparin has been examined as a means of DVT/PE prophylaxis in these patients. Leyvarz et al.[33] showed a reduction in overall DVT from 39% to 14% ($p < 0.01$) and proximal DVT from 32% to 5% in hip replacement patients. The partial thromboplastin time (PTT) of these patients was adjusted between 31.5 and 36 with subcutaneous heparin, when compared to the control group, which had fixed low-dose heparin. This increased protection was not associated with increased perioperative bleeding.

Low-Molecular-Weight Heparin

Another primary prophylactic agent is low-molecular-weight heparin (LMWH). LMWH has been shown to be effective in preventing postoperative thromboembolic complications in patients having elective hip surgery[34] and in general surgery patients.[35,36] As with regular heparin, LMWH is given subcutaneously once or twice daily. When administered to healthy volunteers, subcutaneous LMWH produced peak plasma levels of anti-Xa activity that were at least six times greater than those obtained with conventional heparin given at the same dose.[37] Bleeding complications appeared to be minimal with LMWH. LMWH shows promise as an efficacious prophylactic agent that may be safer than conventional heparin.

Oral Anticoagulants

Prophylaxis with warfarin has been studied in very high risk patients, namely, those undergoing total hip or knee replacement. Institution of warfarin prophylaxis to keep the prothrombin time (PT) 1.5 to 2 times that of the control appears to be associated with a higher frequency of clinically important bleeding.[29] Because of this finding, a two-step warfarin prophylaxis regimen in patients undergoing elective joint replacement was examined by Francis et al.[38] A low dose (on average 3 mg daily) was started 10 to 14 days preoperatively and adjusted to keep the PT 1.5 to 3 seconds above the control. Immediately after operation, the warfarin dosage was increased to keep the PT 1.5 times the control. The overall incidence of venous thrombosis, documented by ascending venography within 2 weeks postoperatively, was significantly less in the 53 patients who were treated with warfarin in comparison to the 37 patients treated with dextran (21% vs. 51%, p <0.005). The incidence of thrombus at or above the knee was decreased with two-step warfarin therapy, declining from 10% to 2%. Measurements of perioperative blood loss were not different between the two groups. Francis et al. concluded that two-step warfarin therapy served as a highly effective prophylaxis against postoperative venous thrombosis in very high risk patients.

Dextran

Dextran is a glucose polymer that was introduced as a volume expander and also has been used for thromboembolism prophylaxis. It reportedly inhibits platelet aggregation. Dextran has not been shown to be effective in the treatment of thromboembolism, but it has been demonstrated as an effective prophylactic agent for venous thrombosis in both general surgical and orthopedic patients. In 8 of 19 studies, there was a statistically significant difference between patients having therapy with dextran 70 and controls in the frequency of postoperative DVT.[29] Because of its cost, unproven efficacy in some studies, and side effects (e.g., volume overload, bleeding, anaphylaxis, and renal failure), dextran has had limited use in the prevention of venous thromboembolism. By comparison with low-dose subcutaneous heparin, dextran is relatively expensive; in addition, it requires intravenous access.

Sequential Compression Devices

Sequential compression devices prevent venous thrombosis by enhancing blood flow in the deep veins of the legs. These devices have been shown to increase fibrinolytic activity systemically.[39-41] In 15 of 22 studies, sequential compression has been demonstrated to significantly reduce the formation of postoperative thrombi. This type of prophylaxis is effective in moderate-risk general surgical patients and in patients undergoing minor surgery, major knee surgery, prostate surgery, and pelvic surgery. It is the method of choice for prophylaxis in patient groups in which low-dose heparin is either contraindicated or ineffective.[29] Sequential compression devices are virtually free of clinically important side effects and offer a valuable alternative in patients who have a high risk of bleeding.

Graduated Compression Stockings

Graduated compression stockings reduce venous stasis by applying compression to the ankle and calf, with greater pressure being applied more distally. Use of these stockings is an effective form of DVT prophylaxis in low-risk general surgery patients. Statistically significant differences between patients wearing graduated compression stockings and controls have been demonstrated in five of seven studies, which involved 547 patients. However, the efficacy of graduated compression stockings in preventing DVT in moderate- to high-risk patients is uncertain.[29] Increased efficacy of DVT prevention occurred when the use of sequential compression devices was combined with graduated compression stockings. Only a 1% incidence of DVT was found when sequential compression was combined with stocking use, vs. a 9% incidence of DVT when sequential compression was used alone.[42]

Special Problems

There are some patients in whom certain prophylactic modalities cannot be employed. Clearly, if there is substantial hemorrhagic risk, one is limited to sequential compression devices as a means of thromboembolism prophylaxis. Patients with ongoing bleeding, those having recent brain, spinal cord, or eye injury, and postoperative neurosurgical or eye surgery patients would fall into this category. Although no significant risk of bleeding has been demonstrated with low-dose heparin, reports indicate a trend toward increased perioperative bleeding.[30,31] Minor amounts of bleeding in these very high risk patients could be extremely dangerous and even fatal. Another difficult patient is the multiply injured individual who has lower extremity trauma that prevents the use of sequential compression devices. Moser[43] has adopted a policy of inserting vena cava filters in such patients to prevent lethal PE because these trauma patients are at very high risk of venous thromboembolism. Another alternative is the application of sequential compression devices to any available extremity, including the upper extremities. These devices have been shown to increase systemic fibrinolysis,[39,41] and their effect may be of benefit in an uninvolved extremity.

The vasa vasorum of arm veins have been shown to contain greater amounts of plasminogen activators compared to leg veins.[44] Also, intermittent compression of the arms during surgery, and for 24 hours postoperatively, has been noted to decrease the incidence of lower extremity DVT by 50%.[45]

Table 12-4 outlines recommendations for venous thromboembolism prophylaxis in surgical patients.

TREATMENT

Anticoagulation therapy remains the mainstay of treatment for venous thromboembolism. Thrombolysis has not yet gained wide acceptance as a first-line therapy. This limitation arises from bleeding risk. Lytic therapy has been reserved for use in unstable patients with massive PE or as part of a study protocol. Surgical thromboembolectomy is reserved for patients with postembolic systemic hypotension who have contraindications to, or have had, unsuccessful thrombolysis.

The ultimate goals of therapy are to prevent morbidity and mortality from PE and to prevent long-term complications of venous thromboembolism. The optimum therapy depends on

TABLE 12-4 Prophylaxis for Venous Thromboembolism

Risk Category	Recommended Approach
Low risk	Graduated compression stocking
Moderate risk	
General abdominal or thoracic surgery	Low-dose heparin or SCD
Penetrating trauma	SCD
Neurosurgery, genitourinary surgery	SCD
High risk	
General abdominal or thoracic surgery	Low-dose heparin and SCD
Elective hip surgery	Two-step warfarin and SCD
Emergency hip surgery	Warfarin and SCD
Major knee surgery	SCD
Multiple trauma	SCD
Multiple trauma with lower extremity injuries	SCD to available extremities or caval filter

SCD, sequential compression device.

the patient's clinical status and cardiopulmonary reserve. It must be remembered that full anticoagulation and caval interruption are forms of prophylaxis designed to prevent further pulmonary embolization. Anticoagulation allows the fibrinolytic system to act unopposed and should limit the size of any embolic material that may be dislodged. Thrombolysis and embolectomy are more definitive therapies that are designed to actively remove pulmonary emboli.

Anticoagulation

Anticoagulation has been shown to be a very effective strategy for managing venous thromboembolism. In fact, the only randomized anticoagulation trial to date was discontinued after use in 35 patients because the investigators thought that withholding heparin in the control group was unethical.[46] Another prospective study examined 144 consecutive patients with angiographically proven PE.[13] All patients received heparin, and no patients were treated with thrombolytic therapy. Twelve patients died of PE, and eight died of other causes.

Continuous intravenous infusion of heparin is more effective than intermittent subcutaneous administration of heparin in preventing recurrent thromboembolism, a consequence of the delay in achieving anticoagulation when heparin is used subcutaneously. Hull et al.[47] reported that the relative risk of recurrent venous thromboembolism was 15 times higher in patients having inadequate anticoagulation therapy during the first 24 hours, whether the heparin was given intravenously or subcutaneously.

Generally, heparin should be given as a bolus to initiate therapy, and the partial thromboplastin time (PTT) should be maintained between 1.5 and 2 times that of the control. Bleeding complications during heparin therapy do not correlate closely with elevated PTT.[48,49] Once the diagnosis of proximal DVT or PE has been made, a rapid approach toward anticoagulation is mandated. I generally initiate heparin therapy with a 5000 to 10,000 U/kg IV bolus and then run a continuous infusion at 500 to 1500 U/hr to maintain the PTT at 1.5 to 2 times that of the control. The risk of major bleeding

with full therapeutic doses of heparin ranges from 1% to 33%, with most studies indicating a frequency of 5% to 10%.[50,51] Continuous infusion results in fewer bleeding complications than intermittent injection.[50]

The following factors have been associated with increased risk of bleeding during heparin therapy:

Dose of heparin
PTT >3 times that of control
Intermittent subcutaneous infusion >continuous infusion
Thrombocytopenia
Vitamin K deficiency
Advanced age
Underlying disease (e.g., malignancy, GI bleeding, renal or hepatic failure)
Use of aspirin, NSAIDs, lytic agents

Early initiation of warfarin therapy shortens both the duration of heparin therapy (from 9.5 to 4.1 days) and the length of hospital stay (by 4 to 5 days).[52,53] In SICU patients, who frequently require surgical or other invasive procedures, early initiation of warfarin therapy may not always be feasible. In these cases the heparin dose can be decreased or stopped temporarily, and the effects will begin to reverse in 1 to 2 hours. Anticoagulation with warfarin can be reversed by the addition of fresh frozen plasma, Vitamin K, or both. If Vitamin K is used for reversal of the effects of warfarin, only 5 to 10 mg should be given *once* since it is very difficult to reanticoagulate the patient for up to 2 weeks after a large dose of vitamin K has been given.[50,51] The patient then would require prolonged heparin therapy until warfarin anticoagulation was again achieved. Initiation of anticoagulation therapy with warfarin alone is not recommended.

In addition to its well-known effect on coagulation factors, warfarin reduces levels of protein C, a naturally occurring antithrombin. Protein C has a half-life of 4 to 6 hours and is depleted early with warfarin therapy. Such depletion creates the potential for a hypercoagulable state. Warfarinization must be initiated with simultaneous infusion of heparin to prevent hypercoagulability. Although the thrombin time (TT) may be in the therapeutic range by the second or third day, the patient is not effectively anticoagulated until factors II, VII, IX, and X have been depleted. The half-life of factor X is about 4 to 5 days.[50]

Generally, warfarin has been given as a once-daily dose to maintain the prothrombin time (PT) at 1.5 to 2 times that of the control. Hull et al.[54] have shown that doses producing a lower PT are just as effective and result in fewer bleeding complications over a 3-month period. In their study the conventional treatment group (average PT of 19 seconds) and the study group (average PT of 15 seconds) had an equal incidence of recurrent DVT. The study group had only two patients with bleeding complications, and the conventional group had 11 bleeding complications.

For uncomplicated venous thromboembolism, 3 months of oral anticoagulation therapy is recommended. Shorter duration of anticoagulation has resulted in excessively high recurrence rates of DVT.[55,56] Reports by Hull and associates[57,58] have shown that providing a dose of warfarin to keep the PT between 1.5 and 2 times that of the control resulted in only a 2% recurrence of proximal DVT. In the subsequent 9 months, there was an additional recurrence of only 4%. Others have reported much higher PE recurrences (17% to 23%) during anticoagulation therapy.[9,59,60] As Hirsch and Hull[61] have suggested, the variability in these recurrence rates may be related to the delay in initiating therapeutic anticoagulation. They recommend that patients with a previous thromboembolic episode or those with persistent risk factors undergo anticoagulation therapy for at least 1 year. Patients who have had more than two thromboembolic episodes should be treated indefinitely.

Heparin-associated thrombocytopenia, an important drug reaction, is discussed in Chapter 45. The most common complication of warfarin therapy is bleeding. In one report, major hemorrhage requiring transfusions or termination of oral anticoagulation therapy occurred in 2% of patients, and minor bleeding occurred in 4.8%.[62] Skin necrosis is another important complication. Warfarin-induced skin necrosis begins as a painful erythematous patch of skin that rapidly progresses to a hemorrhagic area. Necrosis occurs and is followed by infection.

More than 90% of patients affected are women, and necrosis generally begins between the second and fifth days of therapy.[62] A postulated mechanism is microvascular thrombosis secondary to depletion of protein C. Therefore, it has been suggested that warfarin be stopped and heparin restarted as soon as this problem is recognized.

The most important contraindication to warfarin therapy is pregnancy because of warfarin's association with many fetal abnormalities. In a review of 418 pregnancies in which warfarin was given, it was noted that one sixth of the pregnancies resulted in abnormal live-born infants and another one sixth ended in abortion with stillbirths. Complications were seen most frequently when warfarin was used during the first trimester of pregnancy. Pregnant patients should be maintained on subcutaneous heparin or should be considered for vena cava interruption. Heparin is associated with a somewhat higher incidence of prematurity and stillbirths than is warfarin. The overall fetal mortality is approximately 20% in both groups. However, warfarin is associated with a tenfold higher incidence of congenital abnormalities.[63]

The following well-described conditions and drugs potentiate the effects of warfarin:

Conditions:	Amiodarone
Alcoholism	Clofibrate
Cardiac, hepatic, or renal failure	H_2-receptor blockers
	Sulfa drugs
Cholestasis	Danazol
Hypoalbuminemia	Disulfiram
Fever	Glucagon
Malnutrition	Metronidazole
	Quinidine
Drugs:	Tamoxifen
Aspirin	Thyroxine
NSAIDs	

Thrombolytic Therapy

It would seem that rapid clot lysis with plasminogen activators should improve the outcome in treating PE patients. Advocates of lytic therapy observe that the case fatality rate of 15% for PE, which has not improved since the 1960s,[64] is unacceptable but not surprising since the usual treatment for PE continues to be anticoagulation therapy alone.

Thrombolytic therapy can accelerate clot lysis, improve pulmonary reperfusion, and rapidly reverse right heart failure, the usual immediate cause of death in PE.[65] It has been postulated that the high initial recurrence rates with the use of anticoagulation therapy alone that were reported in some studies occurred because of the failure to lyse the embolic source from the pelvic or deep leg veins. Proponents of thrombolytic therapy maintain that recurrence could be averted by aggressive thrombolytic therapy. Initially, it was widely reported that there was no improved long-term survival or reduction in morbidity in PE patients treated with thrombolytic therapy in comparison to those undergoing conventional anticoagulation therapy.[66-68] Longer follow-up may temper this initial pessimistic view of the use of lytic therapy. Follow-up of Urokinase Pulmonary Embolism Trial (UPET) patients, which averages 7 years, has indicated that patients who underwent lytic therapy had more complete resolution of PE.[69] This result was documented by preservation of the normal pulmonary vascular response to exercise. Patients treated with heparin alone demonstrated a markedly abnormal rise in pulmonary artery pressure and pulmonary vascular resistance when undergoing bicycle exercise. In addition, the PE patients assigned to heparin only were in a more symptomatic functional class than those who had initially received thrombolysis followed by heparin.

Recently, recombinant tissue plasminogen activator (rt-PA) has been approved for use in PE thrombolysis. rt-PA lysis is clot-specific rather than systemic. It activates plasminogen without depleting fibrinogen. Thus, rt-PA offers the potential of thrombolytic efficacy with fewer bleeding complications, when compared to streptokinase and urokinase.[70] Trials by Goldhaber and colleagues[70-74] have shown that rt-PA dissolved thrombi more rapidly and with fewer bleeding problems than did urokinase. In these studies lysis was checked with a combination of a 2-hour angiogram and a 24-hour lung scan. The three FDA-approved thrombolytic regimens for PE are listed in Table 12-5.

TABLE 12-5 FDA-Approved Thrombolytic Regimens for Pulmonary Embolism*

Agent	Regimen
Streptokinase	250,000 IU as loading dose over 30 min, followed by 100,000 U/hr for 24 hr
Urokinase	2000 IU/lb as loading dose over 10 min, followed by 2000 IU/lb/hr for 12 to 24 hr
Recombinant-PA	100 mg as continuous peripheral intravenous infusion administered over 2 hr

*From Goldhaber SZ. Recent advances in the diagnosis and lytic therapy of pulmonary embolism. Chest (Suppl) 99:179S, 1991.

The risk of bleeding from lytic therapy is not precisely known but is probably somewhat greater than the risk associated with conventional anticoagulation. In the UPET study,[9] 10% of patients who received urokinase, as opposed to only 4% of patients treated with heparin, had bleeding of sufficient magnitude to require cessation of therapy or transfusion.

Controversy still persists concerning the role of thrombolytic agents in the primary treatment of venous thromboembolism. In 1980, a consensus development conference of the National Institutes of Health suggested that thrombolytic therapy was not being used often enough. Their guidelines recommended the use of thrombolytic therapy for patients with obstruction of blood flow to a lobe or multiple pulmonary segments and for patients with hemodynamic compromise regardless of the anatomic size of the embolus. A multicenter study in the United States recently carried out a 1-year survey in patients with PE diagnosed by high-probability lung scan or positive pulmonary angiogram. This randomized trial, the Thrombolysis in Pulmonary Embolism (TIPE) Patient survey, identified 2539 patients with PE. Overall, 1345 (53%) of these patients would have been acceptable candidates for treatment with thrombolytic therapy.[75]

Thrombolysis has the potential for widespread use as a therapeutic regimen among PE patients rather than being limited to use in patients with massive PE who are hemodynamically unstable. Thrombolytic therapy should help advance the care of patients with venous thromboembolism.

Vena Caval Interruption

In the last 30 years the development of a variety of vena cava interruption devices designed to prevent the occurrence of PE from lower extremity DVT has taken place. Vena cava interruption initially required a laparotomy for either suturing or clipping of the vena cava. Simpler and safer procedures are now available. Inferior vena cava filters or umbrellas may be inserted via the transvenous approach with the patient under local anesthesia. The procedure can be done in the operating room or the radiology suite.

Four major transvenous devices exist. The Hunter detachable balloon may be used in the rare instance in which total caval interruption is required. The Mobin-Uddin filter, developed in 1967, has been a very effective, well-studied device for the prevention of pulmonary emboli. However, its 5-year patency rate is only 47%. The Greenfield filter (MediTech, Inc./Boston Scientific; Watertown, Mass.), currently the most widely used caval interruption device, has a PE recurrence rate of approximately 5%. Long-term caval patency is 97% at 5 years. The Greenfield filter can be placed via the internal jugular vein or the femoral vein approach can be used. The bird's nest filter (Cook, Bloomington, Ind.) is gaining acceptance as another caval interruption technique. However, the long-term patency and efficacy of this device are still not known.[76]

The following are indications for the use of vena cava filters[77,78]:

Recurrent pulmonary emboli despite anticoagulation therapy

PE or proximal DVT in patients with a contraindication to anticoagulation therapy

Development of bleeding or thromboembolic complications secondary to anticoagulation therapy

Progression or extension of an iliofemoral thrombus despite adequate anticoagulation therapy

Demonstration of large, free-floating thrombi in iliac veins or the inferior vena cava

Need for prophylaxis in patients at very high risk for recurrent PE

CNS bleeding and lower extremity fractures in patients with multiple trauma

Treatment following a single massive PE event when a recurrent embolus may prove fatal

Pulmonary Embolectomy

Currently, surgical embolectomy is reserved for patients with postembolic systemic hypotension who have an absolute contraindication to thrombolytic therapy or those who deteriorate despite thrombolytic therapy. The outcome is dependent on surgical skill, interval to surgical intervention, and degree of cardiopulmonary disease. An emergency embolectomy is occasionally truly lifesaving.[79]

Since the advent of cardiopulmonary bypass, the operative mortality for pulmonary embolectomy has steadily fallen from a rate of 60% to approximately 15%. The major sources of morbidity and mortality are severe, prolonged hypoxia, acidosis, and shock, as well as cardiopulmonary arrest prior to angiography or the induction of anesthesia. Patients in such moribund states should be placed on partial cardiopulmonary bypass prior to angiography or induction of anesthesia.[80-82] A few patients have been saved through extracorporeal membrane oxygen support with or without pulmonary embolectomy.[83,84] Most surgeons place a vena cava filter in patients who are undergoing pulmonary embolectomy. Complications of pulmonary embolectomy include hemorrhagic infarction and massive endobronchial hemorrhage after revascularization of ischemic lung tissue. Other complications, such as bleeding, right ventricular failure, cerebral anoxia, or cardiac arrest, are not necessarily a direct result of the procedure; they can be a result of massive PE or lytic therapy.

SUMMARY

- PE should be considered when (1) worsening hypoxemia and respiratory alkalosis occur in a patient being mechanically ventilated, (2) dyspnea in a patient with COPD does not improve with use of a bronchodilator, (3) patient develops atelectasis or a peripheral infiltrate on CXR, or (4) sudden onset of pulmonary hypertension or elevated CVP occurs.
- Pulmonary angiography is the diagnostic standard. Absolute contraindications include allergy to radiocontrast material and severe pulmonary hypertension.
- A normal V/Q scan in itself rules out PE. Only 5% to 10% of V/Q scans are normal.
- Combining V/Q scanning with duplex ultrasound examination of lower extremities improves sensitivity and specificity for PE. See Fig. 12-2, *A*, for an approach to the stable patient.
- Since mortality associated with PE occurs either in the first hour or before a diagnosis is made, prophylaxis, rather than treatment of an established embolus, reduces mortality more effectively.
- Effective prophylactic measures include low-dose heparin, adjusted-dose heparin, LMWH, warfarin, and sequential compression devices.
- Anticoagulation, with continuous heparin infusion, is the standard therapy. Inadequate anticoagulation in first 24 hours is associated with increased recurrent thromboembolism. Administering warfarin early shortens duration of heparin therapy.
- Thrombolytic therapy can accelerate clot lysis, improve pulmonary reperfusion, and reverse right heart failure. Consider using thrombolytic therapy for patients with obstruction of blood flow to lobe or multiple segments. Future indications for thrombolytic therapy are likely to increase.
- Vena cava filters can be used to reduce morbidity and mortality from PE in clinical conditions listed on p. 127.

REFERENCES

1. Newman G. Pulmonary thromboembolism: A historical perspective. J Thorac Surg 4:1, 1989.
2. Kakkar VV, Flank C, Howe CT, et al. Natural history of postoperative deep vein thrombosis. Lancet 2:230, 1969.
3. Carter C, Gent M. The epidemiology of venous thrombosis. In Hirsch J, Marder V, eds. Hemostasis and Thrombosis: Basic Principles and Practice. Philadelphia: JB Lippincott, 1982, p 805.
4. Dalen JE, Paraskos JA, Ockene IS, et al. Venous thromboembolism: The scope of the problem. Chest (Suppl) 89:370S, 1986.
5. Hull RD, Hirsch J, Carter CJ, et al. Pulmonary angiography, ventilation scanning, and venography for clinically suspected pulmonary embolism with abnormal perfusion lung scan. Ann Intern Med 98:891, 1983.
6. Dorfman GS, Cronan JJ, Tuppu TB, et al. Occult pulmonary embolism: A common occurrence in deep vein thrombosis. AJR 148:263, 1987.
7. Moser KM, LeMoine JR. Is embolic risk conditioned by location of deep venous thrombosis? Ann Intern Med 94:439, 1981.
8. Wenger NK, Stein PD, Willis PW. Massive acute pulmonary embolism. The deceivingly non-specific manifestations. JAMA 220:843, 1972.
9. Urokinase Pulmonary Embolism Trial: A national cooperative study. Circulation 47 (Suppl 2):1, 1973.
10. Spence TH. Pulmonary embolization syndrome. In Civetta JM, Kirby RR, Taylor RW, eds. Critical Care. Philadelphia: JB Lippincott, 1988, p 1091.
11. Benotti JR, Dalen JE. Pulmonary embolism. In Rippe JM, Irwin RS, Alpert JS, Dalen JE, eds. Intensive Care Medicine. Boston: Little, Brown, 1985, p 129.
12. Urokinase Pulmonary Embolism Trial. Phase 1 results. JAMA 214:2163, 1970.
13. Alpert JS, Smith R, Carlson CJ, et al. Mortality in patients treated for pulmonary embolism. JAMA 236:1477, 1976.
14. Dalen JE, Haffajee CI, Alpert JS, et al. Pulmonary embolism, pulmonary hemorrhage and pulmonary infarction. N Engl J Med 296:1431, 1977.
15. Goldhaber SZ. Strategies for diagnosis. In Goldhaber SZ, ed. Pulmonary Embolism and Deep Venous Thrombosis. Philadelphia: WB Saunders, 1985, p 79.

16. Goldhaber SZ, Hennekens CH. Time trends in hospital mortality and diagnosis of pulmonary embolism. Am Heart J 104:305, 1982.

17. Robin ED. Overdiagnosis and overtreatment of pulmonary embolism. The emperor may have no clothes. Ann Intern Med 87:775, 1977.

18. Hull RD, Raskob GE, Hirsch J. The diagnosis of clinically suspected pulmonary embolism, practical approaches. Chest (Suppl) 89:417S, 1986.

19. Biello DR, Mattar AG, McKnight RC, Siege BA. Ventilation-perfusion studies in suspected pulmonary embolism. AJR 133:1033, 1979.

20. McNeil BJ. Ventilation-perfusion studies and the diagnosis of pulmonary embolism. J Nucl Med 21:319, 1980.

21. PIOPED Investigators: Value of the ventilation-perfusion scan in acute pulmonary embolism. Results of the prospective investigation of pulmonary embolism diagnosis. JAMA 263:2753, 1990.

22. Hull RD, Hirsch J, Carter C, et al. Diagnostic value of ventilation perfusion in patients with suspected pulmonary embolism and abnormal perfusion scans. Chest 88:819, 1985.

23. Webber MM, Gomes AS, Roe D, et al. Comparison of Biello, McNeil, and PIOPED criteria for the diagnosis of pulmonary emoboli on lung scans. AJR 154:975, 1990.

24. Wheeler AB, Anderson FA. Diagnostic approaches to deep vein thrombosis. Chest (Suppl) 89:407S, 1986.

25. Pollak JE. Doppler ultrasound of the deep leg veins. A revolution in the diagnosis of deep vein thrombosis and monitoring thrombolysis. Chest 99:1655, 1991.

26. Lensing AWA, Prandoni P, Brandjes D. Detection of deep vein thrombosis by real time B-mode ultrasonography. N Engl J Med 320:342, 1989.

27. Montefusco CM, Bakal CW, Sprayregen S, et al. Duplex ultrasonographic venography: The definitive diagnostic tool for thrombophlebitis. In Veith FJ, ed. Current Clinical Problems in Vascular Surgery. St. Louis: Quality Medical Publishing, 1989, p 145.

28. Hull RD, Raskob GE, Coules G, et al. A new noninvasive management strategy for patients with suspected pulmonary embolism. Arch Intern Med 149:2549, 1989.

29. Hull RD, Raskob GE, Hirsch J. Prophylaxis of venous thromboembolism: An overview. Chest (Suppl) 89:374S, 1986.

30. Collins R, Scrimgeour A, Yusuf S, et al. Reduction in fatal embolism and venous thrombosis by perioperative administration of subcutaneous heparin. N Engl J Med 318:1162, 1988.

31. An international multicenter trial: Prevention of fatal pulmonary embolism by low doses of heparin. Lancet 2:45, 1975.

32. Kakkar VV, Corrigan T, Spindler J, et al. Efficacy of low doses of heparin in prevention of deep vein thrombosis after major surgery. A double blind randomized trial. Lancet 2:101, 1972.

33. Leyvarz PF, Bachmann F, Richard J, et al. Adjusted versus fixed dose heparin in the prevention of deep vein thrombosis after total hip replacement. N Engl J Med 309:954, 1983.

34. Turpie ACG. Low molecular weight heparins: Deep vein thrombosis prophylaxis in elective hip surgery and thrombotic stroke. Acta Chir Scand (Suppl) 543:85, 1988.

35. Berqvist D. Prophylaxis of postoperative deep vein thrombosis in general surgery: Experience with fragmin. Acta Chir Scand (Suppl) 543:87, 1988.

36. Hauch O, Jorgensen LN, Kolle TR, et al. Low molecular weight heparin (Logiparin™) as thromboprophylaxis in elective abdominal surgery. Acta Chir Scand (Suppl) 543:90, 1988.

37. Berqvist D, Hedman U, Sjorin E, Holmer E. Anticoagulant effects of two types of low molecular weight heparin administered subcutaneously. Thromb Res 32:381, 1983.

38. Francis CW, Marder VJ, Evarts M, et al. Two-step warfarin therapy, prevention of postoperative venous thrombosis without extensive bleeding. JAMA 249:374, 1987.

39. Allenby F, Pflug JJ, Boardman L, Calvin JS. Effects of external pneumatic compression on fibrinolysis in men. Lancet 2:1412, 1973.

40. Tarnaz TJ, Rohr PA, Davidson AG, et al. Pneumatic calf compression, fibrinolysis, and the prevention of deep venous thrombosis. Surgery 88:489, 1980.

41. Inada K, Koike S, Shirai N, et al. Effects of intermittent pneumatic leg compression for prevention of postoperative deep venous thrombosis with special reference to fibrinolytic activity. Am J Surg 155:602, 1988.

42. Scurr JH, Coleridge-Smith PD, Hasty JH. Regimen for improved effectiveness of intermittent pneumatic compression in deep venous thrombosis prophylaxis. Surgery 102:816, 1987.

43. Moser KM. Venous thromboembolism. Am Rev Resp Dis 141:235, 1990.

44. Pandolfi M, Robertson B, Isaacsson S, Nilsson IM. Fibrinolytic activity of human veins in arms and legs. Thromb Diath Hemorrh 20:247, 1968.

45. Knight MTM, Dawson R. Effect of intermittent compression of the arms on deep venous thrombosis in the legs. Lancet 2:1265, 1976.

46. Barritt DW, Jordan SD. Anticoagulant drugs in the treatment of pulmonary embolism. A controlled trial. Lancet 1:1309, 1960.
47. Hull RD, Raskob GE, Hirsch J, et al. Continuous intravenous heparin compared with intermittent subcutaneous heparin in the initial treatment of proximal vein thrombosis. N Engl J Med 315:1109, 1986.
48. Basu D, Gallus A, Hirsch J, et al. A prospective study of the value of monitoring heparin treatment with the activated partial thromboplastin time. N Engl J Med 287:324, 1972.
49. Deykin D. Regulation of heparin therapy. N Engl J Med 287:355, 1972.
50. Stead R. Clinical pharmacology. In Goldhaber SZ, ed. Pulmonary Embolism and Deep Vein Thrombosis. Philadelphia: WB Saunders, 1985, p 99.
51. Kelton JG, Hirsch J. Bleeding associated with antithrombotic therapy. Semin Hematol 17:259, 1980.
52. Gallus A, Jackman J, Tillet J, et al. Safety and efficacy of warfarin started early after submassive venous thrombosis or pulmonary embolism. Lancet 2:1293, 1986.
53. Rosiello RA, Clan CK, Tencza F, et al. Timing of oral anticoagulation therapy in the treatment of angiographically proven acute pulmonary embolism. Arch Intern Med 147:1469, 1987.
54. Hull RD, Hirsch J, Jay R, et al. Different intensities of oral anticoagulation therapy in the treatment of proximal vein thrombosis. N Engl J Med 307:1076, 1982.
55. O'Sullivan EE. Duration of anticoagulant therapy in venous thromboembolism. Med J Aust 2:1104, 1972.
56. Holmgren K, Andersson G, Fagrelli B, et al. One-month versus six-month therapy and the probabilities of recurrent thromboembolism and hemorrhage. Am J Med 81:255, 1986.
57. Hull RD, Delmore T, Genton E, et al. Warfarin sodium versus low dose heparin in the long-term treatment of venous thrombosis. N Engl J Med 301:355, 1979.
58. Hull RD, Carter C, Hirsch J, et al. Adjusted subcutaneous heparin versus warfarin sodium on the long-term treatment of venous thrombosis. N Engl J Med 306:189, 1982.
59. Wheeler AP, Jaquess RDB, Newman JH. Physician practices in the treatment of pulmonary embolism and deep venous thrombosis. Arch Int Med 148:132, 1988.
60. Monreal M, Ruiz J, Salvador R, et al. Recurrent pulmonary embolism: A prospective study. Chest 95:976, 1989.
61. Hirsch J, Hull RD. Treatment of venous thromboembolism. Chest (Suppl) 89:426S, 1986.
62. Peterson CE, Kwaan HC. Current concepts of warfarin therapy. Arch Int Med 146:581, 1986.
63. Hall JG, Pauli RM, Wilson KM. Maternal and fetal sequelae of anticoagulation during pregnancy. Am J Med 68:122, 1980.
64. Goldhaber SZ. Pulmonary embolism death rates. Am Heart J 115:342, 1988.
65. Come PL, Kim D, Parker JA, et al. Early reversal of right ventricular dysfunction in patients with acute pulmonary embolism after treatment with tissue plasminogen activator. J Am Coll Cardiol 10:971, 1987.
66. Sasahara AA, Sharma GVRK, McIntyre K, et al. A national cooperative trial of pulmonary embolism, phase 1 results of urokinase therapy. J Louisiana State Med Soc 124:130, 1972.
67. Tibbutt DA, Dawes JA, Anderson JA, et al. Comparison controlled clinical trial of streptokinase and heparin in treatment of major pulmonary embolism. Br Med J 1:393, 1974.
68. Ly B, Arnesen J, Eie H, et al. A controlled trial of streptokinase and heparin in the treatment of major pulmonary embolism. Acta Med Scand 203:465, 1978.
69. Sharma GVRK, Folland ED, McIntyre KM, Sasahara AA. Long-term hemodynamic benefit of thrombolytic therapy in pulmonary embolic disease [abstract]. J Am Coll Cardiol 15:65A, 1990.
70. Goldhaber SZ, Vaughan DE, Markis JE, et al. Acute pulmonary embolism treated with tissue plasminogen activator. Lancet 2:886, 1986.
71. Goldhaber SZ, Meyerovitz MF, Markis JE, et al. Thrombolytic therapy of acute pulmonary embolism: Current status and future potential. J Am Coll Cardiol 10:96B, 1987.
72. Goldhaber SZ, Markis JE, Kessler CM, et al. Perspectives in treatment of acute pulmonary embolism with tissue plasminogen activator. Semin Thromb Hemost 13:221, 1987.
73. Goldhaber SZ, Kessler CM, Hert J, et al. A randomized controlled trial of recombinant tissue plasminogen activator versus urokinase in the treatment of acute pulmonary embolism. Lancet 2:293, 1988.
74. Goldhaber SZ. Recent advances in the diagnosis and lytic therapy of pulmonary embolism. Chest (Suppl) 99:179S, 1991.
75. Terren M, Goldhaber SZ, Thompson RO, TIPE investigators. Selection of patients with acute pulmonary embolism for thrombolytic therapy: The Thrombolysis in Pulmonary Embolism (TIPE) survey. Chest (Suppl) 95:279S, 1989.

76. Greenfield L. Vena cava interruption devices and results. In Bergan JJ, Yao JTS, eds. Venous Disorders. Philadelphia: WB Saunders, 1991, p 555.
77. Kempczinski RF. Surgical prophylaxis of pulmonary embolism. Chest (Suppl) 89:384S, 1986.
78. Greenfield LJ. Current indications for, and results of, Greenfield filter placement. J Vasc Surg 1:502, 1984.
79. Hoaglund PM. Massive pulmonary embolism. In Goldhaber SZ, ed. Pulmonary Embolism and Deep Venous Thrombosis. Philadelphia: WB Saunders, 1985, p 179.
80. Mattox KL, Feldman RW, Beall AC, et al. Pulmonary embolectomy for acute massive pulmonary embolism. Ann Surg 195:726, 1982.
81. Sautter R, Myers WO, Ray JF, et al. Pulmonary embolectomy: Review and current status. In Sasahara AA, Sonnenblick EH, Lesch ML, eds. Pulmonary Emboli. New York: Grune & Stratton, 1974, p 143.
82. Masters RG, Koshal A, Higginson LAJ, et al. Ongoing role of pulmonary embolectomy. Can J Cardiol 4:347, 1988.
83. Cooper JD, Tearsdale S, Neems JM, et al. Cardiorespiratory failure secondary to peripheral pulmonary emboli. Survival following a combination of prolonged extracorporeal membrane oxygenation support and pulmonary embolectomy. J Thorac Cardiovasc Surg 761:876, 1976.
84. Krellenstein DJ, Bryan-Brown CW, Fayena AO, et al. Extracorporeal membrane oxgyenation for massive pulmonary thromboembolism. Ann Thorac Surg 23:421, 1977.

CHAPTER 13

Nursing Considerations

Becky Jo Lekander · Beth M. Nelson

Critical care nursing encompasses the diagnosis and treatment of human responses to actual or potential life-threatening health problems. Nursing practice focuses on assisting individuals and families to adapt to health problems and to maintain an optimal level of functioning. This chapter addresses selected topics that require physician-nurse collaboration in order to achieve positive patient outcomes.

In the modern SICU, patient care is frequently complex and involves the collaboration of professionals from many disciplines. The critical care nurse is a vital member of the health care team, offering observations and assessments that are essential in formulating diagnostic and treatment plans. Another vital role of the critical care nurse is that of liaison between the patient and family and the health care team. Conferences with family members are important components of the overall care for patients, and nursing staff can indicate the need for such conferences and organize them. For long-term patients in the SICU, four or five consistent nurses, primary nurses, can be an important resource for the patient, the patient's family, and the health care team during the stress of critical illness.

AIRWAY

Virtually all patients in the SICU setting require aggressive pulmonary support and monitoring. The goal of the critical care nurse is restoration and maintenance of normal, independent respiratory function. Astute assessments and appropriate interventions are required to achieve this goal.

Whether the patient is ventilated or is breathing independently, the nurse will perform several key patient assessments: respiratory effort, breaths per minute, respiratory pattern, breath sounds, and ability to handle secretions. The nurse also assesses the patient's level of pain, restlessness, and fear. Typically, the patient who is in need of intensive nursing care is assessed at least every 2 hours; however, this standard may vary among institutions.

Nonintubated Patients

Nursing interventions are guided by assessment findings and specific physician orders. The objective is to optimize the patient's normal defense mechanisms and respiratory effort. In the nonintubated patient, interventions are focused on maintaining independent respirations by positioning the patient to facilitate breathing and coughing, continuing adequate hydration and humidity to improve secretion removal, and encouraging coughing and breathing exercises. The nurse also must provide analgesics in doses high enough to control pain without suppressing respiratory effort.

Intubated and Tracheostomy Patients

Many patients in respiratory failure require an artificial airway and mechanical ventilation. Usually, patients undergo endotracheal intubation. (A discussion of issues related to tracheostomy is presented in Chapter 11.) Nursing considerations of intubated patients and patients with tracheostomies are summarized in the box.

The basic principles of care for the tracheostomy patient are the following:

Keep stoma clean and dry

Perform tracheostomy care once per shift

Provide adequate humidity

Secure tube with ties or Velcro fasteners

Suction as indicated

Place emergency tracheostomy equipment at bedside

Suctioning

What is routine suctioning? Endotracheal suctioning is performed by nurses to remove secretions from the tracheobronchial tree when a patient cannot cough effectively. Some patients may need to be suctioned as often as every 10 to 15 minutes, whereas others require suctioning only every 4 to 5 hours. Frequently, suctioning is necessary every 1 to 2 hours. The need for suctioning should not be based on policy but on patient assessment.

The most common complication identified with endotracheal suctioning is hypoxemia.[1] Consequently, there are many variations in suctioning techniques aimed at preventing hypoxemia; these include hyperoxygenation, hyperoxygenation/hyperinflation, use of an endotracheal tube adaptor, or use of a closed suction system. A review of the literature demonstrates the need for additional controlled studies to determine the most effective method of preventing hypoxemia.

Communication

Mechanical ventilation is associated with physical and psychologic stress. Pain from the endotracheal tube, suctioning, ventilator alarms, and physical restraints to prevent self-extubation add to the patient's stress level. Loss of speech is a major source of distress in the ventilated patient.[2,3] One of the most important nursing interventions is to find creative ways to help patients communicate their needs and questions. Alphabet boards, paper and pencil, and lipreading are some conventional methods used.

Nursing Care: Intubated Patients With Artificial Airways*

Provide frequent mouth care

Check tube placement often and document position

Secure tube carefully to prevent tracheal damage (tape, twill ties, or Velcro fasteners)

Provide adequate humidity

Move oral tubes side to side at least daily

Suction as indicated

---

*Modified from Neagley SR. The pulmonary system. In Alspach JG, ed. Core Curriculum for Critical Care Nursing. Philadelphia: WB Saunders, 1991, pp 1-131.

EFFECTS OF POSITIONING ON BODY SYSTEMS

Patients in SICUs are restricted to bedrest by virtue of their critical illness. Bedrest has been associated with weakness, muscle atrophy, constipation, urinary retention, decubitus ulcers, thrombophlebitis, pulmonary embolism, atelectasis, pneumonia, osteoporosis, nephrolithiasis, orthostatic intolerance, and depression.

Fluid shift theory provides a basis for understanding the effects of bedrest. During prolonged bedrest, fluid shifts from the lower half of the body to the upper half, resulting in activation of the body's pressure and volume receptors. When the patient stands erect, about 500 ml of blood shifts from the upper body parts to the lower ones because of gravity.[4] This large shift of blood away from the thorax reduces venous return, stroke volume, cardiac output (CO), and arterial pressure. Compensatory mechanisms are then activated to maintain arterial pressure.[5] When the patient is returned to a recumbent position, fluid shifts back to the upper body, activating pressor responses and increasing blood pressure. A reverse Trendelenburg position hastens this response.

Hundreds of studies have been conducted to investigate the effects of bedrest, which are multisystemic and are likely to be more pronounced in criticaly ill persons. Selected systemic effects of bedrest are presented in Table 13-1.

TABLE 13-1 Systemic Effects of Bedrest on Body Systems*

Effect	Clinical Characteristics
Calcium loss	Weight-bearing will reverse this process Exercise and positioning will not prevent calcium loss Urinary calcium excretion begins on day 2 or 3 of bedrest
Blood/plasma volume loss	Diuresis begins 24 hours after bedrest (600 ml within 48 hours) Remaining intravascular volume shifts to upper body, contributing to postural hypotension and tachycardia
Stroke volume reduced	Reduced ventricular filling Results in reduced cardiac output during rest and exercise
Heart rate increased	Increases resting rate 4 to 15 beats/min Heart rate returns to baseline 1 month after patient is mobilized
Orthostatic intolerance	Increased heart rate, decreased pulse pressure, and fainting on sitting Increased risk of falls, fear of changing position or walking, decreased exercise tolerance
Coagulation	Thromboplastin time shortens after 8 days of bedrest Thrombosis is risk due to absence of muscle contraction and weight-bearing in lower extremities Liver synthesizes more fibrinogen
Lung	Abdominal contents push up on diaphragm Inspiratory muscles work in a different plane and gravitational vector All lung volumes except tidal volume are reduced Side-lying position changes blood distribution and flow through lungs
Hormones	Glucose, insulin, and growth hormone peak twice per day rather than once T_3 higher Epinephrine peaks in afternoon rather than morning Aldosterone level drops during midday
Carbohydrate metabolism	Pancreatic function declines Endogenous insulin loses ability to lower serum glucose level
Immune system	Catabolism of immunoglobulin G doubles predisposition to infection Leukocytic activity declines
Gastrointestinal system	Constipation Diarrhea related to impaction
Skeletal muscle	Fatigue due to decreased ATP, decreased glycogen, and increased lactic acid concentration Hypermetabolism potentiates catabolism of skeletal muscle Increased protein degradation Decreased protein synthesis Shortening of muscle fibers, daily loss of 1.3% to 3% of leg strength

*Data from Olson EV, Johnson BJ, Thompsom LF. The hazards of immobility. Am J Nurs 90(3):43-44, 46-48, 1990; Winslow E. Cardiovascular consequences of bed rest. Heart Lung 14:236-246, 1985.

MINIMIZING ADVERSE EFFECTS OF BEDREST

Physiologic responses to turning are highly variable among patients. When prescribing activity therapy, nurses need to consider a patient's individual responses to position changes. Conditions that predispose a patient to adverse reactions from turning include recent surgery (within 12 hours) a cardiac index (CI) of <2.3 L/min/m², use of vasoactive drugs, and mechanical ventilation.

When a patient is being moved from a supine to a sitting position, dangling the patient's legs will help to counterbalance fluid shift and encourage orthostatic stability. Contraindications to this method are hypotension, unstable fractures, acute neurologic events, and hemodynamic instability. Another method aimed at minimizing the negative effects of bedrest is to encourage the patient to assist with repositioning in bed and during transfers from bed to chair. However, it should be noted that such participation may be prohibited by the patient's diminished level of consciousness or labile blood pressure.

Supine and Head-Elevated Positions
Pulmonary artery pressure

Traditionally, critical care nurses obtain pulmonary artery pressure (PAP) measurements with the patient in the flat, supine position to ensure accurate and consistent PAP and pulmonary capillary wedge pressure (PCWP) readings. The flat, supine position may compromise the patient's respiratory or cardiovascular function. Frequent PAP measurements may contribute to sleep disturbances, increased discomfort, and compromised respiratory function. In addition, nursing time may be increased by repositioning a patient if PAP measurements are required several times each hour.

Recent studies suggest that patients need not lie flat for accurate PAP measurements to be obtained. Based on the results of these studies, there is justification for allowing hemodynamically stable patients to remain in a position with the head elevated to 45 degrees for PAP measurements.[6]

Cardiac output

Similarly, in hemodynamically stable patients, correlations have been found between CO measurements involving back-rest elevations of 20 degrees and those obtained with the patient in the flat, supine position. In unstable patients, the flat, supine position can be used for accurate measurement of CO.[7] If the patient cannot tolerate the flat, supine position, a comparison of the patient's CO in both a flat and a slightly elevated (20 degrees) position should be done; the measurements may be similar.

Lateral Position
Pulmonary artery pressure

Practitioners continue to debate the value of using lateral positions for PAP measurements. According to one study, the difficulty in ascertaining the position of the right atrium in this position may account for unreliable PAP measurements.[8] Studies are currently underway to examine the effects of lateral position on phlebostatic axis.

Cardiac output

When compared to the supine position, lateral positions, especially the left lateral position, have been associated with a higher CO. If it is necessary to obtain CO measurements with the patient in a lateral position, it is recommended that these measurements be compared to those obtained with the patient in a flat, supine position.[7,9]

Mixed venous oxygen saturation

Lateral position changes may result in a decrease in S$\bar{v}$o$_2$ of approximately 9% from the baseline and mild changes in heart rate. These changes are usually transient, and a return to baseline can be expected within 5 minutes. If turning triggers excessive or prolonged changes in S$\bar{v}$o$_2$ or heart rate, the patient should be repositioned to prevent adverse effects and evaluated for changes in CO, arterial oxygen content, and oxygen consumption.[10-12]

Oxygenation

Patients who have unilateral lung disease, such as adult respiratory distress syndrome, should be positioned with their unaffected lung down as much of the time as possible.[13]

Prone Position

Prone positioning may prevent the need for mechanical ventilation in patients with acute lung injury and adult respiratory distress syndrome. Other benefits of this position are a lowered oxygen requirement and decreased morbidity.[14] However, the prone position may create difficulties for some patients. Before positioning a patient in this manner, the nurse must consider the patient's physical ability to achieve the position, the patient's acceptance of it, the risks associated with the position, and the difficulties in manipulating tubes and lines.

EARLY MOBILIZATION

The simplest method of combatting the orthostatic and cardiovascular hazards of bedrest is to have the patient sit, stand, and eventually walk. This intervention requires careful nursing assessment and the collaborative efforts of other health team members. One of the greatest nursing concerns is to determine the amount and type of activity that may benefit the critically ill patient. Complications caused by bedrest and premature ambulation are a major concern. Thus nurses monitor such patients for blood pressure, heart rate, oxygenation, pulse quality, and psychologic response to ambulation. After ambulation, nurses continue to monitor hemodynamic and oxygenation measurements as these variables return to baseline. Normal fluctuations of these measurements during ambulation have not been studied to date. Consistent communication and documentation of the patient's response to activity are vital in order to make decisions regarding increasing activity. Studies concerning the timing, distance, and effects of ambulation after surgery have only recently appeared in nursing literature.

WOUND MANAGEMENT

Since wounds can be a major source of morbidity and mortality, wound management is a major concern in the SICU. Almost all patients have some type of wound, whether surgical or traumatic. In wound care, the nurse's primary objectives are promotion of healing and prevention of infection. To accomplish these goals, the nurse must be aware of the common types of wounds, the stages of healing, and the factors affecting wound healing. The types of wounds routinely seen in the SICU are summarized in the box.

Factors Affecting Wound Healing

Nursing care focuses on the numerous factors affecting wound healing, both intrinsic and extrinsic to the patient. Infection is a major cause of impaired healing and may lead to further breakdown of healthy tissue. Treatment of an infected wound includes several therapies administered by the nurse, including dressing changes used to debride necrotic tissue, and systemic antibiotics.

Nutritional status has a major impact on wound healing. Without appropriate amounts of protein, fats, vitamins, and other nutrients, collagen synthesis and other biochemical processes necessary for tissue regeneration will not take place.[15] Poor nutrition also contributes to an increased risk of infection.[16] All members of the health care team must frequently assess the patient's nutritional status throughout the health process and provide appropriate nutritional therapy. Additional factors that may affect the wound healing capability of the body include medications (e.g., steroids or chemo-

---

Types of Wounds*

Clean: Usually a surgical incision uncontaminated by respiratory or gastrointestinal tract flora
Clean contaminated: A surgical incision that involves respiratory, gastrointestinal, genital, or other organs and minimal drainage
Contaminated: A surgical incision contaminated by unavoidable body fluid or by gross error in sterile technique or excessive drainage; also an accidental wound
Infected: A wound with a positive culture or one with gross inflammation or pus

---

*Modified from Martin M. Wound management and infection control after trauma: Implications for the intensive care setting. Crit Care Nurs Q 11(2):43-49, 1988.

therapeutics), diabetes, age, radiation therapy, tissue hypoxia, and renal failure.

Principles of Wound Management

Management of wounds in the SICU can be a difficult and challenging task. Therapy is guided by the following principles: (1) collect and contain drainage; (2) maintain a moist environment; (3) assess the condition of the wound (color, odor, edema); (4) control pain; (5) remove necrotic tissue; (6) protect the wound from harm; (7) maximize potential functional ability of the affected extremity or area; (8) minimize the risk of infection; and (9) protect skin integrity.

Determination of Appropriate Dressing

The correct dressing is essential for optimal healing. The proper dressing serves to protect the wound and create an environment that promotes wound healing.[17] In selecting an appropriate dressing from the many synthetic and conventional therapies available, the type of wound and the features of the dressing technique are important. Table 13-2 summarizes various types of wound dressing techniques.

Frequency of dressing changes depends on an understanding of the dynamics of the wound and the amount of drainage. Frequent changes may slow healing by debriding granulating tissue.

TABLE 13-2 Techniques for Wound Management*

Technique	Description	Advantages	Disadvantages
Dry-dry	Layer of cotton gauze (wide mesh) next to wound surface is covered by second layer Debris and exudate are trapped in gauze and removed when dressing is changed	Good mechanical debridement Absorbs nonviscous exudate Cost-effective	Pain on removal Possible detachment of viable epidermal cells on removal Possible wound desiccation
Wet-dry	Layer of wide mesh gauze is saturated with antibacterial solution (triple antibiotic, amphotericin) or physiologic solution (Dakin's) and placed next to wound surface and covered by second layer of gauze moistened by same solution Necrotic tissue and debris are softened As dressing dries, debris adheres to dressing and is removed via dressing change Contact layer should be completely dry when removed to optimize debridement	Good mechanical debridement Good dilution and absorption of viscous exudate Can be used in conjunction with medications in solution Wound desiccation less likely than with dry/dry Cost-effective	Pain on removal Possible detachment of viable epidermal cells on removal

*Modified from Cuzzell J. Artful solutions to chronic problems. Am J Nurs 85:162-166, 1985. *Continued.*

TABLE 13-2   Techniques for Wound Management—cont'd

Technique	Description	Advantages	Disadvantages
Wet-damp	Variation of wet to dry, but dressing is changed before completely dry	Can be used in conjunction with medications in solution Good dilution of exudate Wound desiccation unlikely Less pain on removal Cost-effective	Less effective mechanical debridement Less absorptive properties than dry dressing Increased possibility of bacterial proliferation Requires accurate timing to prevent bleeding and detachment of viable cells
Wet-wet	Same as wet to dry, but dressing is kept moist with solution Wound surface is continually bathed and viscous exudate is diluted	Least painful Can be used in conjunction with medications in solution Continuous cleansing of wound surface with dilution of exudate No wound desiccation Cost-effective	Less effective mechanical debridement Possible maceration of viable tissue Increased probability of bacterial proliferation Little to no absorptive property
Biologic skin substitutes	Cadaver allograft or porcine heterografts are applied to wound surface Causes local leukocytosis, which is a means of debridement (liquifies necrotic material)	Little pain on removal Most natural covering for open wounds Rapid liquefaction of necrotic debris	Close monitoring of local response that may simulate infection Expensive Requires special storage Requires time-consuming application
Topical enzymes	Proteolytic enzymes derived from plants and bacteria are applied to wound to quicken separation of necrotic tissue	Rapid eschar separation	Expensive Ointments may be difficult to remove from wound surface May elicit local response that simulates infection
Hydrophilic beads, gels, powders	Poured or spread on wound to absorb exudate and cleanse surface	Good absorption of exudate	Expensive Not for dry wounds
Synthetic dressings	Similar to biologic dressings, but made of synthetic material	Rapid softening of necrotic material Little pain when removed	Dressings should remain in place until spontaneous separation occurs Close monitoring is necessary for signs of infection

THERAPEUTIC BEDS AND MATTRESS OVERLAYS

Complicated wound management and complications of immobility may require the use of therapeutic beds and mattress overlays, which vary in cost and effectiveness. The ones most often used in critical care settings are described briefly here.

Air-fluidized beds (Clinitron and Skytron) and low air-loss beds (KinAir, Flexicair, and Mediscus) provide pressure relief. These beds are expensive and should be prescribed only after consideration has been given to less expensive mattress overlays, which may provide adequate pressure relief.

For nonobese patients or patients who may

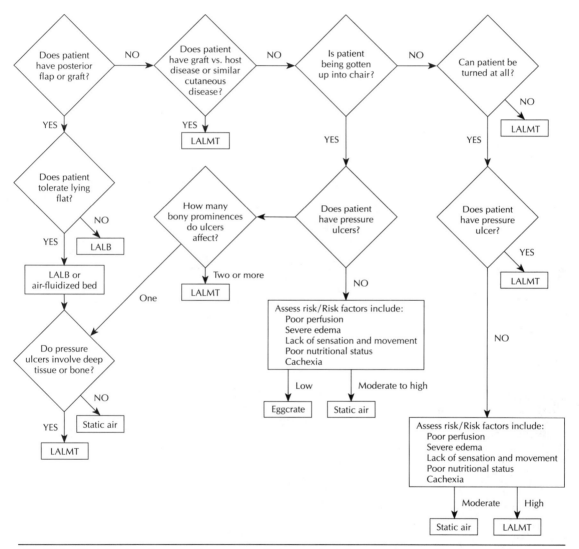

FIG. 13-1 Decision tree for use of pressure-reducing products in management of patients with complicated wounds or complications of immobility. LALMT, low-air-loss topper; LALB, low-air-loss bed. *Note:* Chart does not include RotoRest bed for spinal stabilization or Burke Obese bed for large patients. (Courtesy Kathryn Hoyman, R.N., Minneapolis.)

not need therapy for a long period, a good quality foam pad may offer an excellent means of achieving pressure reduction. As with most mattress overlays, however, foam pads are ineffective if the sheets are tucked so tightly that the patient cannot sink into the foam.

Oscillating beds, such as the RotoRest and Keane mobility beds, are non–pressure-reducing. These beds provide spinal stabilization while rotating the patient to prevent or reduce atelectasis and pneumonia. Clinical studies, however, have failed to prove that oscillating beds prevent orthostatic intolerance, reduced muscle mass, or calcium losses.

Static air mattresses have become increasingly popular in recent years. The mattress is placed on the bed and inflated according to the patient's comfort. Questions have been raised about the safety of this type of mattress during CPR. The speed with which a static air mattress can deflate for CPR should be evaluated before such a mattress is purchased.

Because of the potential costs and variations in effectiveness of therapeutic beds and mattresses, many hospitals have designed systems to determine which ones are best suited to treat specific problems (see Fig. 13-1).

SUMMARY

- Patients who need assessment every 2 hours or more frequently require SICU admission.
- Respiratory assessment includes respiratory effort, respiratory rate, breathing pattern, breath sound variation, and secretion clearance.
- Frequency of endotracheal suctioning depends on patient's state, and suctioning procedures are intended to minimize hypoxemia.
- Use creative means to continue communication with intubated patient.
- Patient mobilization reduces complications of bedrest, including calcium loss, blood volume loss, constipation, and weakness.

- Principles of wound management include control of drainage, prevention of dessication, assessment of wound condition, control of pain, removal of nonviable tissue, protection from noxious factors, preservation of functional ability, and preservation of skin integrity.
- Complicated wound management, prolonged immobility, prolonged use of muscle relaxants, or paralysis may require use of a therapeutic bed or mattress overlay (see Fig. 13-1).

REFERENCES

1. Stone K, Turner B. Endotracheal suctioning. Ann Rev Nurs Res 7:27-49, 1989.
2. Johnson M, Sexton D. Distress during mechanical ventilation. Crit Care Nurse 10(7):48-57, 1990.
3. Saylor J, Stuart BJ. Nurse-patient interaction in the intensive care unit. Heart Lung 14:20-24, 1985.
4. Winslow E. Cardiovascular consequences of bed rest. Heart Lung 14:236-246, 1985.
5. Gauer OH, Thron HL. Postural changes in the circulation. In Hamilton WF, ed. Handbook of Physiology, vol 3, Section 2: Circulation. Washington, D.C.: American Physiological Society, 1965, pp 1409-1439.
6. Cason CL, Lambert CW. Effects of backrest elevation on pulmonary artery pressures. Cardiovasc Nurs 26(1):1-6, 1990.
7. Doering L, Dracup K. Comparisons of cardiac output in supine and lateral positions. Nurs Res 37:114-118, 1988.

8. Kennedy GT, Bryant A, Crawford MH. The effects of lateral body positioning on measurements of pulmonary artery and pulmonary artery wedge pressure. Heart Lung 13:155-158, 1984.

9. Loveys B, Woods S. Current recommendations for thermodilution cardiac output measurement. Prog Cardiovasc Nurs 1:24-32, 1986.

10. Shively M. Effect of position change on mixed venous oxygen saturation in coronary artery bypass surgery patients. Heart Lung 17:51-59, 1988.

11. Tidwell SL, Ryan WJ, Osguthorpe SG, Paull DL, Smith TL. Effects of position changes on mixed venous oxygen saturation in patients after coronary revascularization. Heart Lung 19:574-578, 1990.

12. Winslow EH, Clark AP, White KM, Tyler DO. Effects of a lateral turn on mixed venous oxygen saturation and heart rate in critically ill adults. Heart Lung 19(Pt 2):557-561, 1990.

13. Schmitz T. Fact or myth? Patients with pulmonary disease should be placed in the semi-Fowler's position. Focus on Critical Care–AACN 18(1):58-64, 1991.

14. Langer M, Mascheroni D, Marcolin R, Gattinoni L. The prone position in ARDS patients. A clinical study. Chest 94(1):103-107, 1988.

15. Young ME. Malnutrition and wound healing. Heart Lung 17:60-67, 1988.

16. Martin M. Wound management and infection control after trauma: Implications for the intensive care setting. Crit Care Nurs Q 11(2):43-49, 1988.

17. Meehan P, Mayz E. Nursing management of an open abdominal wound. Crit Care Nurse 8(4):29-34, 1988.

SUGGESTED READINGS

Cuzzell J. Artful solutions to chronic problems. Am J Nurs 85:162-166, 1985.

Hoenig HM, Rubenstein LZ. Hospital-associated deconditioning and dysfunction. J Am Geriatr Soc 39:220-222, 1991.

Lekander BJ, Hoyman K. Improved care of critically ill patients: Contributions of therapeutic beds and mattresses. Perspect Crit Care 1(2):49-68, 1988.

Neagley SR. The Pulmonary System. In Alspach JG, ed. Core Curriculum for Critical Care Nursing. Philadelphia: WB Saunders, 1991, pp 1-131.

Noll ML, Fountain RL. Effect of backrest position on mixed venous oxygen saturation in patients with mechanical ventilation after coronary artery bypass surgery. Heart Lung 19:243-251, 1990.

Olson EV, Johnson BJ, Thompson LF. The hazards of immobility. Am J Nurs 90(3):43-44, 46-48, 1990.

Osborne D. Cardiovascular responses of patients ambulated 32 and 56 hours after coronary artery bypass surgery. West J Nurs Res 6:321-324, 1984.

Tyler DO, Winslow EH, Clark AP, White KM. Effects of a 1-minute back rub on mixed venous oxygen saturation and heart rate in critically ill patients. Heart Lung 19(Pt 2):562-565, 1990.

Waite RM, Parsons D. Measurement of $S\bar{v}o_2$, HR, and MAP in myocardial revascularization patients upon initial postoperative activity. Crit Care Nurse 11(5):87-91, 1991.

Waldhausen JH, Schirmer BD. The effect of ambulation on recovery from postoperative ileus. Ann Surg 212:671-677, 1990.

CHAPTER 14

Role of Rehabilitation

Elizabeth A. Davis

Rehabilitation of the critical surgical patient should begin soon after admission to the hospital. Although bedrest and immobilization are frequently components of patient management in the SICU, inactivity can adversely affect the remaining healthy body functions.

Bedrest has been shown to contribute to the development of contractures, the impairment of muscle strength and endurance, cardiovascular deconditioning, and skin complications.[1]

CONTRACTURES

A contracture may be defined by the lack of full range of motion—active or passive—from joint, muscle, or soft tissue limitations.[2] A variety of conditions may limit the motion, for example, paralysis, level of consciousness, pain, and spasticity. In all of these cases, the problem is lack of mobility. Table 14-1 lists the most common types of contractures affecting joints and methods of prevention.

Prolonged immobilization of joints has been shown to cause contracture of the joint capsule, joint cartilage degeneration, infiltration of fibrofatty connective tissue, and joint ligamentous laxity.[3] Articular connective tissue is continually remodeled with normal activity. When activity is limited, loose areolar connective tissue, which is flexible, reorganizes to form dense connective tissue and restricts motion. Edema, inflammation, and bleeding from trauma may increase the rate of formation of dense connective tissue. This reorganization has been shown to occur in fewer than 7 days.[1] The critical care team should recognize the need for and provide therapy that focuses on the stretching of joints and surrounding muscles and tissues to prevent contracture formation. Motion enhances the flow of synovial fluid, which provides nourishment to cartilage, menisci, and ligaments. Synovial joints require the stimulation of activity to maintain homeostasis.[3] Contractures may interfere with the patient's bed positioning, nursing care, and future mobility. The best treatment of contractures is early prevention through passive or active range-of-motion exercises, positioning, and functional activities.[2,3]

Passive range of motion refers to any movement of an articulation that is produced by an external source.[4] Active range of motion refers to activation of the patient's muscles to move the joint through its complete range. Passive range of motion is used early in prevention of contractures, when the patient cannot actively participate in therapy. When the patient is able, he/she should be encouraged to perform active exercises. Active range of motion will encourage strengthening of supporting muscles, as well as improve the patient's endurance.

A sustained terminal stretch of 20 or 30 minutes during passive or active range of motion should be applied if a contracture has developed.[2,5] The elastic resistance of fibrous tissue is overcome more easily if stretching is done over a long period of time. Serial casting or dynamic splinting may be used for sustained stretching, which is needed with severe spasticity or severe contractures. Heat (e.g., from ultrasonography) also may be applied prior to

| TABLE 14-1 | Common Types of Contractures Affecting Joints |

Joint	Contracture	Prevention
Hip	Flexion	Firm mattress
		Lying prone at least two times a day for 20 min
	External rotation	Trochanter roll
Knee	Flexion	Extended
		Lying prone
		No pillows under hips/knees
Ankle	Flexion	Footboard
		Static splints
Shoulder	Adducted	Firm mattress
	Internally rotated	Pillows or towels to promote abduction, neutral rotation
Elbow	Flexion	Extended
		Static splints
Hands/fingers	Flexion	Resting/functional handsplint

range-of-motion exercises to increase the tissue's elasticity.

To prevent contractures, joints should be taken through their complete range of motion a minimum of twice a day. Proper positioning of the patient in bed is important in minimizing contracture formation. Patients with neurologic involvement (e.g., spinal cord injuries and strokes) need particular attention. Their lack of strength predisposes them to malpositioning. Amputees may develop significant contractures because of muscle imbalance (e.g., hip and/or knee flexion contractures). These contractures, if left untreated, will prevent successful fitting and use of a prosthesis.

Splinting can be used to maintain neutral joint position against the pull of gravity or dominant synergy patterns. Patients at bedrest usually assume a position of comfort, which contributes to the development of flexion contractures.[6] The use of splints can prevent contracture development in patients at prolonged bedrest. Splints are either prefabricated or custom-made and should conform closely to the body surface to prevent pressure breakdown. Skin tolerance determines the length of time a patient may wear a splint. Initial wearing time is usually an interval of 2 hours on and 2 hours off. The cycle should be adjusted in 30-

to 60-minute increments, if skin tolerance allows.

Splints should be serially adjusted to accommodate changes in the joint range of motion. Shortened tendons, ligaments, and muscles may be gradually stretched with serial splinting used to regain the normal range of motion.

The patient should be encouraged to start using the affected extremities as soon as possible to restore function and strength. Each day the critical care team should help to get patients out of bed (if possible), allow them to bear weight, and assist them in ambulation (if possible).

MUSCLE STRENGTH AND ENDURANCE

Immobilization causes muscle fiber atrophy, which directly affects muscle strength and endurance.[7] Fortunately, this process is reversible if no neurogenic etiology, such as paralysis, exists. Muscle fiber atrophy begins after an initial lag and increases in magnitude during the next 5 days.[8]

Prolonged immobilization lowers levels of resting muscle glycogen and ATP and causes more rapid depletion of these substances during work. When compared to normal muscle, immobilized muscle produces a greater increase of lactic acid during work.[9] In 1970, Muller[10] reported that an immobilized muscle will lose approximately 3% of its strength per day. At that rate of loss, a patient who is immobilized for 3 to 4 weeks will lose half of his/her normal muscle strength during that time.

Prevention of loss of muscle strength and endurance involves exercise. Exercise causes hypertrophy of muscle fibers but does not increase the number of fibers. Resumption of normal activities slowly increases muscle strength and endurance. Active exercise accelerates this process.

Exercise can be isometric, isotonic, or isokinetic (see box). The basic goal of strengthening exercises is active recruitment of all the motor units in the muscle. Isometric or isotonic exercises are preferred when the critical care patient can participate in them. Muscle strength can be maintained with isometric contractions of 20% to 30% of maximal tension held for 6 to 10 seconds. These contractions should be performed several times each day.[1] Isometric exercises may be preferred when joint trauma or pain is present. This type of exercise causes little muscle soreness and requires little time. However, isometric exercise can cause a significant increase in blood pressure during exercise. In addition, objective measurement of progress is difficult. Isotonic exercises are performed easily at the bedside when the patient is cooperative and cuff weights are used. Several isotonic training regimens have been developed by DeLorme and Oxford. They recommend five to seven repetitions in three sets of exercise. To activate all the muscle motor units, the weight used should be the maximum for the number of repetitions.[11] Progress with isotonic exercise is followed easily by the

---

Types of Exercise

Isometric
  Static
  Muscle contraction but no movement of load, resulting in no change of muscle length
Isotonic
  Dynamic
  Constant load but uncontrolled speed of movement
Isokinetic
  Dynamic
  Rate of movement controlled but load or force may be variable

---

amount of weight that is used. Muscle soreness is more common after isotonic exercise than after isometric exercise.

Exercise done to increase endurance must improve the overall metabolic capacity of the muscle to sustain work. The actual weight and duration of exercise is not critical for increasing endurance, provided that the muscle is exercised to the point of fatigue. The stimulus to increase the anaerobic or aerobic metabolic capacity of muscle is fatigue of that system.

Cardiovascular deconditioning occurs with bedrest. Stremel et al,[12] measured the $\dot{V}O_2$ max of patients at bedrest with no exercise, static exercise (isometric), and dynamic exercise (isotonic). The least amount of reduction in $\dot{V}O_2$ max was seen during static (4.8%) vs. dynamic (9.2%) exercise. Plasma volume was reduced the least during dynamic exercise. Therefore a combination of static and dynamic exercises is indicated, when possible, to prevent significant cardiovascular deconditioning.

SUMMARY

- Begin rehabilitation soon after patient's admission to SICU.
- Prolonged immobilization causes contractures, loss of muscle strength, and cardiovascular deconditioning.
- Contractures:
  May occur in 7 days or fewer.
  Use passive range of motion twice daily immediately and active range of motion as soon as possible.
  Best treatment is prevention.
- Muscle strength and endurance:
  Maintain muscle strength with isometric contractions of 20% to 30% of maximal tension for 6 to 10 seconds. Repeat several times daily.
  Perform isotonic exercise at bedside with cuff weights if patient is cooperative.
  Exercise patient to point of fatigue.
- Cardiovascular deconditioning:
  Combination of isometric and isotonic exercise minimizes cardiovascular deconditioning.

REFERENCES

1. Kottke FJ. The effects of limitation of activity upon the human body. JAMA 196:117, 1966.
2. Halar EM, Bell KR. Contracture and Other Deleterious Effects of Immobility. In DeLisa JA. Rehabilitation Medicine: Principles and Practice. Philadelphia: JB Lippincott, 1988, p 448.
3. Alkeson WH. Effects of immobilization on joints. Clin Orthop 219:28, 1987.
4. Frank C. Physiology and therapeutic value of passive joint motion. Clin Orthop 185:113, 1984.
5. Kottke FJ. The rationale for prolonged stretching for correction of shortening of connective tissue. Arch Phys Med Rehabil 47:345, 1966.
6. Perry J. Contractures: A historical perspective. Clin Orthop 219:8, 1987.
7. Steinberg FU. The Immobilized Patient: Functional Pathology and Management. New York: Plenum Medical, 1980, p 78.
8. Booth FW. Time course of muscular atrophy during immobilization of hindlimbs in rats. J Appl Physiol 43:656, 1977.
9. Booth FW. Physiologic and biochemical effects of immobilization on muscle. Clin Orthop 219:15, 1987.
10. Muller EA. Influence of training and of inactivity on muscle strength. Arch Phys Med Rehabil 51:449, 1970.
11. Joynt RL. Therapeutic exercise. In DeLisa JA. Rehabilitation Medicine: Principles and Practice. Philadelphia: JB Lippincott, 1988, p 359.
12. Stremel RW, Convertino VA, Bernauer EM, Greenleaf JE. Cardiorespiratory deconditioning with static and dynamic leg exercise during rest. J Appl Physiol 41:905, 1976.

CHAPTER **15**

Optimization of Drug Doses

Pamela K. Borchardt-Phelps · Bruce C. Lohr

The optimization of drug doses in acutely ill patients is a difficult and multifactorial process. The correct dose is one that exerts a desired therapeutic effect while producing a minimal amount of undesirable side effects. Critically ill patients may experience physiologic and pharmacokinetic changes that affect the disposition of medications (e.g., heart failure, renal failure, hepatic failure, trauma, sepsis, burns). To optimize doses, the critical care practitioner first must evaluate these possible physiologic conditions for their effects on the absorption, distribution, metabolism, and excretion of drugs. Other crucial factors to consider include both the condition being treated and other disease states; drug interactions, tolerance, and penetration to the site of action; other drug therapies; the therapeutic index of the drug; toxic effects; and dose-response relationships. These factors are discussed in this chapter in a general way, and a more specific examination is provided for cardiotonic drugs and agents for treating hypertension since use of these classes of drugs is prevalent in the SICU setting.

ABSORPTION

Absorption and bioavailability of a drug are dependent on the drug compound, its vehicle of delivery, its "first-pass" metabolism, and the site of absorption. Bioavailability is defined as the amount of drug that reaches the bloodstream when a drug is given by a chosen route, as compared to the amount of drug reaching the bloodstream when the same drug is given intravenously. Site of absorption depends on route of delivery, which may be oral, rectal, topical, intramuscular, subcutaneous, transdermal, sublingual, or intravenous.

Physiologic changes in a critically ill patient can affect both the first-pass effects and the site of absorption. Drugs absorbed enterically first must be cycled through the portal vein and the liver before reaching the systemic circulation. If a drug is highly metabolized, this enterohepatic cycling results in first-pass metabolism, reducing the bioavailability. If a critically ill patient has severe liver disease, first-pass metabolism may be reduced, resulting in an *increased* bioavailability of the drug. One author advocates a 50% reduction in dosages of highly metabolized ("high-extraction") drugs such as lidocaine, meperidine, metoprolol, morphine, propranolol, and verapamil in patients with chronic liver disease or cirrhosis.[1]

Vasoconstriction and reduced peripheral blood flow in patients with cardiac disease or multisystem organ failure may render the topical, transdermal, IM, or SC routes of administration erratic and ineffective. The presence of ileus or diarrhea may also limit the enteral absorption of drugs given by the oral or rectal route. The presence of enteral feedings can affect the absorption of certain drugs, reducing the bioavailability of phenytoin, for example, by 72%.[2] To ensure adequate drug delivery in SICU patients, the IV route is preferred. Exceptions to this rule include drugs not available in an injectable dosage form (e.g., metolazone, spironolactone, captopril, diltiazem, nifedipine), drugs that exert a local effect (nonabsorbable antibiotics, vancomycin oral solution, nystatin suspension, antacids), drugs whose pharmacodynamic effects are easily measured (transdermal clonidine, antacids, H_2-receptor antagonists), and drugs whose pharmacokinetic changes can be monitored with serum concentrations.

DISTRIBUTION

The volume of distribution (Vd) of a drug is the theoretic volume of serum, tissues, and protein to which a drug is distributed. The Vd is expressed in liters or liters per kilogram. For drugs that remain for the most part in the serum, or central compartment, the Vd may be quite small. For drugs extensively bound to tissues or serum proteins, however, the Vd may be quite large, reaching 100 times the blood volume in some cases. The Vd is used to calculate the effect that an amount of drug administered will have on the serum concentration according to the following equation:

$$\text{Change in concentration} = \text{Dose/Vd}$$

Changes in the volume of distribution can occur in critically ill patients as a result of altered tissue binding, increased or decreased protein binding, or changes in body composition that alter distribution compartments of a drug. For instance, altered body fluid composition has been suggested as a mechanism for increased aminoglycoside Vd in critically ill patients.[3] Critically ill patients frequently need larger-than-usual doses of aminoglycosides to achieve desired therapeutic serum concentrations because of a larger Vd. Likewise, patients

with significant fluid shifts (e.g., with burns, ascites) may also require larger doses of drugs that freely distribute into these fluid compartments. Protein-binding changes frequently occur in critically ill patients. Most acidic drug compounds bind to albumin, and protein binding can be reduced or altered as a result of hypoalbuminemia, malnutrition, or renal disease. Basic drugs such as lidocaine bind to alpha-1 acid glycoprotein, and protein binding can increase as a result of release of acute-phase reactants. The end result is an increase or decrease in the amount of free, or unbound, drug available to exert a therapeutic effect. The impact of an increase or decrease in free drug is probably significant only in drugs whose protein binding is 90% or greater or those with a narrow therapeutic range. The classic examples include phenytoin and warfarin. Phenytoin free concentrations should be monitored if protein-binding changes are suspected. During renal failure, endogenous substances may compete with digoxin for tissue-binding sites, resulting in a 30% to 50% reduction in the Vd.

METABOLISM

Altered metabolism of drugs can occur in critically ill patients as a result of hepatocellular damage or reduced hepatic blood flow. The impact of liver failure on absorption, first-pass metabolism, and protein binding has already been discussed. The point at which altered metabolism of drugs should cause concern is not clear. A reliable indicator of hepatic clearance of drugs is lacking in the clinical setting. High-extraction drugs are those for which the liver has a large metabolic capacity. The rate-limiting step to the metabolism of these drugs is the rate at which the drug is presented to the liver. The metabolism of these drugs, including lidocaine, meperidine, morphine, metoprolol, propranolol, and verapamil, is reduced when hepatic blood flow is reduced, or altered, as in a patient with cirrhosis.[1] Low-extraction drugs are those for which metabolism is more sensitive to hepatic enzyme capacity and protein binding than to hepatic blood flow. Hepatocellular damage may reduce the metabolism of low-extraction drugs such as ampicillin, chloramphenicol, cimetidine, diazepam, furosemide, prednisone, theophylline, and warfarin. Metabolism of certain benzodiazepines through glucuronidation (e.g., lorazepam and oxazepam) is unaffected by chronic hepatic disease.[1] Drugs for which serum concentration monitoring is not routinely available require monitoring for clinical response and signs of toxicity. Drugs of this nature commonly used in the SICU include nitroprusside, fentanyl, midazolam, morphine, calcium channel blockers, meperidine, and beta-blockers. The box lists hepatically cleared drugs commonly used in the SICU that may require dosage reduction in hepatic failure.

EXCRETION

Altered excretion of drugs commonly occurs in critically ill patients. Renal failure can occur as an end result of sepsis, shock, or the administration of nephrotoxic drugs such as amphotericin B, aminoglycosides, and contrast agents. The estimation of the glomerular filtration rate (GFR) and the effects of renal insufficiency on the elimination of drugs presents a challenge to the clinical practitioner. Judging the degree of renal dysfunction on the basis of a serum creatinine level alone could lead to significant dosing errors. In critically ill patients the serum creatinine level is not a reliable indicator of changes in the elimination rate of renally excreted drugs. Fuhs et al.[4] found no correlation between changes in physiologic variables such as serum creatinine and actual body weight or temperature and the measured pharmacokinetic parameters of aminoglycosides. Drug dosages frequently are altered on the basis of creatinine clearance, either estimated or measured. The most accurate determination of a creatinine clearance is through a 24-hour collection of urine for creatinine measurement. Even this method may overestimate actual GFR.[5] Creatinine clearance is estimated by using the methods of Cockcroft and Gault[6] or Jellife.[7,8] These equations take into consideration variables such as body weight, age, and serum creatinine to estimate an individual creatinine clearance.

$$CrCl(ml/min) = (140 - Age)(Weight \ in \ kilograms)/(72)(Serum \ creatinine)$$

For females, multiply the above equation by 0.85.

$$CrCl(ml/min) = 114 - (Age \times 0.8)/Serum \ creatinine$$

For females, multiply the above equation by 0.9.

The assumption made when using these equations is that the elimination of creatinine is at steady state. In a patient with rapidly declining renal function, the assumption is false, and the result is an overestimation of creatinine clearance.

Once an estimated creatinine clearance has been obtained, Table 15-1 can be used for guidance in initiating drug therapy. The drug therapy must be reevaluated on at least a daily basis for changes in renal function, serum concentration monitoring, evidence of drug efficacy, and signs of toxicity. Initial dosages can then be modified to meet the therapeutic needs of individual patients. Hepatically metabolized drugs can also be affected by renal failure. Meperidine's active metabolite, normeperidine, requires elimination by the kidney. Normeperidine has the ability to cause CNS excitation. In the presence of compromised renal function or high doses of meperidine, the accumulation of the active metabolite normeperidine has caused seizures.[9] Procainamide is metabolized to an active metabolite, *N*-acetylprocainamide (NAPA). Although NAPA shares some of the ther-

---

Drugs That May Require Dose Reduction in Patients With Hepatic Failure*

Clindamycin	Procainamide
Chloramphenicol	Disopyramide
Erythromycin	Verapamil
Rifampin	Diazepam
Nafcillin	Midazolam
Lidocaine	Theophylline
Labetalol	Nitroprusside
Metropolol	Fentanyl
Pindolol	Morphine
Prazosin	Meperidine
Propranolol	Dilitazen
Quinidine	Nifedipine

*Modified from Williams RL. Drug administration in hepatic disease. N Engl J Med 309:1616, 1983; McEvoy GK, ed. American Hospital Formulary Service Drug Information. Bethesda, Md.: American Society of Hospital Pharmacists, 1991.

TABLE 15-1   Dosage Modification of SICU Drugs in Patients With Renal Impairment*

Drug	Usual Dose	Dose Adjusted for Creatinine Clearance (ml/min)		
		30-50	10-30	<10
Acyclovir	5 mg/kg IV q 8 hr	5 mg/kg q 12 hr	5 mg/kg q 24 hr	2.5 mg/kg q 24 hr
Amphotericin B†	0.2-1.5 mg/kg IV qd	Unchanged	Unchanged	Unchanged
Ampicillin	1-2 g IV q 4-6 hr	Unchanged	1-2 g q 6-8 hr	1-2 g q 8-12 hr
Ampicillin plus sulbactam (Unasyn)	1.5-3 g IV q 6 hr	1.5-3 g q 8 hr	1.5-3 g q 12 hr	1.5-3 g q 24 hr
Atenolol	50-100 mg po qd	Unchanged	50 mg po qd	50 mg po qod
Aztreonam	1-2 g IV q 6-8 hr	Unchanged	500 mg-1 g q 6-8 hr	250-500 mg q 6-8 hr
Captopril	25-50 mg po bid or tid	Unchanged	Unchanged	12.5-25 mg bid or tid
Cefamandole	1-2 g IV q 6 hr	1-2 g q 8 hr	1 g q 8 hr	1 g q 12 hr
Cefazolin	1 g IV q 8 hr	1 g q 12 hr	500 mg q 12 hr	500 mg q 24 hr
Cefotaxime	1-2 g IV q 6-8 hr	Unchanged	1-2 g q 8-12 hr	1-2 g q 12-24 hr
Cefoxitin	1-2 g IV q 6 hr	1-2 g q 8-12 hr	1-2 g q 12-24 hr	500 mg-1 g q 12-24 hr
Ceftazidime	1-2 g IV q 8 hr	Unchanged	1-2 g q 12 hr	1-2 g q 24 hr
Ceftriaxone	1-2 g IV q 24 hr	Unchanged	Unchanged	Unchanged
Cefuroxime	750 mg-1.5 g IV q 8 hr	Unchanged	750 mg-1.5 g q 12 hr	750 mg-1.5 g q 24 hr
Cimetidine	300 mg po/IV q 6-8 hr	Unchanged	300 mg q 12 hr	300 mg q 12-24 hr
Ciprofloxacin	500-750 mg po q 12 hr	250-500 mg po q 12 hr	250-500 mg po q 18 hr	250-500 mg po q 24 hr
	200-400 mg IV q 12 hr	Unchanged	200-400 mg IV q 18-24 hr	200-400 mg IV q 24 hr
Clindamycin	600-900 mg IV q 8 hr	Unchanged	Unchanged	Unchanged
Clonidine	0.1-0.4 mg po bid	Unchanged	Unchanged	0.05-0.2 mg po bid
Corticosteroids	Variable	Unchanged	Unchanged	Unchanged
Digoxin	0.125-0.375 IV qd	0.125 alternating with 0.25 qd	0.125 qd	0.125 qod
Diltiazem	30-60 mg po q 6-8 hr *or* 60-120 mg slow release po bid	Unchanged	Unchanged	Unchanged

*Modified from McEvoy GK, ed. American Hospital Formulary Service Drug Information. Bethesda, Md.: American Society of Hospital Pharmacists, 1991; Bennett WM, Aronoff GR, Golper TA, et al. Drug Prescribing in Renal Failure. Philadelphia: American College of Physicians, 1987, pp 1-119.
†In a patient with renal failure, the usual dose of amphotericin B is 0.5 mg/kg IV qod.   *Continued.*

TABLE 15-1 Dosage Modification of SICU Drugs in Patients With Renal Impairment—cont'd

Drug	Usual Dose	Dose Adjusted for Creatinine Clearance (ml/min)		
		30-50	10-30	<10
Enalapril	2.5-20 mg po qd or bid	Unchanged	Unchanged	1.25-10 mg qd or bid
Fluconazole	200-400 mg po/ IV qd	100-200 mg qd	50-100 mg qd	50-100 mg qod
Flucytosine	37.5 mg/kg po q 6 hr	37.5 mg/kg q 8-12 hr	37.5 mg/kg q 12-24 hr	37.5 mg/kg q 24-48 hr
Ganciclovir	2.5 mg/kg IV q 8-12 hr	2.5 mg/kg q 12 hr	2.5 mg/kg q 24 hr	1.25 mg/kg q 24 hr
Gentamicin	1.5-2 mg/kg IV q 8 hr	1.5-2 mg/kg q 12-18 hr	1.5-2 mg/kg q 24-48 hr	Follow serum concentrations
Haloperidol	1-4 mg IM q 4-6 hr	Unchanged	Unchanged	Unchanged
Hydralazine	10-100 mg po qid	Unchanged	Unchanged	10-100 mg q 8-24 hr
Imiprenem-cilas-tatin (Pri-maxin)	500 mg-1 g IV q 6 hr	500 mg q 6-8 hr	500 mg q 8-12 hr	250-500 mg q 12 hr
Labetalol	100-200 mg po q 12 hr	Unchanged	Unchanged	Unchanged
Metoprolol	50-100 mg po bid	Unchanged	Unchanged	Unchanged
Metronidazole	500 mg IV or po q 6 hr	Unchanged	Unchanged	500 mg or po q 8 hr
Nafcillin	1-2 g IV 4-6 hr	Unchanged	Unchanged	Unchanged
Nifedipine	10-30 mg po tid-qid *or* 30-60 mg SR qd-bid	Unchanged	Unchanged	Unchanged
Piperacillin	3-4 g IV q 6 hr	3-4 g q 8 hr	3-4 g q 12 hr	3-4 g q 12 hr
Procainamide	250 mg-1 g po q 4-6 hr *or* IV 2-3 mg/ min	750 mg-1 g q 6 hr 2 mg/min	375-500 mg q 6 hr 1 mg/min	375 mg q 8 hr 0.5 mg/min
Propranolol	10-80 mg po q 6 hr	Unchanged	Unchanged	Unchanged
Ranitidine	50 mg IV q 6-8 hr	Unchanged	50 mg q 12 hr	50 mg q 12-24 hr
Rifampin	600 mg po qd	Unchanged	Unchanged	Unchanged
Sulfamethoxa-zole plus tri-methoprim (Bactrim)	2-7.5 mg/kg (TMP) IV q 6-12 hr	Unchanged	2-7.5/kg (TMP) q 18 hr	2-7.5 mg/kg q 24 hr (TMP)
Ticarcillin	3-4 g IV q 4-6 hr	3-4 g q 6-8 hr	2 g q 8 hr	2 g q 12 hr

TABLE 15-1 Dosage Modification of SICU Drugs in Patients With Renal Impairment—cont'd

Drug	Usual Dose	Dose Adjusted for Creatinine Clearance (ml/min)		
		30-50	10-30	<10
Ticarcillin plus clavulanate (Timentin)	3.1 g IV q 4-6 hr	3.1 g q 6-8 hr	2 g q 8 hr	2 g q 12 hr
Tobramycin	1.5-2 mg/kg IV q 8 hr	1.5-2 mg/kg q 12-18 hr	1.5-2 mg/kg q 24-48 hr	Follow serum concentration
Vancomycin	15 mg/kg IV q 12 hr	15 mg/kg q 24-48 hr Follow serum concentrations	15 mg/kg q 2-7 days Follow serum concentrations	15 mg/kg q 7-10 days Follow serum concentrations
Verapamil	80-120 mg po tid or qid *or* 120-240 mg SR po qd or bid	Unchanged Unchanged	Unchanged Unchanged	Reduce dose 50%-75% Reduce dose 50%-75%
Warfarin	1-10 mg po qd	Unchanged (follow PT)	Unchanged (follow PT)	Unchanged (follow PT)

apeutic benefits of the parent drug, it also shares the potential toxicities. Renal failure patients typically accumulate NAPA, even when procainamide serum concentrations alone are "therapeutic."[10] Both procainamide and NAPA serum concentrations must be measured to ensure that the total dose (procainamide plus NAPA) does not exceed 30 to 35 µg/ml.

USE OF SERUM CONCENTRATIONS

Serum drug concentrations can be useful in guiding drug therapy. They are often used for drugs with a narrow therapeutic index; that is, the drug dose or concentrations producing a desirable effect are very close to, or overlap, the dose or concentration producing an undesirable, or toxic, effect. Serum drug concentrations are also used for drugs for which there is a proven benefit to obtaining a certain peak, trough, or average steady-state concentration. In general, it is desirable to wait until a drug reaches steady state before obtaining serum drug concentrations. *Steady state* indicates that

the drug is in equilibrium with the blood and tissue compartments to which it distributes, and it is achieved after approximately five half-lives of a particular drug. Timing of serum drug concentrations is also important. Drug concentrations are usually either at a peak (immediately after a dose) or in a trough (immediately before a dose). For drugs given by a continuous infusion, blood used to determine serum drug concentrations can be drawn at any time once steady state is achieved. Exceptions to these rules include drugs that take a long time to distribute to tissues such as digoxin. Digoxin concentrations should be drawn at least 6 hours after a dose is given to allow for distribution of the drug. Obviously consideration must be given to the timing of a sample when evaluating serum drug concentrations. Evaluating a peak based on dosing recommendations for a trough concentration would lead to gross dosing errors. A serum drug concentration is evaluated based on a desirable therapeutic range. Patient response should be evaluated in conjunc-

TABLE 15-2 Guidelines for Serum Concentration Monitoring*

Drug	Primary Route of Elimination	Half-Life (hr)	Sampling Time	Therapeutic Range	Toxicity and Comments
Phenobarbital	Hepatic	48	Peak or trough	20-40 μg/ml	Ataxia, nystagmus, drowsiness
Procainamide	Hepatic, renal	2.5-4.9	po: trough IV: at steady state	4-10 μg/ml	Accumulation of NAPA in renal failure
N-acetyl-procainamide (NAPA)	Renal	6-8	Same as procainamide	15-25 μg/ml	Procainamide and NAPA total concentrations should not exceed 35 μg/ml
Theophylline	Hepatic	3-12	po: 1-2 hr after dose IV: at steady state	10-20 μg/ml	Dysrhythmias, convulsions at concentrations exceeding 35 μg/ml
Carbamazepine	Hepatic	10-25	Trough	4-12 μg/ml	Induces own metabolism; dose escalation necessary
Valproic acid	Hepatic	8-17	2-4 hr after dose	50-100 μg/ml	Tremor, irritability at concentrations >100 μg/ml
Cyclosporine	Hepatic	12-24	Trough	50-150 ng/ml	Hypertension, nephrotoxicity
Lidocaine	Hepatic	1.2-2.2	Steady state (5-10 hr)	2-5 μg/ml	Metabolite accumulation in renal disease; half-life prolonged after first 24 hr of therapy (dose reduction may be necessary)
Phenytoin	Hepatic	24	Trough	Total: 10-20 μg/ml Free: 1-2 μg/ml	Measure free concentrations in patients with renal failure and hypoalbuminemia
Quinidine	Hepatic	5-7.2	Trough	2-5 μg/ml	Cinchonism at high concentrations
Flucytosine	Renal	3-6	2 hr after dose	50-100 μg/ml	Bone marrow depression at concentrations >100 μg/ml
Gentamicin	Renal	1.5-3	Peak Trough	4-10 μg/ml <2 μg/ml	Nephrotoxicity, ototoxicity
Tobramycin	Renal	1.5-3	Peak Trough	4-10 μg/ml <2 μg/ml	Nephrotoxicity, ototoxicity
Amikacin	Renal	1.5-3	Peak Trough	15-30 μg/ml <10 μg/ml	Nephrotoxicity, ototoxicity

*Modified from Bennett WM, Aronoff GR, Golper TA, et al. Drug Prescribing in Renal Failure. Philadelphia: American College of Physicians, 1987, pp 1-119; Knoben JE, Anderson PO, eds. Handbook of Clinical Data. Hamilton, Ill.: Drug Intelligence Publications, 1988; Melamed AJ, Dristrian A, Muller RJ, Duafala ME. A table for therapeutic drug monitoring. Hosp Pharm 23:743, 1988.

TABLE 15-2	Guidelines for Serum Concentration Monitoring—cont'd				
Drug	Primary Route of Elimination	Half-Life (hr)	Sampling Time	Therapeutic Range	Toxicity and Comments
Disopyramide	Hepatic, renal	5-8	Trough	2-4 μg/ml	
Acyclovir	Renal	2.1-3.8	Peak	40-80 μmol/L	Nephrotoxicity, CNS toxicity
Digoxin	Renal	36-44	Trough (or at least 6 hr after dose)	0.5-2 ng/ml	Dysrhythmias, CNS toxicity; hypokalemia predisposes to digoxin toxicity
Ethosuximide	Hepatic	60 (adult); 30 (children)	Trough	40-80 μg/ml	Nausea, drowsiness, dizziness
Vancomycin	Renal	6-8	Peak Trough	20-40 μg/ml 5-10 μg/ml	Nephrotoxicity, ototoxicity, "red-man" syndrome with rapid infusions (<1 hr)
Chloramphenicol	Hepatic	2-4	po: 2-3 hr after dose IV: 1-2 hr after infusion	10-25 μg/ml	Peaks >25 μg/ml associated with bone marrow depression, anemia

tion with the serum drug concentration, using the lowest dose and concentration that will produce the desirable patient response. Table 15-2 provides recommendations for serum concentration monitoring of drugs used in an SICU.

■ ■ ■

The clinical practitioner must constantly reevaluate the risks vs. the benefits of a drug therapy regimen, especially with drugs exhibiting a narrow therapeutic index. As stated previously, the first step is the evaluation of physiologic processes in a patient having pharmacokinetic disposition of a drug. The box on p. 154 provides a useful summary of pharmacokinetic relations. Although the drug-dosing tables provided give initial guidelines and considerations for acutely ill patients, the therapeutic and toxic effects, serum concentrations, and patient response must be monitored continually to guide further dosage modifications.

■ ■ ■

Certain classes of drugs warrant special consideration because of their frequent use in SICU patients. Helpful dosing guidelines for neuromuscular blocking agents and narcotic analgesic agents are listed in Tables 15-3 and 15-4, Cardiotonic drugs and agents for treating hypertension are examined more thoroughly.

CARDIOTONIC DRUGS

Cardiotonic or positive inotropic agents are drugs that cause an increase in the force of myocardial contraction. The goal of inotropic therapy is to improve cardiac output (CO) and thus improve blood flow to vital areas such as the CNS, liver, heart, and kidneys.

A number of parenteral positive inotropes are used frequently, but no oral inotrope is currently available. Dopamine, dobutamine, and amrinone are the most useful agents and are considered first-line positive inotropes. The older agents, isoproterenol, epinephrine, and norepinephrine, are considered second-line agents and are used mainly as positive inotropic adjuncts in cardiac surgery patients. Table 15-5

Pharmacokinetic Relations*

Volume of distribution

V_d = Amount of drug in body/C

where

V_d = volume of distribution (vol/kg)
C = concentration of drug (mass/vol)

Clearance

CL = Rate of elimination

where

CL = clearance

Concentration

C = Rate of elimination/CL

$$C = \frac{Dose}{V_d} e^{-kt}$$

where

C = concentration of drug
k = rate constant for elimination

Rate constant for elimination

$k = 0.693/T_{1/2}$

where

$T_{1/2}$ = half-life of drug

Half-life

$$T_{1/2} = \frac{0.693}{\lambda_z}$$

where

λ_z (Fig. 15-1)
$T_{1/2} \approx 0.693\, V_d/CL$

Loading dose

$$\text{Loading dose} = \frac{(V_d)\,(Cp)}{(S)\,(F)}$$

where

Cp = Desired plasma concentration
S = Fraction of drug that is active
F = Bioavailability

Maintenance dose

$$\text{Maintenance dose} = \frac{(CL)\,(Cp)\,\tau}{(S)\,(F)}$$

where

τ = Dosing interval

*Modified from Benet LZ, Massoud N. Pharmacokinetics. In Benet LZ, Massoud N, Gambertoglio JG, eds. Pharmacokinetic Basis for Drug Treatment. New York: Raven Press, 1984, pp 1-28.

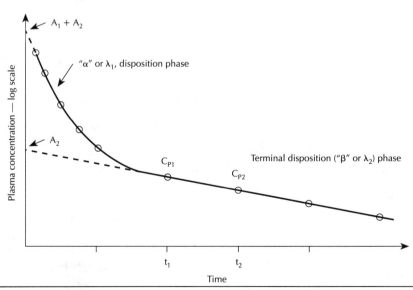

FIG. 15-1 $\lambda_z = \dfrac{\ln (C_{P1}/C_{P2})}{t_2 - t_1}$. This equation allows one to calculate the elimination rate of a drug, given two serum concentrations drawn at two different times; or, once the elimination rate is known, a future concentration can be calculated based on a given concentration at time (t_1). (From Benet LZ, Massoud N. Pharmacokinetics. In Benet LZ, Massoud N, Gambertoglio JG, eds. Pharmacokinetic Basis for Drug Treatment. New York: Raven Press, 1984, pp 1-28.)

summarizes the cardiac and vascular effects of these agents.

Initial Agents
Dopamine

Dopamine is an endogenous catecholamine that is the immediate precursor of norepinephrine. It acts both directly as a beta-1 receptor agonist to increase cardiac contractility and heart rate and indirectly by releasing norepinephrine from storage sites in sympathetic nerve endings. A unique effect of dopamine is its ability to act on postsynaptic dopamine-1 receptors located in the renal and mesenteric arterial blood vessels to cause vasodilation. Dopamine also acts on alpha-1 and alpha-2 receptors to cause vasoconstriction in arterial and venous vascular beds. Vasoconstriction gener-

Text continued on p. 160.

TABLE 15-3 Neuromuscular Blocking Agents*

Pancuronium	Vecuronium	Atracurium
Type		
Nondepolarizing	Nondepolarizing	Nondepolarizing
Loading dose		
0.03-0.1 mg/kg	0.08-0.1 mg/kg	0.3-0.5 mg/kg
Continuous infusion		
0.3-0.6 μg/kg/min	1.25 μg/kg/min	2-9 μg/kg/min
Half-life		
4 hr	1 hr	20 min
Duration		
30-40 min (12-24 hr with continuous infusion)	20-25 min	20-25 min
Elimination		
Renal	Hepatic (25% renal)	Enzymatic
Cardiovascular effects		
Tachycardia, increased blood pressure, increased pulmonary vascular resistance	None	Slight
Special considerations		
Prolonged effect in renal insufficiency	Prolonged effect in hepatic failure	May be used in the presence of renal or hepatic failure
Reversal with atropine, neostigmine, edrophonium, pyridostigmine	Reversal with atropine, neostigmine, edrophonium, pyridostigmine	Reversal with atropine, neostigmine, edrophonium, pyridostigmine
Potentiated by local anesthetics, quinidine, phenytoin, propranolol, aminoglycosides, tetracyclines	Potentiated by local anesthetics, quinidine, phenytoin, propranolol, aminoglycosides, tetracyclines	Potentiated by local anesthetics, quinidine, phenytoin, propranolol, aminoglycosides, tetracyclines

*Modified from McEvoy GK, ed. American Hospital Formulary Service Drug Information. Bethesda, Md.: American Society of Hospital Pharmacists, 1991; Dubaybo BA, Piskorowski TJ, Carlson RW. Use of sedatives and muscle relaxants in acute respiratory failure. Hosp Formulary 26:278, 1991.

TABLE 15-4   Narcotic Analgesic Agents*

	Morphine	Meperidine	Fentanyl	Buprenorphine	Nalbuphine
Class	Opiate agonist	Opiate agonist	Opiate agonist	Partial antagonist and agonist	Partial antagonist and agonist
Dosage	Bolus dosing: 2-5 mg IV q 3-4 hr IV infusion: load, 0.1 mg/kg; infusion, 0.05-0.3 mg/kg/hr	Bolus dosing: 25-100 mg IM q 4-6 hr IV infusion: load, 1.4 mg/kg; infusion 0.3-0.4 mg/kg/hr	Bolus dosing: 50-100 µg IV or IM q 1-2 hr IV infusion: load 3 µg/kg; infusion 0.02-0.05 µg/kg/min	0.3-0.6 mg IV or IM q 4-6 hr	10-20 mg IM or IV q 3-6 hr
Duration of effect	2-6 hr	2-4 hr	30-60 min	6-8 hr	3-6 hr
Half-life	2-4 hr	3-6 hr	1.5-6 min	3 hr	5 hr
Elimination	Hepatic	Hepatic	Hepatic	Hepatic	Hepatic
Relative potency	1	0.1	200	30	1

Side effects	Respiratory depression, sedation, euphoria, cough suppression, decreased gut motility, potentiation of cardiovascular and respiratory effects of other sedatives and analgesics, increased tone of anal and biliary sphincters, urinary retention, nausea, vomiting	Same as morphine; less nausea and vomiting	Sedation, dizziness, headache, nausea, vomiting, hypotension, respiratory depression, hypoventilation, miosis, diaphoresis	Sedation, dizziness, vertigo, miosis, headache, nausea, vomiting, dry mouth, cardiovascular effects <1%, respiratory depression
			Can produce withdrawal in opioid-dependent patients; large doses of naloxone required for reversal	Can produce withdrawal in opioid-dependent patients
Special considerations	Metabolite can accumulate with renal failure, causing prolonged sedation	Same as morphine; vagolytic action; use with caution in supraventricular tachycardia; anticholinergic effects	Normeperidine metabolite accumulates with renal failure and can cause seizures; not recommended in renal failure	Highly lipophilic, accumulates with prolonged use; skeletal and thoracic muscle rigidity and hypotension can be caused by rapid infusions; available as a transdermal system, delivering 25 μg/hr, 50 μg/hr, 75 μg/hr, or 100 μg/hr

*Modified from McEvoy GK, ed. American Hospital Formulary Service Drug Information. Bethesda, Md.: American Society of Hospital Pharmacists, 1991; Dubaybo BA, Piskorowski TJ, Carlson RW. Use of sedatives and muscle relaxants in acute respiratory failure. Hosp Formulary 26:278, 1991.

TABLE 15-5   Relative Cardiac and Vascular Effects of Positive Inotropic Drugs

Drug and Usual IV Dose	Relative Receptor Activity Effects					Hemodynamic Effects					Remarks
	Beta-1 (inotropic)	Beta-1 (chronotropic)	Alpha (vasoconstriction)	Beta-2 (vasodilation)	Dopaminergic (vasodilation)	CO	SVR	MAP	PCWP	HR	
First-line agents *Dopamine (Intropin)*											
Low dose: 0.5-3 µg/kg/min	0/+	0/+	0	0/+	+++	0	−	−	0	0	May induce or exacerbate supraventricular and ventricular dysrhythmias; extravasation may produce tissue necrosis similar to that of norepinephrine
Medium dose: 4-10 µg/kg/min	+++	+	+	+	+	+	−	+	+	+	
High dose: 11-20 µg/kg/min	+++	++	+++	0	0	+	+	+	+	+	
Dobutamine (Dobutrex)											
2-15 µg/kg/min	+++	+	+	+	0	+	−	0/+	−	0/+	Ventricular dysrhythmias and increased HR may occur but less likely than with other catecholamines
Amrinone (Inocor)											
0.75 mg/kg loaded over 5 min, then 5-10 µg/kg/min	0	0	0	0	0	+	−	0/−	−	0/+	Side effects: thrombocytopenia (2%-3%), fever, GI upset, hypotension, worsening of dys-

										Comments
	++	+	0	0	0	+	−	−/+	0	+	rhythmias; invasive hemodynamic monitoring recommended
Second-line agents											
Epinephrine (Adrenaline)											
Low dose: 0.01-0.06 μg/kg/min	+++	++	+	0	++	+	+	−/+	0	+	May induce or exacerbate ventricular ectopy, especially in patients receiving digoxin
High dose: >0.06 μg/kg/min	+++	++	+++	0	+++	++	++	+	0	+	
Norepinephrine (Levophed)											
0.03-0.2 μg/kg/min	++	++	+	0	++	0	+++	+	+	−/+	Administer into a central vein; avoid extravasation; if it occurs, infiltrate area with 5-10 mg of phentolamine diluted in 10 ml of normal saline solution
Isoproterenol (Isuprel)											
0.01-0.1 μg/kg/min	+++	0	+++	0	+++	+++	0	0/−	−	+	Avoid use in patients with ischemic heart disease; may exacerbate tachyarrhythmia from digoxin toxicity or hypokalemia

Receptor effects: +++, pronounced effect; ++, moderate effect; +, slight effect; 0, no effect. Hemodynamic effects: +, increase; −, decrease; 0, no change. CO, cardiac output; SVR, systemic vascular resistance; MAP, mean arterial pressure; PCWP, pulmonary capillary wedge pressure; HR, heart rate.

ally affects blood vessels in skeletal muscle, mesentery, and kidneys. Dopamine has little or no action on beta-2 receptors. Dopamine produces markedly different hemodynamic and renal effects, depending on the infusion rate at which it is administered. Although patient response is highly variable, infusion-dosing guidelines are available for obtaining the appropriate effect.

Precautions. Dopamine should be administered through a central line, if possible, or through a large vein (antecubital or femoral) because of its potent alpha-vasoconstrictor effects. In the event of extravasation of dopamine, phentolamine, an alpha-blocker, should be infiltrated throughout the ischemic area. Concurrent administration of large doses of metoclopramide (Reglan) and other dopamine antagonists such as chlorpromazine (Thorazine) and haloperidol (Haldol) could attenuate the dopaminergic effects of dopamine. In addition, beta-adrenergic blockers such as propranolol (Inderal) can attenuate dopamine's beta-1 effects and cause an increase in systemic vascular resistance (SVR).

Low-dose range. Dopamine-1 receptors are activated in the low-dose range of 0.5 to 3 $\mu g/kg/min$. Blood pressure may be lowered slightly, but heart rate does not change or decrease. Low-dose dopamine frequently is used to improve renal perfusion and promote diuresis.

Medium-dose range. In the medium-dose range of 4 to 10 $\mu g/kg/min$, beta-1 adrenergic stimulation is obtained in addition to the dopaminergic stimulation. This infusion range is used for treatment of heart failure. CO increases, and further improvement in renal blood flow generally occurs. SVR decreases, and pulmonary capillary wedge pressure (PCWP) usually does not change. Heart rate may increase, decrease, or remain unchanged, depending on the patient's sensitivity to beta-1 chronotropic stimulation. Dopamine is commonly used in conjunction with vasodilators such as nitroprusside or nitroglycerin. The vasodilator enhances the hemodynamic effects of dopamine by reducing afterload.

High-dose range. In doses of 10 to 20 $\mu g/kg/min$ the alpha-1 and alpha-2 receptors are recruited, and SVR and blood pressure increase. However, the range of doses for increasing blood pressure can be extremely variable. Rates of up to 50 $\mu g/kg/min$ rarely have been used in patients with shock. Preload deficit must be corrected before starting dopamine therapy in order to to prevent excessive vasoconstriction, necrosis, and gangrene.

■ ■ ■

Dopamine, an agent with unique dose-related pharmacologic effects, remains one of the most commonly used agents for inotropic support. Effects on heart rate are less pronounced than those of epinephrine and isoproterenol but are more than those of dobutamine and amrinone.

Dobutamine

Dobutamine mediates its effects by stimulation of beta-1, beta-2, and alpha receptors. Dobutamine does not cause release of endogenous norepinephrine as dopamine does. The predominant effects of dobutamine are an increase in myocardial contractility, stroke volume, and CO without significant increases in heart rate and blood pressure. Because of competing peripheral alpha and beta-2 stimulation, pulmonary vascular resistance is also reduced. At doses of 5 to 15 $\mu g/kg/min$, dobutamine improves CO by 45% to 55%. Dobutamine increases myocardial oxygen consumption, but it also improves myocardial oxygen delivery by increasing coronary blood flow as a result of decreased coronary vascular resistance.

Precautions. Use of dobutamine is contraindicated in patients with idiopathic hypertrophic subaortic stenosis and other obstructive hypertrophic cardiomyopathies. Dobutamine should be used with caution in patients with severe dysrhythmias because it can induce or exacerbate these conditions.

Dosing. Dobutamine is administered as a continuous IV infusion, with a volumetric infusion pump used. Unlike dopamine, dobutamine may be administered through a peripheral IV line. The starting dose is 3 to 5 $\mu g/kg/min$. The usual range is 3 to 20 $\mu g/kg/min$. Doses of 40 $\mu g/kg/min$ or higher have been reported.

■ ■ ■

Dobutamine is a very effective inotropic agent that directly increases CO, decreases left ventricular filling pressures, and indirectly decreases SVR without significantly increasing heart rate or dysrhythmogenicity. The drug is useful in treating patients with acute ventricular dysfunction from myocardial infarction, ischemia, pulmonary embolism, and chronic congestive heart failure (CHF).

Amrinone

Unlike the other positive inotropic agents, amrinone's activity is not related to sympathomimetic stimulation. Amrinone acts by raising intracellular levels of cyclic adenosine monophosphate (cAMP) through selective inhibition of phosphodiesterase. Enhanced myocardial contractility is a result of modulation of intracellular calcium. The vasodilatory effect of amrinone is believed to be secondary to increased cAMP levels in smooth muscle, with a resultant reduction in SVR and PCWP. Amrinone-mediated increases in CO usually are associated with unaltered or decreased myocardial oxygen consumption. Amrinone is approved for use in adults with all causes of severe CHF. However, patients with restrictive cardiac disease may respond poorly to amrinone because of preload reduction.

Precautions. Amrinone is contraindicated in patients with a history of hypersensitivity reactions to the drug or to sodium metabisulfites. As is true with other inotropic agents, amrinone may worsen hemodynamics in patients with hypertrophic obstructive cardiomyopathy and may enhance atrioventricular (AV) nodal conduction, leading to an increased ventricular response rate in patients with supraventricular tachyarrhythmias. The drug should be used cautiously in patients with hypotension and thrombocytopenia. Transient hypotension occurs in approximately 2% of patients and can be managed by lowering the rate of infusion or administering IV fluids. Thrombocytopenia, which is dose related, develops in approximately 2% to 3% of patients.

Dosing. Amrinone must be diluted to a concentration of 1 to 3 mg/ml in saline solution before administration. Dextrose-containing solutions are not compatible. To hasten the onset of activity, an IV loading bolus of 0.75 mg/kg over 2 to 3 minutes is generally given. The maintenance infusion is administered at a rate of 5 to 10 μg/kg/min. To minimize the potential for severe hypotension from the loading bolus, the drug can be infused at a rate of 40 μg/kg/min for 1 hour and the loading bolus omitted. After 1 hour the infusion can be reduced to the maintenance rate of 5 to 10 μg/kg/min.

■ ■ ■

Amrinone is an effective alternative or adjunct to other inotropes in the treatment of severe CHF. The drug increases CO and reduces preload and afterload and pulmonary vascular resistance. Tachyphylaxis does not occur short term with amrinone, and the drug is minimally dysrhythmogenic.

Secondary Agents
Epinephrine

Epinephrine, a naturally occurring catecholamine, is used as an adjunct to dopamine or dobutamine for improvement of myocardial contractility. In the lower dosage range of 15 to 60 ng/kg/min or 1 to 4 μg/min, epinephrine acts on beta-1 and beta-2 receptors to increase CO and heart rate and to lower SVR. In the dosage range >60 ng/kg/min or 4 μg/min, the alpha-vasoconstrictive effects become more predominant, and tachycardia occurs. Epinephrine is not used as a first-line inotrope because of the availability of dobutamine, dopamine, and amrinone, which have fewer chronotropic and vasoconstrictor effects.

Isoproterenol

The pure beta-1 and beta-2 agonist isoproterenol has positive inotropic and chronotropic effects on the myocardium. It also has pulmonary and peripheral vasodilating properties. Its usefulness as an inotrope has been surpassed by the newer agents, which are less prone to increase heart rate and myocardial oxygen consumption and to cause ventricular dysrhythmias. Isoproterenol is currently used for its chronotropic effects in certain clinical situations, including atropine refractory bradycardia, the overdrive pacing of torsade de pointes and acute cardiac tamponade, and third-degree AV block. Isoproterenol is administered as an IV infusion at a rate of 2 to 10 μg/min.

Norepinephrine

Norepinephrine, a naturally occurring cate-cholamine also known as levarterenol, acts on beta-1 and alpha-adrenergic receptors. Its usefulness as a positive inotrope is limited by its potent alpha-vasoconstrictive effect, which negates any improvement in myocardial contractility. Norepinephrine primarily is used in clinical situations such as sepsis in which peripheral vascular resistance is depressed and vasoconstrictive effects are believed beneficial. The usual IV infusion rate for norepinephrine is 0.03 to 0.2 μg/kg/min. The drug should be administered through a central line to minimize the risk of extravasation.

Combination inotropic therapy

There are many situations in clinical practice in which it is advantageous to use two or more positive inotropic agents concurrently. For instance, low-dose dopamine can be combined with dobutamine. A beneficial effect on renal blood flow and urinary output is obtained from dopamine and improvement in CO from dobutamine. Amrinone and dobutamine, which act through different pharmacologic mechanisms, can be used together to obtain a greater inotropic response than may be achieved with either agent alone. A combination of norepinephrine, low-dose dopamine, and dobutamine may be advantageous in a patient in whom it is desirable to increase mean arterial pressure (MAP), renal blood flow, and CO. Inotropic agents may also be combined with the vasodilators nitroprusside and nitroglycerin to achieve desired hemodynamic effects. Dopamine commonly is combined with nitroprusside to achieve the renal and inotropic effect of dopamine and a reduction in SVR from the nitroprusside.

ANTIHYPERTENSIVES

The ideal drug for treating hypertension should have a rapid onset, a short elimination half-life in case of undesirable side effects, and a re-sponse that is titratable. Choice of agent requires a careful assessment of each patient's medical condition, the urgency of lowering blood pressure, and the hemodynamic and pharmacologic effects that may be troublesome for the patient. (See also Chapter 23.) Tables 15-6 and 15-7 compare the pharmacodynamics of parenteral and oral antihypertensive agents, respectively.

Nitroprusside

Nitroprusside possesses characteristics that make it an ideal agent for lowering high blood pressure. Its onset of action is within seconds, and its duration of action is 3 to 5 minutes. With careful monitoring and titration, blood pressure can be smoothly regulated to a desired range with minimal side effects. The drug directly relaxes the smooth muscle of both arteriolar and venous vasculature. The disadvantages of nitroprusside include the need to administer it by continuous IV infusion, its degradation from light exposure, and the potential for thiocyanate and cyanide toxicity.

Precautions. Nitroprusside is metabolized by red blood cells to hydrocyanic acid, which is further metabolized in the liver to thiocyanate and excreted by the kidneys. Both cyanide and thiocyanate have the potential for accumulating and causing toxicity under certain circumstances. In the presence of renal failure, thiocyanate can accumulate and cause toxic symptoms such as mental status changes, nausea, abdominal pain, tinnitus, hyperreflexia, and seizures. Thiocyanate toxicity is rare when infusion rates are kept below 3 μg/kg/min for periods of 72 hours or less. Measurement of serum levels of thiocyanate is advisable when high or prolonged dosage regimens are used or renal failure is present. Thiocyanate serum levels below 10 mg/dl indicate that continued use of nitroprusside is usually safe. Thiocyanate levels, however, do not reflect cyanide toxicity. Toxic levels of thiocyanate can be managed by stopping the nitroprusside infusion, switching to a different antihypertensive agent, and using hemodialysis for removing thiocyanate.

Cyanide toxicity is a rare complication from nitroprusside but is potentially fatal. It occurs in patients with severe hepatic dysfunction, in sulfur-depleted patients, or in patients with excessive doses of nitroprusside. Early cyanide toxicity is manifested as metabolic acidosis and increasing tolerance to the drug. Toxicity is associated with or followed by dyspnea, headache, vomiting, dizziness, and loss of consciousness. Other signs of cyanide poisoning are coma, imperceptible pulse, absent reflexes, widely dilated pupils, and a pink color. Oxygen therapy alone will not reverse the poisoning. If cyanide toxicity is suspected, the nitroprusside infusion is discontinued, a blood sample is obtained for determination of cyanide level, and treatment is instituted. Treatment consists of administering amyl nitrite inhalations for 15 to 30 seconds each minute until a 3% sodium nitrite solution can be prepared for IV administration. This solution is injected at a rate not exceeding 2.5 to 5 ml/min up to a total dose of 10 to 15 ml. Blood pressure is monitored for hypotension. Then sodium thiosulfate (12.5 g in 50 ml of 5% dextrose in water IV over 10 minutes) is administered and the patient is observed for several hours. If signs of cyanide toxicity reappear, sodium nitrite and sodium thiosulfate injections are repeated using one half of the previous doses.

Dosing. Nitroprusside should be started at an infusion rate of 0.25 to 0.5 μg/kg/min IV via a volumetric infusion pump. The infusion can be titrated by increments of 0.5 μg/kg/min every 5 to 10 minutes until the desired blood pressure control is obtained. The therapeutic dosage range for nitroprusside is 0.25 to 8 μg/kg/min. Most patients are controlled with an average dose of 1.5 μg/kg/min. If adequate blood pressure reduction is not obtained within 10 minutes at an infusion rate of 10 μg/kg/min, the nitroprusside should be terminated and an alternative antihypertensive drug administered.

■ ■ ■

Nitroprusside is a potent vasodilator and has been used in the treatment of hypertensive emergencies, acute valvular insufficiency, low cardiac output states, and congestive myocardial failure.

Nitroglycerin

Nitroglycerin acts on smooth muscle to cause relaxation and vasodilation. It primarily dilates venous vessels but also dilates arterial vessels. Nitroglycerin is a less potent antihypertensive agent than nitroprusside, but it is useful in patients with hypertension associated with myocardial ischemia or infarction. The drug acts within seconds to lower systemic blood pressure and pulmonary vascular resistance. The drug also maintains or improves collateral coronary circulation.

Precautions. Nitroglycerin is generally well tolerated, but side effects related to vasodilation do occur. They include hypotension, headache, and reflex tachycardia. Rare, but potentially dangerous, is paradoxical bradycardia.

Dosing. Nitroglycerin is administered as a continuous IV infusion through a volumetric infusion pump. The starting dose is 0.25 to 0.5 μg/kg/min, with titration done every 5 to 10 minutes by 0.25 to 0.5 μg/kg/min increments to achieve the desired response. The normal therapeutic dosing range is 0.5 to 3 μg/kg/min.

■ ■ ■

Although not as effective an antihypertensive agent as nitroprusside, nitroglycerin is a useful agent for lowering blood pressure when ischemia is present.

Labetalol

Labetalol is a nonselective beta-receptor blocker that also has peripheral alpha-receptor blocker activity. This combination of beta- and alpha-receptor blockade makes it an ideal agent for lowering SVR and blood pressure acutely.

Precautions. Hypotension and dizziness are dose related, and the patient should remain in a supine position during administration. Other precautions with labetalol are releated to its beta-blocking effects. The drug should not be used in patients with asthma, heart block greater than first degree, sinus bradycardia, or severe heart failure. The drug should be used with caution in patients with intermittent claudication or Raynaud's syndrome.

Dosing. The initial IV bolus dose is 5 mg slowly over 2 minutes, followed by repeated

Text continued on p. 168.

TABLE 15-6 Comparative Pharmacodynamics of Parenteral Antihypertensive Agents

Drug and Usual Dose	Mechanism of Action	Onset	Duration	Hemodynamic Effects					Major Side Effects	Remarks
				CO	SVR	MAP	PCWP	HR		
Nitroprusside (Nipride)										
0.25-8 µg/kg/min IV	Arteriolar and venous vasodilator	Seconds	3-5 min	+/−	−	−	−	+	Hypotension, nausea, cyanide toxicity, thiocyanate toxicity	Use cautiously in patients with liver and/or renal failure
Nitroglycerin (Tridil)										
10-40 µg/min IV 50-250 µg/min IV	Venous and arteriolar vasodilator	Seconds	Minutes	0 +	0 −	0 −	− −	0 +	Hypotension, headache Tachycardia	Less potent than nitroprusside as antihypertensive
Hydralazine (Apresoline)										
10-40 mg IV bolus repeated as necessary	Arteriolar vasodilator	20-40 min	2-4 hr	+	−	−	0	+	Tachycardia, headache	Avoid use or use with caution in patients with angina, myocardial infarction, and aortic dissection
Labetalol (Trandate, Normodyne)										
Initial: 20 mg IV over 2 min, then 40-80 mg q 10-15 min until desired response	Alpha blockade and nonspecific beta blockade	5 min	3-6 hr	0	−	−	0/−	−	Hypotension, nausea, vomiting	Avoid use in patients with asthma, CHF, bradycardia, and heart block greater than first degree

Esmolol (Brevibloc)

Dose	Classification	Onset	Duration						Side Effects	Comments
Initial*: 0.25 mg/kg IV over 30 sec, then 25-50 µg/kg/min infusion for 4 min. If necessary, increase infusion by increments of 50 µg/kg/min q 4 min up to maximum of 300 µg/kg/min. Continuous infusion has been used for up to 48 hr	Beta-blocker	Minutes	10-30 min	—	0	—	—	0	Hypotension, bradycardia	Not FDA approved for treatment of hypertension. Contraindicated in patients with second- or third-degree heart block, sinus bradycardia, cardiogenic shock, or overt cardiac failure

Enalaprilat (Vasotec IV)

Dose	Classification	Onset	Duration						Side Effects	Comments
0.625-1.25 mg IV q 6 hr over 5 min	ACE inhibitor	15 min	6-8 hr	0/+	—	—	—	0	Hypotension, dizziness, angioedema, rash, headache	Use lower dose for first dose for patients receiving diuretics to avoid hypotension

+, increase; —, decrease; 0, no change; CO, cardiac output; SVR, systemic vascular resistance; PCWP, pulmonary capillary wedge pressure; HR, heart rate.

*The initial loading bolus of 0.25 mg/kg may be omitted; however, maximal response may be delayed.

TABLE 15-7   Comparative Dosing and Pharmacologic Effects of Oral Antihypertensive Agents

Drug	Initial Oral Dose (mg)	Maintenance Oral Dose (mg)*	Onset (min)	Peak Effect (hr)	Duration (hr)	Hemodynamic Effects				Remarks
						RBF	PVR	CO	HR	
ACE inhibitors										
Captopril (Capoten)	6.25-12.5 tid	25-50 tid	15-30	1-1½	6-12	+	−	0/+	0	Except for fosinopril, start with lower doses in patients receiving diuretics and in renal failure patients.
Enalapril (Vasotec)	2.5-5 qd	2.5-10 bid	60-120	4-8	12-24	+	−	0/+	0	
Lisinopril (Prinivil)	2.5-10 qd	10-20 qd	60	6-8	24	+	−	0	0	
Fosinopril (Monopril)	10 qd	20-60 qd	60-120	2-6	24	0	−	0	0	
Calcium channel blockers										
Verapamil (Calan)	40-80 tid	120 tid	30	1-2	2-6	0	−	−/+	−	Use verapamil and diltiazem cautiously in patients with poor left ventricular function.
Nifedipine (Procardia)	10 tid	20-30 tid or qid	10-20	1	3-5	+	−	+	0/+	
Diltiazem (Cardizem)	30 qid	90 tid or qid	30-60	3	6-10	0	−	0/+	−	Avoid use in patients with second- or third-degree block or sick sinus syndrome.
Beta-blockers										
Metoprolol (Lopressor)	50 bid or tid	100-200 bid	30	1-2	12-19	0/−	0/−	−	−	Metoprolol and atenolol are beta-1 specific.
Atenolol (Tenormin)	50 qd	100 qd	60	2-4	24	0/−	0	−	−	

Drug	Initial dose	Maintenance dose*								Comments
Propranolol (Inderal)	40 bid	80 bid or tid	60	2-4	8-12	0/−	0/−	0/−	−	Avoid use in patients with asthma, CHF, bradycardia, and heart block greater than first degree.
Alpha-1 blockers										
Prazosin (Minipress)	1 bid or tid	2-5 tid	30-60	1-3	6-12	0	−	0/+	0	Dizziness, headache, drowsiness, weakness, palpitations, and nausea occur frequently.
Doxazosin (Cardura)	1 qd	4-8 qd	120	6	24	0	−	0/+	0	
Alpha-2 central agonists										
Clonidine (Catapres)	0.1 bid	0.1-0.3 bid or tid	30-60	2-4	6-12	0/−	−	0/−	−	Dry mouth, drowsiness, dizziness, fatigue, and headache occur frequently. Avoid abrupt discontinuation.
Guanfacine (Tenex)	1 qd	1-3 qd	60	1-4	24	0	−	0	−	
Alpha-1 blocker plus beta-blocker										
Labetalol (Trandate)	100 bid	200-400 bid	30-60	1-3	8-12	0/+	−	0	−	Beta-blocker activity is nonspecific. Follow same precautions as with other beta-blockers.

+, increase; − , decrease; 0, no change; RBF, renal blood flow; PVR, peripheral vascular resistance; CO, cardiac output; HR, heart rate.

*Maintenance oral-dose recommendations represent extended ranges. Dosages should be titrated to effect and to minimize side effects. Few patients are likely to require maximum maintenance dose.

injections of 10 mg, 20 mg, 40 mg, and 80 mg at 10-minute intervals until a desired blood pressure is achieved or a total cumulative dose of 300 mg has been given. The peak effect of each bolus is usually seen in 10 minutes. The duration of effect with bolus administration is usually several hours. Labetalol may also be administered as a continuous IV infusion using a volumetric infusion pump starting at 2 mg/min. The dose can then be titrated to the blood pressure response. If an adequate response is obtained and oral administration is possible, oral labetalol can be instituted upon discontinuing parenteral labetalol. An initial oral dose is 200 mg, followed by 200 to 400 mg 6 to 12 hours later, depending on blood pressure response. Then titration can proceed at 1-day intervals.

■ ■ ■

Labetalol combines the advantages of alpha- and beta-blockers while lowering the unwanted effects of both types of agents. Many reports support its use in patients with severe hypertension and during hypetensive emergencies.

Enalaprilat

Enalaprilat (Vasotec IV) is the active form of enalapril. It is currently the only angiotensin-converting enzyme (ACE) inhibitor available in the United States in a parenteral form. It is approved for the treatment of hypertension when oral therapy is not practical. Enalaprilat reduces blood pressure by lowering SVR by suppression of the renin-angiotensin-aldosterone system. The drug also lowers blood pressure in patients with low renin levels.

Precautions. Severe hypotension is the most common adverse effect of enalaprilat therapy, and patients should be monitored closely after starting therapy. Patients taking diuretics or those with renal failure need an initial dose of 0.625 mg IV to avoid significant hypotension.

Dosing. The initial IV dose of enalaprilat is 1.25 mg over 5 minutes every 6 hours. A clinical response is usually seen within 15 minutes. Peak effects may not occur for up to 4 hours after administration.

■ ■ ■

Parenteral enalaprilat is a useful alternative antihypertensive agent. It is particularly useful in patients who have contraindications for using other agents or who have not had an adequate response.

Esmolol

Esmolol is a beta-1 selective beta-blocker having an ultrashort duration of action. It was approved in 1986. The drug has been used for prompt control of ventricular rate in patients with supraventricular tachycardias. Esmolol has been used for the treatment of postoperative hypertension, a nonapproved use. The drug has a half-life of approximately 9 minutes. Upon discontinuation of esmolol, the drug's pharmacologic effects are reversed within 20 to 30 minutes.

Precautions. Severe hypotension is the most common adverse effect seen with esmolol. Hypotension will generally resolve with dose adjustments or termination of the infusion.

As with other beta-1 selective blockers, esmolol should be used with caution in patients with bronchospastic disease. The drug is contraindicated in patients with heart block greater than first degree, sinus bradycardia, or severe heart failure.

Dosing. Esmolol is administered as an IV continuous infusion using a volumetric infusion pump. An IV loading bolus may be given to provide a quicker onset of activity. The loading dose is 0.25 to 0.5 mg/kg over 30 to 60 seconds. If too rapid a response in blood pressure is a concern, the loading dose can be eliminated and the normal maintenance continuous infusion started at 25 to 50 μg/kg/min and titrated by increments of 25 to 50 μg/kg/min every 4 minutes to the desired response or a maximal dose of 300 μg/kg/min. It may take 20 to 30 minutes to achieve the desired response by this dosing scheme vs. 5 to 10 minutes using the bolus dose. The continuous infusion has been used for up to 48 hours.

■ ■ ■

Esmolol is an ultrashort-acting beta-1 receptor blocker that has proved useful in controlling the rapid ventricular response in supraventricular tachycardias. It may be a useful antihypertensive in postoperative patients with tachycardia and hypertension secondary to increased catecholamine release.

SUMMARY

- The correct dose of a drug is one that produces the desired therapeutic effect and minimal side effects.
- The dynamic course of critically ill patients affects absorption, distribution, metabolism, and excretion of drugs. These effects vary with time, and doses need revision as a patient's condition changes.
- Serum drug concentrations can help guide therapy, especially for drugs with a narrow therapeutic index.
- Positive inotropic agents include dopamine, dobutamine, epinephrine, and isoprotenerol, which are beta-agonists, and amrinone, which increases intracellular cAMP, modulates intracellular calcium, and produces vasodilation.
- Antihypertensive agents include nitroprusside, nitroglycerin, labetalol, enalaprilat, and esmolol. Nitroprusside relaxes arteriolar and venous smooth muscle. Nitroglycerin primarily dilates venous vessels and is especially useful in patients with myocardial ischemia. Labetalol has both alpha- and beta-blocker activity. Enalaprilat is an ACE inhibitor. Esmolol is an ultra-short-acting beta-blocker.

REFERENCES

1. Williams RL. Drug administration in hepatic disease. N Engl J Med 309:1616, 1983.
2. Krueger KA, Garnett WR, Comstock TJ, et al. Effect of two administration schedules of an enteral nutrient formula on phenytoin bioavailability. Epilepsia 28:706, 1987.
3. Hassan E, Ober JD. Predicted and measured aminoglycoside pharmacokinetic parameters in critically ill patients. Antimicrob Agents Chemother 31:1855, 1987.
4. Fuhs DW, Mann HJ, Kubajak CAM, Cerra FB. Inpatient variation of aminoglycoside pharmacokinetics in critically ill surgery patients. Clin Pharm 7:207, 1988.
5. Robert S, Zarowitz BJ. Is there a reliable index of glomerular filtration rate in critically ill patients? DICP Ann Pharmacother 25:169, 1991.
6. Cockcroft DW, Gault MH. Prediction of creatinine clearance from serum creatinine. Nephron 16:31, 1976.
7. Jelliffe RW. Creatinine clearance: A bedside estimate. Ann Intern Med 79:604, 1973.
8. Jelliffe RW, Jelliffe SM. A computer program for estimation of creatinine clearance from unstable serum creatinine levels, age, sex, and weight. Math Biosci 14:17, 1972.
9. Szeto HH, Inturrisi CE, Houde R, et al. Accumulation of normeperidine, an active metabolite of meperidine, in patients with renal failure or cancer. Ann Intern Med 86:738, 1977.
10. Drayer DE, Lowenthal DT, Woosley RL, et al. Accumulation of N-acetylprocainamide, an active metabolite of procainamide, in patients with impaired renal fuctions. Clin Pharmacol Ther 22:63, 1977.

SUGGESTED READINGS

Bottoro PP, Ruttledge DR, Pieper JA. Evaluation of intravenous amrinone: The first of a new class of positive inotropic agents with vasodilator properties. Pharmacotherapy 5:227, 1985.

Chiarello M, Gold HK, Lienbach RC, et al. Comparison between effects of nitroprusside and nitroglycerin on ischemic injury during acute myocardial infarction. Circulation 54:766, 1976.

Cressman MD, Gifford RW. Labetalol—The first combined alpha blocker and beta blocker. J Cardiovasc Med 9:593, 1984.

DeMarco T, Daly PA, Liu M, et al. Enalaprilat, a new parenteral angiotensin converting enzyme inhibitor: Rapid changes in systemic and coronary hemodynamics and humoral profile in chronic heart failure. J Am Coll Cardiol 9:1131, 1987.

Di Sea UJ, Gold JA, Shemin RJ, et al. Comparison of dopamine and dobutamine in patients requiring postoperative circulatory support. Clin Cardiol 9:253, 1986.

D'Orio V, El Allaf D, Juchmes J, et al. The use of low doses of dopamine in intensive care medicine. Arch Int Physiol Biochem 92:511, 1986.

Gage J, Rutman H, Lucido D, et al. Additive effects of dobutamine and amrinone on myocardial contractivity and ventricular performance in patients with severe heart failure. Circulation 74:367, 1986.

Goldstein RE. Coronary vascular response to vasodilator drugs. Prog Cardiovasc Dis 24:419, 1982.

Gray RJ, Bateman TM, Czer LSC, et al. Comparison of esmolol and nitroprusside for acute post-cardiac surgical hypertension. Am J Cardiol 59:887, 1987.

Herling IM. Intravenous nitroglycerin: Clinical pharmacology and therapeutic considerations. Am Heart J 108:141, 1984.

Konstam MA, Cohen SR, Weiland DS, et al. Relative contribution of inotropic and vasodilator effects to amrinone-induced hemodynamic improvement in congestive heart failure. Am J Cardiol 54:242, 1986.

Lowenthal DT, Porter RS, Saris SD, et al. Clinical pharmacology, pharmacodynamics and interactions with esmolol. Am J Cardiol 56:14F, 1985.

Palmer RF, Lasseter KC. Drug therapy: Sodium nitroprusside. N Engl J Med 300:294, 1975.

Scholz H. Inotropic drugs and their mechanisms of action. J Am Coll Cardiol 4:389, 1984.

Weiner N. Norepinephrine, epinephrine, and the sympathomimetic amines. In Goodman Gilman A, Goodman LS, Rall TW, Murad F, eds. Goodman and Gilman's The Pharmacological Basis of Therapeutics, ed 7. New York: Macmillan, 1985, pp 145-180.

Wilson DJ, Wallin JD, Vlachakis ND, et al. Intravenous labetalol in the treatment of severe hypertension and hypertensive emergencies. Am J Med 75:95, 1983.

PART THREE

PATHOPHYSIOLOGIC CONDITIONS

CHAPTER 16

Evaluation of the Comatose Patient

Martha A. Fehr · David S. Knopman

CONSCIOUSNESS vs. COMA

Consciousness is the state of awareness of self and environment. It depends on the normal functioning of two regions of the central nervous system. The first is the reticular activating system (RAS), which is a collection of neurons in the brainstem extending from the medulla to the thalamus. The RAS sends inhibitory projections to nonspecific thalamic nuclei, which, in turn, are inhibitory and project diffusely to the cerebral cortex. Thus the RAS maintains arousal indirectly. The second region, composed of the cerebral hemispheres, is responsible for the integration of multiple inputs that allow meaningful understanding of self and environment, as well as appropriate motor and verbal responses to the environment.

Coma refers to the total absence of awareness of self and environment, even when external stimulation is applied. Different levels of impaired consciousness produce varying degrees of interaction with the environment.

ETIOLOGY

Coma is caused by the destruction of the RAS, the presence of lesions in both hemispheres (anatomic coma), or diffuse disruption of brain metabolic processes (metabolic coma).

Lesions in the cerebral hemispheres may cause coma in several ways:

1. Bilateral diffuse lesions prevent the expression of arousal even when the RAS is functioning.
2. Large unilateral lesions may compress the contralateral hemisphere and effectively create bilateral lesions.
3. Large unilateral or bilateral lesions may cause coma indirectly by compressing the brainstem RAS (transtentorial herniation).

Lesions in the cerebellum also may cause coma indirectly by compressing the brainstem RAS (cerebellar herniation). Lesions in the brainstem itself may directly interfere with RAS function. Table 16-1 outlines the common causes of anatomic and metabolic coma seen in surgical patients and lists suggestions for laboratory evaluation.

DIAGNOSIS

With the comatose patient, the history is extremely important and may help to clarify the temporal onset of symptoms, preceding neurologic symptoms, history of medical illness, drug and alcohol use, medications, and psychiatric history (Table 16-2). A general physical

TABLE 16-1   Common Causes of Coma and Suggested Laboratory Evaluation

Cause	Evaluation
Anatomic coma	
Vascular disease	Head CT or MRI
1. Infarct	
a. Atherosclerotic (carotid)	Carotid Doppler examination
b. Nonatherosclerotic (embolization from heart)	Echocardiogram
c. Vasculitis	Cerebral angiography
2. Intracerebral hemorrhage	Head CT or MRI
a. Hypertensive crisis	
b. Ruptured aneurysm with intraparenchymal hemorrhage	Cerebral angiography
c. Arteriovenous malformation	Cerebral angiography
d. Coagulopathy	PT, PTT, TT, platelets
Trauma	Head CT or MRI
1. Subdural hematoma	
2. Epidural hematoma	CT plus skull x-ray
3. Concussion	
4. Contusion	
Infection	
1. Abscess	
2. Meningitis	CT plus lumbar puncture (if head CT shows no mass lesions)
3. Encephalitis	
Neoplasm	
1. Metastatic	
2. Primary CNS	Head CT or MRI
Metabolic coma	
Metabolic encephalopathy	Electrolytes, BUN, creatinine, blood sugar,
1. Hepatic encephalopathy	liver function, calcium, magnesium,
2. Uremia	phosphorus
3. Hypoglycemia	
4. Diabetic ketoacidosis	
5. Hyponatremia	
6. Hypercalcemia, hypocalcemia	
7. Myxedema	
8. Vitamin deficiency (e.g., Wernicke's encephalopathy)	
Hypoxic/ischemic encephalopathy	ECG, CXR, ABG, cardiac enzymes
1. Cardiac or respiratory failure	
2. Severe congestive heart failure	
Toxic encephalopathy	Urine/serum toxic screen
1. Drugs (e.g., opiates, cocaine, barbiturates)	
2. Alcohol	
3. Carbon monoxide	
4. Heavy metals	
Postictal/ictal (epilepsy)	EEG, anticonvulsant levels

TABLE 16-2   Features of Patient's History Suggesting Anatomic vs. Metabolic Coma*

Suggests Anatomic	Suggests Metabolic
Sudden observed onset	History of major medical illness:
Preceding "hard" neurologic symptoms:	Liver
Aphasia	Renal
Diplopia	Pulmonary
Vertigo	Cardiac
Hemiparesis	Previous history of overdose or severe depression
Coagulopathy	Known drug abuse
Chronic alcoholism	Use of sedative medication
Previous anatomic brain lesion:	
Stroke	
Tumor	
Subdural hematoma	

*Modified from Ropper AH. Coma in the emergency room. In Earnest MP, ed. Neurologic Emergencies. New York: Churchill Livingstone, 1983, p 83.

examination should be done, with special attention given to the following areas:

1. Vital signs. Ventilatory and circulatory status should be assessed promptly in any comatose patient. Several respiratory patterns are useful in neuroanatomic localization:
   a. Cheyne-Stokes respiration which is characterized by periods of hyperventilation that diminish to apnea, indicates bilateral deep hemispheric dysfunction.
   b. Apneustic breathing, which is characterized by a prolonged inspiratory phase followed by apnea, is seen in pontine dysfunction.
   c. Ataxic breathing is characterized by chaotic respirations. This type of breathing is agonal and indicates damage to the respiratory centers in the medulla.
   d. Breathing patterns seen in metabolic coma include depressed breathing, which is characterized by shallow, ineffective breathing. Depressed breathing is often caused by drugs that lead to medullary depression. Coma with hyperventilation can be seen in metabolic disorders that lead to metabolic acidosis or respiratory alkalosis.

2. Evidence of trauma to the head or spine should be sought. Helpful localizing findings include:
   a. Battle's sign suggests mastoid fracture
   b. "Racoon's eyes" suggest orbital fracture
   c. Hemorrhage from ears or nostrils suggests basilar skull fracture
   d. Neck stiffness may suggest infection, subarachnoid hemorrhage, or trauma (if cervical spine fracture is suspected, the neck should not be manipulated)

3. The skin should be examined for evidence of systemic embolization, infection, and trauma. Comatose patients who are brought to the emergency department also should be examined for needle marks.

The neurologic examination will help in differentiation of anatomic from metabolic coma and determination of the region(s) of the nervous system involved (hemispheres vs. RAS vs. diffuse). The assessment should focus on depth of coma, presence of asymmetric movements, general nature of movements, Babinski's sign, funduscopic examination, and brainstem reflexes. A clinically important description is the depth of coma. Because terms such as "obtundation" and "lethargy" are not consistently used, it is important to describe the patient's response to various stimuli. The Glasgow Coma Scale score (see Chapter 18) provides a clinically useful description.

First, the patient is observed while undisturbed. Natural positions reminiscent of normal sleep suggest a lighter coma, from which the patient may be easily aroused. Unnatural positions suggest a deeper coma, from which arousal may be difficult. Next, painful stimulation is applied (e.g., to nailbed) and the patient is observed for evidence of arousal. Responses may vary from complete arousal and verbal response (i.e., patient was not comatose) to no response at all. The patient's response should be described and recorded.

Next, the patient's movements are observed. With the patient in the resting posture, any asymmetries are noted. An externally rotated leg may suggest a hemiparesis. Then the patient is observed for spontaneous movements. A persistent lack of spontaneous movement on one side indicates hemiparesis. Spontaneous rhythmic twitching of the face and/or extremities may be the only indication of seizure activity.

Decerebrate or decorticate posturing also may be observed (Fig. 16-1). Posturing has poor localizing value and may be seen in both anatomic and metabolic coma. Unilateral posturing is more suggestive of a structural abnormality. Posturing may coexist with purposeful movements, a finding that suggests incomplete damage to the motor system. If spontaneous movements have been observed, response to painful stimulation applied to the limbs is checked. Observations are made for asymmetries, posturing, and purposeful movements.

The presence or absence of Babinski's sign is noted. A unilateral upward-pointing toe is a

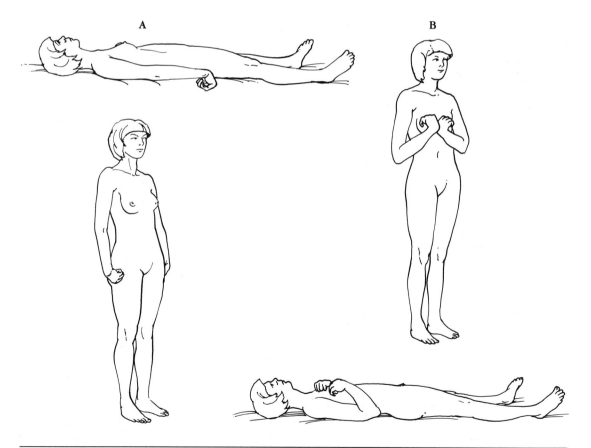

FIG. 16-1 Decerebrate and decorticate posturing. **A,** Decerebrate. Arms are extended; wrist and fingers are flexed with thumb trapped in palm. Arm is internally rotated. Legs are extended. **B,** Decorticate. Arm, wrist, and fingers are flexed; thumb is trapped in palm. Arm is adducted and internally rotated on chest. Legs are extended.

sign of asymmetric damage to the central nervous system. Bilateral upward-pointing toes may be seen with metabolic disease. A funduscopic examination should be performed. Papilledema is suggestive of increased intracranial pressure. A subhyaloid hemorrhage is often seen in subarachnoid hemorrhage. Brainstem reflexes are an important part of the evaluation of a comatose patient. When brainstem reflexes are being evaluated, pupillary reaction and eye movements are emphasized. Examination of the pupils is done first. Pupillary size and equality in reaction to direct and consensual light are checked (Fig. 16-2). Reactive pupils indicate that the midbrain and the third cranial nerve are intact. In the presence of unresponsiveness, absent extraocular movements, and corneal reflexes, reactive pupils are suggestive of metabolic coma. With metabolic encephalopathies, the pupillary light reflex is preserved until the end stage, whereas destructive lesions of the midbrain negate the light reflex.

Small but reactive pupils are indicative of pontine damage, although small pupils also may be caused by the use of certain drugs (e.g., opiates, pilocarpine). Midposition (3 to 5 mm), nonreactive pupils are indicative of midbrain damage. A unilaterally dilated and nonreactive pupil in a comatose patient is indicative of compression of the third cranial nerve from temporal lobe (uncal) herniation. Less frequently, a dilated, nonreactive pupil can be caused by symmetric midbrain damage. Bilaterally dilated and nonreactive pupils indicate severe midbrain compression of the third cranial nerve. Drugs with atropinic activity may cause these findings.

Next, eye movements are observed. Horizontal eye movements, which are controlled by the pons and the midbrain (third nerve), are the key to determining if a brainstem lesion is the cause of coma. Spontaneous eye movements are observed first, if present. The presence of conjugate side-to-side eye movements

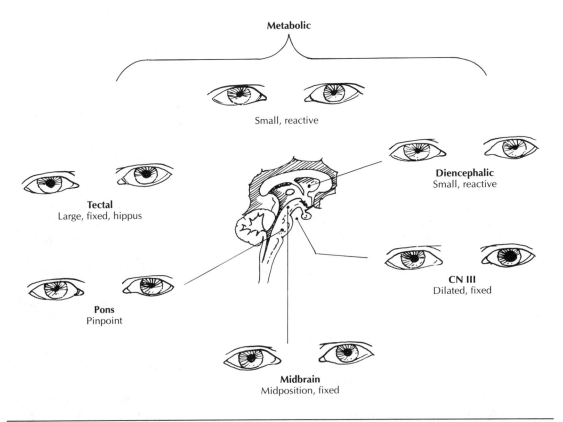

FIG. 16-2 Pupils in comatose patients. (Redrawn from Plum F, Posner JB. The Diagnosis of Stupor and Coma, 3rd ed. Philadelphia: FA Davis, 1980.)

suggests that the pons and the midbrain are intact. Spontaneous dysconjugate eye movements are always abnormal and indicative of midbrain-pontine damage. Spontaneous conjugate roving eye movements indicate that the cerebral hemispheres are depressed or disconnected from the brainstem (i.e., coma is caused by bilateral hemispheric or diffuse process). Conjugate eye deviation toward the side of the lesion can be seen with unilateral hemispheral lesions. Conjugate eye deviation away from the side of the lesion also can be seen in unilateral thalamic and pontine lesions.

In patients who do not exhibit spontaneous eye movements, the integrity of the pathways must be checked by head turning (oculocephalic response) or caloric stimulation (oculovestibular response). Caloric stimulation is used when no response with head turning is observed.

Abnormalities of elicited horizontal eye movements are interpreted as follows:

1. Normal response consists of conjugate eye movements in the opposite direction of the head turn. The normal response to cold water caloric stimulation is conjugate deviation of the eyes toward the irrigated ear.
2. Abnormal abduction (outward movement) of one eye is caused by a sixth cranial nerve lesion.
3. Abnormal adduction (toward nose) of one eye is cause by a third cranial nerve or midbrain-pontine lesion.
4. Conjugate gaze paresis, as a consequence of a hemispheric lesion, usually can be overcome with caloric stimulation, whereas conjugate gaze paresis from brainstem lesions cannot. The corneal reflexes are reliable indicators of pontine function and therefore should be tested.

MANAGEMENT

In all patients in a state of coma, an airway is established and maintained (see Chapters 11 and 27). Care is taken to remove dentures. An oropharyngeal airway may prove adequate. If ventilation is unsatifactory, intubation will be necessary. Thiamin, 100 mg IV, should be given if Wernicke's encephalopathy is suspected; glucose, 1 A D_{50}W IV, should be given if hypogly-

cemia is suspected; and naloxone, 2 to 4 mg IV, is useful for narcotic overdose. Once the patient is stable and has an adequate airway, further evaluation includes head CT or MRI and routine screening for metabolic causes of coma (see Table 16-1).

Management of the patient with increased intracranial pressure is an emergency. Proper management optimizes brain perfusion with oxygenated, nutrient-containing blood. Since the adult skull fixes the volume available for the brain, edema of the brain can increase cerebral perfusion pressure (CPP). CPP is given by the following relation:

$$CPP = MAP - ICP$$

where MAP is the mean arterial pressure and ICP is the intracranial pressure. Normal ICP is approximately 10 mm Hg. If a patient has a MAP of 90 mm Hg, CPP = 80 mm Hg.

Cerebral blood flow (CBF) is described by:

$$CBF = \frac{CPP}{CVR}$$

where CVR is cerebral vascular resistance. In the general population, autoregulation changes CVR to maintain constant CBF over a wide range of MAP.

In general, CPP between 65 and 80 mm Hg allows satisfactory brain perfusion; CPP between 50 and 65 mm Hg provides borderline perfusion; and CPP <50 mm Hg produces cerebral ischemia. Usually, the clinician can increase CPP by decreasing ICP through a series of interventions.

Maneuvers that help to reduce ICP can be as simple as elevating the head of the bed 30 to 45 degrees. Cerebral vessels are sensitive to changes in $Paco_2$, and hyperventilation to a $Paco_2$ of 28 to 30 mm Hg causes short-term cerebral vasoconstriction. The use of hyperventilation as standard treatment is controversial. Mannitol has been used to treat cerebral edema by increasing plasma oncotic pressure. The dosage remains controversial. Unless a dire neurosurgical emergency is unfolding, mannitol, 0.25 g/kg body weight, is administered intravenously over 60 to 90 minutes. Serum osmolality should be followed routinely and not allowed to increase above 315 to 320 mOsm. Barbiturate administration causes cerebral vasoconstriction. Because of danger with such administration, expert assistance is necessary. Finally, intractable cerebral edema may require surgical decompression.

Increasing CPP by increasing MAP is successful only if MAP is low. With normal MAP, autoregulation increases CVR. If MAP is low, the clinician can use colloid solutions to correct hypovolemia, dopamine to raise MAP, or neosynephrine to increase MAP. Neosynephrine is acceptable in the case of isolated head injury because cerebral vessels do not respond to α-agonists.

Further management, which includes nutrition formulation of appropriate metabolic support, depends on the clinical presentation (see Chapter 3). Diarrhea, constipation, and impaction can occur. These abnormalities of GI function can present significant risk. Careful attention is given to bowel function and the need for stool softeners as necessary. An indwelling catheter is often required. The catheter should be clamped intermittently to maintain bladder tone. Measures to acidify the urine, such as continuous irrigation with 0.25% acetic acid, will prevent stone formation. For the obtunded patient, the use of methylcellulose eyedrops and taping the eyelids closed will minimize corneal injury.

Unnecessary sedation is avoided. If agitation is severe, a short-acting benzodiazepine (e.g., lorazepam, 1 to 2 mg IV q 12 hr) or a potent neuroleptic (e.g., haloperidol, 1 to 5 mg IM q 12 hr) is used. Usually, elderly patients require a smaller dose than younger patients. Oversedation is a common cause of prolonged impairment of consciousness in hospitalized patients, especially the elderly. Formal neurologic consultation should be considered when coma is encountered in patients in the SICU.

SUMMARY

- Coma may result from anatomic or metabolic causes. Glasgow Coma Scale score (see Chapter 18) provides a clinically important description of coma. Sudden onset (preceding neurologic symptoms), coagulopathy, previous anatomic brain lesion, or chronic alcoholism favors anatomic coma.
- Major medical illness, history of drug abuse, history of drug overdose, depression, or use of sedative medication favors metabolic coma.
- Patterns of breathing may be helpful in neuroanatomic diagnosis.
- Battle's sign, raccoon's eyes, or hemorrhage from ears or nose suggests trauma.

- Neck stiffness suggests infection, subarachnoid hemorrhage, or trauma.
- Posturing may occur in both anatomic and metabolic coma.
- Evaluation of coma should include test of Babinski's sign, fundoscopic examination, pupillary reaction, and eye movements.
- Management:
  Always establish and maintain airway.
  Elevated intracranial pressure is an emergency.
  Monitor bowel function closely.
  Acidify urine.
  Avoid unnecessary sedation.

BIBLIOGRAPHY

Lassen NA, Christenson MS. Physiology of cerebral blood flow. Br J Anaesth 48:719-731, 1976.

Plum F, Posner JB. The Diagnosis of Stupor and Coma, 3rd ed. Philadelphia: FA Davis, 1980.

Ropper AH. Coma in the Emergency Room. In Earnest MP, ed. Neurologic Emergencies. New York: Churchill Livingstone, 1983, p 83.

Ward JD, Choi A, Moulton R, Muizelaar JP, DeSalles A, Becker DP, Kontos HA, Young HF. Effect of prophylactic hyperventilation on outcome in patients with severe head injury. In Hoff JT, Betz AL, eds. Proceedings of Seventh International Symposium on Intracranial Pressure. New York: Springer-Verlag, 1988, pp 630-633.

Wilkinson HA. Intracranial Pressure. In Youmans JR, ed. Neurological Surgery. Philadelphia: WB Saunders, 1989, pp 661-695.

CHAPTER 17

Seizures

Fernando Torres

According to Webster's dictionary, one definition of a seizure is "a sudden attack (as of disease): fit." "Fit" is defined as "a stroke of a disease producing convulsions or unconsciousness." The following discussion uses this definition. Only in passing, as necessary for understanding this presentation, is the more narrowly defined concept of epilepsy used. Epilepsy has been defined as the condition in which repeated epileptic seizures occur chronically. This definition excludes the isolated seizure that may occur in an acute state of intoxication or metabolic imbalance and even repeated seizures that recur within the few days or weeks that this general toxic or metabolic abnormality persists. Since this discussion deals with critical care, the latter situation will be considered primarily, but it also includes the management of the patient with epilepsy who, for any reason, develops seizures that become frequent or severe enough to warrant admission to an SICU.

In most instances, the diagnosis of epileptic seizures is rather easy. It is based mainly on the history taken from the patient and, whenever possible, from someone who has observed the seizures. However, in some cases, even the best description may not make it possible to distinguish between a primarily generalized seizure and a partial one with or without secondary generalization. Because of this difficulty, performance of an EEG is necessary in most cases and desirable in all cases. Table 17-1 shows a simplified version of the international classification of epileptic seizures. Obviously, a complete physical and neurologic examination is an important part of the diagnostic evaluation of patients with suspected seizures. In patients with epilepsy that is a chronic condition, the neurologic examination usually shows no abnormalities. Most of these cases correspond to idiopathic epilepsy. In some patients there will be neurologic findings that may be caused either by primary CNS involvement or a neurologic dysfunction that is secondary to systemic disease.

In the SICU the physician may encounter a patient with continuous or repeated abnormal movements. This symptom may be the primary cause for admission to the unit, or it may develop in a patient who was admitted for a systemic or nonneurologic condition and developed the symptom during the course of the primary disease process. In either case an accurate diagnosis and prompt treatment are essential because the convulsive condition can be fatal independently of what the primary illness may be.

SEIZURES AND MYOCLONUS

If the abnormal movements consist of repeated jerks of one or more extremities, with or without involvement of state of consciousness, the more likely differential diagnosis must be between epileptic seizures and myoclonus. Table 17-2 shows the major categories of myoclonus. Generally, a preliminary impression may be obtained from clinical observation. In seizures, whether or not they include tonic and clonic components, there is an evolution manifested

TABLE 17-1   Classification of Epileptic Seizures*

Clinical	EEG Seizure	EEG Interictal
Focal seizures (partial local)		
Simple partial or focal seizures (consciousness not impaired) With motor signs With somatosensory symptoms With autonomic symptoms	Local contralateral seizure discharge (not always recordable from scalp)	Local contralateral epileptiform discharge
Complex partial or focal seizures (with impairment of consciousness; may sometimes start as simple focal) Simple partial onset followed by impairment of consciousness With impairment of consciousness at onset	Unilateral or bilateral discharge, diffuse or focal in temporal or frontotemporal regions	Unilateral or bilateral generally asynchronous focus; usually in temporal or frontal regions
Partial or focal seizures evolving to secondary generalized seizures	Discharges become secondarily and rapidly generalized	Background activity usually normal
Generalized seizures (convulsive or nonconvulsive)		
Absence seizures Impairment of consciousness only With various mild brief motor or autonomic components	Usually regular, bilateral, and symmetric 3 Hz (sometimes 2 to 4 Hz) spike and slow-wave complexes	
Atypical absence seizures More pronounced changes in tone than with typical absence seizures Onset or cessation, which is not abrupt	More heterogeneous; may include irregular spike and slow wave, polyspike and wave, or other paroxysmal activity; bilateral but may be asymmetric	Background usually normal but with some paroxysmal activity of spikes or spike and slow wave
Myoclonic seizures (single or multiple myoclonic jerks)	Polyspike and wave	Irregular with spikes or spike and slow waves
Clonic seizures	Rhythmic fast activity and slow waves; irregular spike and slow wave or flattening	Irregular; spike and wave or polyspike and wave discharges
Tonic seizures	Rhythmic fast activity decreasing in frequency and increasing in amplitude	Abnormal background with discharges of spikes and slow waves
Tonic-clonic seizures	Similar to above	Similar to above
Atonic seizures	Polyspike and wave or flattening	Similar to above

*Modified from Commission on Classification and Terminology of the ILEA. Proposal for revised clinical and electroencephalographic classification of epileptic seizures. Epilepsia 22:489-501, 1981.

TABLE 17-2 Classification of Myoclonus			
	Major Clinical Manifestation	EEG Spike Synchronized*	Induced by Stimulus or Movement
Spontaneous cortical myoclonus	Generalized or partial jerks	+	−
Stimulus-sensitive (reflex) cortical myoclonus	Generalized or partial jerks	+	+
Subcortical myoclonus			
Reticular myoclonus	Partial jerks involving muscles distal and proximal to brainstem	±	±
Segmental myoclonus	Partial jerks involving various limbs	−	±

*EEG spike synchronized shown by backaveraging. (For explanation of technique of backaveraging, see Shibasaki H, Kuroiwa Y. Electroencephalographic correlates of myoclonus. Electroencephalogr Clin Neurophysiol 39:455-463, 1975.)

by a change in the frequency and severity of the clonic contractions. Myoclonus is generally more monotonous, continuous, and dysrhythmic. However, in all instances, the appropriate differentiation between myoclonus and epileptic seizures requires the use of the EEG, preferably with additional polygraphic recordings.

If the EEG shows spikes, it is important to determine their temporal correlation (or lack of correlation) with the jerky muscle contractions. This determination can help in deciding whether one is dealing with segmental, reticular, or cortical myoclonus or with seizures. Unfortunately, the distinction between myoclonus and epilepsy becomes more blurred the closer to the cerebral cortex the origin of the myoclonus is located. Although segmental myoclonus is clearly a different entity, reticular myoclonus may or may not affect cerebral cortical activity, and cortical myoclonus may become indistinguishable from partial simple seizures, including epilepsia partialis continua (Fig. 17-1).

The handling of a patient presenting with either myoclonus or epileptic seizures will vary depending on the history. In general, patients with myoclonus that is not associated with systemic disease do not need admission to an SICU. Treatment of this condition is not necessary if it can be established that one is dealing with physiologic or benign myoclonus. If the condition is persistent and incapacitating, the patient should be admitted and an effective airway should be established. Intravenous clonazepam may be helpful. For adults, the dose should be 0.5 to 1 mg every 1 to 2 minutes to a maximum of 4 to 5 mg (less if respiration becomes compromised). The blood level of clonazepam rises rapidly, and its half-life is about 20 to 25 hours. For longer effects, sodium valproate can be given by mouth if the condition is not controlled with the clonazepam.

Myoclonus that is part of other neurologic or general systemic syndromes may be difficult to control, and the treatment should be oriented toward correcting the metabolic condition. Myoclonic epilepsy falls under the general category of seizures.

In the case of seizures, if a history of epilepsy can be obtained, the most likely cause for sudden exacerbation is lack of compliance with the treatment or, in some cases, recurrence of seizures after discontinuation of medication by the treating physician. In such cases the patient does not need to be admitted to the SICU unless he/she is having repeated seizures or status epilepticus. After a single seizure or two, the patient will probably be handled in the emer-

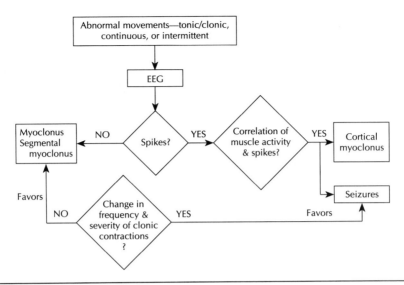

FIG. 17-1   Differentiation between myoclonus and epileptic seizures in patient demonstrating abnormal movements.

gency room. The situation will be explained to the patient and a determination will be made that he/she is receiving his/her usual antiepileptic medication. The proper instructions for taking the medication will be reviewed, and the patient will be reminded to be sure to see a physician regularly. If, on the other hand, the patient has never had seizures before, a careful and complete investigation of the cause of this first seizure or series of seizures must be done. If the patient is in good general condition, both physically and mentally, this investigation may be done on an outpatient basis. If not, he/she may need to be admitted to a regular inpatient unit. If the seizures are repetitive and constitute status epilepticus, admission to the SICU is necessary.

STATUS EPILEPTICUS

Status epilepticus has been defined by the World Health Organization as "a condition characterized by an epileptic seizure that is sufficiently prolonged or repeated at sufficiently brief intervals so as to produce an unvarying and enduring epileptic condition."[1] However, the most frequent definition used at the present time is "any seizure lasting 30 minutes or more."[2] This definition is based on the rationale that after about 30 minutes of seizures there is

a critical systemic transition from relatively benign conditions to those that will likely result in brain damage.[3] Because this is a life-threatening situation that is a relatively common mode of presentation of seizures in the SICU, the following discussion focuses mainly on it.

In the above-mentioned definition, the key word is "seizure." It must be recognized that repeated or prolonged seizures constituting status epilepticus can include any of those listed in the classification of seizures (see Table 17-1). Therefore, the spectrum of state of consciousness, may range from no alteration (e.g., at the beginning of partial simple seizures) to slight confusion, to deep coma.

How can the diagnosis of status epilepticus be made? With the simple partial variety, there should be no problem, if the definition given for status epilepticus is used. In complex partial status epilepticus, the situation becomes more difficult because of the absence or paucity of clinical findings other than the involvement of state of consciousness. In those cases fluctuations in consciousness will occur since the seizure episodes will be followed by a postictal state involving confusion, which, in turn (and before recovery), will be followed by one more seizure. Treiman and Delgado-Escueta[4] give a very good description of the sequences that can be encountered. Therefore, in any patient who presents with an alternation between unresponsivity and automatisms at one moment and simple confusion at the next, the suspicion of complex partial status epilepticus should arise.

Among the generalized types of status epilepticus is the absence type. The most frequently described (but not most frequently seen) absence status epilepticus occurs in children who suffer from absence seizures. Status epilepticus ensues when the absence seizures occur repeatedly and frequently enough to qualify for the general definition of status epilepticus. In this situation there is, at least for the first few hours, no postictal alteration or confusion, as seen with complex partial status epilepticus. After each absence the patient suddenly becomes alert and normally responsive for a few minutes before the next absence. Children and the few adults who present with this kind of status epilepticus may be seen in the emergency room but usually will not need admission to the SICU.

Diagnosis in the other form of generalized status epilepticus should not be difficult since the clinical picture is so dramatic that no other condition should come to mind. The patient will show repeated generalized tonic, clonic, or tonic-clonic seizures without recovery of consciousness between attacks.

NONCONVULSIVE STATUS EPILEPTICUS

Nonconvulsive status epilepticus, including partial complex and absence status, constitutes a problem if the physician does not keep it in mind as a possible cause for either episodic changes in state of consciousness or sustained unconsciousness arising in a patient who has been brought to the SICU fully conscious or with decreased state of alertness for known causes such as recovery from anesthesia. In the former situation, the various possible causes for loss or altered state of consciousness must be considered. In the latter, a slow recovery or no recovery should alert the physician to new developments generally not related to anesthetic effect. In these situations an EEG should be ordered and consultation with a neurologist should be arranged (Fig. 17-2).

Nonconvulsive status epilepticus may be caused by partial complex or absence seizures. There is, in addition, a third type of seizure, which has not been well defined because its EEG manifestations do not correspond to either of those two conditions that are well known as causing nonconvulsive seizures. In this situation the patient will be in a coma, not showing any kind of movements or, on occasion, may have subtle manifestations such as rhythmic grimacing, chewing or sucking, or slight rhythmic movements of the fingers that are not easily detectable. There also may be subtle changes in the depth of coma if there are intervals between the seizures.

In many cases a previous history of seizures is not present. In a recent series of 45 patients seen in the SICU by neurologists who diagnosed status epilepticus, only 12% had a history of previous seizures.[5] Fifty percent had nonconvulsive status, either as the only manifestation of status epilepticus or alternating with clinical convulsions.

How is nonconvulsive status epilepticus diagnosed? The only sure way is by means of an EEG. This test will show recurrence of electrical seizures without concomitant clinical convulsions. In cases with typical absence status epilepticus, which is rare in adults, the EEG will show generalized spike and wave discharges. In partial complex status, a focal involvement will continue or become generalized secondarily. If the EEG does not capture the onset of one seizure, it may be difficult to determine its "partial" characteristic. The third type of convulsive status mentioned earlier and one that is most often seen in patients without a history of previous seizures may show many different forms of abnormality in the EEG, most of them clearly of seizure type but some not so typical. In these cases the diagnostic use of benzodiazepines in conjunction with the EEG is most helpful.

When electrical seizures are seen or suspected in the EEG, the intravenous injection of diazepam at a rate of approximately 1 mg every 2 to 3 minutes, up to a total of 5 mg in adults, or lorazepam, 0.5 mg every 2 minutes up to 2 mg, will show clear changes in the EEG, usually stopping the electrical seizure activity and thus helping in diagnosis. A result that is most sat-

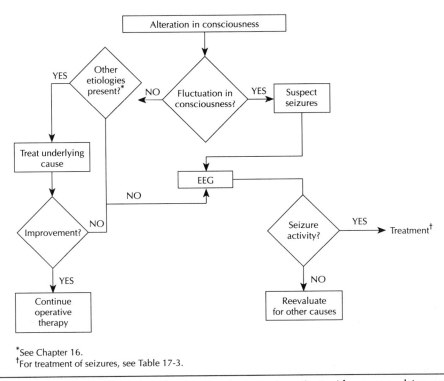

FIG. 17-2 Treatment approach to alteration in consciousness in patient with nonconvulsive status epilepticus.

isfactory and confirmatory of the diagnosis takes place when the patient's state of consciousness changes dramatically after the injection, as he/she becomes alert and responsive from a confusional state or waking up from a coma. The benzodiazepines are given in this situation as a diagnostic method to confirm the EEG findings, which, in certain cases, may not be those clearly indicative of an ongoing seizure. For this reason the recommended doses are low compared to those used for treatment. In effect, if larger doses are given at the diagnostic stage, they may induce sleep, which will cause less specific changes in the EEG and prevent the clinical manifestation of recovery from the seizure that makes the diagnosis more dramatic and certain.

GENERAL EFFECTS OF SEIZURES

Pathologic lesions in epilepsy have been described since 1880, when Sommer[6] noted selective loss of pyramidal neurons in the hippocampus of patients with chronic epilepsy.

However, although it is well recognized that hippocampal sclerosis occurs in patients with epilepsy, its exact cause is still not well understood. It has been postulated, among other causes, that the sclerotic lesions are caused by hypoxia that is secondary to herniation of the uncus with compression by the edge of the cerebellar tentorium. The fact that hypometabolism occurs between seizures in brain areas corresponding to EEG epileptogenic foci has been shown by positron emission tomography (PET) studies.[7] PET studies also have shown, at the other extreme, increased metabolic rates during a seizure. Experimental work on primates has shown that neuronal death occurs after prolonged seizures even under paralyzing agents and with pure oxygen ventilation,[8] indicating that the seizure per se, without convulsions or systemic anoxia, may be lethal to neurons. In humans, prolonged, even very localized seizures may produce focal brain damage, as reported in a case of epilepsia partialis continua.[9]

There is thus important, although sometimes incomplete, evidence of brain damage caused by seizures, whether because of secondary decrease in oxygen and/or glucose to the neuron or resulting from a mechanism more directly related to the excessive neuronal discharge. Whatever damage may be caused by isolated seizures is obviously multiplied by many factors in cases of status epilepticus.

TREATMENT OF SEIZURES

The treatment of chronic seizures or epilepsy is not the task of critical care physicians. If a patient is admitted to the SICU with epilepsy or if a patient develops epilepsy as a consequence of the condition that brought him/her to the SICU, a neurologist should be called in consultation to determine the type and dose of medication to be prescribed at the time of discharge. On the other hand, in the case of isolated seizures occurring during the patient's stay in the SICU, and especially if such a situation develops into status epilepticus, the critical care physician should be able to adequately treat the patient. Status epilepticus is an emergency situation and thus should become a high priority to be treated intensively, regardless of other underlying systemic conditions.

In general, the goal should be to completely control the seizures without endangering the patient by depressing respiratory or cardiac function. Therefore, whether the patient is brought to the SICU with status epilepticus or develops seizures during a stay in the unit, the first thing to do (if it has not been done previously because of the patient's general condition) is to be sure that ventilation is adequate. If the patient is in coma, intubation should be performed. At the same time, the EEG laboratory should be called. In some cases an EEG is performed as one of the first procedures to verify the diagnosis of seizures. In all cases involving seizures it is done to monitor the effect of treatment. If an IV line has not been placed, one should be established and kept open with normal saline. Blood should be drawn for serum chemistries. In a new patient with either known epilepsy or unavailable history, antiepileptic drug concentrations should be determined.

If the patient continues to have seizures or does not recover consciousness, immediate treatment should be started without waiting for EEG verification of persistent seizures. After direct push of 50 ml of 50% glucose IV, a benzodiazepine injection should be started. Diazepam is very effective, but lorazepam may be preferred. Either drug may cause respiratory depression and the effective cerebral action of both is relatively short. Therefore respirations should be watched and, if necessary, assisted and a second drug with a longer half-life should be started immediately after the completion of the benzodiazepine injection. Table 17-3 presents the sequence of actions to follow in the treatment of status epilepticus. After the benzodiazepine injection, intravenous loading with phenytoin should be done. The loading dose is 18 to 20 mg/kg. Injection should be slow, no faster than 50 mg/hr, to avoid a sudden drop in blood pressure. After the dose of phenytoin has been completed, if seizures continue, a loading dose of phenobarbital should be given; if this is still insufficient, anesthesia becomes necessary and is best accomplished with intravenous pentobarbital. Doses and speed of injections are given in Table 17-3.

In order to determine whether the electrical status epilepticus is controlled, it is necessary to continuously monitor cerebral activity with the EEG. The desired state of anesthesia is also determined by the induction of the burst-suppression pattern in the EEG.

Since electrical seizures may recur after temporary control, it is necessary to continuously monitor cerebral electrical activity for days or weeks. Also, if burst-suppression pattern is to be maintained, its continuation must be verified by EEG recording. Continuous EEG monitoring, however, is very inconvenient and inefficient. Large amounts of paper accumulate, interpretation by an expert electroencephalographer is necessary, a competent technician must be continuously available to run the record, and it is difficult to determine trends with such voluminous records.

In order to perform continuous cerebral monitoring in a practical way, it is possible to record the EEG on magnetic tape, which can be viewed on-line on a television screen and selected parts of which may be printed. Video EEG can be used in this fashion. However, this method still needs the continuous collaboration of an electroencephalographer and an EEG technician. More practical methods can be used, but they involve data reduction at the expense of some of the information obtainable with standard EEG. Special instruments are available that compress time and give quantitative values of amplitude or frequency (or both) of EEG activity in an easily interpretable form, which also simplifies patterns corresponding to seizures or decreases in general electrical cerebral output[10] (Fig. 17-3). With only minimal instruction, interns and nurses are able to detect abnormalities. A regular EEG

TABLE 17-3 Treatment of Status Epilepticus

Medication	Speed of Delivery	Total Dose	Possible Complications
Initial			
Diazepam	2 mg/min	10 to 20 mg	Respiratory
Lorazepam	<2 mg/min	4 to 8 mg	Respiratory
Additional (even if seizures are controlled with benzodiazepines)			
Phenytoin	No faster than 50 mg/min	20 mg/kg	Hypotension
If no response to A and B			
Phenobarbital	100 mg/min	10 mg/kg	Respiratory
If no response to A, B, or C			
Pentobarbital (anesthetic)	2 mg/min	5 mg/kg initially and continue to induce EEG burst-suppression pattern	Respiratory Cardiac

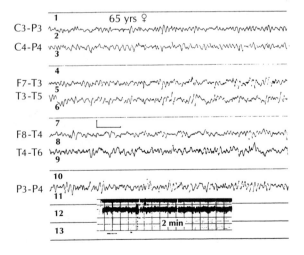

FIG. 17-3 Seven-channel EEG for comparison of its time base with that of cerebral function monitor (CFM) shown at bottom. Time calibration in EEG is 1 second. In CFM, time between two consecutive vertical divisions is 2 minutes. One-channel CFM, taken from derivation P3-P4 of EEG, represents maximal amplitudes in upper edge of second black, ragged tracing and minimal amplitudes in its lower edge. Upper, more regular black tracing of CFM gives rough indication of changes in frequency.

is still necessary to make it possible to interpret the record produced by these instruments, but only at the beginning of the recording and later with spot checks for interpretation of some changes in the data-reduced tracings. The two instruments I have used most often for the data-reduced continuous monitoring of cerebral function are the cerebral function monitor (Cerebral Function Monitor; Critikon, Ascot Berks, England), which mainly measures amplitude, and a monitor that produces a compressed spectral array (Neurotrac; Interspec, Ambler, Pa.). There are, however, other suitable machines commercially available.

SUMMARY

- Seizures typically demonstrate a change in frequency and severity of clonic contractions.
- Myoclonus typically is more monotonous, continuous, and dysrhythmic than epileptic seizures.
- Differentiation of seizures from myoclonus in the SICU usually requires an EEG.
- Clonazepam may be effective in controlling myoclonus.
- Status epilepticus, defined as any seizure lasting 30 minutes or more, is a medical emergency.

- Suspect complex partial status epilepticus in any patient who alternates among automatisms, simple confusion, and unresponsivity.
- Episodic changes in state of consciousness or sustained unconsciousness may represent nonconvulsive status epilepticus. EEG is required for diagnosis. Since electrical seizures may recur, continuous cerebral monitoring may be required in the SICU.

REFERENCES

1. Lotham E. The biochemical basis and pathophysiology of status epilepticus. Neurology (Suppl 2)40:13-23, 1990.
2. Gastaut H. Dictionary of Epilepsy. I. Definitions. Geneva: World Health Organization, 1973.
3. Hauser WA. Status epilepticus: Frequency, etiology and neurological sequelae. In Delgado-Escueta AV, Westerlain CG, Treiman DM, Porter RJ, eds. Advances in Neurology, vol 34. Status Epilepticus: Mechanisms of Brain Damage and Treatment. New York: Raven Press, 1983, pp 3-14.
4. Treiman DM, Delgado-Escueta AV. Complex partial status epilepticus. In Delgado-Escueta AV, Westerlain CG, Treiman DM, Porter RJ, eds. Advances in Neurology, vol 34. Status Epilepticus: Mechanisms of Brain Damage and Treatment. New York: Raven Press, 1983, pp 69-81.
5. Altafullah I, Asaikar S, Torres F. Status epilepticus: Clinical experience with two special devices for continuous cerebral monitoring. Acta Neurol Scand 84:374-381, 1991.
6. Sommer W. Erkrankungen des Ammonshorns als aetiologisches Moment der Epilepsie. Arch Psychiatr Nervenkr 10:631-675, 1880.
7. Sperling MR, Gur RC, Alavi A, Gur RE, Resnick S, O'Connor MJ, Reivich M. Subcortical metabolic alterations in partial epilepsy. Epilepsia 31:145-155, 1990.
8. Meldrum BS, Briesley JB. Prolonged epileptic seizures in primates: Ischaemic cell change and its relation to ictal physiologic events. Arch Neurol 28:10-17, 1973.
9. Knopman D, Margolis G, Reeves AG. Prolonged focal epilepsy and hypoxemia as a cause of focal brain damage: A case study. Ann Neurol 1:195-198, 1977.
10. Talwar D, Torres F. Continuous electrophysiologic monitoring of cerebral function in the pediatric intensive care unit. Pediatr Neurol 4:137-147, 1988.

CHAPTER 18

Head Injury

Anthony Bottini

BASIC CONCEPTS

The competent management of a patient with severe head injury is a demanding task, one that requires the expertise of not only neurosurgeons but also allied surgical and medical specialists who can provide the multidisciplinary approach necessary in this critically ill population. Head injury is among the most common life-threatening conditions treated in a critical care setting. Approximately 50% of all deaths from trauma are associated with a significant head injury, and over 60% of deaths from motor vehicle accidents are caused by head injury. A patient dies of a head injury every 12 minutes in the United States. These observations indicate that the problem is both significant and common. The optimal care of patients with head injury is not fully defined, and management is constantly evolving.

The brain does not respond well to injury. It is infinitely better to prevent CNS injury than to attempt to repair it because the damage that occurs at the time of the patient's brain injury is largely irremediable. The focus of all therapeutic efforts subsequent to brain injury is to prevent secondary insults that will limit survival or increase the neural deficits resulting from the primary injury. Efficient, accurate assessment and appropriate, timely intervention are essential in caring for patients with head injury.

NEUROANATOMIC AND PATHOLOGIC SUBSTRATES

The initial rapid assessment of the patient with head injury centers around those elements in-cluded in the Glasgow Coma Scale (GCS) (see box) and includes the presence of eye opening, level of responsiveness, and movement of the extremities. This scale, initially developed as a research tool, has found wide acceptance because of good inter-observer reliability and strong correlation with prognosis. The GCS

Glasgow Coma Scale*

Eye opening (E)

Spontaneous	4
To speech	3
To pain	2
None	1

Best motor response (M)

Obeys commands	6
Localizes pain	5
Withdraws	4
Abnormal flexion	3
Extensor response	2
None	1

Best verbal response (V)

Oriented	5
Confused conversation	4
Inappropriate words	3
Incomprehensible sounds	2
None	1

TOTAL (E + M + V) = (3-15)

---

*From Teasdale B, Jennett B. Assessment and prognosis of coma after head injury. Acta Neurochir (Wien) 34:45-55, 1976.

score should serve as the fundamental measure of injury at presentation and as a means of serial comparison throughout the acute clinical course.

The neuroanatomic substrate for consciousness resides primarily in the reticular activating system (RAS). The RAS is diffusely distributed throughout the posterior portion of the brainstem and extends from the superior pons as far rostral as the thalamus and the hypothalamus. Injury to this area, through direct impact, concussion, or distortion by an intracranial mass, will produce coma. Discrete injuries elsewhere in the cerebrum also will cause coma, although these areas are less commonly responsible for loss of consciousness following trauma (see box).

A more in-depth neurologic examination is done to assess those systems that may have localized intracranial pathologic conditions. These systems include the pupillary light reflex, motor system, and respiratory pattern. The pathway for the pupillary light reflex originates at the retina. The afferent limb includes the optic nerve and the dorsal midbrain. The efferent parasympathetic reflex arc, which acts to constrict the pupil, originates in the Edinger-Westphal nucleus of the midbrain, proceeds with the third cranial nerve to the ciliary ganglion, and finally probes through the short ciliary nerve to the iris. The efferent sympathetic supply, which dilates the pupil, passes from the hypothalamus through the lateral tegmentum of the brainstem to synapse in the intermediolateral cell column of the spinal cord from C8-T2 and then through the sympathetic chain to the stellate ganglion. Sympathetic fibers travel with the carotid artery to the orbit and then pass through the long ciliary nerve to innervate the pupillodilatory mechanism of the iris.

In uncal herniation following head injury, the uncus of the temporal lobe is forced into the tentorial incisura, compressing the ipsilateral third cranial nerve. The parasympathetic supply to the pupil is interrupted, and the unbalanced sympathetic tone produces dilation of the ipsilateral pupil. Conversely, although far less commonly, trauma to the region of the stellate ganglion or the carotid sheath may in-

---

Anatomic Substrates of Alertness

Reticular activating system (RAS): extends from superior half of pons through midbrain to hypothalamus and thalamus

Bilateral cerebral hemispheric lesions: produce transient unresponsiveness, especially if lesion involves mesial frontal region

Large unilateral lesions of dominant hemisphere: occasionally cause transient unresponsiveness

Posterior hypothalamic lesions: produce prolonged hypersomnia

Paraventricular thalamic nuclei: acute bilateral lesions that produce transient unresponsiveness and permanent severe amnestic dementia

---

terrupt the sympathetic supply to the pupil and produce unbalanced parasympathetic tone. Pupillary constriction and ipsilateral miosis then occur. In this situation the resulting anisocoria may be misinterpreted as contralateral pupillary dilation.

Motor control originates in the primary motor cortex in the posterior frontal region, condenses into the internal capsule, and forms the corticospinal tract, which subsequently decussates in the lower medulla. This pathway, within the pyramidal tract, is found laterally at the level of the midbrain. In this area the tract is susceptible to compression by either the herniating uncus of the temporal lobe or the free edge of the tentorium contralateral to the intracranial mass (Fig. 18-1). In the case of direct uncal compression of the pyramidal tract, the motor deficit is found contralateral to the intracranial mass. When the motor pathways are compressed by the free edge of the tentorium, paresis is found ipsilateral to the mass lesion (Fig. 18-2). This false lateralizing finding, or Kernohan's notch phenomenon, is found in approximately 15% of patients with an asymmetric motor examination following closed head injury. In comparison to the pupillary light reflex, motor findings following head injury are less reliable as a lateralizing indication. If there is doubt, it should be remembered that the mass lesion is usually on the side of the pupillary

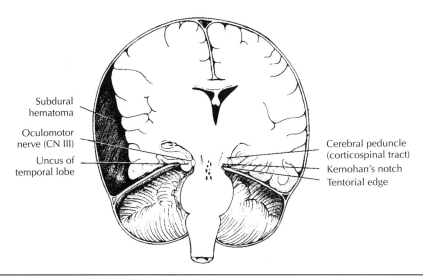

FIG. 18-1   Uncal herniation in a coronal plane.

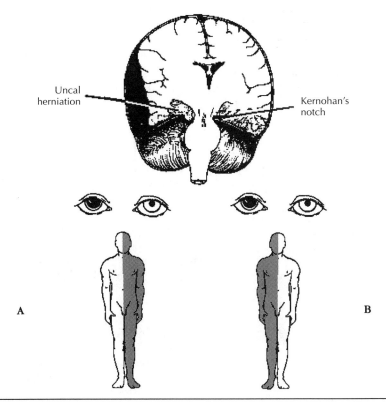

FIG. 18-2   Lateralizing signs in uncal herniation. **A,** Expected signs. **B,** Kernohan's notch phenomenon.

abnormality. Respiratory irregularities also have some value for localizing injury in the setting of progressive rostral-to-caudal brainstem herniation (Table 18-1).

SKULL FRACTURES

Skull fractures are a common finding after a severe head injury, although they in themselves do not constitute a mechanism for neurologic injury. The search for a skull fracture should never become a primary objective in evaluation of the patient and should certainly never delay appropriate initial management of a patient with evidence of neurologic deterioration.

Linear Nondisplaced Skull Fractures

A linear, nondisplaced fracture is a stellate-appearing break of the cranial vault seen on plain radiographs of the skull. It is a direct effect of physical contact with the skull and reflects the amount of energy the skull has absorbed in the traumatic event. Not uncommonly, patients with skull fractures demonstrate little or no underlying neurologic injury because the energy of the impact has been expended in fracturing the skull; therefore accelerational injury imparted to the underlying brain is minimized. The most worrisome part of a linear skull fracture is that disruption of the inner table of the skull also may disturb dural vascular structures. The most important of these structures, and the one most frequently injured, is the middle meningeal artery. This vessel is a branch of the external carotid artery, which enters the skull under the temporal lobe through the foramen spinosum, and is contained intracranially within a shallow bone channel on the inner surface of the skull that runs laterally and anteriorly from the foramen spinosum. Although the vessel is located within this channel, it is highly susceptible to injury when the skull is fractured. Near the lateral termination of the greater wing of the sphenoid bone, just anterior to and above the ear, the vessel leaves the bony channel to run between the leaves of the dura and branches widely to supply the lateral expanse of the supratentorial dura. Other vascular structures that may be imperiled by a linear skull fracture are the sagittal sinus and the lateral or sigmoid sinuses. Disruption of either a dural artery or vein may produce an epidural hematoma. A linear skull fracture in a conscious patient increases the risk of intracranial hematoma by a factor of 400 and increases the probability that the patient will require a craniotomy by a factor of 20.[1,2]

TABLE 18-1   Respiratory Patterns in Coma

Pattern	Possible Cause
Cheyne-Stokes respiration	Brief hyperpnea alternating with even shorter periods of apnea; represents loss of forebrain "smoothing" of respiratory response to Pco_2; found with bilateral thalamic lesions or lesions from cerebral hemispheres down to upper pons; also found with uremia or diffuse anoxia
Sustained regular hyperventilation	Lesions of midbrain or pons may produce rapid hyperpnea
Apneustic respiration	Lesions in lateral tegmentum of caudal pons may result in long periods of inspiration with breathholding followed by expiration
Cluster respiration	Lesions in lower pons or upper medulla may produce irregular pattern of clusters of respiration
Ataxic respiration	Damage to dorsomedial medulla may produce a completely irregular pattern of gasps and episodes of tachypnea; found in agonal patients as precursor to complete respiratory failure

Identifying patients with linear fractures also specifies a patient population at greater risk for a major intracranial disaster. As a general principle, all patients with skull fractures should undergo CT scanning and close observation.

Depressed Skull Fractures

A depressed skull fracture occurs when a skull fragment is displaced one bone width below the surrounding skull. Such fractures are more common after severe or focal cranial impact than after the type of impact that produces linear fractures. In general, depressed fractures result from direct blows to the head, frequently those with small impact areas, and are more commonly associated with underlying brain and vascular injury than are linear skull fractures.

An open, depressed skull fracture always requires surgical management. This type of injury represents a potential for bacterial contamination of the CSF pathways and the brain. It requires prompt and meticulous debridement, repair of any dural lacerations, and removal of contaminated skull fragments. Closed depressed skull fractures may be treated conservatively, depending on the location, underlying structures, and depth of the depressed fragments. Some neurosurgeons strongly argue that a depressed skull fracture represents a powerful predisposition to a posttraumatic seizure disorder and that elevation of these fractures is always indicated. Others have advocated a more conservative approach to the majority of these injuries.[3,4] A depressed skull fracture, whether open or closed, necessitates neurosurgical consultation.

Basilar Skull Fractures

A basilar skull fracture is generally a clinical diagnosis rather than a radiographic one. Occasionally, a basilar fracture may be imaged on a CT scan, but such a fracture is most commonly diagnosed through physical findings (e.g., hemotympanum, ecchymosis in mastoid region (Battle's sign), periorbital ecchymoses ("raccoon eyes"), or a CSF leak from ear or nose).

Fractures that cross the cribriform plate, paranasal sinuses, or mastoid cells of the petrous temporal bone and breach the underlying dura may produce CSF leaks. Patients with suspected basilar skull fracture should be questioned closely for signs or symptoms of CSF otorrhea or rhinorrhea and examined serially to detect a leak or facial nerve paralysis. In patients who develop a CSF fistula following a closed head injury, approximately 85% will have cessation of leakage with a week of conservative, expectant treatment alone.[5] During this time the patient should remain in an upright position as much as possible because the pressure of the brain over the area of dural disruption may help to seal the fistula. Consideration also may be given to lumbar drainage of CSF to permit closure of the basilar CSF fistula. A persistent CSF leak disposes the patient to late infectious complications, such as meningitis or brain abscess, and surgery may be necessary if leakage has not stopped after 1 week.

The use of prophylactic antibiotics in patients with basilar skull fractures, with or without evidence of a CSF leak, is controversial. Little clear, objective evidence exists to show that prophylactic antibiotics are effective, but data are available that demonstrate that prophylactic antibiotics may change the nasopharyngeal flora to more pathogenic organisms, principally Gram-negative enteric bacteria.[6,7] Nasotracheal or nasogastric tubes should be used with great caution in patients with clinical signs of a basilar skull fracture because they may penetrate the fracture and pass into the intracranial cavity. These patients also should not have cotton swabs or other instrumentation (except the otoscope) placed in their external acoustic meatus.

Cranial nerve dysfunction, especially of the facial nerve, also may result from a basilar skull fracture. Fractures that are transverse to the long axis of the petrous portion of the temporal bone are associated with a higher risk of facial nerve palsy because they cross the path of the facial nerve in a transverse direction. Facial nerve palsies that are present immediately following trauma have a poorer prognosis than those that occur as a delayed complication because an immediate facial palsy may indicate that the facial nerve was transected when the temporal bone was fractured. A delayed facial weakness, caused by nerve edema or the presence of a hematoma within the facial canal, has important implications for management. The paresis may be improved with surgical decompression of the facial nerve. This consideration emphasizes the need for close and careful observation of facial nerve function in a patient suspected of sustaining a basilar skull fracture.

HEMATOMAS
Epidural Hematoma

An epidural hematoma (EDH) represents the greatest threat and the greatest challenge to clinicians who care for patients with brain injury. This type of hematoma most commonly results when the middle meningeal artery is lacerated along its course from its entrance into the intracranial cavity through the foramen spinosum to its eventual distribution and ramifications over the broad expanse of the supratentorial dura. The epidural space, usually only a potential space, is very distensible and is limited only by the attachment of the dura along the suture lines. Because the injury is arterial and the clot dissects the dura from the inner surface of the brain, the resulting lesion appears convex on axial imaging studies. Epidural hematomas are uncommon in elderly patients because the dura is often strongly adherent to the underlying surface of the skull. In the elderly the epidural space may not exist.

The challenge involved in treating patients with EDH is early recognition. Most patients who suffer from an EDH have sustained little or no brain injury at the time of the trauma. The expanding hematoma in the epidural space represents a secondary injury that quickly may prove fatal. No one should ever die of an epidural hematoma. Because the neurologic prognosis is good in this group of patients, it is a needless tragedy if a patient suffers irreversible brain injury or death as a result of a delay in recognizing this type of lesion. Confounding this situation, which is anxiety-producing for the clinician, is the recognition that EDHs are most commonly found in a patient population younger than 40 years of age. Thus this potentially fatal, but easily treatable condition, is an affliction of people who are in the prime of their lives.

A common clinical presentation for the patient with an EDH is a brief loss of consciousness in an accident, recovery of consciousness at the scene, and a near-normal neurologic examination on initial presentation to the paramedics or the emergency room. The patient subsequently undergoes a delayed, and sometimes rapidly progressive, neurologic deterioration. The pathophysiologic reason for this clinical course is that although the patient suffers a minor cerebral contusion at the time of impact, the impact also produces a skull fracture and vascular laceration. Consciousness is soon regained because of the minimal cerebral contusion, but the hematoma within the epidural space begins to expand.

Initially, the brain shifts toward midline to accommodate this new intracranial mass, and CSF is displaced from the ventricles into the lumbar thecal sac to accommodate the growing extra-axial mass. As the dura is stretched, the patient complains of headache; as the mass outgrows the brain's ability to accommodate it, intracranial pressure begins to rise and the midline structures become distorted. The patient becomes less responsive, increasingly somnolent, and, finally, comatose. This clinical presentation of EDH is often described as the "lucid interval." Relatively early in this progression, the ipsilateral third cranial nerve may be compressed and initially may produce an oval pupil ipsilateral to the EDH. With further expansion of the hematoma, a widely fixed and dilated ipsilateral pupil occurs. (Patients who have a dilated, nonreactive pupil because of uncal herniation always have lost consciousness first.) With continued brainstem compression, the herniation syndrome becomes complete and the patient may develop bilateral pupillary abnormalities. Incomplete expressions of this syndrome may occur. The clinical findings may progress more slowly or to a lesser degree, and the predominant clinical complaint is increasing headache.

Any patient with a linear skull fracture or with the progression of symptoms described above should be suspected of having an EDH or another type of space-occupying intracranial mass until proven otherwise.

The treatment of EDH almost always demands immediate surgical management. Definitive treatment consists of a limited craniotomy with evacuation of the clot and control of the bleeding source. The presence of an epidural hematoma in a patient with signs of neurologic compromise is the paramount neurosurgical emergency. In recent years, some authors have advocated nonoperative management of small epidural hematomas in patients who have no or minimal symptoms.[8,9] The decision not to operate may initiate a precarious clinical course. Such a decision should be made only by a neurosurgeon.

Acute Subdural Hematoma

An acute subdural hematoma (ASDH) is the most commonly noted lesion in patients who present to the emergency department with severe head injury. It is also the most common injury that produces a fatal outcome following trauma. Whereas epidural hematomas are not usually associated with underlying brain injury, ASDHs are usually a reflection of the amount of injury the brain has sustained. In severe injury, the brain suffers serious contusion, multiple small cortical veins are ruptured, and an ASDH is usually formed by venous bleeding from the cortical surface. The mortality of acute subdural hematoma is extremely high, approximately 40%, and the outcome is related to two factors: the speed with which the clot is removed in a patient who is deteriorating and the degree of associated underlying brain injury. In a classic clinical study of patients with ASDH, severe morbidity and mortality was three times greater in patients who had an ASDH removed more than 4 hours following trauma compared to those patients who were operated on within 4 hours.[10] Speed is of the essence in diagnosing and treating ASDHs.

Subdural hematomas form in the subdural space, the space between the brain or arachnoid membrane and the dura. Unlike the situation with epidural hematoma, the subdural space is not limited by suture lines. For this reason, subdural hematomas tend to spread widely over the convexity of the brain and form a concave appearance on axial imaging. Clinical findings in a patient with an ASDH range from a patient who is deeply comatose from the time of injury to one who experiences a lucid interval comparable to that described with epidural hematomas. Although the lucid interval of presentation is common among patients with EDH, it is a less common clinical course for patients with subdural hematomas. Because ASDHs have a much higher incidence than that of EDHs, the majority of patients with a lucid interval will suffer from a subdural hematoma. Because both the EDH and the ASDH tend to occur over the lateral, frontal, or temporal regions, the mass effect from these lesions tends to be directed toward the midline. The ASDH produces a midline shift of the frontal and temporal lobes and, if not controlled, leads to uncal herniation by forcing the medial portion of the temporal lobe into the incisura.

The surgical treatment of ASDH is similar to that of EDH. In both, a temporal trauma flap is fashioned and a free bone flap is elevated over the frontal and temporal regions. For treatment of an ASDH, the dura must be opened before the hematoma can be removed. An ASDH is usually several centimeters thick, spreads out over the entire convexity of the brain, and is clotted and semifirm rather than liquid. The ASDH must be removed with a combination of suction and irrigation. The usual source of subdural bleeding is the small venules over the surface of the brain. It is unusual to find a discreet or major bleeding source when a subdural hematoma is removed. A major exception is the removal of a subdural clot produced by injury to a major venous structure such as the sagittal or lateral sinus.

Following the successful removal of an ASDH, the dura is closed, the bone flap is replaced, and an intracranial pressure monitor is customarily placed to aid in the management of intracranial hypertension as cerebral edema develops.

Traumatic Intracerebral Hematoma

A hematoma may form within the brain parenchyma itself as a result of trauma. Such hematomas are relatively uncommon and have an incidence ranging from 4% to 12% in patients who suffer severe closed head injury.[11] Intracerebral hematomas are far less common than subdural hematomas; they occur with a frequency approximately equal to that of epidural hematomas. Intracerebral hematomas result from severe disruption of the deep white matter and may occur at the time of injury. Alternatively, they may represent a coalescence of multiple smaller contusions contained within an injured lobe. Characteristically, these contusions, and thus the eventual hematoma, are found as a contrecoup accompaniment to trauma. Therefore frontal intracerebral hematomas are most commonly found in patients who fall and strike the occiput. These hematomas are expanded masses surrounded by edematous brain. They may elevate intracranial pressure and distort adjacent brain tissue sufficiently to mandate surgical removal. Most patients with large intracerebral hematomas resulting from trauma will have a profoundly altered state of consciousness and must be managed with close monitoring of intracranial pressure and neurologic status.

Hematomas in proximity to the tentorial incisura, for example, those in the posterior frontal or anterior temporal lobes, are particularly dangerous. They may produce uncal herniation and brainstem injury with only a minimum of warning.[12] Some neurosurgeons remove such hematomas prophylactically.

Delayed Traumatic Intracerebral Hematoma

A delayed traumatic intracerebral hematoma (DTICH) is found in patients with head trauma who had no evidence of such a blood clot on admission CT scanning. This type of hematoma develops hours to days following head injury and is more common in older patients.

Following the removal of an extra-axial mass lesion such as a subdural hematoma, the brain underlying the hematoma reexpands. This portion of the brain has been severely traumatized by a combination of concussion and compression. Cerebral contusions frequently appear in the white matter upon reexpansion and then

may coalesce to form a DTICH.[13] Those patients who develop disseminated intravascular coagulopathy and fibrinolysis following a head injury may be at increased risk of developing a delayed intracerebral hematoma.

The clinical presentation of DTICH is neurologic deterioration in a patient who has been stable or shown improvement following the initial phases of head injury. DTICH may be heralded by an unexpected rise in the patient's intracranial pressure. Such deterioration should always prompt a search for a surgical intracranial lesion. A repeat CT scan is the most efficient means of diagnosing these hematomas. In patients who develop evidence of coagulopathy following head injury, serial CT scans may allow the early detection of a DTICH. As a matter of practice, CT scans of patients with severe head injury should be repeated routinely on postinjury days 1 and 3. The yield on these "routine" studies is high and helps lessen the possibility of an unwelcome surprise.

PATHOPHYSIOLOGY

Trauma produces a wide variation in the type of injury that the brain and its surrounding structures sustain. All of these injuries, edema, contusions, and hematomas, can be discussed in the context of the Monro-Kellie doctrine. This doctrine states that the intracranial capacity is a fixed volume occupied by brain, blood, CSF, and any other masses that may develop within this closed space. Because the space cannot expand, there is a limited amount of compliance within the system before pressure begins to elevate dramatically in response to an increasing mass. The intracranial mass that follows a head injury may comprise cerebral edema, hyperemia that increases cerebral blood flow, an extra-axial or intra-axial hematoma, air, a penetrating object, or any combination of these elements. The initial response of the system in terms of compliance is to displace CSF from the ventricles into the spinal thecal sac. This mechanism provides approximately 50 to 70 cc of additional intracranial volume to accommodate the mass. A second mechanism that affords additional intracranial compliance is the collapse of venous capacitance vessels in response to rising intracranial pressure. When this space has been filled by an enlarging mass, the system's response to the addition of any further intracranial mass is rapidly increasing intracranial pressure.

The goal of management of the patient with head injury is to preserve cerebral blood flow, minimize the formation of cerebral edema, and control intracranial pressure. Cerebral blood flow cannot be measured in most SICUs but must be inferred from a measurement of cerebral perfusion pressure (CPP), defined clinically as the difference between mean arterial pressure (MAP) and intracranial pressure (ICP). The formula to determine cerebral perfusion pressure is:

$$CPP = MAP - ICP$$

Under most circumstances, the cerebral blood flow will remain fairly constant within the limits of autoregulation (CPP = 60 to 150 mm Hg). Autoregulation is a physiologic accommodation that maintains near-constant cerebral blood flow over a wide range of perfusion pressures. Within the limits of cerebral autoregulation, cerebral ischemia will not occur. This mechanism is operant only in intact brain. Autoregulation is largely disrupted in edematous, traumatized, or ischemic brain, and cerebral blood flow may vary directly with changes in cerebral perfusion pressure.

As ICP rises, CPP generally falls. If CPP falls below the lower limits of cerebral autoregulation, the traumatized brain becomes ischemic. This ischemia produces a secondary and sometimes devastating insult to vulnerable traumatized neural tissue. The actual incidence and relative contribution of cerebral ischemia that follows closed head injury has been vigorously debated by authorities in the field. Cerebral ischemia may affect only a minority of patients with severe head injury, although these patients tend to be more severely injured and have a worse prognosis.[14]

The more common response of cerebral blood flow to severe head injury is moderate to extreme hyperemia, particularly in children and young adults. Such a finding probably reflects a failure of autoregulation and makes the cerebral capillary system vulnerable to hemorrhage or transudation of edema fluid into the interstitium.

MANAGEMENT OF INTRACRANIAL PRESSURE

A plan to manage intracranial hypertension is based on the Monro-Kellie doctrine and attempts to favorably affect each of the components that occupy intracranial volume (Fig. 18-3). The first line of defense is to remove those masses—epidural, subdural, or intracerebral hematomas—that are present when the patient arrives at the hospital. There is little or no place for medical treatment of intracranial mass lesions. Usually, surgery for this indication has been performed before the patient arrives in the SICU, and the responsibility of the SICU physician is to monitor the patient carefully to detect the late development or recurrence of such a mass. At least 15% of patients who have undergone surgical removal of an intracranial hematoma will develop a delayed or recurrent hematoma after arriving in the SICU. The detection of such a lesion is the primary objective of all neurologic and clinical monitoring. Any unexplained deterioration in the patient's neurologic status or an abrupt rise in ICP must alert the clinician to the possibility of a delayed development of a mass lesion. A corollary to this principle is that an unexplained rise in blood pressure may be a physiologic response to a narrowed cerebral perfusion pressure as the brain struggles to maintain adequate cerebral blood flow. The possibility of a delayed mass lesion should always be considered when systolic hypertension occurs in patients with head injury, especially those who do not have ICP monitoring.

In those patients who have continuing ICP elevations following the evacuation of all surgical lesions, management is directed at increasing the compliance of the system through one of several manipulations. First, and most effective, is hyperventilation, which serves to constrict venous capacitance primarily and to decrease the amount of intracranial volume taken by systemic blood. Hyperventilation also decreases the hyperemia that commonly fol-

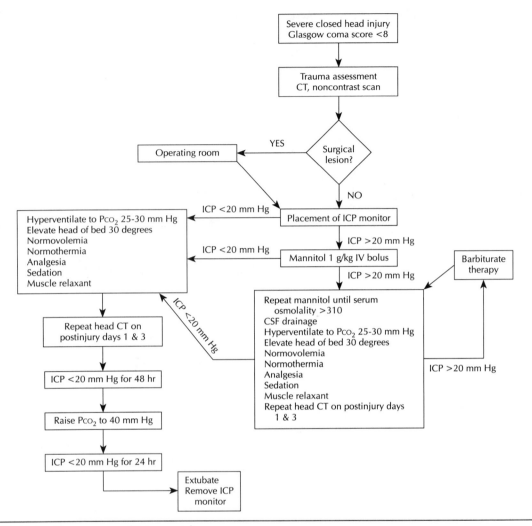

FIG. 18-3 Management of intracranial pressure.

lows head injury and has a direct and profound effect on intracranial pressure. The target P_{CO_2} is 25 to 29 mm Hg. Positive end expiratory pressure may be used in patients with head injury at levels of 5 to 10 cm H_2O without significantly affecting ICP.

A second strategy for decreasing ICP is to treat the patient with a hyperosmotic agent, which decreases the amount of cerebral interstitial volume and cerebral edema. Mannitol is the drug of choice in most centers and is administered in a dose of 1/2 to 1 g/kg as a bolus injection over several minutes. Mannitol is most

effective in decreasing ICP when given as a bolus, although some physicians use this agent in a drip form to maximize serum osmolarity. Mannitol may be infused until the serum osmolarity is in the range of 305 to 310. Increasing the osmolarity beyond this point does not significantly affect intracranial edema and potentiates serious electrolyte imbalances. The goal of mannitol therapy is to render the patient hyperosmotic but not hypovolemic. Hypovolemia may compromise the brain, and in patients with multiple trauma such manipulation may limit the chance of survival. Nonosmotic diuretics also may be used to assist in the control of intracranial hypertension. Furosemide is the drug that has been used most often for this indication, and there is evidence that it acts synergistically with mannitol.[15] The clinician should use caution because combined therapy may produce profound dehydration far faster than either agent does alone and may lead to circulatory collapse. In its effect on ICP, furosemide appears to be less reliable as a sole agent than mannitol.

The next portion of the Monro-Kellie doctrine that can be manipulated is the intracranial volume occupied by CSF. Production of CSF will continue in the ventricles until very high ICP is reached. The development of posttraumatic hydrocephalus can be a terminal event. Compliance in the system may be increased by providing an alternative outlet for CSF drainage through placement of a ventriculostomy catheter, which can serve the dual role of providing ICP monitoring and an outlet for CSF flow.

In patients who are intubated, muscle relaxants used in conjunction with analgesics and/or sedatives are another useful adjunct to lowering ICP. Doses of these agents should be reduced or interrupted on a regular basis every few hours to permit monitoring of neurologic function. In those patients with continuous ICP monitoring, sedatives and muscle relaxants can be used with slightly more confidence.

Elevation of the head of the patient's bed to control ICP is controversial in the literature, although in practice it is a nearly universal management technique. Typically, the patient's head is elevated approximately 30 degrees to facilitate venous drainage and to diminish the formation of cerebral edema.

High-dose barbiturate therapy also has been used as a management option in patients with increased ICP.[16-18] Most centers reserve this type of therapy for those patients who are hemodynamically stable and have intracranial hypertension that has proven refractory to conventional management. High-dose barbiturate therapy has the dual purpose of protecting the brain metabolically while decreasing cerebral blood flow and volume. The initiation and maintenance of pentobarbital coma is complex and

dangerous and should be considered only in patients who (1) are not neurologically devastated, (2) are young and not volume depleted, and (3) have arterial pressure monitoring and Swan-Ganz monitoring catheters in place. The greatest risk with the initiation of barbiturate therapy is profound and refractory hypotension. Hemodynamic monitoring and optimization is necessary. Pentobarbital loading should be performed with a dose of 10 mg/kg over 30 minutes followed by a maintenance dose of 5 mg/kg/hr for the next 3 hours. Long-term maintenance is then begun at 1 to 2 mg/kg/hr and titrated to achieve ICP control. If ICP is not controlled, additional boluses of pentobarbital (100 to 200 mg) should be administered intravenously at a slow rate. Serum pentobarbital levels should be checked every 12 hours for 48 hours and subsequently at least every 24 hours. Serum concentrations should be maintained at 3 to 4 mg/dl. The endpoint for pentobarbital therapy is ICP control; pentobarbital is frequently a therapy of last resort, the drug should be used aggressively until ICP is controlled or the patient displays signs of significant drug toxicity, such as refractory hypotension.

The use of steroids in patients with severe head injury is also controversial. Despite many clinical studies, not a single controlled study has shown evidence that administration of steroids improves patient outcome. New agents are under development and may be more effective in reducing cerebral edema and less likely to produce side effects. Presently, no indication for the use of steroids in head injury exists.[19]

Table 18-2 summarizes the pharmacologic control of ICP.

POSTTRAUMATIC SEIZURES

Posttraumatic seizures are relatively common among patients with severe head injury, having an estimated incidence of 20% to 50%. Higher rates are found in patients with depressed skull fractures or penetrating brain injuries and in children with severe head injuries.

Seizures are common from several hours to several days following severe head injury. Termed "early" seizures, they are a direct re-

TABLE 18-2 Pharmacologic Control of Intracranial Pressure		
Drug	**Administration**	**Notes**
Mannitol (osmotic diuretic)	Bolus IV dose: 1 g/kg	Effective until serum osmolality >320
Furosemide (loop diuretic)	Bolus IV dose: 10-20 mg (adult)	Less effective than mannitol; may potentiate electrolyte abnormalities if used in conjunction with osmotic diuretics
Vecuronium (paralyzing agent)	0.1 mg/kg IV dose or 1 μg/kg/min continuous IV infusion	Must be used in conjunction with a sedative
Lorazepam (sedative)	1-4 mg IV dose	Effect lasts 6-8 hours, includes both sedation and relative amnesia
Pentobarbital (cerebral protective agent)	Loading dose: 10 mg/kg over 30 min Maintenance dose: 1-2 mg/kg/hr	Hypotension is a common complication; drug is used until ICP is controlled or patient becomes refractorily hypotensive

flection of the injury to the brain and are not, in themselves, considered epileptic. It is clear that early seizures are a predisposing factor to the development of late seizures or posttraumatic epilepsy. However, the occurrence of early seizures following trauma does not mean that posttraumatic epilepsy is inevitable.

The rationale for the use of anticonvulsants for early seizure prophylaxis is to decrease the incidence of these seizures, reduce the likelihood of late seizures, prevent acute complications of ictal events, and avoid further brain injury secondary to epileptiform discharge. In multiple double-blinded controlled studies, the most commonly used prophylactic anticonvulsant, phenytoin, has been shown to have an effect on the frequency of early seizures but no effect on that of late seizures. The use of phenytoin for patients with head injury is somewhat controversial.[20] A conservative recommendation is that phenytoin be used as prophylaxis in all patients with acute severe head injury

characterized by intracranial hematoma, contusion, depressed skull fracture, or open or penetrating injury. Anticonvulsants should be administered routinely to those patients who have suffered an early seizure.

If anticonvulsants are used, they must be administered in an adequate dosage. Patients with head injury are hypermetabolic, and serum phenytoin concentrations are almost always subtherapeutic in the acute stage of management. Phenytoin is the drug of choice in this clinical setting because it can be administered parenterally and has a relatively short half-life. When phenytoin is used in a critical care setting for a patient with head injury, serum drug concentrations should be followed at least daily to ensure that adequate blood concentrations are attained. Those patients who develop early seizures should be treated as though they were in status epilepticus, with the intravenous administration of diazepam or lorazepam (see Table 18-2).

SUMMARY

- All therapeutic efforts following brain injury attempt to prevent or reduce additional brain injury.
- Early, accurate diagnosis and therapy are essential to decrease morbidity and mortality.
- Initial assessment of patients with head injury must include Glasgow Coma Scale, pupillary light reflex, motor system evaluation, and respiratory pattern.
- A linear nondisplaced skull fracture indicates increased risk for development of intracranial hematoma.
- An open depressed skull fracture requires surgical management. Any depressed skull fracture mandates neurosurgical consultation.
- Basilar skull fractures are diagnosed clinically. Prophylactic antibiotic therapy for basilar skull fracture is controversial.

- Epidural hematomas are common in young patients, most likely are caused by injury to the middle meningeal artery, and require emergency surgical evaluation. A lucid interval is characteristic of the patient's history.
- ASDHs are lesions most commonly associated with severe head injury. Rapid evacuation can decrease morbidity and mortality. ASDHs also may be characterized by a lucid interval.
- Development of systolic hypertension following head injury may indicate development of a new intracranial mass lesion.
- Management of increased ICP attempts to remove space-occupying masses, improve compliance with hyperventilation or mannitol, or decrease the volume of CSF with a ventriculostomy catheter.

REFERENCES

1. Jennett B, Teasdale G. Early assessment of the head injured patient. In Management of Head Injuries. Philadelphia: FA Davis, 1981.
2. Dacey R, Alves W, Rimel R, et al. Neurosurgical complications after apparently minor head injury—Assessment of risk in a series of 610 patients. J Neurosurg 65:203, 1986.
3. Brackman D. Depressed skull fracture: Data, treatment and follow-up in 225 consecutive cases. J Neurosurg Psychiatry 34:106, 1971.
4. Van den Heever H, Van der Merwe J. Management of depressed skull fractures: Selective conservative management of nonmissile injuries. J Neurosurg 71:186, 1989.
5. Jacobs J, Persky M. Traumatic pneumocephalus. Laryngoscope 90:515, 1980.
6. Ignelzi R, VanderArk G. Analysis of the treatment of basilar skull fractures with and without antibiotics. J Neurosurg 43:721, 1975.
7. Hoff J, Brewin A. Antibiotics for basilar skull fractures. J Neurosurg 44:649, 1976.
8. Illingworth R, Shawdon H. Conservative management of intracranial extradural haematoma presenting late. J Neurol Neurosurg Psychiatry 46:558, 1983.

9. Bullock R, Smith R, van Dellen J. Nonoperative management of extradural hematoma. Neurosurgery 16:602, 1985.
10. Seelig J, Becker D, Miller J, et al. Traumatic acute subdural hematoma. Major morbidity reduction in comatose patients treated within four hours. N Engl J Med 304:516, 1981.
11. Eisenberg H, Gary H Jr, Aldrich E, et al. Initial CT scan findings in 753 patients with severe head injury: A report from the NIH traumatic coma bank. J Neurosurg 73:688, 1990.
12. Andrews B, Chiles B III, Olsen W, et al. The effect of intracerebral hematoma location on the risk of brain-stem compression and on clinical outcome. J Neurosurg 69:518, 1988.
13. Fukamachi A, Kohno K. Nagaseki Y, et al. The incidence of delayed traumatic intracerebral hematoma with extradural hemorrhages. J Trauma 25:145, 1985.
14. Robertson CS, Grossman RG, Goodman JC, et al. The predictive value of cerebral anaerobic metabolism with cerebral infarction after head injury. J Neurosurg 67:361, 1987.
15. Pollay M, Fullenwider C, Roberts P, et al. Effect of mannitol and furosemide on blood-brain osmotic gradient and intracranial pressure. J Neurosurg 59:945, 1983.

16. Rockoff M, Marshall L, Shapiro M. High-dose barbiturate therapy in humans: A clinical review of 60 patients. Ann Neurol 6:194, 1979.

17. Rea G, Rockswold G. Barbiturate therapy in uncontrolled intracranial hypertension. Neurosurgery 12:401, 1983.

18. Eisenberg H, Frankowski R, Contant C, et al. High-dose barbiturate control of elevated intracranial pressure in patients with severe head injury. J Neurosurg 69:15, 1988.

19. Marion DW, Ward JD. Steroids in closed-head injury. Perspect Crit Care 3(1):19, 1990.

20. Temkin N, Dikmen S, Winn H. Posttraumatic seizures. Neurosurg Clin North Am 2:425, 1991.

CHAPTER 19

Spinal Cord Injury

Anthony Bottini

Critical care of patients with spinal cord injuries is a unique clinical challenge. These patients are usually young, recently healthy adults who have suffered a devastating injury that has dramatically altered their physiology, function, independence, and self-image. They are vulnerable to a variety of insults and complications that may contribute to serious, life-long disability. Optimal management requires the physician to accurately assess and stabilize the cervical spinal injury, carefully monitor neurologic function, support the patient's homeostatic and recuperative mechanisms, and initiate physical and psychologic rehabilitation.

CLINICAL ASSESSMENT

Assessment begins with a clear and detailed history of the patient's trauma and subsequent course. Important details include the mechanism of injury (e.g., flexion, extension, rotation), the patient's realization of his/her deficit, and some understanding of the evolution of the neurologic deficit since the time of injury. The examiner should note whether the injury was complete initially or incomplete with subsequent progression. Details of the patient's extrication and transport to the hospital are also significant. Precautions undertaken to protect the patient's neurologic function during transport should be detailed, and a description of the patient's positioning, level of neurologic function, and immobilization measures in use at the time of unit admission should be documented.

The key element in assessment is a precise, complete, and carefully documented neurologic examination.[1] Neurologic examination on admission is critical to establish the baseline with which subsequent physicians may compare their evaluations and determine the patient's neurologic course.

The patient's head and neck should be immobilized. Any cervical orthosis obscuring the clinician's view should be removed and the neck examined. Obvious signs of injury to the neck should be noted, and carotid palpation should be performed alternately. Superficial temporal pulses should also be palpated and any signs of trauma representing a threat to the airway noted. Careful palpation over the spinous processes may also enable the clinician to narrow his/her search for evidence of injury on plain radiographs. The patient's head and neck should be maintained in a neutral position during the examination and not manipulated in any fashion. Typically patients with spinal cord injuries do not have observable surface deformities, except those who have suffered a unilaterally locked facet with forced rotation of the head to one side. The Philadelphia collar or other stabilizing orthosis should be replaced after examination of the patient's neck.

Motor Examination

The motor examination is of prime importance. All major muscle groups in each of the four extremities should be serially examined, and the strength of muscle contraction carefully documented. A grading system such as the one suggested in the box on p. 204 is objective and allows different clinicians to make meaningful comparisons. A standard motor examination in spinal cord–injured patients should test those muscle groups listed in Table 19-1. The reader is referred elsewhere for a description of the techniques for performing this examination.[2] Special care should be taken to determine if the muscles examined have any contractile function, even that which does not exceed the threshold for movement.

Grading System for Motor Examination of Patient With Spinal Cord Injury*

5   Contraction against powerful resistance (normal power) = 100%

4   Contraction against gravity and some resistance = 75%

3   Contraction against gravity only = 50%

2   Movement only possible with gravity eliminated = 25%

1   Flicker of contraction but no movement = 10%

0   Complete paralysis = 0%

---

*From Clain A, ed. Hamilton Bailey's Demonstrations of Physical Signs in Clinical Surgery. Bristol: John Wright & Sons, 1980, p 402. With permission of Butterworth-Heinemann Ltd.

Sensory Examination

The sensory examination, performed next, should be a careful, systematic examination with a variety of modalities, including pinprick, light touch, and proprioception. Multimodality testing is essential because the structures within the spinal cord that conduct sensation decussate at different levels in the CNS and travel in different quadrants of the spinal cord (Fig. 19-1). Incomplete cord lesions may produce a combination of sensory findings, depending on the tracts involved. Below the level of a complete lesion, all sensory modalities will be absent. Radicular pain or paresthesias may be present at the level of the injury and may have localizing value.

Pain sensation (nociception), as tested by pinprick, is primarily mediated in the lateral spinothalamic tract. This modality is tested with a disposable pin proceeding in a systematic fashion from the lower extremities up the trunk to the upper extremities. Left and right extremities should always be examined in serial fashion and compared. The chest and abdomen should also be examined, both over the anterior surfaces and as far posteriorly as possible.

Light touch, carried through the spinal cord's posterior columns, may be tested either with manual touch or with a tissue or some other minimal stimulus. To further refine this ex-

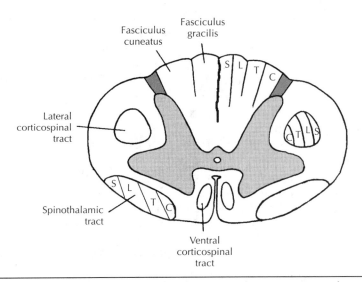

FIG. 19-1   Cervical spinal cord anatomy. *S,* sacral; *L,* lumbar; *T,* thoracic; *C,* cervical.

TABLE 19-1 Testing of Muscle Groups in Standard Motor Examination of Patient With Spinal Cord Injury*

Action	Muscle(s)	Root(s)	Peripheral Nerve
Upper extremities			
1. Abduct (initial) arm and extend rotation of arm	Supraspinatous, infraspinatous	C5, C6	Suprascapular
2. Abduct arm (hold at 90 degrees against resistance)	Deltoid	C5	Axilliary
3. Flex arm (hand supine)	Biceps	C5, C6	Musculocutaneous
4. Flex arm (hand midway between supine and prone)	Brachioradialis	C5, C6	Radial
5. Extend arm	Triceps	C7	Radial
6. Extension of wrist			
a. Hand abducted (toward thumb)	Extensor carpi radialis longus	C5, C6	Radial
b. Hand adducted (toward fifth finger)	Extensor carpi ulnaris	C7, C8	Posterior interosseous
7. Flexion of wrist	Flexor carpi radialis	C6, C7	Median
8. Flexion of fingers	Flexor digitorium superficialis (proximal)	C7, C8, T1	Median
	Flexor digitorum profundus (distal)		
a. First and second digits		C7, C8	Anterior interosseous
b. Third and fourth digits		C7, C8	Ulnar
9. Palmar abduction of thumb	Abductor pollicis brevis	C8, T1	Median
10. Opposing thumb to base of fifth finger	Opponens pollicis	C8, T1	Median
11. Spreading and adducting fingers	Interossei	C8, T1	Ulnar
Lower extremities			
1. Flexion of hip	Iliopsoas	L1, L2, L3	Direct branches from root
2. Extension of hip	Gluteus maximus	L5, S1	Inferior gluteal
3. Adduction of thigh	Adductors	L2, L3, L4	Obturator
4. Extension of leg (lower)	Quadriceps femoris	L2, L3, L4	Femoral
5. Flexion of knee	Hamstrings	L5, S1, S2	Sciatic
6. Plantar flexion of foot	Gastrocnemius and soleus	S1, S2	Tibial
7. Dorsiflexion of foot	Anterior tibial	L4, L5	Deep peroneal
8. Inversion of foot	Posterior tibial	L4, L5	Tibial
9. Extension of toes	Extensor digitorum longus and extensor hallucis longus	L5, S1	Deep peroneal
10. Eversion of foot	Peroneal longus and brevis	L5, S1	Sciatic

*Reprinted with permission from Weisberg L, Strub RL, Garcia CA. Essentials of Clinical Neurology, 2nd ed. Rockville, Md.: Aspen Publishers, 1989, pp 12-13.

Note: Underscoring indicates principal spinal nerve supply.

amination, two-point discrimination may also be tested to detect more subtle loss of sensation. A dermatomal diagram, in which the upper cervical dermatomes drape over the base of the neck and shoulders in a capelike fashion, is shown in Fig. 19-2. These determinations should be remembered in interpreting both the nociceptive and light-touch portion of the sensory examination; sensation in this capelike distribution may be misinterpreted as a preserved sensory level below an observed cervical motor level. In a patient with a cervical motor level, preservation of sensation over the clavicular regions should not be regarded as evidence of incomplete cervical spinal cord injury.

Proprioception should also be carefully tested over the patient's upper and lower extremities. Take care that the patient is not able to see the direction of digit deflection. In performing this examination, the examiner's thumb and forefinger are best positioned on the lateral aspects of the digit being tested. This position removes the additional pressure or light-touch sensation differential that may result when the digit is alternatively deflected upward or downward. Both light touch and proprioception are mediated through the posterior sensory columns.

Deep tendon reflexes should be tested over the biceps, triceps, brachioradialis, patella, gastrocnemius, and soleus tendons. This examination should then be recorded as a traditional stick-figure diagram for later comparison. In addition to deep tendon reflexes, other reflexes should also be tested in patients suspected of having spinal cord injury, including the abdominal, cremasteric, bulbocavernosus, anal wink, and crossed adductor reflexes.

A rectal examination should always be performed in a patient with a spinal cord injury. Preservation of perirectal sensation is an important finding in a patient who appears to have an otherwise complete spinal cord injury. This so-called sacral sparing of sensation results because of the onion skin–like lamination of fibers within the spinothalamic tract. Sacral fibers run in the ventrolateral portion of the tract and may be spared, even with deep intraparenchymal lesions. The distinction between an incomplete and a complete cord syndrome has great significance for further diagnostics, therapeu-

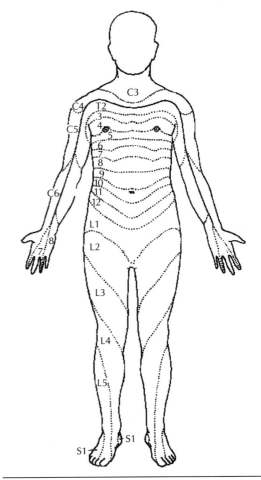

FIG. 19-2 Dermatomal diagram for examination of patient with spinal cord injury.

tics, and prognostication for the patient and family. The patient should also be carefully examined for sphincter tone and anal reflexes for these same reasons.

RADIOGRAPHIC ASSESSMENT

Radiologic evaluation of a spinal cord injury must always begin with plain cervical spine films. The single most useful view is a lateral radiograph, which includes at least C1 through C7 and preferably T1 as well. The examiner must develop and consistently use a systematized approach in studying cervical spine films. The most practical way to review cervical spine radiographs is to work from one direction to another; for example, in an anterior-to-posterior, then cephalad-to-caudal direction. The clinician should initially study the retropharyngeal soft tissue to determine if a hematoma, swelling, or other soft tissue sign provides a clue to the existence of a cervical spine injury. Study the anterior vertebral line to be certain that each of the vertebral bodies is properly aligned in a normal cervical lordotic configuration. Additionally, the examiner should look for avulsion fractures from the anterior endplates of these bodies, which might indicate that the patient has suffered an unstable hyperextension injury. The vertebral bodies are next examined and counted. A cervical spine film that does not include C7 is judged inadequate for further study. The heights of the vertebral bodies are studied for evidence of compression fractures, and their posterior margins are evaluated for a normal cervical lordotic configuration. Any subluxation or abrupt displacement of bone or vertebral bodies into the spinal canal should be noted. The spinal canal itself can be visualized as existing between the posterior margin of the vertebral bodies and the anterior margin of the spinous process. The normal diameter of an adult spinal cord is approximately 11 mm. Any smaller distance suggests cervical spinal canal stenosis of critical proportion. The spinous processes should be examined for fractures or spacing irregularities. A flexion injury that disrupts the interspinous ligament is frequently noted by an increase in the interspinous distance between the two levels involved in the injury. This "fanning" of the spinous processes may be the only radiographic indication of a potentially unstable flexion injury.

The next area of focus should be the C1-C2 complex. The base of the odontoid process should be carefully studied for evidence of fracture, angulation, or displacement anteriorly or posteriorly. Additionally, the preodontoid space, that is, the space between the posterior aspect of the anterior arch of C1 and the anterior portion of the odontoid process, should be less than 3 mm in an adult. A widened preodontoid space suggests atlantoaxial instability. The relationship of the occiput and the foramen magnum to the odontoid process and C1 also should be noted. In severe trauma, craniospinal dislocation may occur and carries a grim prognosis for the patient.

An anteroposterior cervical spine radiograph has limited usefulness in cervical spinal trauma. Careful inspection of the spinous processes may disclose abnormal rotation between two levels. With forward displacement and locking of the superior facet, the spinous process of the vertebra cephalad to the dislocated level rotates toward the affected facet. This finding is pathognomonic for a unilaterally locked facet. An anteroposterior projection may also show irregular spacing of the spinous processes after a flexion injury or disruption of the lateral border of the column of facets after a rotational injury.

Other radiographic projections add further dimensions to the radiographic examination. In a cooperative patient, an open-mouth odontoid view is useful in studying the atlantoaxial complex and searching for a burst fracture (Jefferson fracture) of C1. Oblique views show the neural foramen and facet joints well and are useful in searching for unilaterally locked facets. Flexion and extension lateral cervical spine films are invaluable in determining spinal stability, but they should never be obtained in patients who are intoxicated, have a diminished level of consciousness, or have any evidence of neurologic impairment. Lateral tomography is valuable in diagnosing odontoid fractures. CT scanning of the cervical spine without intrathecal contrast enhancement is useful in studying Jefferson fractures or any vertebral body fracture or dislocation. The standard for studying cervical spinal cord injury remains myelography with water-soluble contrast material, followed by CT scanning. This study reliably demonstrates bony injury; masses within the spinal canal, including hematomas or herniated disks; the contour and configuration of the spinal cord; and any degree of canal or foraminal stenosis. MRI has limited usefulness in the evaluation of acute spinal cord injury. Problems with patient stability, incompatible ancillary equipment such as ventilators, the presence or suggestion of contained metal fragments, inadequate bone detail, and the inability of trauma patients to cooperate with a prolonged study in the small confines of the gantry all limit use of MRI in the acutely injured patient.

Once they are stabilized, all patients with spinal cord injury should undergo either myelography or MRI to ensure that the spinal cord is not suffering residual compression by disk material, bone fragments, or hematomas.

NEUROLOGIC SYNDROMES FOLLOWING SPINAL CORD INJURY

Spinal cord injury may be divided into complete and incomplete syndromes. With complete spinal cord injury, there is no motor or sensory function below the affected level. In making this distinction, it is important that the patient be carefully examined for evidence of preserved perianal sensation or sphincter tone. All sensory modalities, including pain, light touch, proprioception, and vibration, should be tested before determining that a patient has a complete spinal cord injury. In acute spinal cord lesions, the muscles innervated below the level of a complete injury are flaccid and areflexic. In male patients, priapism accompanies spinal cord injury. With more chronic spinal cord injury, muscle tone is increased or spastic below the injury level. Hyperreflexia and upgoing toes are found. Common radiographic correlates of complete spinal cord injury are bilaterally locked facets or compression fractures of cervical vertebrae suffered in flexion or axial loading injuries.

Incomplete spinal cord injuries require a greater understanding of spinal cord anatomy. Three incomplete cord injury syndromes deserve special attention. Rarely are these syndromes present in a pure form; more commonly an incomplete spinal cord injury shares elements of these syndromes (Fig. 19-3).

Brown-Sequard Syndrome

A Brown-Sequard syndrome follows hemisection of the spinal cord. Because of the different levels of decussation of the anterior spinothalamic tract and the posterior sensory columns, a dissociation is noted between the sides of the sensory impairment occurring after this unilateral cord lesion. The lateral spinothalamic tract, which conveys pinprick and temperature sensation, enters the spinal cord through the dorsal roots and ascends one or two levels in the substantia gelatinosa before crossing through the ventral commissure to the opposite side of the spinal cord. In contradistinction, the posterior columns continue ipsilaterally until they decussate at the brainstem. If half of the cord is disrupted, loss of pain and temperature sensation begins approximately two dermatomal segments below and contralateral to the side of the lesion and extending caudally. Proprioception and light touch is lost beginning at the dermatomal segment just below and ipsilateral to the level of injury. Corticospinal tracts decussate at the level of the pyramids in the medulla and continue ipsilateral to the muscle groups they supply throughout the length of the spinal cord. Motor loss is therefore ipsilateral to the side of hemisection. At the level of the lesion, segmental lower motor neuron findings and sensory loss may be found ipsilaterally, a consequence of damage to the anterior horn cells and roots. A pure Brown-Sequard syndrome after trauma is rare. More commonly, a partial Brown-Sequard pattern is noted with ipsilateral weakness and contralateral loss of pain and temperature sensation.

Central Cord Syndrome

A central cord syndrome is produced when the deepest regions of the cervical spinal cord are injured, producing distal weakness of the upper extremities with relative sparing of motor function in the lower extremities. Variable sensory and bladder findings may also be present. This syndrome is most commonly seen after extension injuries when the gray matter of the cervical spinal cord enlargement is damaged. Complete recovery is possible; significant recovery is almost invariable.

Anterior Cord Syndrome

An anterior cord syndrome may occur after trauma when disk or bone fragments are driven into the spinal canal and compress the ventral cord. On examination, these patients suffer profound motor loss, as well as loss of pain and temperature sensation below the affected level. Only posterior column function, light touch, and proprioceptive sensation may remain intact. Patients who suffer an anterior cord syndrome should be carefully evaluated for the

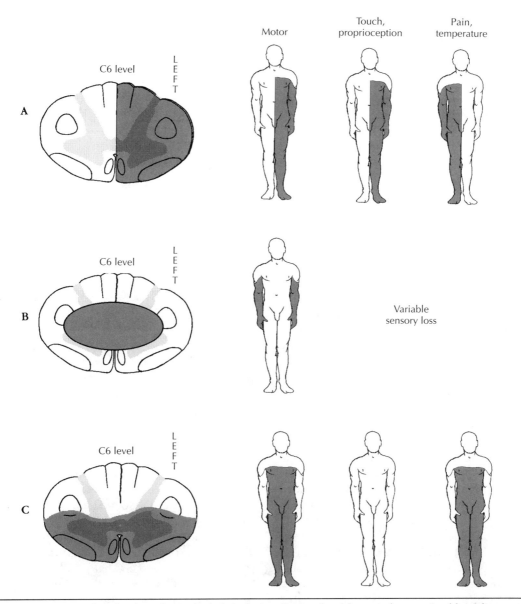

FIG. 19-3 Incomplete lesions of spinal cord. **A,** Brown-Sequard syndrome, characterized by (1) contralateral loss of pain and temperature sensation; (2) ipsilateral loss of proprioceptive sensation and variable degrees of loss of light touch sensation; and (3) ipsilateral loss of motor function. **B,** Central cord syndrome. Predominant weakness of arms is characteristic of central cord injury. **C,** Anterior cord syndrome, characterized by (1) loss of motor function below level of lesion; (2) loss of pain and temperature sensation; and (3) relative preservation of proprioception and light touch.

presence of a ventral, extra-axial mass such as a large-disk herniation. Establishing the presence or absence of such a mass is necessary if a deficit persists after realignment of the cervical spine. An anterior cord syndrome is uncommon after trauma; more commonly it is produced by an anterior spinal artery infarct.

STABILIZATION AND PROTECTION OF INJURED SPINE

All patients with known or suspected spinal injury require stabilization. A wide range of ancillary orthotics are used in a critical care setting to immobilize an injured spinal column. These range from soft or semisoft cervical collars, such as the foam collar or Philadelphia collar, to more reliable and complicated orthoses such as the Gardner-Wells tongs, halo vest, and thoracolumbosacral brace.

A cervical foam collar does not provide any measure of immobilization or security for a patient with known or suspected spinal cord injury. They should never be used in an SICU. A Philadelphia collar, if properly applied, is more effective, particularly in preventing extremes of flexion and extension. However, this collar is difficult to tolerate over extended periods, becomes progressively less effective with use, and cannot be used to place traction or other distracting forces on the cervical spine.

The standard for acute immobilization of the unstable cervical spine remains the Gardner-Wells tongs. These tongs are placed in the temporal region, after shaving and anesthetizing an area immediately superior to the external acoustic meatus and slightly below the superior temporal line. Patient anxiety may be reduced during application if the practitioner takes several minutes to explain the procedure to the patient. The patient should be reassured that although initial placement of the tongs may cause discomfort, pain at the pin sites is short lived, and the patient usually notes a significant decrease in neck pain after traction is applied. Proper application of these tongs places the pins in a direct axial line above the external acoustic meatus and approximately 0.5 to 1 cm below the superior temporal line. Application in this area avoids the thin temporosquamosal skull and minimizes painful trauma to the tem-

poralis muscle. Insertion of the tongs through a great bulk of the temporalis muscle produces significant discomfort for the patient both at rest and on opening the mouth to talk or chew. It is important that the points not be placed at or above the superior temporal line, or they may slip during traction and produce a scalp laceration. The tong points may be placed either more anterior or posterior than the direct axial line above the external acoustic meatus, if the practitioner wishes to place the patient's cervical spine in either flexion or extension, respectively. However, the indications for such a maneuver are uncommon.

An alternative to rigid skull fixation and traction is a halo ring placed early in the patient's hospital course. A halo system may be used as either an acute or long-term orthosis for an unstable cervical spine. Generally, halo immobilization is used as a long-term measure in those patients who have a vertebral fracture that does not require surgical stabilization. Initial placement of a halo ring as a means of providing skeletal traction, rather than Gardner-Wells tongs, may save the patient a second application of skull fixation if any consideration is given to treating the injury with long-term immobilization. A halo ring is applied in much the same fashion as Gardner-Wells tongs. After shaving the scalp and injecting a local anesthetic, four pins are placed, two over the sides of the forehead and two over the parieto-occipital region. The remainder of the halo vest may or may not be initially connected to the halo ring. The ring alone may be used as a fixation device for axial skeletal traction. In the event that a satisfactory alignment is produced with this traction, the remainder of the vest and halo system may then be applied and normal anatomic alignment preserved while the patient heals.

Every SICU physician should have at least a passing acquaintance with halo vests, since their use may produce special problems in managing a patient's airway or during resuscitation efforts. Intubation of a patient immobilized in a halo can be problematic at best and requires extra skill and some prior planning. If possible, this intubation should be attempted only by or in the presence of someone with demonstrated expertise in intubation and only when other alternative measures such as fiberoptic laryngoscopy, bronchoscopy, or cricothyroidotomy are available. Electively, a fiberoptic technique is the procedure of choice. In a true emergency, when such a device is unavailable, blind nasal intubation should be attempted. Cricothyroidotomy should follow if intubation attempts are unsuccessful. Loosening of the halo device to permit cervical extension runs a distant third as an option. Such a manuever might be considered in a life-or-death situation in a patient with a complete cord injury.

Intensive care practitioners should inspect the patient's halo system upon admission to the SICU to determine how to remove the chest component quickly in the event CPR is required. The majority of systems have hinges built into the sternal portion of the vest that allow the practitioner to swing the anterior part of the vest away from the remainder of the halo device after disconnecting the abdominal straps. The vertical uprights remain in place so that cervical traction and stabilization may be maintained through resuscitation. For some older vest types, it may be necessary to loosen the vertical upright supporting the head ring. Because manipulation or removal of a halo orthosis may be necessary in an emergency, each patient in a halo must have a wrench that fits his/her hardware. This wrench should always be taped to the halo and should accompany the patient during any transports.

MEDICAL MANAGEMENT
Monitoring

Careful, detailed, serial neurologic examinations at regular intervals are absolutely essential. These examinations are invaluable in monitoring the course of the patient's injury to detect ongoing injury to the spinal cord and to formulate a rational treatment plan. The clinicians' findings and the time of examination should be legibly and accurately recorded on the chart. The need for careful documentation of care and patient condition cannot be overemphasized.

Nursing orders should also include frequent neurologic checks. Ideally, these should be performed every hour in a patient with acute spinal cord injury and no less than twice in an 8-hour

period in any patient with spinal cord compromise. Patients who are in cervical traction or those patients with a known unstable fracture or dislocation should have daily lateral cervical spine films to detect change in alignment. Additionally, plain films should be repeated after any major event in the patient's hospital care, for example, an extended transport to another portion of the hospital, a change in traction alignment or weights, placement in a halo vest, or adjustment of any orthotic device. Patients with spinal cord injury should also be routinely monitored with oxygen saturation monitors, careful fluid balance worksheets, and daily weights. In the acute setting, all patients with spinal cord injury should have a nasogastric tube placed to low continuous suction, and gastric aspirate should be monitored for pH levels. ECG monitoring, arterial pressure monitoring, and Swan-Ganz catheterization may also be indicated, depending on the clinical situation.

Steroids

The pharmacologic treatment of acute spinal cord injury has been an area of intense research for at least two decades. Recently, a randomized, controlled, double-blinded trial of methylprednisolone and naloxone demonstrated a significant improvement in motor and sensory recovery in patients treated with methylprednisolone. This beneficial response was found in patients with both incomplete and complete injuries, but only in those patients who received the steroid within 8 hours of injury.[3]

Methylprednisolone was administered as an initial intravenous bolus dosage of 30 mg/kg, followed by a maintenance dose of 5.4 mg/kg/hr for a total of 24 hours of treatment. There was no increase in mortality or any significant difference in the incidence of infectious or gastrointestinal complications in the steroid-treated group.

The cellular mechanisms that underlie this steroid effect are not presently clear. Dosages of methylprednisolone used in this study are much greater than those necessary to activate corticosteroid receptors. Methylprednisolone may act directly to preserve membrane integrity by limiting lipid peroxidation and hydrolysis in injured spinal cord tissue.[4] Steroid analogs that have virtually no glucocorticoid activity and are more effective in stabilizing membranes and suppressing lipid peroxidation are currently under development.

HEMODYNAMICS

A patient with cervical or thoracic spinal cord injury suffers a loss of sympathetic outflow with preservation of vagal afferents and efferents. Sympathetic supply originates in the hypothalamus and travels through the periaqueductal gray matter, pons, and posterolateral medulla to synapse within the intermediolateral cell column of the thoracic spinal cord. A complete spinal cord injury in the cervical region effectively removes all preganglionic sympathetic fibers. In contrast, the parasympathetic system retains input and output supplied through the vagus nerve. In the acute phase, patients with spinal cord injury have unbalanced parasympathetic action, because they lose sympathetic mediated reflexes. A patient with an acute injury usually is brought to the emergency room with moderate hypotension and bradycardia. In the absence of associated injuries these patients are not hypotensive as a result of hypovolemia. The loss of sympathetic tone may cause mean arterial pressures in the range of 70 to 80 mm Hg to persist even after 4 to 6 L of resuscitation fluid. Invasive cardiac monitoring in young quadriplegic patients has demonstrated that they have an acutely elevated cardiac index: loss of sympathetic tone results in low systemic vascular resistance.[5] Loss of peripheral vasoconstriction produces hypoperfusion of the renal and splanchnic beds by shunting blood flow to skin and skeletal muscle beds. Heat dissipation increases, and shivering occurs. Oliguria is commonly found in patients with acute spinal cord injury and, like hypotension, may be refractory to continued fluid administration. When pulmonary artery occlusion pressures exceed 18, administration of further volume may result in pulmonary edema or congestive heart failure. A patient with marginal pulmonary reserve may then require intubation and ventilatory support.

In the past many clinicians commonly used alpha-agonists, such as phenylephrine or nor-epinephrine, to treat hypotension after spinal cord injury. Although these agents are effective in producing vasoconstriction in the periphery, they may decrease renal blood flow. Use of these agents may also elevate systemic blood-pressure sufficiently to produce a reflex bradyarrhythmia. Most young patients with spinal cord injury have some degree of hypotension, but it rarely becomes symptomatic or requires treatment with alpha-agents. In the young oliguric patient, a better drug choice might be dopamine in renal dosages (<5 μg/kg/min). The clearest indications for treatment of moderate hypotension are change in mentation, evidence of myocardial ischemia, or urine output less than 0.5 ml/kg/hr.

Hemodynamic management is far more difficult when the quadriplegic patient is elderly or has preexistent coronary disease. In these patients, symptomatic bradyarrhythmias are common and may be severe enough to produce profound hypotension or asystole. The treatment of choice is an anticholinergic drug, such as atropine. Dopamine may also be used for its beneficial chronotropic effect. If bradycardia persists or has profound consequences, transvenous pacing may be necessary. In elderly patients or in patients experiencing congestive heart failure, pulmonary artery catheterization is essential to direct hemodynamic management. Clinicians should also recognize that many patients with spinal cord injury arrive in the SICU after vigorous fluid resuscitation in the field and during the initial stage of evaluation and resuscitation in the emergency room. A great imbalance in intake compared to output during the initial hospitalization inevitably leads to fluid mobilization several days after admission. Failure to recognize and manage this expected diuresis may compromise patients with marginal respiratory function.

RESPIRATORY SYSTEM

The phrenic nerve arises from the C3 through the C5 level of the cervical spinal cord and innervates the diaphragmatic muscles. The intercostal nerves and accessory muscles of respiration also take their origin from the low cervical and thoracic spinal cord. Therefore a lesion above C4 disrupts the diaphragm, as well as the accessory muscles of respiration. A lower cervical spinal cord lesion leaves the diaphragmatic function intact, while taking accessory muscle function away. Patients without phrenic nerve function cannot survive without ventilatory support. Those patients who sustain an injury above the C4 level require intubation in the field, or they will not survive to reach the hospital. The great majority of these patients remain ventilator dependent for the remainder of their lives. It is the larger group of patients, those with injuries at C5 or below, who have lost their accessory muscles of respiration and their intercostal muscles, who occupy the majority of this discussion.

The inability to fix the thoracic cage during inspiration and to forcibly diminish its capacity during expiration through the use of intercostal muscles greatly diminishes the efficiency of the respiratory effort. Patients with acute spinal cord injury have flaccid accessory muscles and a compliant thoracic cage, in effect, a functional flail chest. With time, the intercostal muscles redevelop tone and although they may not regain innervation, they will contribute to the efficiency of respiration by producing a more rigid chest wall. Acutely, respiratory function is poor. If respiratory indicators are measured, they commonly fall below those levels which would produce an elective intubation in other patients. Of primary importance, the patient's tidal volume is notably reduced, a consequence of the loss of the intercostal muscles. Atelectasis is the immediate result of this inefficient respiratory mechanism and is exacerbated by the lack of deep breathing or an effective cough. Initially, these atelectatic changes may not be audible on auscultation or visible on chest radiographs. The first indication of the process may be a subtle decrease in lung compliance. Decreasing compliance increases ventilatory dead space, further reduces the efficiency of respiration, and increases atelectasis in an accelerating downward spiral. Respiratory failure in these patients is usually heralded by increasing tachypnea; blood gas measurements may appear relatively normal until the late stages of respiratory decompensation. Then, hypocapnea is supplanted by hypoxia as the patient progresses to respiratory arrest. Providing supplementary oxygen as the patient becomes hypoxemic may, paradoxically, hasten respiratory failure by producing "absorption atelectasis." This phenomenon occurs when the gas mixture within the alveoli is composed of a high proportion of oxygen. In high concentrations, oxygen, which is rapidly absorbed from the alveoli, displaces nitrogen, which is not absorbed. Alveolar volume becomes proportionately less, and atelectasis increases.[6]

Patients with spinal cord injuries may suffer other injury-associated pulmonary problems such as aspiration, near-drowning, pulmonary edema, pulmonary contusion, and hemopneumothorax. Any or all of these problems may progress to the adult respiratory distress syndrome (ARDS). The morbidity and mortality of ARDS is extremely high. At best, the progression of a quadriplegic patient to ARDS greatly prolongs the period of mechanical ventilation and hospitalization. Diminished pulmonary reserve substantially delays rehabilitation and impedes neurologic recovery. Preventing ARDS is clearly a high priority in the initial care of these patients. Most interventions consist of maintaining the patient's functional residual capacity. Cough and deep breathing instruction ("quad coughing") may be used, although the patient's functional limitations may minimize the efficacy of these interventions in the acute setting. Intermittent use of a continuous positive airway pressure (CPAP) mask may be the single most effective intervention in nonintubated, quadriplegic patients. Continuously oscillating beds have been shown to decrease the incidence of pulmonary complications in this patient group by diminishing atelectasis, minimizing ventilation/perfusion mismatches, and draining secretions. Pulmonary secretions should be managed using orotracheal, nasotracheal, or endotracheal suctioning. Control of airway humidity using warm mist nebulizers facilitates mobilization of secretions and should not be neglected. Bronchodilator therapy may also be helpful in keeping small airways open.

Spinal cord–injured patients should be observed closely for evidence of pulmonary infection. Daily chest radiographs and frequent chest auscultation should be routine for these patients. Appropriate antibiotics should be administered immediately, if clinical or radiographic evidence of an incipient pneumonia is observed. Antibiotic therapy should start while cultures are pending. The decision to continue these agents should be based on the nature of the organisms cultured, sputum characteristics, chest films, and clinical picture. Colonization of the tracheobronchial tree is an inevitable occurrence in these patients, and a distinction must be drawn between these organisms and true pathogens. Prophylactic antibiotics have no place in this setting.

Finally, endotracheal intubation should not be delayed in those patients who show signs of respiratory failure. Timely intubation may prevent unnecessary pulmonary or neurologic complications. An elective intubation in these patients with difficult airways is always preferred to an unplanned, emergency intubation. Patients who have been intubated and have failed extubation trials or patients who have marginal weaning ability should be considered for a tracheostomy. Tracheostomy may improve respiratory efficiency, allow a ventilator-dependent patient to become independent, provide better airway access for pulmonary toilet, allow more effective use of intermittent CPAP to minimize atelectasis, and provide ready airway control in the event of respiratory failure.

DEEP VENOUS THROMBOSIS AND PULMONARY EMBOLI

Pulmonary embolism is one of the most feared complications of spinal cord injury. A great many measures are in widespread clinical use as prophylaxis for this problem, but none have proven efficacy in this population. Interventions that are probably at least partially effective include hydration, antiplatelet therapy with aspirin, sequential compression devices for lower extremities, continuously oscillating beds and vena cava filter devices. These measures should be used in the order just listed. Sequential compression stockings must be used continuously—even while transporting the patient or in the operating room—to be effective. Ade-

quate hydration and some form of anticoagulation therapy, such as aspirin, or a mini-dose of heparin, have widespread applicability in this patient population and should probably be employed as a minimum standard of prophylaxis.[7] Oscillating-bed therapy may also diminish clot propagation into the proximal venous system of the legs.[8,9] In a patient with an established deep venous thrombosis or antecedent pulmonary embolus who cannot receive anticoagulation therapy, percutaneous placement of a caval filter is a safe and effective procedure.

AUTONOMIC DYSREFLEXIA

Autonomic dysreflexia refers to an exaggerated sympathetic response to afferent stimulation, resulting in hypertension, reflex bradycardia, sweating, cutaneous flushing above the level of the neurologic injury, and headaches. This condition follows the resolution of spinal shock in about 70% of patients with spinal cord injuries above the T6 level and is usually triggered by visceral stimulation.[10] The classic cause of this response is bladder distention, although skin stimulation and bowel distention may also produce the syndrome. This problem has also been described as a response to endoscopic and urodynamic studies.

Autonomic dysreflexia may cause hypertension severe enough to produce myocardial infarction and subarachnoid or intracerebral hemorrhage. Emergency, temporary blood pressure control may be achieved by using nifedipine 10 mg sublingually or phentolamine 5 mg intravenously. The clinician should also immediately determine and eliminate the source of the dysreflexic response. Patients undergoing endoscopic or urodynamic procedures should be premedicated with 10 mg of oral nifedipine just before the procedure.

Stool softeners should also be routinely used to prevent obstipation, rectal distention, or fecal impaction, which may also precipitate dysreflexia.

GASTROINTESTINAL MANAGEMENT

Gastric atony and ileus of both the small and large bowel are an almost invariable consequence of spinal cord injury. This complication usually takes several days to develop. Continuous nasogastric drainage is necessary to minimize aspiration of stomach contents. Gastric atony with dilation may also compromise respiration as a result of subdiaphragmatic pressure. The ileus may persist for days or weeks and delay enteral nutrition for some patients for extended periods. In patients who require prolonged nasogastric suction or in those who have copious gastric secretions, a metabolic alkalosis may develop.

Stress ulceration may occur in these patients unless preventive measures are taken (see Chapter 33). H_2 blockers or antacids should be administered by protocol to keep the gastric pH >4.5. In those patients who develop gastric ulceration (or any other intra-abdominal complication), the usual clinical symptoms and signs may be obscured because of the patient's spinal cord injury. A high index of suspicion of an intra-abdominal process should be maintained in the presence of persistent fevers, an unexplained sepsis, an unstable hemoglobin concentration, or recurrent autonomic dysreflexia.

POIKILOTHERMIA

Patients with a cervical or high thoracic injury suffer a functional sympathectomy and temporarily lose the capacity for peripheral vasoconstriction below the involved level. Because of their decreased ability to preserve heat, they shiver as a means of producing heat. These patients are not able to regulate body temperature effectively, are thermally dependent on their environment (poikilothermic), and are easily chilled. They may become hypothermic in an SICU unless appropriate care is provided.

SKIN BREAKDOWN

Patients who are immobile as a consequence of their neurologic deficit, cervical traction, pain, or spinal instability are at high risk of developing decubitus ulcers. In the spinal cord–injured patient the usual sites of breakdown are the sacral region and the posterior aspects of the heels. An established decubitus ulcer can be a source of significant morbidity, delayed rehabilitation, prolonged hospitalization, and occasionally death. Prevention of this complication assumes a high priority in the nursing care of these patients.

In the acute care setting, continuously oscillating beds are the best method of prevention. These devices allow greater patient motion than even the most conscientiously applied program of logrolling and positioning, provide safety while the patient is stabilized with traction, and add pulmonary benefits as well. Air-cushion beds may be used with stable patients to minimize skin breakdown. Special care should be taken to ensure that the patient's heels do not rest on the mattress for prolonged periods. Small, soft rolls under the calves elevate the heels and prevent ulceration.

URINARY TRACT MANAGEMENT

After an acute spinal cord injury, the urinary bladder is flaccid, and normal detrusor reflexes are abolished. The initial goals in management are to prevent distention and to monitor urinary output. These goals are best accomplished initially with a continuous indwelling urinary catheter. A secondary goal should be to remove this catheter as soon as possible and use intermittent bladder catheterization. With the intermittent technique, urinary bladder volumes should not be allowed to exceed 400 to 500 ml. Routine urinalysis should be monitored and cultures obtained if evidence of urinary tract infection exists. The use of prophylactic antibiotics is controversial. We do not recommend such prophylaxis.[11,12]

In the chronic phase of spinal cord injury, the bladder becomes hypertonic and spastic. Autonomic reflexes are reestablished, and bladder distention may trigger autonomic dysreflexia. Meticulous bladder management is necessary to prevent autonomic dysreflexia and to minimize the incidence of infection, vesicoureteral reflux, hydronephrosis, calculi, and renal dysfunction in this patient population.

PREPARATION FOR REHABILITATION

Physical therapy should be initiated as soon as the patient is medically stable. Early goals are passive range-of-motion exercises, avoiding contractures, and establishing a relationship with the providers who may be responsible for later substantive rehabilitation. The psychologic effects of this therapy are of great positive benefit.

PSYCHOLOGIC FACTORS

For many patients quadriplegia is feared more than death and is without equal in psychologic stress for the affected individual, family, and friends. Acceptance of quadriplegia is achieved only after terrible suffering, a profound sense of loss, and grieving for that loss. Just as every individual expresses any profound emotion differently, just as every family communicates and copes in its special manner, so do individuals and families differ in their responses, adjustment, and management of quadriplegia. The profundity of the loss and the wide range of response, more than anything, must be remembered by the clinician caring for the quadriplegic patient and family. Psychologic support and effective communication frequently become the greatest challenge for health care providers after several days of hospitalization.

The initial frenetic pace of care after a spinal cord injury serves the dual psychologic purpose of convincing the patient and family that something is being "done" and allows them to concentrate on procedures, tests, and technology. This phase of care initiates the denial response to the injury. Denial may last hours to days, or longer. The patient may make tentative, limited exploration of the prognosis attendant to his/her injury but generally is reluctant to ask "the question" directly. Occasionally, "the question" becomes almost palpable, underlying every turn of conversation with care providers. The physician should be sensitive to the patient's readiness and desire to turn to this most serious issue.

Timing is important, and a discussion of prognosis should not be forced on the patient. Every conscious quadriplegic is acutely aware of his/her level of dysfunction and most have already assumed the worst. The patient may wait to choose the setting, company, and health care provider before opening the discussion. This communication is critical to the patient and should be conducted as an unhurried private conversation in which the patient is free to assume control. Based on the facts, the clinician should determine the essential information to impart and then make certain that it is communicated effectively to the patient and family. They will remember little beyond the physician's estimate of the chances of recovery; further information should be provided as the patient directs. The patient should be advised frankly of the uncertainty of any clinical estimation of outcome, particularly in the complex setting of an incomplete spinal cord injury. He/she should be assured of receiving complete, honest answers to questions. A degree of denial has its merits early in the patient's clinical course, and no attempt should be made to force him/her to accept "the truth." Physicians should learn to prevent their emotional concerns about quadriplegia from becoming an added burden to the patient. Be cautious not to remove all hope, even if the situation appears hopeless. Allow the patient to cling to whatever level of denial he/she chooses early in the course. The skilled clinician's task is to allow the patient to replace denial with determined rehabilitation and a realistic view of what is possible, rather than what is impossible. This transition is more easily made when the patient has rehabilitation and functional goals to concentrate on, not when he/she is lying immobile in the SICU.

As the patient's denial begins to falter, frustration, anger, and then depression often supervene. During these phases, the patient requires continued emotional support, communication, and understanding. In some communities, rehabilitated quadriplegic patients may be available as a source of support and can be helpful after the patient has progressed at least through the phases of denial and anger. Acceptance usually occurs during the rehabilitation process, long after the patient has left the critical care setting.

Family communication is another matter of great importance. Family members almost always ask the physician for an estimation of the chances of neurologic recovery early in the hospital course and commonly wish to withhold the full import of the injury from the patient.

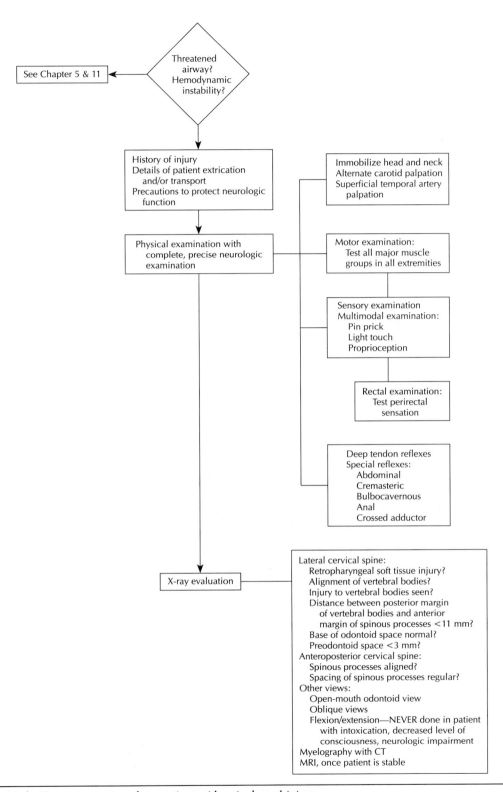

FIG. 19-4 Treatment approach to patient with spinal cord injury.

Be as open, forthcoming, and complete as possible in communicating with the family. Communication can be a complicated process in a critical care unit, and family members tend to compare statements made by different staff members. They become disconcerted by discrepancies, real or imagined. Understanding may be facilitated early in the clinical course by clearly identifying the principal provider and arranging periodic meetings to convey clinical information and to resolve uncertainties or conflicts. The process of grieving for the patient, accepting disability, and preparing realistic options must be accelerated for the family and friends, if they are to be available as a source of support.

Families cope in a variety of ways. Initially, they tend to focus on the details of the injury or on the patient's care. This effort may also be a form of denial and lasts until it is displaced by a second phase, anger and frustration. Usually the anger is directed at a specific target, commonly the nursing or medical staff. The family insists that an individual or individuals not participate in the care of the patient. The inciting event for this anger is usually trivial, but the emotion is real and may lead to strained relations, a hospital transfer, or litigation, if not dealt with effectively. Rarely does this hostility extend to include the primary physician, and frequently the primary physician is in the best position to defuse the situation. When these situations arise, as they almost inevitably do with every quadriplegic patient, the solution is usually to narrow the circle of staff members providing information, not to enlarge it.

SUMMARY

- Optimal management of patients with spinal cord injury requires immediate stabilization of unstable spinal segment, accurate and well-documented neurologic assessment, and timely recognition and management of medical complications that may limit patient's degree or probability of recovery.
- Special anatomic and physiologic circumstances peculiar to patients with spinal cord injury must be remembered so that intervention is both appropriate and effective.

- Principles of acute management include close neurologic monitoring, spinal immobilization, and maintenance of effective respiration, body temperature, and blood pressure.
- Invasive hemodynamic monitoring should be instituted in patients with extensive systemic injuries to reinstate patients by oxygen transport criteria (see Chapter 2) and to optimize specific oxygen function, cardiac or renal.

REFERENCES

1. Brazis PW, Biller J. The localization of lesions affecting the spinal cord. In Brazis PW, Masden JC, Biller J, eds. Localization in Clinical Neurology. Boston: Little, Brown, 1985.
2. Riddoch G. Aids to the Examination of the Peripheral Nervous System. London: Baillière-Tindall, 1986.
3. Bracken M, Shepard MJ, Collins WF, et al. A randomized, controlled trial of methylprednisolone or naloxone in the treatment of acute spinal-cord injury. Results of the Second National Spinal Cord Injury Study. N Engl J Med 322:1405-1411, 1990.
4. Braughler JM, Hall ED, Means ED, Waters TR, Anderson TK. Evaluation of an intensive methylprednisolone sodium succinate dosing regimen in experimental spinal cord injury. J Neurosurg 67:102-105, 1987.
5. Mackenzie CF, Shin B, Krishnaprasad D, McCormack F, Illingworth W. Assessment of cardiac and respiratory function during surgery on patients with acute quadriplegia. J Neurosurg 62:843-849, 1985.
6. Rosner M. Medical management of spinal cord injury. In Pitts LH, Wagner FC, ed. Craniospinal Trauma. New York: Thieme Medical Publishers, 1990.
7. Casa ER, Sanchez MP, Arias CR, et al. Prophylaxis of venous thrombosis and pulmonary embolism in patients with acute traumatic spinal cord lesions. Paraplegia 14:178, 1976.
8. Becker D, Gonzalez M, Gentile A, Green B, Eismont F. Prevention of deep venous thrombosis in acute spinal cord injury: Use of rotating table. In Green BA, Summer WR, eds. Continuous Oscillation Therapy: Research and Practical Applications. Miami: University of Miami Press, 1986.
9. Brackett T, Cordon N. Comparison of the wedge turning frame and kinetic treatment table in the acute care of spinal cord injury patients. Surg Neurol 22:53, 1984.
10. Kurnick N. Autonomic dysreflexia and its control in patients with spinal cord lesions. Ann Intern Med 44:678, 1956.
11. Stickler DJ, Dphil MA, Chawla JC. An appraisal of antibiotic policies for urinary tract infection in patients with spinal cord injuries undergoing long-term intermittent catheterization. Paraplegia 26:215, 1988.
12. Stover SL, Lloyd LK, Waites KB, et al. Urinary tract infection in spinal cord injury. Arch Phys Med Rehabil 70:47, 1989.

CHAPTER 20

Altered Cardiac Physiology

Vivian L. Clark · James A. Kruse · Richard W. Carlson

Knowledge of the physiology and manifestations of altered cardiac function is essential to the clinical management of critically ill patients. It is equally important for the clinician to be aware of the potential effects of critical illness itself on cardiac physiology. Anticipation and recognition of these effects allows the rational selection and titration of therapy to optimize cardiac function, restore vital organ perfusion, and aid in preventing or minimizing organ system failure.

NORMAL PHYSIOLOGY

Cardiac performance and myocardial oxygen demand are dependent on four major factors: heart rate, preload, afterload, and myocardial contractility.[1,2] Since cardiac output (CO) is the product of *heart rate* and stroke volume, it can be adversely affected by both bradyarrhythmias and tachyarrhythmias. The ability to tolerate abnormal cardiac rhythms is largely dependent on the patient's underlying level of ventricular function. For example, an individual with chronic heart failure or marked left ventricular hypertrophy may tolerate atrial fibrillation poorly, even when heart rate is increased only modestly. On the other hand, the otherwise normal resting individual may tolerate supra-

ventricular rhythms with rates of up to 200 min^{-1} or more without substantial hemodynamic consequences. Although abnormal rhythms, including sinus tachycardia, may result in hemodynamic compromise, it should be recognized that sinus tachycardia never occurs as a primary dysrhythmia. Rather, this rhythm represents a compensatory response to either a physiologic or pathologic condition, such as exercise, fever, hypoxia, hypovolemia, anemia, heart failure, agitation or pain, or as an effect of certain drugs (e.g., beta-adrenergic agonists). Therefore in a patient with sinus tachycardia, it is important to search diligently for an underlying cause. Efforts to slow this rhythm with digoxin or beta-blockers are rarely appropriate; instead, treatment should focus on correcting the underlying cause.

Preload refers to ventricular end-diastolic volume and thus is a measure of myocardial fiber stretch just prior to contraction. The Frank-Starling principle expresses the relationship between preload and CO generated during subsequent systole. This relationship is depicted in Fig. 20-1. End-diastolic myocardial fiber stretch is indicated by the point at which ventricular volume is maximal. Although the Frank-Starling principle is based on myocardial fiber length or ventricular volume, for clinical purposes preload is frequently estimated by ventricular filling pressure since volume measurements are not readily obtainable at the bedside.[2,3] The relationship between ventricular pressure and ventricular volume during diastole is termed "compliance" (also referred to by its reciprocal, "stiffness"). Ventricular stiffness can be represented graphically by the slope of the diastolic portion of the pressure-volume loop (Fig. 20-2). If chamber compliance is assumed to be constant, then changes in intracavitary pressure will be proportional to changes in chamber volume. However, myocardial compliance is altered in a number of disease states. For example, in a low-compliance (stiff) ventricle, such as that observed in the patient with hypertrophy, a given change in ventricular volume will result in a greater change in ventricular pressure compared to that seen in the individual with normal compliance.[4,5] Certain drugs also can affect ventricular compliance; for example, catecholamines decrease ventricular compliance (increase stiffness), whereas beta-blockers and calcium channel blockers produce the opposite effect.

In the absence of valvular stenosis, atrial pressure is in equilibrium with ventricular pressure at end-diastole. Right atrial pressure (RAP) (or central venous pressure [CVP]) is therefore commonly used to assess right ventricular filling pressure. Except in certain postcardiac surgery patients, left atrial pressure is not accessible to the clinician. However, the balloon-tipped pulmonary artery (PA) catheter allows left atrial pressure to be estimated.[3,5] During balloon inflation a continuous static column of fluid exists between the monitoring orifice at the tip of the catheter and the left atrium. Thus pulmonary capillary wedge pressure (PCWP) and right atrial pressure serve as indirect estimates of left ventricular and right ventricular preload, respectively.

Inadequate preload, such as occurs with hypovolemia, results in decreased CO, according to the Frank-Starling relationship. If the degree of hypovolemia is severe, this condition will lead to hypotension and frank circulatory shock.[6] Factors that can lead to increased preload include volume overload and both systolic and diastolic ventricular dysfunction. Patients with abnormal ventricular function generally require higher filling pressures to maintain optimal CO.[3] Increasing right- and left-sided preload eventually can lead to peripheral and pulmonary vascular congestion, respectively. Severe increases in left ventricular pressure can increase PCWP sufficiently to cause pulmonary edema with attendant hypoxemia and possibly respiratory failure.

Afterload can be defined as the resistance to ejection of blood by the ventricles.[2] Blood pressure is the simplest measure of afterload. Thus mean arterial pressure (MAP) can be used to estimate left ventricular afterload, and mean pulmonary arterial pressure (MPAP) can be used to estimate right ventricular afterload. Afterload also can be represented as the ventricular pressure at the end of isovolumic contraction (see Fig. 20-2). As this pressure increases, the resistance to ventricular ejection rises and the ventricle must exert a greater force during systole. Increases in afterload therefore are associated with increases in myocardial oxygen consumption (MvO_2). The added work imposed by an elevation in afterload also can precipitate heart failure in the patient with underlying car-

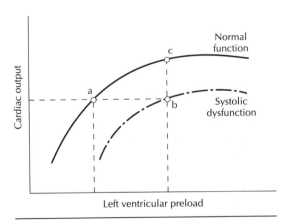

FIG. 20-1 Relationship between preload and CO in normal cardiac function and systolic dysfunction. At similar levels of CO, normal heart *(a)* requires lower preload than heart with impaired systolic function *(b)* to maintain normal resting CO. Similar preload results in higher CO in normal heart *(c)* compared to heart with impaired systolic function *(b)*.

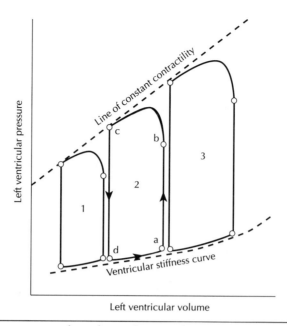

FIG. 20-2 Left ventricular pressure-volume loops showing changes in preload and afterload. Loop 2 represents normal cardiac cycle. During diastole (segment *d-a*), ventricle fills and pressure increases until end-diastolic pressure and end-diastolic volume are attained *(a)*, representing preload. Slope of curve *d-a* is measure of ventricular stiffness. During isovolumic contraction (both valves closed), pressure rapidly increases while volume remains the same (segment *a-b*). When intraventricular pressure exceeds central aortic pressure, aortic valve opens and systole ensues *(b)*. Point *b* represents afterload. As ventricle empties, ventricular pressure falls until it is below aortic pressure and aortic valve then closes *(c)*. Stroke volume is indicated by distance between points *b* and *c* along X-axis. During isovolumic relaxation period (both valves closed), ventricular pressure falls rapidly (segment *c-d*) until it is below left atrial pressure; mitral valve then opens (point *d*), beginning a new cycle. Changes in preload and afterload are evident in loops 1 and 3. Note that point *c* of each loop falls along line of constant contractility, indicating same inotropic state for all three loops. Changes in contractility would be indicated by a change in slope of this line.

diac disease. Vascular resistance represents another method of quantifying afterload.[2] Systemic vascular resistance (SVR) and pulmonary vascular resistance (PVR) can be calculated at the bedside from CO, which is obtained by the thermodilution PA catheter, and the pressure gradient across the respective vascular bed (Table 20-1). Factors that lead to increased left ventricular afterload include systemic hypertension (both essential and secondary varieties), use of vasoconstricting agents, and conditions leading to obstruction of ventricular outflow such as aortic valvular stenosis. Right ventricular afterload is increased by positive pressure ventilation (PPV), use of positive end-expiratory pressure (PEEP), pulmonary embolism, and pulmonary hypertension (both pri-

mary and that secondary to left ventricular dysfunction or mitral valvular disease). Left ventricular afterload is decreased by systemic vasodilation (which commonly occurs in sepsis and cirrhosis), arteriovenous shunting, and a variety of drugs, including nitroprusside and other antihypertensive and vasodilating agents.

Contractility refers to the intrinsic inotropic property of the myocardium that is independent of the effects of preload, afterload, and heart rate. Although the position of the pressure-volume loop changes as preload, afterload, and ventricular stiffness are varied, the position of the end-systolic pressure-volume point (Fig. 20-2) is constrained to move along a given straight line as long as contractility is constant. An increase in contractility results in

TABLE 20-1 Formulas and Normal Ranges for Commonly Measured Hemodynamic Variables

Variable/Formula	Range	Unit
Right atrial pressure (RAP) or central venous pressure (CVP)	2-8	mm Hg
Right ventricular pressure (RVP) [s/d]	15/2-30/8	mm Hg
Pulmonary artery pressure (PAP) [s/d/m]	15/4/8-30/12/15	mm Hg
Pulmonary capillary wedge pressure (PCWP)	5-12	mm Hg
Mean arterial pressure (MAP) [= d + {(s − d) ÷ 3}]	85-100	mm Hg
Cardiac output (CO)	4.5-6	$L \cdot min^{-1}$
Cardiac index (CI) [= CO ÷ BSA]	2.6-3.8	$L \cdot min^{-1} \cdot M^{-2}$
Stroke volume (SV) [= 1000 × CO ÷ HR]	60-90	ml
Stroke index (SI) [= 1000 × CO ÷ HR ÷ BSA]	35-50	$ml \cdot M^{-2}$
Right ventricular stroke work index (RVSWI) [= SI × (mean PAP − CVP) × 0.0136]	8-12	$g \cdot M \cdot M^{-2}$
Left ventricular stroke work index (LVSWI) [= SI × (MAP − PCWP) × 0.0136]	40-60	$g \cdot M \cdot M^{-2}$
Systemic vascular resistance index (SVRI) [= (MAP − CVP) × 80 ÷ CI]	1400-2100	$dyne \cdot sec \cdot cm^{-5} \cdot M^2$
Pulmonary vascular resistance index (PVRI) [= (mean PAP − PCWP) × 80 ÷ CI]	180-400	$dyne \cdot sec \cdot cm^{-5} \cdot M^2$
Ejection fraction (EF) [= SV ÷ EDV]	55-75	%

s, Systolic; d, diastolic; m, mean; BSA, body surface area; EDV, end-diastolic volume (ventricular).

an increase in the slope of this line, whereas a decrease in contractility results in a more shallow slope. Clinically, ejection fraction (Table 20-1) is sometimes used as a gauge of contractility, although in reality this variable also is influenced to some degree by both preload and afterload.[4] Contractility may be increased in hypertrophic myopathy, in some hypermetabolic states (e.g., thyrotoxicosis) and by inotropic agents such as beta-adrenergic agonists and cardiac glycosides (e.g., digoxin). Contractility is diminished in myocardial ischemia or infarction, in cardiomyopathic processes, in sepsis, and by a variety of drugs, including beta-blockers and calcium channel blockers.

The overall work performed by the ventricle is the product of pressure and volume, represented by the area within the pressure-volume loop. Calculated stroke work index thus can be used to assess the total contractile work generated by the left or the right ventricle (see Table 20-1).

PATHOPHYSIOLOGY OF HEART FAILURE

Abnormal systolic function, one of the most frequently encountered cardiac disorders, is a common cause of postoperative complications. There are many underlying etiologies, but the most common causes are ischemic heart disease, hypertensive heart disease, valvular heart disease, and dilated cardiomyopathy. The hallmark of systolic dysfunction is impaired contractility, which is usually secondary to myocardial ischemia, necrosis, or fibrosis. In an effort to maintain adequate CO, several compensatory responses occur, including salt and water retention.[2,4] Fluid retention leads to ventricular dilation, and, as a consequence, preload is elevated. This increase in preload serves as

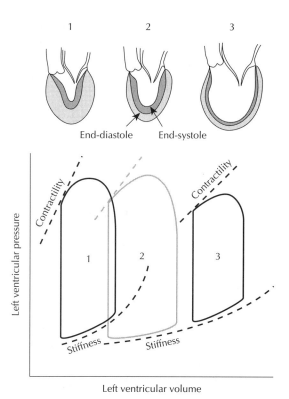

FIG. 20-3   Left ventricular pressure-volume loops comparing normal ventricular function (loop 2) with pure diastolic dysfunction (loop 1) and pure systolic dysfunction (loop 3). Note that left ventricular volume is lower than normal in diastolic dysfunction but higher than normal in systolic dysfunction. End-diastolic pressure is increased and stroke volume may be decreased in both disorders. Increased slope of diastolic (bottom) portion of loop 1 indicates increased intrinsic stiffness (decreased compliance) characteristic of diastolic dysfunction. In systolic dysfunction, ventricular stiffness curve is normal, but stiffness is increased because ventricle is distended. Slope of respective contractility lines demonstrates diminished contractility characteristic of systolic dysfunction and augmented contractility that may be seen in diastolic dysfunction.

a compensatory mechanism that helps maintain a normal level of cardiac work by way of the Frank-Starling relationship (see Fig. 20-1). The pressure-volume relationship in systolic dysfunction is depicted in Fig. 20-3 (loop 3). Stroke volume is impaired, but in mild cases near-normal CO may be maintained by compensatory tachycardia.

The elevated filling pressures and low CO resulting from systolic dysfunction are associated with a variety of clinical manifestations[4] (Table 20-2). In addition to tachycardia, these include neck vein distention, peripheral edema, and presence of rales (indicating pulmonary congestion). If systolic function is severely impaired, hypotension and signs of impaired end-organ perfusion, such as oliguria or changes in mental status, may be observed. Many patients with systolic dysfunction are asymptomatic under normal circumstances, but clinical symptoms may be precipitated by the stress of infection, trauma, or surgery. Multiple uptake gated acquisition (MUGA) nuclear scanning, and two-dimensional echocardiography usually demonstrate a diminished ejection fraction and increased ventricular volume.

Fig. 20-1 demonstrates the relationship between filling pressure and CO in a normal heart and a heart with abnormal systolic function. Patients with systolic dysfunction can be quite sensitive to changes in preload, and they may deteriorate clinically if subjected to either hypovolemia or fluid overload. In addition, increased afterload may lead to cardiac decompensation. This condition can occur as a result of increasing Mvo_2 in the face of coronary artery disease or simply because of the greater workload imposed on an already failing heart. Perioperative use of the balloon-tipped thermodilution PA catheter for hemodynamic monitoring in patients with known systolic dysfunction may allow early recognition and prevention of cardiac decompensation.[3]

A number of pharmacologic agents are useful for treating systolic dysfunction.[2] In cases where there is pulmonary congestion without compromise of CO, diuretic therapy alone may be effective. Loop diuretics, such as furosemide or bumetanide, are the agents of choice. Nitrates, which also reduce preload, are a useful adjunct, particularly in patients with coronary artery disease. If low CO accompanies congestion, then digoxin, combined with diuretics, may be of benefit. Digoxin is particularly useful in patients with atrial dysrhythmias, such as atrial flutter or fibrillation, but also has been shown to be of some value in patients with sinus rhythm.[1] Afterload-reducing agents are being used with increasing frequency in the treatment

TABLE 20-2 Clinical Findings
Frequently Present in Heart Failure

Mechanism	Finding
Elevated filling pressures	Rales, rhonchi
	Distended neck veins
	Hepatic congestion
	Peripheral edema
	Pulmonary congestion
	Hypoxemia
	Pleural effusions
	Ascites
Low cardiac output	Tachycardia
	Low pulse pressure
	Oliguria
	Altered sensorium
	Cold extremities
	Anorexia

of systolic dysfunction with low CO, and they have been shown to improve life expectancy in patients with heart failure.[7] In emergency situations, sodium nitroprusside is often the agent of choice since it is administered by intravenous infusion, has a rapid onset of action and a short half-life, and can be titrated easily. However, nitroprusside can be used for only a short duration since cyanide and thiocyanate toxicity can develop with high-dose or prolonged infusions, particularly in patients with renal insufficiency. For long-term treatment, angiotensin-converting enzyme inhibitors are the agents of choice, but they, too, must be used cautiously in patients with renal dysfunction. Other afterload-reducing agents that may be of value include hydralazine, prazosin, and high-dose, intravenously administered nitroglycerin.

Patients with severe compromise of systolic function, particularly when accompanied by hypotension, may require inotropic agents, such as dobutamine, dopamine, or amrinone, for short-term hemodynamic support.[1] Dobutamine, a beta-adrenergic catecholamine, can increase CO without significantly increasing Mvo_2, and it often lowers PCWP. Since dobutamine has peripheral vasodilating properties, it may not increase blood pressure. Dopamine has both alpha- and beta-adrenergic properties

and may be effective in increasing both CO and blood pressure in hypotensive patients. The improvement in blood pressure, however, may occur at the expense of increasing both Mvo_2 and PCWP. Dopamine also stimulates dopaminergic receptors in the splanchnic and renal vasculature; at low doses it may augment renal perfusion and improve urine output. Amrinone has both inotropic and vasodilating properties, and although it is not a catecholamine, its hemodynamic effects are similar to those of dobutamine.

Diastolic dysfunction is becoming increasingly recognized as an important cause of cardiac decompensation. Patients generally have reduced myocardial compliance with impaired ventricular filling, but they often have normal or even hypercontractile systolic function.[8-10] The pressure-volume loops in Fig. 20-3 illustrate some of the physiologic characteristics of diastolic dysfunction compared to normal function and systolic dysfunction. Most notable are the increased stiffness of the ventricle, as shown by the steeper slope of the diastolic portion of the loop, and the relatively low ventricular volumes.

Diastolic dysfunction is seen most often in the patient with severe left ventricular hypertrophy, which may be idiopathic, secondary to long-standing hypertension, or may result from outflow obstruction, such as that caused by aortic stenosis.[10] It also may occur in ischemic heart disease, in which it is frequently combined with systolic dysfunction. Hypertrophy and ischemia both impair myocardial relaxation and alter ventricular compliance, leading to inadequate ventricular filling.[11] Increased chamber stiffness also results in elevation of filling pressure for any given level of ventricular volume or preload. This disturbance in the pressure-volume relationship in diastolic dysfunction can be seen in Fig. 20-3 (loop 1). The increase in filling pressures provides some degree of compensation by increasing the driving pressure for diastolic filling, but the higher pulmonary and systemic venous pressures also lead to congestive manifestations. Left ventricular diastolic dysfunction thus manifests clinically as symptoms of pulmonary congestion and hemodynamically through elevated PCWP.

It is important to distinguish this form of

heart failure from systolic dysfunction since it may have important implications in terms of management (Table 20-3).[9-11] Patients with diastolic dysfunction usually have a normal cardiac size on physical examination and CXR. Although a third heart sound is frequently present in patients with systolic dysfunction, patients with diastolic dysfunction often have an S_4 gallop. Echocardiography can prove extremely useful in identifying these patients by demonstrating significant ventricular hypertrophy and normal ventricular size along with normal or hyperdynamic systolic function.[8]

Appropriate treatment of pure diastolic dysfunction may differ markedly from that of patients with pure systolic dysfunction. Inotropic agents such as beta-adrenergic agonists and digoxin actually can worsen cardiac failure due to diastolic dysfunction. This effect also may be true of preload- and afterload-reducing drugs, such as diuretics, nitrates, and vasodilators, although some reduction in preload with diuretics may be necessary if there is significant edema or pulmonary congestion present. Patients generally respond to agents such as beta-blockers and calcium channel blockers, which improve myocardial relaxation and thereby enhance ventricular compliance.[11,12] These drugs also can be used to treat associated hypertension. When hypotension occurs in patients with isolated diastolic dysfunction, pure alpha-ago-

nists, such as phenylephrine, may be more effective than catecholamines that combine both alpha and beta effects. This use is particularly important in patients with diastolic dysfunction caused by idiopathic hypertrophic subaortic stenosis. As with patients with systolic dysfunction, individuals with diastolic dysfunction have high resting filling pressures and tend to be sensitive to changes in preload. Even relatively mild degrees of hypovolemia or hypervolemia should be avoided since they can lead to marked clinical deterioration. Acutely decompensated patients and those at high risk for major shifts in intravascular volume may benefit from invasive hemodynamic monitoring with the balloon-tipped thermodilution PA catheter. Such monitoring allows for early detection of such volume shifts and assists with titrating intravenous fluids and diuretics.

PERICARDIAL TAMPONADE

Pericardial tamponade is a clinical syndrome characterized by peripheral venous congestion and low CO due to impaired cardiac filling from accumulation of fluid in the pericardial sac. If severe, this condition can lead to extreme hemodynamic compromise and frank circulatory shock. Ventricular compliance is decreased in tamponade, not because of increased intrinsic myocardial stiffness, as occurs in ischemia or hypertrophy, but because of the constraint to

---

TABLE 20-3   Characteristics and Pharmacotherapy of Systolic vs. Diastolic Dysfunction

	Systolic Dysfunction	Diastolic Dysfunction
Ventricular size	Dilated	Normal, hypertrophied
Contractility	Decreased	Increased
Cardiac output	Low	Low
Clinical findings	Pulmonary congestion Peripheral congestion S_3	Pulmonary congestion Peripheral congestion S_4
Treatment	Diuresis Afterload reduction Inotropes	Beta-blocker Calcium channel blocker

normal diastolic filling imposed by the surrounding pericardial effusion.[13] Thus tamponade resembles a form of diastolic dysfunction. Its development and severity are dependent on both the volume of pericardial fluid and the rapidity with which it accumulates.[13] For example, patients with end-stage renal disease may develop very large pericardial effusions over a long period without progressing to tamponade, whereas a patient with a stab wound to the chest may develop tamponade with only 50 ml of blood in the pericardial sac. This effect is due to the lack of distensibility of the pericardium unless tension is applied over a prolonged time.

Pericardial effusion leading to tamponade can result from a number of causes. The most common is pericarditis (either idiopathic or secondary to infection), radiation therapy, collagen-vascular disease, uremia, or open heart surgery. Hypothyroidism and malignancy are also common causes, and effusions associated with the latter are particularly likely to progress to tamponade. Hemopericardium, a common cause of tamponade encountered in the SICU, can occur as a consequence of blunt or penetrating thoracic trauma, aortic dissection, or myocardial rupture.

As fluid accumulates within the pericardial sac, right atrial pressure rises and limits venous return. This limitation results in peripheral venous congestion and decreased CO, which in turn results in the typical signs and symptoms of tamponade. The patient usually will complain of dyspnea and chest discomfort, both of which are often aggravated by assuming a supine position. Other common symptoms include nausea, anorexia, fatigue, and malaise; these symptoms may occur acutely or have an insidious onset. Important findings on physical examination include hypotension with pulsus paradoxus (defined as an inspiratory drop in systolic pressure of at least 10 mm Hg), elevated jugular venous pressure, tachycardia, tachypnea, a quiet precordium on auscultation, and dullness of the posterior chest just below and medial to the left scapula (Ewart's sign). A pericardial friction rub may or may not be present. If the accumulation of fluid has occurred slowly,

there may be evidence of chronic venous congestion, including ascites and lower extremity edema. The EEG commonly shows sinus tachycardia with reduced QRS voltage. Electrical alternans (beat-to-beat alteration in QRS amplitude) and diffuse ST-segment elevation characteristic of pericarditis also may be present. The CXR typically shows an enlarged cardiac silhouette with a globular shape but no evidence of associated pulmonary congestion. The cardiac silhouette may be normal in those patients with a small but rapidly accumulating pericardial effusion.

Pericardial tamponade causing hypotension can be difficult to distinguish from other causes of shock. The finding of jugular venous distention is important and should alert one to the possibility of tamponade while helping to exclude hypovolemia. Central venous catheterization will reveal a correspondingly elevated right atrial pressure. PA catheterization will show equalization of diastolic pressures and reduced CO (Figs. 20-4 and 20-5). Echocardiography can confirm or exclude the presence of pericardial fluid. In addition, the echocardiogram may reveal visual evidence of tamponade, such as inspiratory collapse of the right heart chambers, which may be present even before there are obvious clinical findings of tamponade.[14]

Pericardial tamponade is a medical emergency and requires prompt intervention. Volume loading may be useful as a temporizing measure by increasing mean systemic vascular pressure and thus improving right heart filling and CO. Definitive treatment includes needle or catheter pericardiocentesis or pericardial window placement. For medical causes of pericardial effusion, the latter has the advantage of providing tissue for diagnosis and also prevents reaccumulation of fluid (see box, p. 229).

CARDIAC FUNCTION IN SEPSIS AND SEPTIC SHOCK

A distinct hemodynamic pattern occurs in patients with sepsis and septic shock. Characteristic findings include a low systemic vascular resistance secondary to peripheral vasodilation and often increased CO. In addition, some patients experience a potentially reversible im-

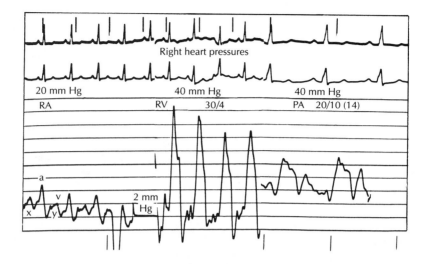

FIG. 20-4 Normal pulse pressure recordings from right heart structures. Scale for RA is 20 mm Hg; normal a and v waves with x and y descents are shown. Scale form RV and PA is 40 mm Hg. *RA,* right atrium; *RV,* right ventricle; *PA,* pulmonary artery. (From Warren JV, Lewis RP. Diagnostic Procedures in Cardiology. Chicago: Year Book Medical, 1985, p 265.)

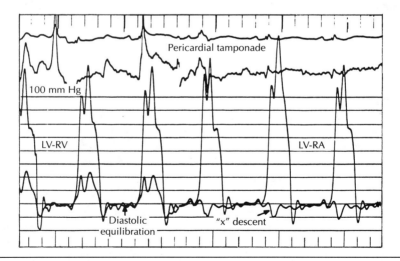

FIG. 20-5 Pulse pressures demonstrate hemodynamic characteristics of pericardial tamponade. Diastolic equilibration between LV, RV and RA, x descents of RA pressure, and failure of early diastolic pressure of ventricles to reach baseline. Scale is 100 mm Hg. *LV,* left ventricle; *RV,* right ventricle; *RA,* right atrium. (From Warren JV, Lewis RP. Diagnostic Procedures in Cardiology. Chicago: Year Book Medical, 1985, p 280.)

pairment in systolic function.[15,16] This impairment is associated with acute left ventricular dilation, reduced contractility, and diminished ejection fraction. Decreased contractility in the face of increased CO may seem contradictory, but it can occur because of marked decrease

Pericardial Tamponade

Mechanism

Pericardial fluid limits ventricular filling, a form of diastolic dysfunction

Symptoms

Dyspnea
Chest discomfort } Worse in supine position

Signs

Hypotension
Pulsus paradoxus
Jugular venous distention
Tachycardia
Tachypnea
Distant heart sounds
Ewart's sign
Friction rub

ECG

Sinus tachycardia, ↓ QRS complex voltage
Electrical alternans
Diffuse ST-segment elevation

CXR

Enlarged, globular heart; no pulmonary congestion

Echocardiogram

Pericardial fluid
Collapse of right heart chambers on inspiration

Hemodynamic monitoring

Equalization of right and left diastolic pressures

Treatment

An emergency
Volume loading as temporizing measure
Pericardiocentesis or pericardial window placement

in afterload, increase in preload, and tachycardia, all of which serve to counter the negative inotropic effect. This abnormality affects approximately half of patients with septic shock and appears to be mediated by a circulating myocardial depressant factor.[16] Paradoxically, patients who do not develop these changes appear to have a higher mortality rate. For survivors, abnormalities in ventricular function gradually reverse as resolution of the sepsis occurs.

Although the mainstay of treatment for sepsis is appropriate antibiotic therapy and drainage of closed-space infections, measures to maintain adequate perfusion and reverse the shock state are also important.[17] Initial management should include fluid resuscitation to restore and optimize preload.[6] Clinical investigations have shown that, in general, the optimal PCWP for patients with septic shock is approximately 12 mm Hg.[17] This level is lower than the optimal PCWP for patients with cardiogenic shock due to acute myocardial infarction; the difference probably relates to the increased ventricular stiffness that occurs with myocardial ischemia. It is not uncommon for patients with severe sepsis to require several liters of isotonic fluid administered intravenously over only a few hours. Patients with severe sepsis are susceptible to pulmonary edema on the basis of several factors. The vigorous fluid resuscitation that is often required increases the risk of overhydration; impaired cardiac function increases the risk of cardiogenic pulmonary edema. In addition, these patients are at high risk for developing adult respiratory distress syndrome. PA catheterization is therefore helpful in titrating fluid therapy and assessing cardiac function in critically ill patients with sepsis.

In addition to optimization of preload, many patients will require administration of sympathomimetic agents (e.g., dopamine and/or norepinephrine) to treat hypotension.[15] These agents are generally employed only in patients who remain hypotensive or exhibit other signs of impaired organ perfusion despite optimization of left ventricular preload.

SUMMARY

- Cardiac performance and myocardial oxygen demand depend on heart rate, preload, afterload, and contractility.
- Sinus tachycardia is a compensatory response to either a physiologic or pathologic condition.
- Preload is left ventricular end-diastolic volume.
- Ventricular compliance is approximated by the slope of diastolic portion of ventricular pressure-volume loop.
- PCWP and right atrial pressure are indirect estimates of left ventricular and right ventricular preload, respectively. An assumption about compliance is implicit when volume is inferred from pressure measurements.
- Patients with abnormal ventricular function usually require higher filling pressures.
- MAP and MPAP provide simple estimates of left ventricular and right ventricular afterload, respectively.
- SVR and PVR are useful estimates of left ventricular and right ventricular afterload, respectively, when CO and pressure gradients across the system and pulmonary vascular beds are available.

- Clinically, ejection fraction is an estimate of contractility, although ejection fraction depends on preload and afterload.
- External work of the heart is the area contained in the ventricular pressure-volume loop.
- Impaired contractility is characteristic of systolic dysfunction.
- Patients with systolic dysfunction are sensitive to changes in preload.
- Use inotropic agents in severe compromise of systolic function.
- Diastolic dysfunction can be an important cause of cardiac decompensation. The clinician must distinguish systolic from diastolic dysfunction (see Table 20-3).
- Use agents that improve myocardial compliance to treat diastolic dysfunction.
- Pericardial tamponade is a form of diastolic dysfunction. Diagnosis and treatment comprise an emergency (see box, p. 229).
- Cardiac function in sepsis is associated with low SVR and increased CO. Transient systolic dysfunction is common. Patients need volume resuscitation to restore and optimize preload and sympathomimetic drugs.

REFERENCES

1. Braunwald E, ed. Heart Disease, 4th ed. Philadelphia: WB Saunders, 1992.
2. Little RC, Little WC. Cardiac preload, afterload, and heart failure. Arch Intern Med 142:819, 1982.
3. Marini JJ. Pulmonary artery occlusion pressure: Clinical physiology, measurement and interpretation. Am Rev Resp Dis 128:319, 1983.
4. McElroy PA, Shroff SG, Weber KT. Pathophysiology of the failing heart. Cardiol Clin 7:25, 1989.
5. Wiedermann HP, Matthay MA, Matthay RA. Cardiovascular-pulmonary monitoring in the intensive care unit. Chest 85:537, 1984.
6. Bressack MA, Raffin TA. Importance of venous return, venous resistance, and mean circulatory pressure in the physiology and management of shock. Chest 92:906, 1987.
7. The SOLVD Investigators. Effect of enalapril on survival in patients with reduced left ventricular ejection fractions and congestive heart failure. N Engl J Med 325:293, 1991.
8. Echeverria HH, Bilsker MS, Myerburg RJ, et al. Congestive heart failure: Echocardiographic insights. Am J Med 75:750, 1983.
9. Dougherty AH, Naccarelli GV, Gray EL, et al. Congestive heart failure with normal systolic function. Am J Cardiol 54:778, 1984.
10. Topol EJ, Traill TA, Fortuin NJ. Hypertensive hypertrophic cardiomyopathy in the elderly. N Engl J Med 312:277, 1985.
11. Harizi RC, Bianco JA, Alpert JS. Diastolic function of the heart in clinical cardiology. Arch Intern Med 148:99, 1988.
12. Setaro JF, Zaret BL, Schulman DS, et al. Usefulness of verapamil for congestive heart failure associated with abnormal left ventricular diastolic filling and normal left ventricular systolic performance. Am J Cardiol 66:981, 1990.
13. Reddy PS, Curtiss EI. Cardiac tamponade. Cardiol Clin 8:627, 1990.

14. Levine MJ, Lorell BH, Diver DJ, et al. Implications of echocardiographically assisted diagnosis of pericardial tamponade in contemporary medical patients: Detection before hemodynamic embarrassment. J Am Coll Cardiol 17:59, 1991.

15. Natanson C, Hoffman WD, Parillo JE. Septic shock: The cardiovascular abnormality and therapy. J Cardiothorac Anesthesia 3:215, 1989.

16. Parker MM, Shelhamer JH, Bacharach SL, et al. Profound but reversible myocardial depression in patients with septic shock. Ann Intern Med 100:483, 1984.

17. Packman MI, Rackow EC. Optimum left heart filling pressure during fluid resuscitation of patients with hypovolemic and septic shock. Crit Care Med 11:165, 1983.

CHAPTER 21

Dysrhythmias

John W. McBride

The patient with the dysrhythmia, not the dysrhythmia itself, is the object of treatment. Appropriate treatment includes proper identification of the dysrhythmia, recognition of the underlying pathologic or pathophysiologic state, and recognition of any hemodynamic consequences produced by the dysrhythmia.

Proper identification of dysrhythmias implies the application of a method of ECG or rhythm strip interpretation that allows complete identification and reduces or eliminates errors of omission. Frequently two or more leads are required to be certain. Most modern bedside ECG monitors allow standard leads I, II, III, aVR, aVL, aVF, and a V lead.

SINOATRIAL NODE AND ATRIUM

The sinoatrial (SA) node ordinarily acts as a primary pacemaker or impulse generator. The impulse escapes from the SA node and electrically depolarizes atrial muscle, resulting in the P wave on the ECG.

Normal sinus rhythm (NSR) (Fig. 21-1) is characterized by the following:
- P waves in a given lead of a constant configuration
- P waves in the frontal plane of +45 degrees ± 15 degrees
- Atrial rate of 60 to 100 beats/min (bpm)
- Usually a consistent PP interval (if the latter varies, usually rhythmically with inspiration, the rhythm is *sinus dysrhythmia*)

Sinus Tachycardia

Sinus tachycardia fulfills the criteria for NSR, but the rate is >100 bpm (Fig. 21-2). Sinus tachycardia occurs during exercise or other states of catecholamine discharge, fever, congestive heart failure (CHF), thyrotoxicosis, anemia, or intravascular volume depletion. It occurs postoperatively for a number of reasons, including inadequate ventilation or hypoxemia. Primary treatment is that of the underlying condition causing the sinus tachycardia. If the patient is hemodynamically compromised by the tachycardia, it may be necessary to slow the rate medically. Calcium channel blockers have a negative chronotropic effect in the SA node (Table 21-1). Digoxin usually does not have a significant effect on the SA node but may be helpful in combination with diltiazem. Digoxin plus verapamil can approximately double the plasma concentration of digoxin and lead to digitalis toxicity. Beta-inhibitors, especially short-acting agents such as esmolol with a $t_{1/2}$ of 7 to 11 minutes, can be given by both bolus and infusion to control sinus rate. Contraindications to the use of beta-blockers include bronchospastic pulmonary disease or moderate to severe CHF (see Table 21-1).

Sinus Bradycardia

Sinus bradycardia (Fig. 21-3) fulfills the criteria for NSR except the rate is <60 bpm. In the absence of clinical evidence of tissue underperfusion (i.e., cold or pale extremities, bradycardia-dependent altered mentation, decreased urinary output, or bradycardia-dependent ST-T segment change on the ECG suggesting ischemia), sinus bradycardia does not require treatment. A search for causation (e.g., pharyngeal suction–stimulated reflex bradycardia, hypothyroidism, hypothermia, elevated intracranial pressure [Branham's sign], or chronotropic incompetence in the elderly) should be conducted.

Other Tachycardias

Supraventricular tachycardia should be considered as a general category that does not specify the exact name or mechanism. The astute clinician should try to identify the dysrhythmia more specifically. SA or atrial reentry tachycardias are not common, but *AV nodal reentry tachycardia* (Fig. 21-4), formerly known as *PAT,*

is common. The rate is usually 150 to 250 bpm. Characteristically, the rate is such that P waves are buried in the T wave and cannot be identified. The rhythms are paroxysmal and are characterized by a narrow QRS complex. Mechanical maneuvers such as carotid sinus massage may be effective as therapy. Carotid sinus massage need not be painful. While the ECG paper is running, the middle finger is placed on the thyroid cartilage and moved laterally over the carotid artery. The forefinger and fourth fingers may also be used to apply gentle but firm rotational pressure over the carotid artery while the ECG monitor is watched. Massage of the left side may be more effective than that of the right. As soon as the rhythm breaks, massaging is stopped. If this maneuver is unsuccessful, it is repeated after a few seconds on

Text continued on p. 238.

TABLE 21-1 Useful Medications for Dysrhythmias

Class	Agent	Dose	Route	Interval
Calcium channel blockers	Verapamil	80-120 mg	po	tid or qid
	Verapamil SA	120, 180, 240 mg	po	qd or bid
	Verapamil	2.5-5 µg/kg/min	IV	Constant infusion
	Diltiazem	60-120 mg	po	tid or qid
	Diltiazem SR	90-120 mg	po	qd or bid
	Diltiazem CD/XL	180, 240, 300 mg	po	qd
Digitalis	Digoxin	0.25-0.75 mg	IV	Reevaluate 2-6 hr
	Digoxin	0.25-0.5 mg	po	qd
Beta-inhibitors	Propranolol	30 mg/kg	IV	At 1 mg/min
	Propranolol	10-40 mg	po	qid
	Metoprolol	5 mg	IV	To 15 mg at 5-min interval
	Metoprolol	25-100 mg	po	bid or tid
	Atenolol	25-50 mg	po	qd
	Esmolol	500 µg bolus	IV	Titrate as required
		50 µg/min	Infusion	
Antidysrhythmics	Quinidine	200-300 mg	po	qid
	Procainamide	250-1250 mg	po	qid
	Procainamide	0.75-2 mg/min	IV	Constant infusion
	Lidocaine	50-100 mg	IV	Bolus
		1-4 mg/min	IV	Constant infusion
	Adenosine	6, 12 mg	IV	Bolus plus fast flush
	Epinephrine or isoproterenol	1-5 mg/min	IV	Constant infusion

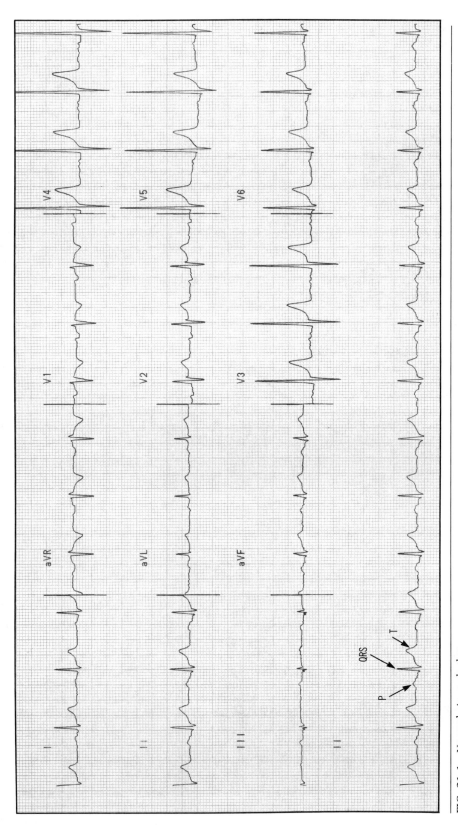

FIG. 21-1   Normal sinus rhythm.

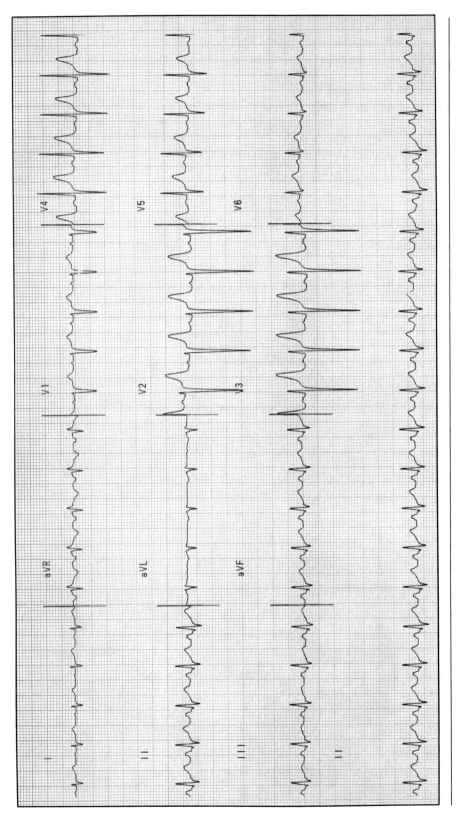

FIG. 21-2   Sinus tachycardia.

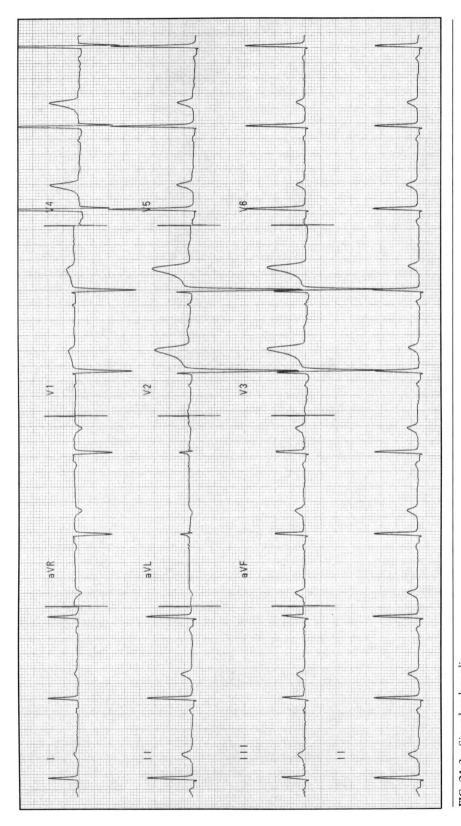

FIG. 21-3 Sinus bradycardia.

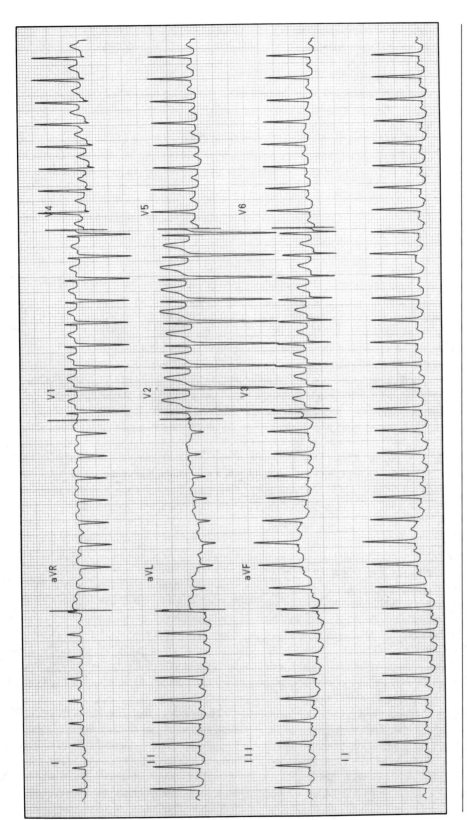

FIG. 21-4   AV nodal reentry tachycardia.

the other side. Occasionally a combination of Valsalva maneuver and carotid massage is effective. The recurrence of transient neurologic abnormalities mandates stopping. The medication of choice, if required, is adenosine, with a $t_{1/2}$ of 7 to 11 seconds. The usual dose is 6 mg by rapid IV infusion and immediate fluid flush because of the short half-life. If the 6 mg dose is unsuccessful, an attempt with 12 mg should be tried as soon as possible. Complete block may occur, but blockage usually lasts fewer than 6 to 10 seconds.

Atrial Fibrillation

Atrial fibrillation (Fig. 21-5) is characterized by the absence of organized atrial activity with the presence of an undulating baseline. The atrial rate is 350 to 600 bpm and is ineffective in filling the ventricle. The ventricular response may be slow (<60 bpm), controlled (60 to 100 bpm), or rapid (>100 bpm) and should be totally irregular. Whether the QRS configuration is wide or narrow depends on conduction through the right and left bundles and the His-Purkinje system to the ventricular muscle. Depolarization of ventricular muscle is represented on the ECG by QRS.

Atrial fibrillation may be caused by thyrotoxicosis, mitral valve stenosis, acute alcoholic ingestion, arteriosclerotic heart disease (especially with left ventricular failure), acute cor pulmonale such as with pulmonary embolus, postoperative effect of open heart surgery, pericarditis, mitral valve regurgitation, or systemic hypertension, especially if associated with acute or chronic left ventricular failure.

Primary treatment is that of the underlying disease state. Control of AV node conduction, however, may be necessary for symptomatic or hemodynamic decompensation. Traditionally digoxin has been the most widely used medication. Although digoxin may reduce the ventricular response at rest to <100 bpm, recent studies using 24-hour ambulatory ECG monitoring have suggested that achieving ventricular rate control during activity or exercise is uncommon. Better control of the ventricular rate occurs with the use of calcium channel blockers or beta-blockers alone or in combination with digoxin (see Table 21-1). If atrial fibrillation

lasts beyond 3 to 5 days, anticoagulation therapy with heparin acutely and coumadin for 4 to 6 weeks is indicated before chemical conversion with, for example, quinidine or procainamide or electric conversion.

Atrial Flutter

Atrial flutter (Fig. 21-6) is characterized by inferiorly directed atrial activity with a sawtooth baseline evident, usually in leads II, III, aVF, and occasionally V_1 to V_2. The atrial rate is 220 to 350 bpm but is usually 300 bpm with a 2:1, 3:1, or 4:1 ratio and often with varying AV block. Atrial flutter with an odd number:1 block >4:1 (e.g., 5:1, 7:1) suggests possible digitalis toxicity. Atrial flutter is usually an unstable rhythm and converts to normal sinus rhythm or to atrial fibrillation.

Therapy includes digoxin, beta-blockers, or calcium channel blockers for rate control or conversion to normal sinus rhythm. Oral quinidine sulfate (200 to 300 mg qid), oral procainamide (500 to 1250 mg qid), or IV procainamide at 1 to 2 mg/min may chemically convert the rhythm. Electric conversion is often successful at low energies (e.g., 5 to 50 joules).

Multiform Atrial Tachycardia

Multiform atrial tachycardia (Fig. 21-7) is characterized by at least three different P configurations in a given lead with (1) a varying PP interval, (2) usually a varying PR interval, and (3) often nonconducted P waves caused by the P wave's falling in the AV nodal refractory period. This rhythm is seen in any circumstance in which atrial fibrillation occurs (see discussion of atrial fibrillation). It has occurred as an intermediate rhythm in patients whose rhythm was varying between atrial fibrillation and normal sinus rhythm. It commonly is associated with an acute exacerbation of chronic pulmonary disease or an acute pulmonary complication.

The underlying disease is treated. Digoxin, beta-blockers, and calcium channel blockers are useful in the appropriate situation, but each may be contraindicated in patients with specific causes of multiform atrial tachycardia. Oxygenation, ventilation, and bronchodilators are useful when the cause is pulmonary.

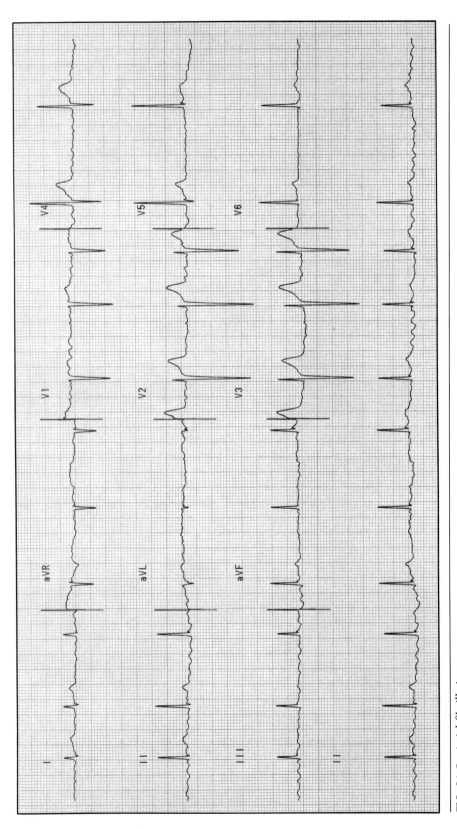

FIG. 21-5   Atrial fibrillation.

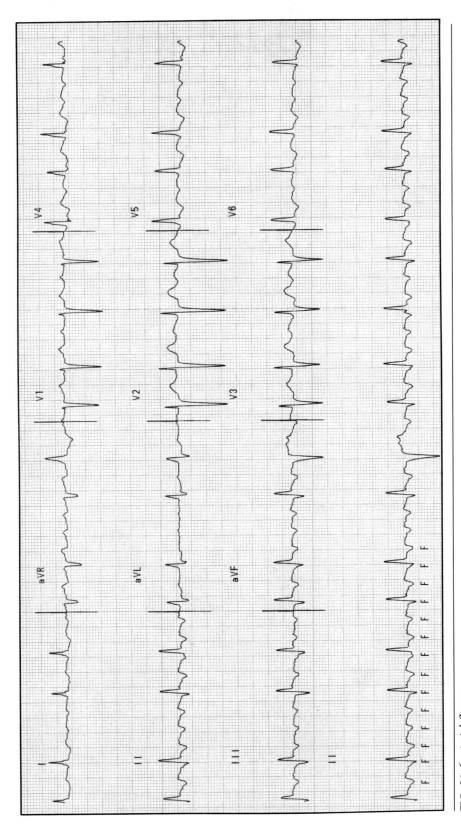

FIG. 21-6   Atrial flutter.

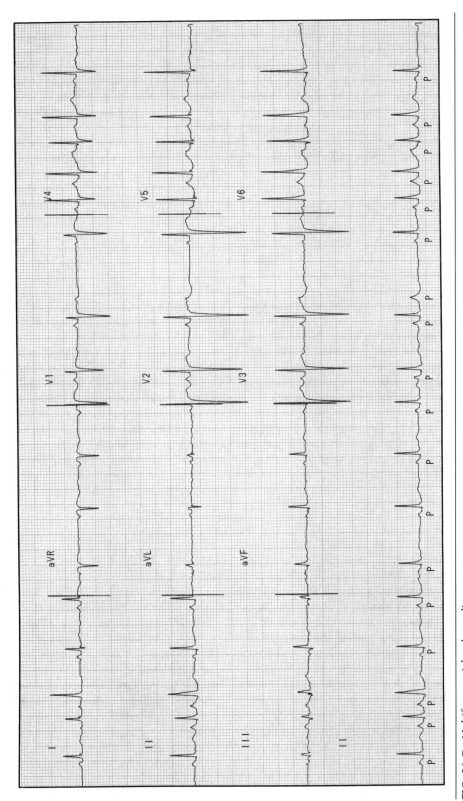

FIG. 21-7 Multiform atrial tachycardia.

Sick Sinus Syndrome

Sick sinus syndrome may be present with one of the following conditions:

- Sinus bradycardia in the absence of medication that slows SA nodal automaticity; chronotropic incompetence may also manifest itself as an inadequate increase in sinus rate during anemia, volume depletion, catecholamine discharge, or a postoperative state
- Second-degree or third-degree SA block (i.e., sinus pauses or sinus arrest)
- Rapid atrial fibrillation with intermittent bradycardic episodes or slow atrial fibrillation with intermittent bursts of supraventricular tachycardia. Symptoms usually occur during sudden changes in rate as from fast to slow or slow to fast; this is the one form that can predispose to cerebral emboli and warrants consideration of using anticoagulation therapy
- Atrial fibrillation with a slow ventricular response in the absence of medication that slows conduction through the AV node
- Atrial fibrillation treated by electric conversion that results in ventricular asystole

The last two forms of atrial fibrillation may be related to AV node function but have been considered with SA node disease since approximately 17% to 30% of patients with SA node disease also have AV node conduction disorders.

Treatment of most forms of sick sinus syndrome is aimed at increasing the atrial or ventricular rates. Therapies include transcutaneous or transvenous temporary pacing or permanent pacemaker implantation. Medical treatment includes medications that increase the rate of firing of the SA or AV nodes. Epinephrine and isoproterenol infusion rates are identical. Epinephrine has the advantage of raising blood pressure, whereas isoproterenol as a vasodilator may result in decreasing pressure or perfusion. These drugs are usually infused at 1 to 5 μg/min, with increases as clinically necessary. The advantage over atropine is the shorter duration of action of the constant IV infusion of catecholamine. If tachycardia occurs and the infusion is stopped, the tachycardia will last only 5 to 10 minutes.

ATRIOVENTRICULAR NODAL BLOCK
First-Degree and Third-Degree AV Block

The SA node fires, the atrium responds, *but* is there a QRS complex for each P wave? If yes, is the PR interval normal (i.e., <0.2 to 0.22 second)? If it is this long or longer, there is first-degree AV block (Fig. 21-8). If there is no relationship, but regular PP intervals and independent and regular QRS complexes with a regular RR interval are present, the block is a complete or third-degree atrioventricular (AV) block. The clinician should determine whether the pacemaker for the ventricle is either at the AV node, with a narrow QRS (Fig. 21-9) and a rate of 40 to 60 bpm, or below the His bundle in the His-Purkinje system where the QRS is wide and the rate is <40 (Fig. 21-10). These two situations identify first-degree AV block and third-degree AV block with an AV nodal or junctional rhythm or third-degree AV block with an idioventricular rhythm.

Second-Degree AV Block

All other rhythms with normal atrial activity with fewer QRS complexes than P waves and with irregular RR intervals are second-degree AV block. The four varieties of second-degree AV block include the following:

- *Mobitz type I or Wenckebach block* (Fig. 21-11). The PR interval becomes progressively longer until a P wave occurs so early that it is not conducted to the ventricle. The pattern repeats itself, resulting in "group beating." The ratio of P waves to QRS complexes vary, with one more P wave than QRS complexes for each group (e.g., 5:4, 3:2, 6:5). The QRS complex is usually narrow since the block occurs above the His bundle unless a bundle branch block or other interventricular conduction (IVCD) is present.
- *Mobitz type II block* (Fig. 21-12). Usually located below the His bundle, the PR interval is within the normal range, possibly close to the upper range of normal. The PR interval remains constant until a P wave is not followed by a QRS complex. Again, a form of group beating is present, with ratios of 3:2, 4:3, 5:4, 6:4. The QRS configuration is usually, but not always, wide.

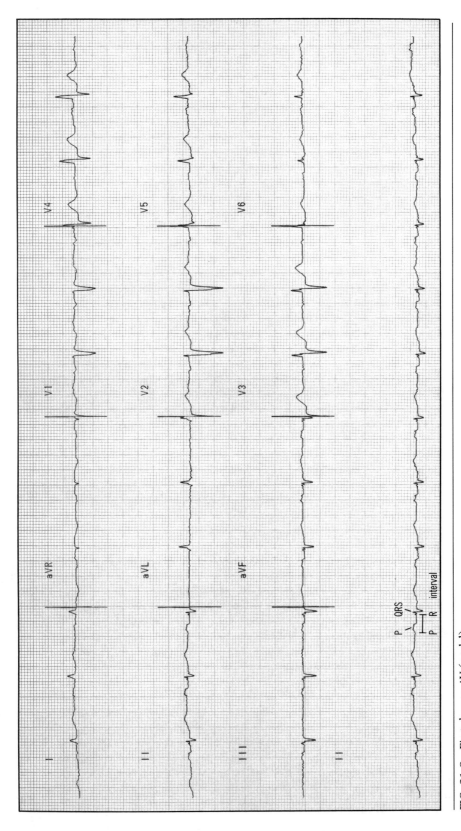

FIG. 21-8   First-degree AV (nodal).

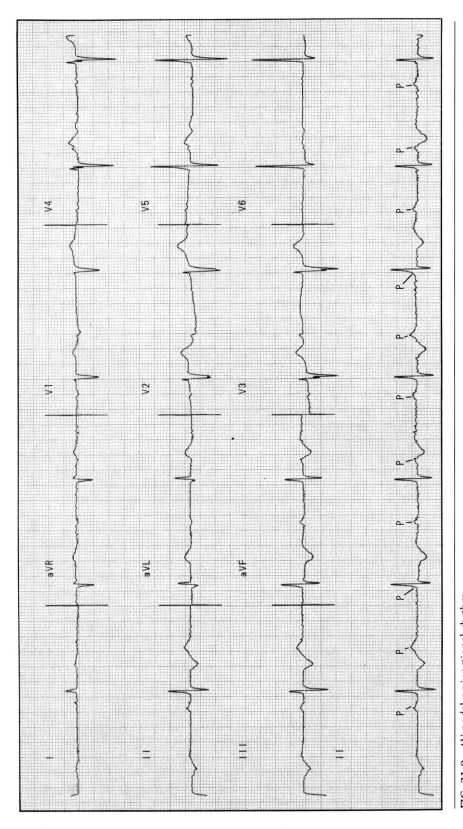

FIG. 21-9   AV nodal or junctional rhythm.

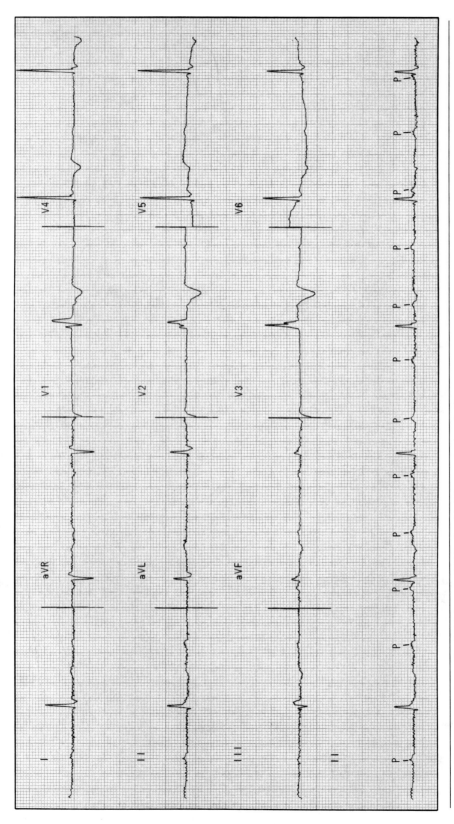

FIG. 21-10 Sinus rhythm with third-degree AV block with idioventricular rhythm.

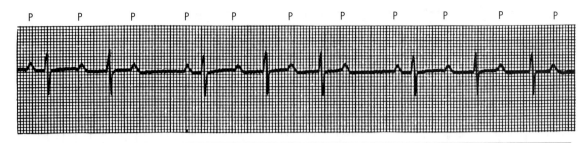

FIG. 21-11 Second-degree AV block, Mobitz type I or Wenckebach.

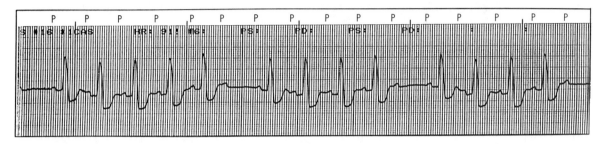

FIG. 21-12 Second-degree AV block, Mobitz type II.

- *2:1 AV block* (Fig. 21-13). Only the rhythm strip or ECG reveals a ratio of two P waves: 1 QRS, and the rest of the ECG rhythm strip precludes a definite differential between either Mobitz type I or Mobitz type II.
- *Advanced form of second-degree AV block* (Fig. 21-14). With this variety, there are at least two consecutively nonconducted P waves.

■ ■ ■

First-degree AV block and Mobitz type I second-degree AV block may be due to ischemia (especially inferior ischemia), digitalis excess, calcium channel blockers, and primary conduction system disease. Treatment involves addressing the underlying condition.

Mobitz type II second-degree AV block, or the advanced form, more likely will be seen in patients with anterior ischemia or primary conduction disease. If symptomatic, these forms are likely to require permanent cardiac pacing. With the initial appearance of symptoms, patients may require temporary transcutaneous or transvenous pacing. If it is not immediately available, 2 to 3 mg of epinephrine in 500 ml of normal saline solution is infused at 1-5 μg/min, increasing as necessary.

Interventricular Conduction Defects

The three basic types of IVCDs are right bundle branch block (RBBB), left bundle branch block (LBBB), and nonspecific IVCD. In patients with these blocks the impulse has been transmitted to the atrium and has depolarized it and has passed through the AV node and the His bundle. The block occurs below the His bundle in the right bundle, left bundle, or one of the two divisions of the left bundle. In patients with *nonspecific IVCD* ("normal complexes" in Fig. 21-15) the QRS is >0.12 second without the configuration of either typical right or left bundle branch block.

Right bundle branch block. RBBB (Fig. 21-16) results in abnormalities in the impulse depolarizing the septum in the usual fashion from left to right. Because two thirds to three fourths of the septum is functionally part of the left ventricle, a normal initial q wave in standard lead I, aVL, and V_6—the normal *septal q*—occurs. Likewise, a normal *septal r* is seen in aVR and V_1. The middle forces are also normal—a tall R wave in I, aVL, and V_6 and a deep S wave

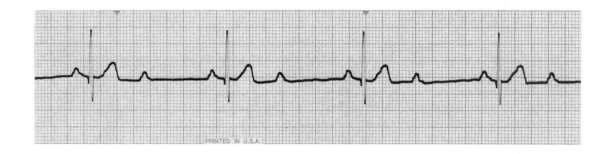

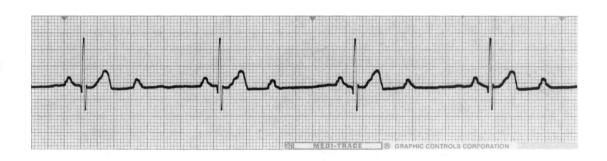

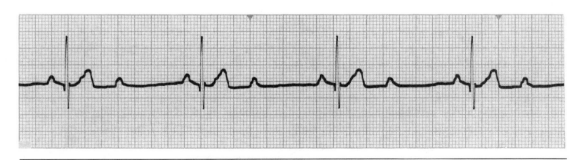

FIG. 21-13   2:1 AV block; continuous tracing, lead II.

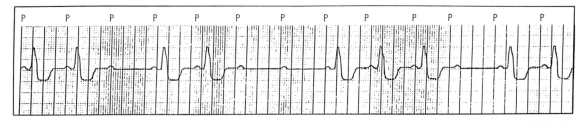

FIG. 21-14 Advanced form of second-degree AV block.

in aVR and V_1. However, terminal conduction through muscle that has not been depolarized in the right ventricle occurs. The terminal forces are slow and slurred and cause a wide slow S wave in I, aVL, and V_6 and a slow, slurred R′ in aVR and V_1. Since initial and middle forces are normal, a myocardial infarction can be diagnosed in RBBB. The T wave is in the direction opposite the terminal conduction delay. The shape of the ST-T segment is that of a long sloping descending limb, with convexity upward in I, aVL, and V_6 and concavity downward in aVR and V_1. There is a brisk return to baseline in the terminal portion of the T wave. The result is an asymmetric T wave. Symmetry in T waves suggests ischemia or hyperkalemia.

Left bundle branch block. LBBB (Fig. 21-17) results in the impulse leaving the right bundle branch and depolarizing the septum from right to left, opposite the usual direction. The result is conduction toward the left ventricle and the loss of the usually expected small r in aVR and V_1 and also the loss of the normal q in I, aVL, and V_6—the so-called septal q waves. The QRS is 0.12 second or longer, and the T wave is opposite in direction to the QRS. Since the initial forces, middle forces, and terminal forces are all abnormal, a myocardial infarction cannot be diagnosed in the presence of a LBBB.

■ ■ ■

IVCDs of all three types can occur because of underlying ischemic heart disease, cardiomyopathy, primary conduction system disease, or metabolic disorder or hypoxemia. Treatment is that of the underlying heart disease. No treatment is needed if the IVCD is stable or old. If associated with other forms of electric instability such as changing RBBB and first-degree

AV block plus left axis deviation (left anterior fascicular block or hemiblock) or right axis deviation (left posterior hemiblock), temporary transcutaneous or transvenous pacing may be required. LBBB plus changing AV conduction (e.g., first-degree or second-degree AV block) may also require pacing. Otherwise, attention should be paid to electrolyte and blood gas values and the underlying disease.

PREEXCITATION SYNDROMES

Lown-Ganong-Levine syndrome. Lown-Ganong-Levine (LGL) syndrome is a group of signs and/or symptoms. LGL is characterized by (1) normal sinus rhythm, (2) a short PR interval, (3) normal QRS duration, and (4) paroxysms of supraventricular tachycardia (SVT). An ECG with normal sinus rhythm, short PR interval, and narrow QRS but the absence of SVT should not be labeled LGL.

Treatment is necessary only to prevent or break the SVT and generally includes a beta-blocker or calcium channel blockers, which will decrease the rate of SA or AV nodal pacemakers and slow AV conduction or SA to atrial conduction.

Wolff-Parkinson-White syndrome. In a patient with Wolff-Parkinson-White syndrome (Fig. 21-18) normal sinus and atrial activity is expected, but conduction to the ventricles proceeds through an accessory pathway. Early ventricular excitation occurs. This syndrome is characterized by a delta wave on the ECG and a wider-than-normal QRS.

Episodes of SVT can occur from reentry mechanisms, with antegrade or orthodromic conduction through the AV node and retrograde conduction to the atrium through the accessory pathway. ST-T changes cannot be in-

Text continued on p. 253.

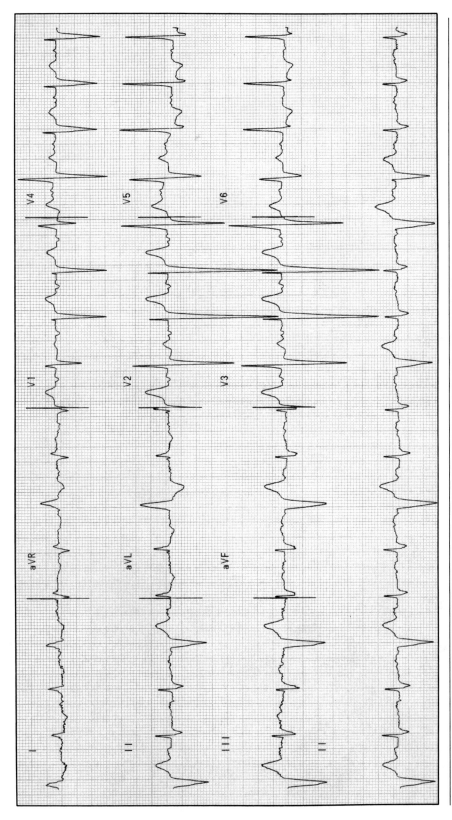

FIG. 21-15   Nonspecific interventricular conduction defect (plus ventricular premature complexes).

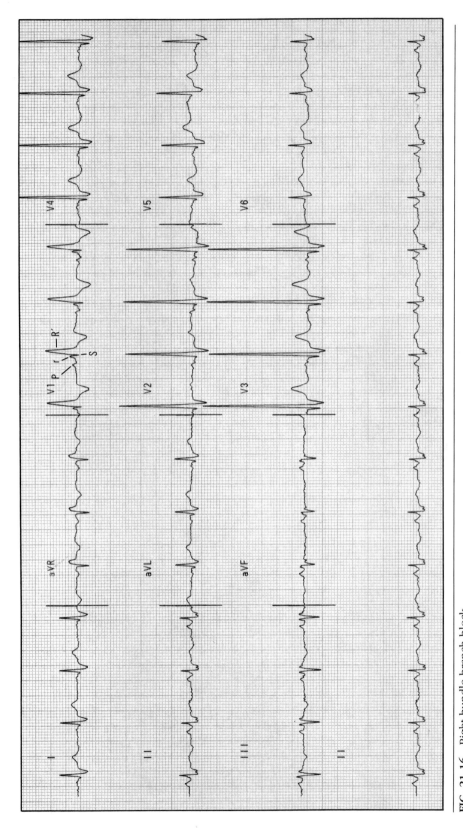

FIG. 21-16 Right bundle branch block.

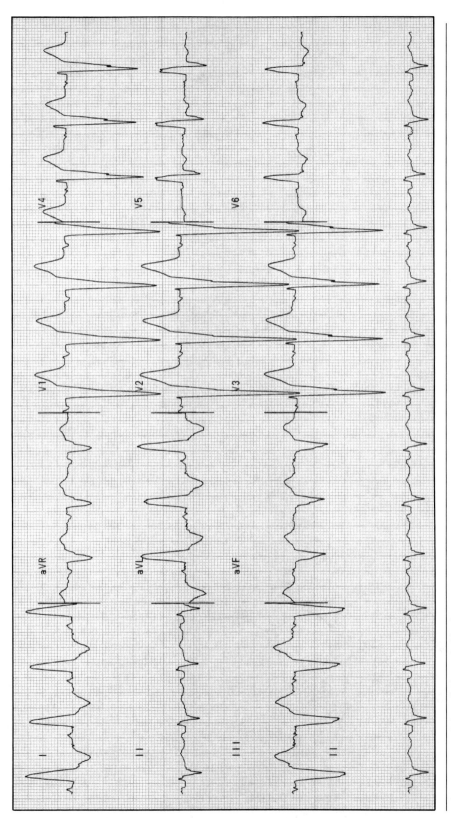

FIG. 21-17 Left bundle branch block.

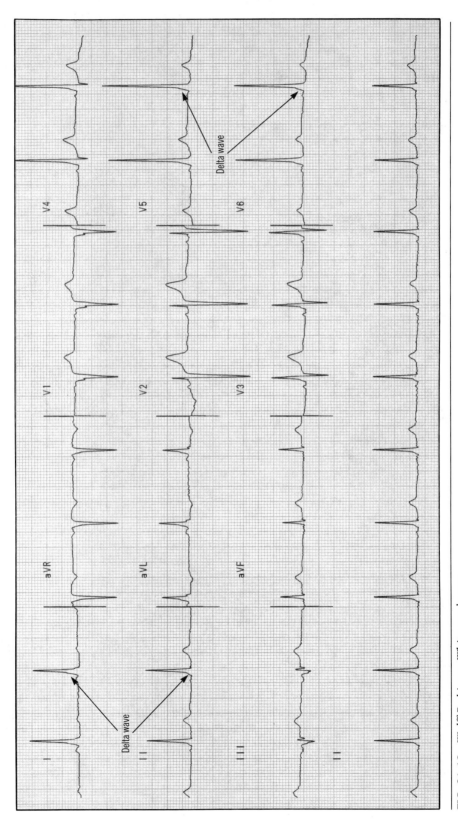

FIG. 21-18   Wolff-Parkinson-White syndrome.

terpreted in patients with Wolff-Parkinson-White syndrome since abnormal depolarization results in abnormal repolarization. Treatment depends on the hemodynamic stability of the patient. SVT with hemodynamic instability requires urgent cardioversion. The most serious situation is atrial fibrillation in patients with this syndrome because atrial fibrillation conducted to the ventricle can result in ventricular fibrillation. This is an emergency that requires electric defibrillation. Occasionally atrial fibrillation with a long accessory pathway refractory period does not result in ventricular fibrillation. Such cases should be referred to an electrophysiologist for evaluation.

VENTRICULAR DYSRHYTHMIAS

SA, AV nodal, and bundle branch block system conduction may or may not be normal. Function at those locations should be evaluated before evaluation of the ventricular dysrhythmia, if possible, to avoid errors of omission or commission.

Ventricular premature complexes. Ventricular premature complexes (VPCs), or ectopy, arise below the AV node and result in wide bizarre QRS complexes. *Uniform VPCs* (Fig. 21-19) refer to several premature ventricular contractions (PVCs) in a rhythm strip or ECG that are not consecutive but are of the same configuration. *Multiform VPCs* (Fig. 21-20) show more than one form. *Couplets* are two consecutive VPCs and *triplets* are three consecutive VPCs, whether they are uniform or multiform (as in Fig. 21-20). *Bigeminy* (Fig. 21-19) refers to repetition of a normal P-QRS/T-VPC, with fixed intervals between the two. *Trigeminy* currently means normal-normal-VPC, whereas trigeminy used to refer to repetitive patterns of normal-VPC-VPC. Some VPCs occur so early that they land on the descending limb of the T wave of the previous P-QRS/T complex. That descending limb of the T wave is the so-called vulnerable period. A VPC landing there can precipitate ventricular tachycardia or ventricular fibrillation.

Ventricular escape complex. This complex occurs when the supraventricular mechanism—sinus or AV nodal—slows down to a rate of less than the rate of a ventricular focus, usually a rate of 30 to 40 bpm. Ventricular escape complexes can occur as individual complexes or as a series, for example, as a ventricular escape rhythm (see Fig. 21-10).

Ventricular tachycardia. Ventricular tachycardia (Fig. 21-21) refers to three or more consecutive VPCs at a rate >100. Ventricular tachycardia is sustained if it lasts >30 bpm or 2 minutes (author dependent) or is nonsustained if it does not. Sustained VT more likely is reproducible by electrophysiologic studies, and treatment more likely is predictable by the results of such studies.

Ventricular fibrillation. Ventricular fibrillation (Fig. 21-22) is that rhythm whereby the electric activity in the ventricle is identical to that in the atrium during atrial fibrillation. The ineffective ventricular activity results in the absence of effective cardiac contractility and therefore of cardiac output. In the absence of electric defibrillation (recommended therapy is 200 to 360 J) or immediate chemical conversion using, for example, procainamide, lidocaine, or bretylium, the patient will die. Thus ventricular fibrillation is a medical emergency. It may degenerate into ventricular asystole (see Fig. 21-22).

Results from the Cardiac Arrhythmia Suppression Trial (CAST) show that treatment of VPCs in patients who have had a previous myocardial infarction resulted in reduced LV function and is likely to cause an increased rather than a decreased mortality rate. The cardiologist's approach to ventricular ectopic activity has changed greatly. Cardiologists rarely consider treating VPCs, even in the presence of nonsustained ventricular tachycardia in the absence of hemodynamic compromise. A search for underlying correctable pathophysiologic abnormalities such as hypokalemia or hyperkalemia, hypomagnesemia, hypoxemia, other fluid or electrolyte disorders, or ischemia is recommended. Ectopy per se, however, is not treated. Suppression of symptomatic or hemodynamically compromising ectopy can be accomplished by administering lidocaine (50 to 100 mg bolus to a total dose of 225 to 325 mg). Conservative treatment is indicated in patients with CHF or liver disease in whom lidocaine metabolism may be abnormal. Once control is achieved, 1 to 2 mg/min lidocaine drip is given. If lidocaine does not work, pro-

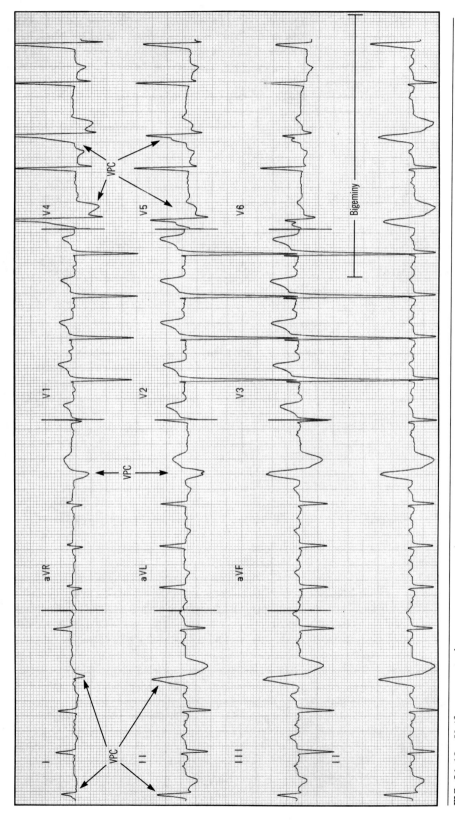

FIG. 21-19   Uniform ventricular premature complexes.

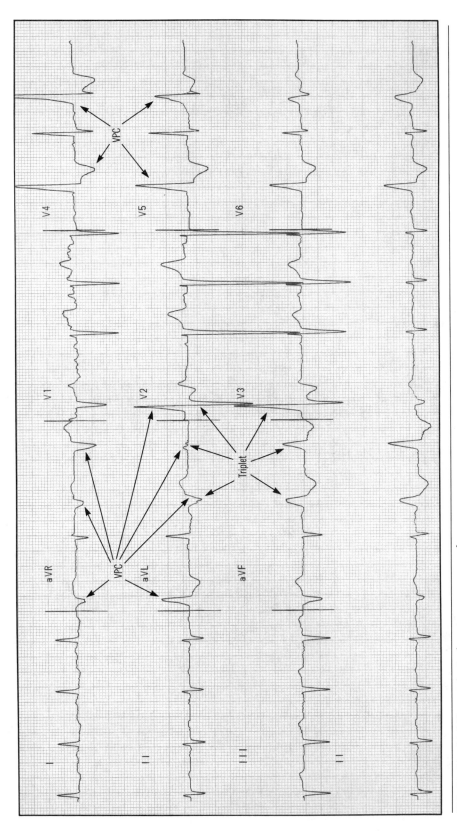

FIG. 21-20   Multiform ventricular premature complexes.

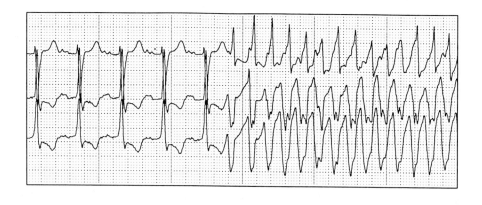

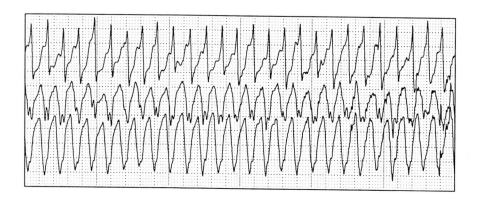

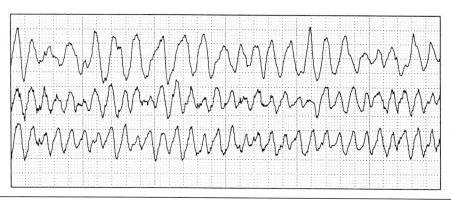

FIG. 21-21   Ventricular tachycardia.

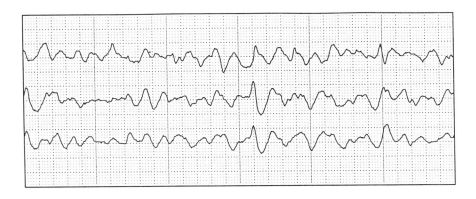

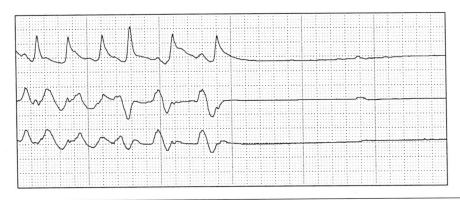

FIG. 21-22   Ventricular fibrillation.

cainamide can be used. Pharmacologists as consultants are helpful in pharmacokinetically predicting loading and maintenance doses determined by lean body weight, age, and liver and kidney function. If such doses are unavailable, procainamide boluses of 20 to 50 mg/min to a total dose of 1000 to 1200 mg may be given, but less safely. Maintenance infusion of 0.75 to 2 mg/min after VPC control may be less safe than using pharmacokinetic planning but is sometimes necessary. Bretylium bolus, 5 to 10 mg/kg up to 30 mg/kg, and maintenance infusion of 1 to 2 mg/min may be necessary. Esmolol may also be considered for acute treatment. Chronic treatment of ectopy may require a cardiologist or a knowledgeable internist.

Of major importance is the ability to differentiate ectopy from supraventricular complexes with aberration. Table 21-2 presents criteria for such distinction.

TABLE 21-2 Differentiation Between Ectopy and Supraventricular Complexes With Aberrant Conduction

	Ectopy	Complexes With Aberrant Conduction
P waves	Unrelated to QRS	Precede QRS by reasonable interval
Initial QRS	Abnormal in direction in several leads	Normal direction in all leads
Middle QRS	Abnormal	Normal direction
Terminal QRS	Abnormal	Terminal slurring; RBBB pattern
Number phases	Monophasic or diphasic	Triphasic
	Often one less than usual complexes	Usually one more than usual complexes
	If rSR', first "rabbit ear" is greater than second	If rSR', second "rabbit ear" is greater than first
Coupling interval	Fixed; rule of begeminy (or trigeminy)	Variable
Undue prematurity	So early it cannot be conducted normally	No
Fusion complexes	A combination of supraventricular plus ventricular	No
Previous anomalous complexes	If similar to complexes seen in the same lead in a prior ECG and they were clearly ventricular then, they still are	If similar to complexes seen in the lead in a prior ECG and they were clearly aberrant, they still are
QRS duration	>0.16 sec	<0.12 sec
Frontal plane axis	> −60 degrees −90 to −180 degrees	Normal
Aberrant beats	Precordial concordant positive (negative); all QRS complexes in horizontal plane are positive (negative)	
Reversal of usual pattern	V_6 resembles normal V_1; and V_1 resembles normal V_6	None
Ashman's phenomenon and cycle sequencing*		Ashman's phenomenon and cycle sequencing

*Ashman phenomenon states that the complex that ends a short cycle that is preceded by a longer cycle probably is supraventricular with aberrancy. Unfortunately, ventricular bigeminy (see Figure 21-19) fulfills that criterion. Cycle sequencing carries this phenomenon one step further. Cycle sequencing states that as the heart slows or accelerates, conduction slows or accelerates. The abnormal complex that ends a short cycle, preceded by a sequence of cycles in which the heart is slowing as is conduction, probably will be supraventricular with aberrancy. If the sequence of cycles is such that the heart rate is accelerating, conduction is also accelerating. The abnormal complex that ends a sequence of cycles in which the heart rate is accelerating more likely will be ventricular.

SUMMARY

- Appropriate dysrhythmia treatment requires identification of dysrhythmia, recognition of underlying pathophysiologic condition, and assessment of hemodynamic consequences.
- SA node is normally the primary pacemaker. Rhythms associated with SA node function are normal sinus, sinus tachycardia, and sinus bradycardia.
- Supraventricular tachycardia includes AV nodal reentry tachycardial, atrial fibrillation, atrial flutter, and multiform atrial tachycardia.
- Treatment of sick sinus syndrome attempts to increase atrial or ventricular rates. Pacemaker therapy may be necessary.
- AV nodal block:
  First-degree AV block has a PR interval >0.22 second with a QRS for each P.
  Third-degree AV block demonstrates no relationship between P and QRS complexes but has regular PP intervals and regular RR intervals because of an idionodal or idioventricular rhythmn.

Second-degree AV block comprises all other rhythms, with normal atrial activity and fewer QRS complexes than P waves with irregular RR intervals.
Second-degree AV block includes Mobitz I or Wenckebach, Mobitz type II, 2:1 AV block, and advanced second-degree AV block.
- Interventricular conduction defects (IVCDs), QRS ≥ 0.12 second, are right bundle branch block, left bundle branch block, and nonspecific block.
- Preexcitation syndrome includes the Lown-Ganong-Levine and Wolff-Parkinson-White syndromes. Atrial fibrillation in Wolff-Parkinson-White syndrome requires emergency cardioversion.
- Ventricular dysrhythmias include ventricular premature complexes, ventricular escape complex, ventricular tachycardia, and ventricular fibrillation. Ventricular fibrillation requires emergency conversion.

BIBLIOGRAPHY

Marriott HJL. Practical Electrocardiography, 8th ed. Baltimore: Williams & Wilkins, 1988.

Textbook of Advanced Cardiac Life Support. Dallas: American Heart Association, 1987.

CHAPTER 22

Acute Myocardial Infarction

Robert E. Cunnion · Steven M. Hollenberg

Myocardial infarction in surgical patients can be subtle. Aftereffects of surgery and medication can mimic or mask the classic features of myocardial infarction (substernal chest pain radiating to the jaw and arm, shortness of breath, diaphoresis, nausea). Therefore the vigilant surgeon must maintain a high index of suspicion and a low threshold for obtaining a 12-lead ECG. The symptoms of myocardial infarction may also be mimicked by dissecting aortic aneurysm, pericarditis, pulmonary embolism, and biliary or gastroesophageal processes.

More than 90% of myocardial infarctions result from thrombus formation, usually at a site of atherosclerotic plaque. When a thrombus is large enough to occlude coronary artery flow, the myocardium distal to the occlusion develops ischemia and then, unless prompt reperfusion takes place, becomes infarcted. The consequences of an infarct depend on its size and location (see box).

DIAGNOSIS

In most cases the diagnosis of myocardial infarction is apparent from serial ECG tracings. Classically, the initial ST-segment elevation is accompanied by tall, peaked T waves. Within the first few hours, the T waves become flattened and then inverted, the ST segments return toward baseline, and, in transmural infarctions, Q waves begin to develop. When these diagnostic ECG findings are present, cardiac enzymes serve a confirmatory role. In many cases, though, the ECG is nondiagnostic, with equivocal ST-segment elevation or ST-seg-

ment depression and without development of Q waves. In such cases cardiac enzymes are key to the diagnosis.

The creatinine phophokinase (CPK) concentration peaks in 12 to 24 hours and then falls rapidly. CPK fractionation reveals elevation of the MB isoenzyme released from necrotic cardiomyocytes. When the total CPK concentration is elevated but consists entirely of the MM isoenzyme, then myocardial infarction is unlikely, and surgery, muscle trauma, or intramuscular injections are more likely causes. It has become conventional practice to serially measure not

---

Distributions of Major Coronary Arteries

Right coronary artery

ECG leads II, III, and aVF
Supplies most of right ventricle and inferior portion of left ventricle
Sole blood supply of posterior papillary muscle of mitral valve

Left circumflex coronary artery

ECG leads aVL, V_5, V_6
Gives off obtuse marginal branches
Supplies lateral and posterolateral aspects of left ventricle

Left anterior descending coronary artery

ECG leads V_1 to V_5
Gives off diagonal and septal branches
Supplies anterior and anterolateral left ventricle

only the CPK concentration but also the aspartate aminotransferase (AST) and lactate dehydrogenase (LDH) concentrations. AST usually peaks 36 to 60 hours and LDH 3 to 6 days after an infarct; both of these enzymes are nonspecific and therefore are of limited clinical use.

INITIAL THERAPY

All patients with suspected myocardial infarction should be prescribed bed rest, with supplemental oxygen and IV access, in a critical care or telemetry unit. Unless he/she is hypotensive, the patient with ongoing chest pain should receive sublingual nitroglycerin (0.4 mg q 5 min × three doses), followed by aliquots of IV morphine sulfate (2 mg q 5 min), until relief is obtained or hypotension supervenes. Morphine tends to be underused in myocardial infarction, and its use should be encouraged; the drug relieves anxiety, decreases sympathetic tone, diminishes myocardial oxygen demand, and lowers preload. The patient should suck or chew an aspirin tablet (325 mg) to achieve an immediate antiplatelet effect. Lidocaine should be reserved for symptomatic ventricular dysrhythmias and should not be given prophylactically. Thrombolytic therapy should be considered (see upper box). Recent surgery contraindicates thrombolytic therapy in the majority of patients. Emergency coronary arteriography and angioplasty may be considered as an alternative when thrombolytic therapy is contraindicated (see lower box). Angioplasty can achieve coronary recanalization in up to 90% of myocardial infarction patients.

The data currently available indicate that streptokinase, which is inexpensive, reduces mortality to levels comparable with more expensive thrombolytic agents and carries a comparable rate of hemorrhagic complications. Streptokinase causes a transient hypotensive response in up to 10% of recipients and in rare cases causes anaphylaxis. Tissue plasminogen activator (t-PA) is clearly the agent of choice only for those who have received streptokinase previously and might have neutralizing antibodies to streptokinase. Thrombolytic therapy might be considered 6 to 12 hours after the onset of symptoms, especially in a patient with

a "stuttering" pain pattern suggestive of ongoing infarction, although such therapy has not been shown to improve outcome. The features of streptokinase, t-PA and anisoylated plasminogen-streptokinase activator complex (APSAC) are summarized in Table 22-1.

Aspirin, Heparin, Nitrates, and Beta-Blockers

All patients should receive aspirin 325 mg daily whether or not thrombolytic therapy and heparin are given. Data on the use of heparin with thrombolytic therapy are inconclusive. Heparin should be given after t-PA. Although the optimal timing and dosage are not well established, we recommend a 5000 unit bolus at the time the t-PA infusion is completed, followed by 1000

Indications for Thrombolytic Therapy
Fewer than 6 hours elapsed from onset of symptoms
Definite ST-segment elevation (*not* ST-segment depression) or new bundle branch block
Beneficial in both anterior and inferior infarctions
Beneficial whether or not patient has had previous infarctions
No age limit

Contraindications to Thrombolytic Therapy
Any active or recent bleeding other than menstruation
Intracranial or intraspinal neoplasm, arteriovenous malformation, or aneurysm
Stroke, neurosurgery, or head injury within past 2 months
Major surgery or trauma within past month
Diabetic retinopathy
Pregnancy
Bacterial endocarditis
Known bleeding diathesis
Uncontrolled hypertension (>200/110)
Prolonged or traumatic cardiopulmonary resuscitation

TABLE 22-1 Comparison of Thrombolytic Agents

	Streptokinase	t-PA	APSAC
Dose	1.5 million U	100 mg	30 U
Administration	1-hr infusion	3-hr infusion	5-min bolus
Systemic fibrinolysis	High	Low	High
Risk of hemorrhage	High	High	High
Antigenicity	Yes	No	Yes
Hypotensive responses	Yes	No	Yes
Coronary patency at 90 min	50%-60%	60%-80%	60%-70%
Half-life	Long	Short	Long
Improved survival rates	Yes	Yes	Yes

units/hr for 24 to 48 hours. Heparin may not be needed after streptokinase and does not appear to enhance outcomes after APSAC.

An IV nitroglycerin infusion should be started, titrating the dose to normalize the arterial pressure of a hypertensive patient or to reduce the systolic pressure of a normotensive patient by 10% to 20% (but not to less than 100 mm Hg), regardless of whether a patient has ongoing chest pain. Given in this manner, nitroglycerin has been shown to limit infarct expansion, preserve ventricular function, and reduce mortality. After the first 24 hours, the infusion may be slowly tapered. Oral or topical nitroglycerin need not be introduced unless the patient has heart failure or recurrent angina.

The role of acute beta-blockade is less well-defined. Patients who have heart failure should not be given beta-blockers. Unquestionably, in patients who have persistent tachycardia, hypertension, or chest pain and who do not have congestive heart failure, acute IV beta-blockade (e.g., metoprolol 5 mg q 5 min × three doses) is indicated. However, it is not clear, despite several randomized studies, that immediate IV beta-blockade improves outcome in patients who are normotensive and pain free. We generally do not use IV beta-blockers in such patients.

For the patient with Q-wave infarction (usually transmural) without congestive heart failure, long-term oral beta-blockade (e.g., metoprolol 50 mg bid) is clearly beneficial. For the patient with non–Q-wave infarction (usually subendocardial) without congestive heart failure, long-term oral calcium channel blockade

(specifically, diltiazem 60 mg qid) may be beneficial. We evaluate patients with uncomplicated infarcts 24 to 36 hours after presentation and start beta-blockers or diltiazem at that time.

EVALUATION AFTER UNCOMPLICATED MYOCARDIAL INFARCTION

The management strategies outlined thus far apply primarily to patients whose infarcts are uncomplicated by congestive heart failure or recurrent chest pain. Once they recover from their surgical procedures and their myocardial infarctions, these patients customarily undergo submaximal treadmill testing (with or without concomitant thallium imaging) before discharge. If there are no signs of ischemia, they are generally discharged to outpatient follow-up with aspirin and beta-blockers or diltiazem. With signs of ischemia, coronary arteriography is usually appropriate. Depending on the findings, a decision can be made to continue with pharmacologic therapy, to attempt coronary angioplasty, or to perform elective bypass surgery.

COMPLICATIONS OF MYOCARDIAL INFARCTION

The management of supraventricular and ventricular dysrhythmias after myocardial infarction is addressed in Chapter 21. The remainder of this chapter discusses the diagnosis and management of the other complications of myocardial infarction (see box, p. 263).

Postinfarction Ischemia

In general, recurrence of chest pain or of asymptomatic ECG changes ("silent ischemia")

Complications of Myocardial Infarction

Atrial and ventricular dysrhythmias
Postinfarction ischemia and infarct extension
Congestive heart failure
Cardiogenic shock
Conduction disturbances
Pericarditis
Acute mitral regurgitation
Acute ventricular septal rupture
Acute ventricular free-wall rupture
Ventricular aneurysm
Right ventricular infarction
Thrombosis and embolism

in the wake of a myocardial infarction is a sign that additional myocardium is in jeopardy and that the original infarct might be extending. Recurrent ischemia should be managed aggressively. The physician should address any correctable causes of decreased myocardial oxygen supply or increased myocardial oxygen demand (i.e., hypertension, fever, hypotension, anemia, hypoxemia, dysrhythmias). Pharmacologic measures must be individually tailored, depending on blood pressure, the presence or absence of congestive heart failure, and overall clinical status, but typically include IV nitroglycerin, beta-blockade, aspirin, and heparin (unless contraindicated). If chest pain remains refractory, consideration should be given to intra-aortic balloon counterpulsation, which enhances coronary perfusion while decreasing afterload. Virtually all patients with recurrent ischemia after infarction should undergo semi-emergency coronary arteriography.

Congestive Heart Failure

The patient who develops congestive heart failure after myocardial infarction usually fits one of three categories: preexisting myocardial damage before the infarct, large infarct, or mechanical complication of the infarct (e.g., acute mitral regurgitation or ventricular septal rupture). Aggressive management is in order both diagnostically and therapeutically.

Physical examination will establish whether the patient is well perfused or hypotensive and going into cardiogenic shock; whether the signs

of failure are left-sided, right-sided, or biventricular; and whether telltale murmurs or other signs exist. Emergency echocardiography can be extremely helpful in showing, for example, a large akinetic segment of myocardium, a flail mitral valve leaflet, or evidence of a left-to-right intracardiac shunt.

The pharmacologic management of congestive heart failure is highly individualized. The patient who is normotensive or hypertensive can readily be managed with diuretics (and perhaps digitalis and vasodilators, such as nitrates or angiotensin-converting enzyme inhibitors). However, the patient with congestive heart failure and borderline blood pressure is problematic. Diuretics and vasodilators may relieve the congestion but are likely to induce hypotension. The management of such patients can be facilitated by insertion of a thermodilution pulmonary artery catheter. With that device, the preload can be carefully manipulated, the cardiac index quantified, and pharmacologic therapy optimized. Such patients often benefit from simultaneous titration of positive inotropic agents (e.g., dopamine, dobutamine, amrinone) and vasodilators (e.g., nitroprusside, nitroglycerin).

Coronary arteriography and reperfusion therapy in patients with postinfarction congestive heart failure should generally be aggressive. Even without evidence of recurrent ischemia, such patients have little physiologic reserve; any opportunity to revascularize and protect the remaining myocardium by angioplasty or bypass surgery should be considered.

Cardiogenic Shock

Cardiogenic shock, which occurs in 5% to 10% of cases, is the leading cause of inpatient death in myocardial infarction. It is characterized by arterial hypotension, peripheral vasoconstriction, lactic acidosis, oliguria, and obtundation. Cardiogenic shock is defined hemodynamically as a cardiac index <2.2 L/min/m^2 with a pulmonary capillary wedge pressure >18 mm Hg. With pharmacologic treatment alone, its mortality exceeds 90%; with aggressive management (intra-aortic balloon counterpulsation, coronary arteriography, and angioplasty or bypass surgery), its mortality may be reduced to 50%. Cardiogenic shock usually is caused by necrosis of 40% or more of the left ventricle, extensive right ventricular infarction, or an infarct-related mechanical defect, such as septal, free-wall, or papillary muscle rupture.

Initial management of cardiogenic shock depends in large part on the patient's appearance. If the patient is hypotensive but does not have rales or other signs of left ventricular failure, then resuscitation with crystalloid or colloid solutions may succeed in restoring an adequate blood pressure. If the patient is hypotensive and also has signs of congestive heart failure, then neither fluids nor diuretics can readily be administered. In such a situation (while waiting for the cardiac catheterization laboratory to prepare for the patient) we favor the insertion of a pulmonary artery catheter to guide pharmacologic therapy and an intra-aortic balloon pump to assist the failing heart. If necessary, even before the insertion of a pulmonary artery catheter, dobutamine can be started (initially 5 μg/kg/min, titrating upward to as much as 30 μg/kg/min). Dopamine or norepinephrine may be necessary for persistent hypotension. Thrombolytic therapy may be considered, despite the likelihood of difficulties with hemostasis during catheterization or surgery. Acidosis, hypoxemia, and electrolyte derangements should be corrected. If the patient is tachypneic, endotracheal intubation and mechanical ventilation permit sedation, decrease the work of the respiratory muscles, and reduce the body's oxygen consumption.

Conduction Disturbances

Anterior and inferior myocardial infarctions can disrupt normal conduction of electrical impulses through the atrioventricular node, the bundle of His, and the distal portions of the conducting system. These conduction abnormalities may lead to symptomatic bradycardias, and certain types are statistically associated with a risk of progression to complete heart block. Accordingly, temporary transvenous ventricular pacing for the conduction abnormalities listed in the box is reasonable therapy. Placement of

---

Indications for Temporary Pacing in Acute Myocardial Infarction
Bradyarrhythmias with hypotension, ventricular ectopy, angina, left ventricular failure, or syncope
Complete atrioventricular block
Mobitz type II second-degree atrioventricular block
New LBBB or bifascicular block (RBBB + LAHB, RBBB + LPHB, alternating RBBB/LBBB)

LBBB, left bundle branch block; RBBB, right bundle branch block; LAHB, left anterior hemiblock; LPHB, left posterior hemiblock.

an external demand pacing system may be an alternative in certain settings (e.g., after thrombolysis, when wire insertion carries increased risk of hemorrhage).

Pericarditis

Up to 25% of large transmural infarctions are complicated by pericardial inflammation, manifested by chest pain, friction rub, fever, elevation of the erythrocyte sedimentation rate, and pericardial effusions (which are rarely hemodynamically significant). The treatment of postinfarction pericarditis consists of nonsteroidal anti-inflammatory agents (e.g., ibuprofen) or, in refractory cases, corticosteroids. Distinguishing between the pain of pericarditis and the pain of ischemia can be difficult.

Acute Mitral Regurgitation

The right coronary artery is the sole blood supply of the posterior papillary muscle of the mitral valve. Right coronary artery infarctions are often associated with an apical systolic murmur that is caused by ischemic papillary muscle dysfunction. This common and hemodynamically benign situation is in sharp contrast to actual papillary muscle rupture, which leads to acute catastrophic mitral regurgitation with acute pulmonary edema. Papillary muscle rupture may not be accompanied by an audible murmur. Its diagnosis may have to rely on echocardiography or on the visualization of giant "v" waves on a pulmonary capillary wedge tracing. The treatment of papillary muscle rupture consists of stabilization with pharmacologic agents (especially nitroprusside), intra-aortic balloon counterpulsation, and definitive surgery.

Acute Ventricular Septal Rupture

In 1% to 3% of anterior myocardial infarctions, enough septal necrosis occurs to cause perforation and shunting of blood from the higher pressure left ventricle to the lower pressure right ventricle. Depending on the size of the shunt, acute pulmonary edema and cardiogenic shock can develop. As a rule a loud pansystolic murmur with a parasternal thrill will be present. Echocardiography is helpful in establishing the diagnosis. In right-sided heart catheterization a step-up in oxygen saturation from the right atrium to the pulmonary artery will be evident. As in acute mitral regurgitation, therapy for acute ventricular septal rupture generally consists of medical stabilization followed by definitive surgical correction.

Acute Ventricular Free-Wall Rupture

In approximately 1% of transmural infarctions, the wall of the left ventricle ruptures. Ventricular rupture typically happens during the first week after infarction. Classically, the patient is elderly, female, and hypertensive. Blood leaks into the pericardium, producing tamponade, and the patient develops electromechanical dissociation. Survival is possible, but only if the situation is promptly recognized, the pericardial blood is drained by pericardiocentesis or thoracotomy, and the myocardial defect is closed surgically.

Ventricular Aneurysm

As it heals, a large infarct can leave a large fibrotic, dyskinetic area that can contribute to congestive heart failure, decrease cardiac output, become a nidus for thrombus formation, and serve as a dysrhythmogenic focus. Such a ventricular aneurysm, which generally evolves weeks to months after infarction, may require palliative surgical aneurysmectomy.

Right Ventricular Infarction

Approximately 30% of inferior infarctions involve the right ventricle; the right ventricular involvement is clinically significant in 10% of the cases. ST elevations are sometimes appreciable only in specially placed right-sided precordial ECG leads. Sizable right ventricular infarctions are classically manifested by signs of right-sided heart failure (e.g., jugular venous distention, hepatic distention, and edema) in the absence of rales. When right ventricular dysfunction is severe, arterial hypotension may supervene. The therapy of choice is volume expansion; if hypotension persists, positive inotropic drugs (e.g., dobutamine or amrinone) produce more hemodynamic benefit than nitroprusside. Pulmonary artery catheterization may be useful diagnostically. In right ventricular infarction, elevated right atrial and right ventricular diastolic pressures are present. Yet, pulmonary capillary wedge pressure measurements may be misleading. When the right ventricle is infarcted, left ventricular compliance becomes abnormal. Normal wedge pressure may not indicate adequate filling pressure.

Thrombosis and Embolism That Complicate Infarction

Infarctions are sometimes attended by the formation of mural thrombi and by arterial thromboembolism. Long-term prophylactic warfarin (Coumadin) is beneficial after large anterior infarctions. Most cardiologists use warfarin for patients with chronic or paroxysmal atrial fibrillation and for patients with echocardiographically documented intracardiac thrombi. When infarctions are small or other than anterior, no firm consensus regarding the role of warfarin exists. Most postinfarction patients take aspirin, which confers some benefit as thromboembolic prophylaxis.

SUMMARY

- *Uncomplicated infarction—day 1:*
  Transfer patient to monitored unit; give supplemental oxygen.
  Prescribe sublingual nitroglycerin and IV morphine for initial pain relief.
  Give aspirin 325 mg immediately.
  Consider thrombolytic therapy (if contraindicated, consider primary angioplasty).
  Administer IV nitroglycerin to reduce systolic pressure 10% to 20% but not to <100 mm Hg.
  Check cardiac enzymes at 0, 12, and 24 hours and perform serial ECGs.
- *Uncomplicated infarction—day 2:*
  Continue aspirin 325 mg daily.
  Begin tapering of IV nitroglycerin.
  Start oral beta-blockers (for Q-wave infarcts).
  Start oral diltiazem (for non–Q wave infarcts).

- *Treatment recommendations for complications of infarction:*
  Supraventricular dysrhythmias: pharmacologic treatment
  Symptomatic ventricular dysrhythmias: pharmacologic suppression
  Conduction disturbances: prophylactic pacing in selected cases
  Recurrent ischemia: antianginal treatment and coronary arteriography
  Congestive heart failure: stabilization and coronary arteriography
  Cardiogenic shock: stabilization, intra-aortic balloon, coronary arteriography, and reperfusion
  Right ventricular infarction: volume loading and, in selected cases, inotropic agents
  Rupture of papillary muscle, ventricular septum, or ventricular free wall: stabilization and surgery
  Thrombosis and embolism: prophylaxis with aspirin and, in selected cases, warfarin
  Pericarditis: palliation with NSAIDs

BIBLIOGRAPHY

American College of Cardiology/American Heart Association Task Force. Guidelines for the early management of patients with acute myocardial infarction. J Am Coll Cardiol 15:249, 1990; Circulation 82:664, 1990.

Beta-Blocker Heart Attack Trial Research Group. A randomized trial of propranolol in patients with acute myocardial infarction. JAMA 247:1707, 1982.

European Cooperative Study Group. Intravenous tissue plasminogen activator and size of infarct, left ventricular function, and survival in acute myocardial infarction. Br Med J 297:1374, 1988.

Gruppo Italiano per lo Studio della Streptochinasi nell'Infarto Miocardico (GISSI). Effectiveness of intravenous thrombolytic treatment in acute myocardial infarction. Lancet 1:397, 1986.

Held AC, Cole PL, Lipton B, et al. Rupture of the interventricular septum complicating acute myocardial infarction: A multicenter analysis of clinical findings and outcome. Am Heart J 116:1330, 1988.

Isner JM. Right ventricular myocardial infarction. JAMA 259:712, 1988.

Lee L, Erbel R, Brown TM, Laufer N, Meyer J, O'Neill WW. Multicenter registry of angioplasty therapy of cardiogenic shock: Initial and long-term survival. J Am Coll Cardiol 17:599, 1991.

MacMahon S, Collins R, Peto R, Kostor RW, Yusuf S. Effects of prophylactic lidocaine in suspected acute myocardial infarction: An overview of results from the randomized, controlled trials. JAMA 260:1910, 1988.

Multicenter Diltiazem Postinfarction Trial Research Group. The effect of diltiazem on mortality and reinfarction after myocardial infarction. N Engl J Med 319:385, 1988.

Schreiber TL, Miller DH, Zola B. Management of myocardial infarction shock: Current status. Am Heart J 117:435, 1989.

Second International Study of Infarct Survival (ISIS-2) Collaborative Group. Randomised trial of intravenous streptokinase, oral aspirin, both, or neither among 17,187 cases of suspected acute myocardial infarction. Lancet 2:349, 1988.

Shapira I, Isakov A, Burke M, Almog C. Cardiac rupture in patients with acute myocardial infarction. Chest 92:219, 1987.

Theroux P, Ouimet H, McCans J, et al. Aspirin, heparin, or both to treat acute unstable angina. N Engl J Med 319:1105, 1988.

Thrombolysis in Myocardial Infarction (TIMI) Study Group. Comparison of invasive and conservative strategies after treatment with intravenous tissue plasminogen activator in acute myocardial infarction. N Engl J Med 320:618, 1989.

Tofler GH, Muller JE, Stone PH, et al. Pericarditis in acute myocardial infarction: Characterization and clinical significance. Am Heart J 117:86, 1989.

CHAPTER 23

Hypertensive Emergencies

John W. Hoyt

A common description of a hypertensive emergency includes the patient's having a diastolic blood pressure of at least 120 to 130 mm Hg along with complications such as hypertensive encephalopathy, intracranial hemorrhage, aortic dissection, pulmonary edema, and myocardial ischemia.[1] It is rare to see a patient with a combination of these findings in the hospital because, although over 60 million Americans have hypertension, only 1% to 2% develop a hypertensive crisis.[2]

In contrast, potentially dangerous elevations of blood pressure occur on a daily basis in the operating room, recovery room, SICU, emergency room, and hospital ward. These elevations of blood pressure may or may not be associated with symptoms but, depending on past medical history, may put the patient at increased risk for cardiovascular and CNS complications. The physician evaluating a patient with acutely elevated blood pressure often feels compelled to "do something" to correct the problem. This chapter deals with physiologic reasons why it is important to do something and provides guidelines on when to treat, what to use for treatment, and how to monitor treatment.

SYMPATHETIC STORM

First, the common hospital event, that is, sympathetic storm, must be managed. Many hospitalized patients are candidates for episodes of hypertension and tachycardia when facing the anxiety and stress of invasive procedures

and surgery. Patients with a history of hypertension are particularly likely to develop substantial elevations of blood pressure and heart rate in the hospital. These abnormalities are true even when their blood pressure has been well controlled in the ambulatory setting. Stress and anxiety before surgery and pain and fear after surgery can trigger a hypertensive crisis, or sympathetic storm.

When a sympathetic storm occurs, it is the physician's responsibility to determine the role of pain and anxiety. Short-acting analgesics such as fentanyl, administered intravenously in doses of 50 to 100 μg, and anxiolytics such as midazolam, given parenterally in doses of 1 to 2 mg, frequently will resolve the hypertensive crisis. No other treatment is needed except for instituting a better program of pharmacologic pain and anxiety management.

Other patients will not respond to sedation and analgesia, and this therapy should not be pushed to the point that level of consciousness is altered just to lower blood pressure. An antihypertensive must be selected if there is concern about cardiac or CNS complications of the elevated blood pressure.

CARDIAC COMPLICATIONS

Cardiac complications represent the greatest concern for patients in hypertensive crises. Coronary artery disease and ischemic heart problems are ubiquitous in hospitalized patients. Hypertension puts a special stress on cardiac patients because of alterations of myocardial oxygen supply and demand. The determinants of myocardial oxygen demand include systolic blood pressure, heart rate, and cardiac wall tension. Myocardial oxygen supply is governed by hemoglobin levels, oxygen saturation of hemoglobin, and flow of blood through the coronary arteries.

Unlike in most organs in the body, blood flow to the heart does not, for the most part, occur during systole. Cardiac blood vessels go from an epicardial position with the main coronary arteries to an endocardial position with terminal vessels. When the heart is in systole, high chamber and muscle pressures preclude blood flow. As a result, blood flow to the myocardium must occur during diastole. Diastolic blood pressure and diastolic time become essential determinants of myocardial oxygen supply.

The primary compromising factor for diastolic time is tachycardia. When heart rate increases, systole stays essentially the same, but there is a progressive shortening of diastolic time. At a heart rate of 60, there is more time spent in diastole than systole, and the myocardium is well perfused as long as there is adequate diastolic pressure and minimal coronary occlusion. At a heart rate of 90, the times in systole and diastole are largely equal. At a heart rate of 120, significant compromise of diastolic time has occurred.

At some point in the elevation of heart rate the balance of myocardial oxygen supply and demand will tip into the range of ischemia. If ischemia persists, muscle will die, and usually a subendocardial myocardial infarction will occur. It is this scenario of ischemia that prompts most physicians to act in lowering blood pressure for the hospitalized patient with a hypertensive crisis.[3]

The issue of heart rate must be emphasized. The patient with a normal heart rate and elevated blood pressure has increased myocardial oxygen demand and is at risk of ischemia. If tachycardia is added to hypertension, the problem is much worse since tachycardia increases myocardial oxygen demand and decreases myocardial oxygen supply by its effect on diastole. The tachycardia can be endogenous to the patient or exogenous, created by the pharmacologic choice of the physician since many antihypertensive agents (e.g., nitroprusside, hydralazine, nifedipine) are associated with reflex tachycardia. In either case of tachycardia, gains made in reducing myocardial oxygen demand by lowering systolic blood pressure may be lost by the effects of tachycardia.

CENTRAL NERVOUS SYSTEM CONCERNS

CNS concerns represent a second justification for lowering blood pressure in a hypertensive crisis.[4] Blood flow to the brain is controlled by the process of autoregulation. Between mean blood pressures of 50 and 150 mm Hg, CNS blood flow remains approximately the same. With pathologic alterations to the brain such as head trauma, surgery, and encephalopathy, there may be a loss of autoregulation and substantial increases in blood flow to the brain during hospitalization, which can worsen cerebral edema markedly and elevate intracranial pressure.

Evaluating the hospitalized patient with an acute elevation of blood pressure and deciding to treat with an antihypertensive agent is difficult and many times arbitrary. Clearly young people with normal cardiac and CNS function can tolerate substantial elevations of blood pressure without risk. On the other hand, the patient with a history of angina, cardiac ischemia, and/or previous myocardial infarction is at significant risk if systolic blood pressure is >200, diastolic blood pressure is >110, and heart rate is >100. Ideally it would be best to treat this patient before symptoms develop. On most occasions the physician will be notified by the nurse that blood pressure is elevated, only to find the patient symptom-free. A decision to treat must be based on a knowledge of the patient's history, particularly the cardiac and central nervous systems, and a knowledge of the physiologic impact of hypertension with or without tachycardia on important body systems.

Treatment becomes essential if patient evaluation suggests complications of the acutely elevated blood pressure.[5] Chest pain consistent with angina may be present but many times is a poor indicator of significant ischemia. Diabetic patients in particular are known to develop prominent ischemia by various indicators and be free of chest pain. New ST depression or T-wave inversion is a good indicator of cardiac complications of hypertension. The absence of these findings does not mean the absence of ischemia, which is a dangerous imbalance of myocardial oxygen supply and demand. Left ventricular wall motion abnormalities determined by transesophageal echocardiography are earlier indicators of ischemia but provide an unlikely evaluative tool for the usual elevation of blood pressure. Other findings such as a new cardiac gallop or rales in the chest revealed by auscultation of the lung likely indicate a decompensating hypertensive state that must be treated immediately. On many occasions it is appropriate for the physician to begin treatment in the absence of signs and symptoms because of the known cardiac and CNS problems of hypertension.

TYPES OF HYPERTENSIVE CRISES

Hypertensive crises can be divided into three categories that allow for discussion of appropriate therapy and monitoring: (1) a simple but significant hypertensive episode without signs or symptoms of complications; (2) a complicated hypertensive crisis in which there is evidence of cardiac and/or CNS involvement; and (3) a decompensated hypertensive crisis in which life support is required to reverse the sequelae of elevated blood pressure (Table 23-1).

Simple Compensated Crisis

A simple compensated hypertensive episode commonly is detected in a non–critical care environment in which no or minimal monitoring is available. The patient's blood pressure is elevated, with a systolic pressure of 200 mm Hg or greater and a diastolic pressure of 100 mm Hg or greater. The patient is free of symptoms but may have a significant history of coronary artery disease. The elevation of blood pressure is at least 25% to 50% above normal and apparently is not associated with pain or anxiety. Concerns about cardiac complications should motivate the physician to treat the condition if the elevated blood pressure has persisted for more than 10 to 15 minutes. If this hypertension is associated with a tachycardia of 90 beats/min or greater, there is increased justification for treatment.

At this point there is little justification for transfer to an SICU. At least two oral medications and three parenteral agents can be used safely on the regular hospital floor with monitoring by automated noninvasive blood pressure (NIBP) cuff. Frequent monitoring of blood pressure by the Riva-Rocci technique, listening for Korotkoff sounds with a stethoscope, is very time-consuming for the floor nurse. An oscillotonometer technique, which cycles automatically every 5 minutes and detects trends, is significantly more convenient and probably safer because of its accuracy and alarm system, and it frees the nurse to monitor other aspects of the patient's response to medication.

| TABLE 23-1   Hypertensive Crises |

Type of Hypertension	Clinical Findings	Therapeutic Agents
Simple compensated	None	Clonidine Nifedipine
Complex compensated	Cardiac symptoms Neurologic symptoms	Hydralazine Labetalol Enalaprilat
Complex decompensated	Myocardial infarction Shock Coma	Nitroprusside Trimethaphan camsylate

There is substantial experience with the use of both oral clonidine and nifedipine for treating patients with hypertensive crises. Clonidine, a centrally acting antihypertensive agent, should be given in starting oral doses of 0.1 to 0.2 mg, followed by hourly doses of 0.1 mg until the desired blood pressure is achieved.[6] Maximal correction of blood pressure normally occurs in 2 to 3 hours. Blood pressure should be monitored every 5 minutes by NIBP cuff for at least the first hour and then every 10 to 15 minutes for subsequent hours. Onset of action is within 30 minutes, and the duration of action of oral clonidine is 6 to 8 hours.

Likewise oral nifedipine can be used for a hypertensive crisis without complications in the hospital floor setting.[7] Nifedipine, a dihydropyridine calcium channel blocker, is a direct arteriolar vasodilator that often creates significant reflex tachycardia. The starting dose of nifedipine is 10 mg. Nifedipine is a liquid inside a capsule and can be given orally by aspirating the liquid from the capsule or rupturing the capsule by biting it before swallowing, thus accelerating absorption and resulting in a 10- to 15-minute onset of action and a 3- to 5-hour duration of action.

Parenteral agents that can be safely used outside the critical care environment include hydralazine, labetalol, and enalaprilat. These agents are rapid acting and predictable, but response to therapy should be monitored with the NIBP cuff. Hydralazine is an old drug with a long history of safety and efficacy.[8] The onset of action of a starting IV dose of 5 mg is within 10 minutes, and the duration of action is 2 to 4 hours. After the initial dose has been administered to assess patient response, subsequent doses of 10 to 20 mg can be administered every 15 to 30 minutes until the desired lowering of blood pressure is achieved. Hydralazine acts as a direct arteriolar vasodilator and is associated with reflex tachycardia.

Labetalol is also safe and predictable and is both a nonselective beta-blocker and a selective alpha$_2$-blocker.[9] A starting parenteral dose of labetalol is 5 mg, with subsequent doses of 10 and then 20 mg when patient response has been clearly determined. Labetalol acts within 5 minutes and has a 3- to 6-hour duration of action. This agent is not indicated when the patient has active wheezing and bronchospasm, a significant history of reactive airway disease, low cardiac output syndrome, or heart block. There is no reflex tachycardia with this agent because of the beta-blocking properties. Labetalol would be the parenteral agent of choice when a hypertensive crisis is associated with a heart rate of 90 to 100 or greater.

Finally, enalaprilat, a converting enzyme inhibitor, can be administered safely outside the SICU in starting IV doses of 0.625 mg. Onset of action for enalaprilat is 10 to 15 minutes, with an 8- to 12-hour duration of action. Minimal change in heart rate occurs with this agent. Follow-up doses can be 1.25 to 2.5 mg q 8 hr when patient response has been determined.[10]

Complicated Compensated Crisis

A second class of hypertensive crises is associated with complications such as cardiac and/or CNS problems. The patient with elevated blood pressure may complain of chest pain, the ECG may demonstrate signs of ischemia, auscultation of the chest may reveal rales not previously present, or there may be a decrease in level of consciousness. If these signs and symptoms persist after initiation of therapy outside the SICU, the patient must be transferred immediately to a critical care area.

Monitoring with the NIBP cuff is no longer adequate for this type of patient. An arterial catheter should be inserted to permit beat-to-beat assessment of blood pressure, and use of a triple-lumen central venous line should be considered for administration of medication and fluid if there should be a precipitous drop in blood pressure with the initiation of treatment.

Continuous infusion parenteral agents such as nitroprusside or trimethaphan camsylate should be considered if the previously discussed parenteral agents have failed or the patient is deteriorating rapidly.[11] Nitroprusside has been the first-line antihypertensive agent for hypertensive crises for the last 10 years of critical care. It is a direct arteriolar vasodilator with an onset of action within seconds and a 3-

to 5-minute duration of action. Complications of nitroprusside include reflex tachycardia and cyanide toxicity. The latter complication is associated with administration of large doses (>3 to 4 µg/kg/min) and prolonged administration (>3 to 4 days). The usual starting dose of nitroprusside is 0.25 µg/kg/min, titrating to effect. Often, use of a simultaneous beta-blocker such as esmolol or metoprolol will prevent the reflex tachycardia and optimize the antihypertensive effect.

Trimethaphan camsylate is a ganglionic blocker that is not associated with reflex tachycardia; like nitroprusside, it has a rapid onset of action (1 to 5 minutes) and a very short duration (5 to 10 minutes). It must be given by continuous infusion, starting at 0.5 mg/min and titrating until the desired antihypertensive effect is achieved.

Complex Decompensated Crisis

The third and last type of hypertensive crisis is the decompensated state. Cardiac ischemia decreases the compliance of heart muscle and can precipitate an episode of pulmonary edema that is not related to volume overload. If this state persists untreated, hypoxia, respiratory failure, and myocardial infarction with cardiogenic shock will ensue. Immediate attention must be given to restoring oxygen transport and providing life support. Nitroprusside usually would be the agent of choice for management of blood pressure. Monitoring should include use of an arterial catheter and may include use of a fiberoptic pulmonary artery catheter for a more complete assessment of cardiac function. In this setting pulmonary capillary wedge pressure (PCWP) may be a poor indicator of vascular volume and a good indicator of ventricular function.

Cardiac ischemia will elevate PCWP despite normal or even low left ventricular end-diastolic volume (LVEDV), precipitating pulmonary edema, which is best treated by lowering blood pressure rather than by diuresis. If after a reduction in blood pressure and restoration of oxygen transport, an elevated PCWP persists, diuresis is indicated. Initial aggressive diuresis makes nitroprusside very difficult to use since the patient likely will be hypovolemic and extremely sensitive to small doses of medication.

ANTIHYPERTENSIVE AGENTS

Guidelines are provided to assist in choosing the antihypertensive agent for various types of hypertensive crisis. Heart rate is used as the discriminator (Table 23-2). Three clinical situations can guide the choice of drug: (1) hypertension with a heart rate of 90 or below (good diastolic time); (2) hypertension with a heart rate of 90 to 110 (borderline diastolic time); and (3) hypertension with a heart rate of 110 or greater (inadequate diastolic time).

The first clinical situation permits the physician to use agents that clearly cause reflex tachycardia. Nifedipine (oral), hydralazine (par-

TABLE 23-2 Hypertension and Heart Rate

Heart Rate	Diastolic Time	Therapeutic Agents	Route of Administration
<90	Good	Nifedipine Hydralazine Nitroprusside	Oral IV bolus IV infusion
90-110	Borderline	Clonidine Enalaprilat Trimethaphan camsylate	Oral IV bolus IV infusion
>110	Poor	Metoprolol Labetalol Esmolol	Oral IV bolus IV infusion

enteral bolus), and nitroprusside (parenteral continuous infusion) used as direct arteriolar vasodilators are well known for causing reflex tachycardia. These agents are all potent anti-hypertensives that will quickly and safely lower blood pressure, but their use simultaneously leads to a 10% or greater increase in heart rate, depending on dose of medication.

Second is a clinical situation (heart rate, 90 to 110) in which there is a matching of diastolic and systolic times but further increases in heart rate may lead to ischemia. Agents at this time

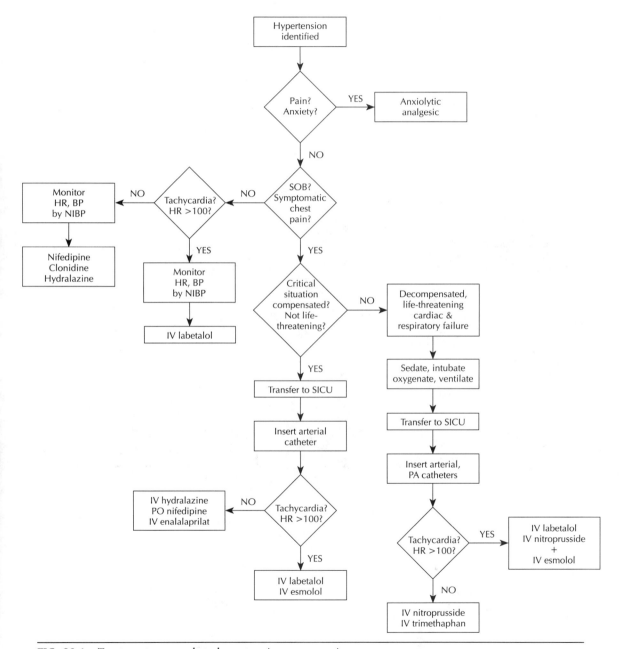

FIG. 23-1 Treatment approach to hypertensive emergencies.

should have a neutral effect or slow the heart rate. An oral agent would be clonidine, a parenteral bolus agent would be enalaprilat, and a parenteral continuous infusion agent would be trimethaphan camsylate.

When heart rate exceeds 110, there is significant opportunity for ischemia, based on the increase in myocardial oxygen consumption secondary to tachycardia and the reduction in myocardial oxygen supply from reduced diastolic time. Appropriate antihypertensive agents in this setting require some beta-blocking property. Oral agents include metoprolol or atenolol, both cardioselective beta-blockers with both an antihypertensive effect and a

negative chronotropic effect. The best parenteral bolus medication would be labetalol. A recommended continuous infusion parenteral agent is esmolol.[12]

Esmolol is a rapid-acting (5 to 10 minutes), ultra-short acting (half-life, 7 minutes), cardioselective beta-blocker. It originally was developed for treating various types of supraventricular tachycardia but has not been as commonly used as verapamil. In a patient with sinus tachycardia associated with hypertension, esmolol becomes the drug of choice in the absence of low cardiac output syndrome, bronchospasm, or heart block.

SUMMARY

- In a hypertensive crisis diastolic blood pressure is at least 120 to 130 mm Hg. Other complications include hypertensive encephalopathy, intracranial hemorrhage, aortic dissection, pulmonary edema, and myocardial ischemia.
- Sympathetic storm:
  Patients with a history of hypertension are likely to have substantial blood pressure increase and tachycardia.
  Analgesia and anxiolytics may provide adequate treatment.
  Choice of an antihypertensive is based on the likelihood of cardiac or CNS complications from the hypertension.
- Cardiac complications:
  Hypertension alters myocardial oxygen supply and demand and may cause ischemia.

  Heart rate must be noted carefully.
  Tachycardia may reduce myocardial oxygen supply more than lowering blood pressure reduces myocardial oxygen demand.
- Central nervous system:
  Head trauma, surgery, and encephalopathy may deregulate blood flow to the brain. Hypertension can worsen loss of autoregulation and increase intracranial pressure.
  Hypertension should be treated when complications of elevated blood pressure are present.
  Hypertensive crises may be simple compensated, complex compensated, or complex decompensated. Antihypertensive therapy differs for each category (see Table 23-1).

REFERENCES

1. Calhoun DA, Oparil S. Treatment of hypertensive crisis. N Engl J Med 323:1177-1183, 1990.
2. Houston MC. Pathophysiology, clinical aspects, and treatment of hypertensive crises. Prog Cardiovasc Dis 32:99-148, 1989.
3. Smith CB, Flower LW, Reinhardt CE. Control of hypertensive emergencies. Hypertensive Emerg 89:111-119, 1991.
4. Rahn KH. How should we treat a hypertensive emergency? Am J Cardiol 63:48C-50C, 1989.
5. Ferguson RK, Vlasses PH. Hypertensive emergencies and urgencies. JAMA 255:1607-1613, 1986.
6. Houston MC. Treatment of hypertensive emergencies and urgencies with oral clonidine loading and titration. Arch Intern Med 146:586-589, 1986.
7. Houston MC. Treatment of hypertensive urgencies and emergencies with nifedipine. Am Heart J 111:963-969, 1986.
8. Koch-Weser J. Drug therapy: Hydralazine. N Engl J Med 295(Suppl 6):320, 1976.
9. Cressman MD, Vidt DG, Gifford RW, et al. Intravenous labetalol in the management of severe hypertension and hypertensive emergencies. Am Heart J 107:980, 1984.
10. Strauss R, Gavras I, Vlahakos D. Enalaprilat in hypertensive emergencies. J Clin Pharmacol 26:39, 1986.
11. Drugs for hypertensive emergencies. Medical Lett 31:32-34, 1989.
12. Cucchiara RF, Benefiel DJ, Matteo RS, et al. Evaluation of esmolol in controlling increases in heart rate and blood pressure during endotracheal intubation in patients undergoing carotid endarterectomy. Anesthesiology 65:528, 1986.

CHAPTER 24

Cardiopulmonary Interactions

Michael R. Pinsky

The primary goal of the cardiorespiratory system is to continually deliver adequate amounts of oxygen to meet the metabolic demands of the tissues. Oxygen delivery (Do_2) is a function of arterial oxygen content (Cao_2) and cardiac output (CO). Alterations in both Cao_2 and CO occur routinely during spontaneous ventilation and can be quite abnormal and life-threatening in patients with either cardiovascular instability or respiratory insufficiency. Furthermore, artificial ventilation and ventilatory maneuvers (e.g., bag sigh suctioning) can profoundly alter not only gas exchange (Cao_2) but also CO. Only with an understanding of these interactions during both spontaneous and artificial ventilation can the physician comprehend the impact that application and withdrawal of ventilatory therapies have on the patient's overall cardiovascular homeostasis.

CARDIOPULMONARY PHYSIOLOGY

To understand these heart-lung interactions, the baseline cardiorespiratory function of the patient first must be determined, followed by the method of ventilation. Ventilation alters cardiovascular function in four primary ways:

- Determines intrapulmonary gas exchange and work of breathing: Determines partial pressure of oxygen in arterial blood (Pao_2) and partial pressure of carbon dioxide in arterial blood ($Paco_2$)
- Changes lung volume: Alters pulmonary vascular resistance (PVR)
- Alters intrathoracic pressure (ITP): Alters pressure gradients for venous return and left ventricular (LV) ejection
- Determines ventricular interdependence: Alters LV diastolic compliance

By determining intrapulmonary gas exchange and the work-cost of breathing, ventilation modulates the levels of carbon dioxide and oxygen in the blood. Although mild hypoxemia and hypercarbia stimulate sympathetic tone, producing increased blood pressure and CO,[1,2] profound hypoxemia (Pao_2 <35 torr) and hypercarbia, if associated with acidosis (pH <7.25), blunt the vascular response to sympathetic stimulation.[2] In patients with markedly increased work-costs of breathing, even adequate intrapulmonary gas exchange does not decrease the metabolic load imposed by this increased energy expenditure.[3] In some critically ill patients the work-cost of breathing exceeds the body's ability to deliver oxygen to the respiratory muscles and still carry on its normal metabolic functions.

Changing lung volume alters PVR through a variety of mechanisms. As compared to the left ventricle, the ability of the right ventricle to adapt to increasing ejection pressure loads is markedly limited because its muscular free wall is relatively thin. Varying the ejection pressure load can profoundly affect the right ventricular (RV) performance.

By its very nature, ventilation alters ITP. Gas moves between the lungs and the airway opening during ventilation by varying the pressure gradients between these two regions. Since the heart is acted upon by ITP as its surrounding pressure, while the rest of the systemic vasculature is outside the chest, changes in ITP alter the pressure gradients for both venous return to the heart and LV ejection from the heart, independent of the heart itself.

Since the two ventricles share a common septum, acute dilation of the right ventricle will shift the intraventricular septum into the LV cavity (ventricular interdependence), decreasing LV diastolic compliance.

In patients with normal cardiopulmonary function, positive-pressure ventilation decreases CO by decreasing the pressure gradient for venous return to the heart. In contrast, spontaneous ventilation increases CO by increasing venous return when compared to an apneic baseline.[4-10] These findings occur because patients with normal cardiopulmonary function have a highly preload-sensitive heart, compliant lungs that transmit a majority of the increased airway pressure to the pleural surface, and PVR that is very low.

Most critically ill patients do not have normal cardiopulmonary function. Varying degrees of cardiac, systemic vascular, pulmonary vascular, pulmonary parenchymal, and effective circulating blood volume abnormalities exist in most critically ill patients, and all these factors are modified by ventilation. Although the issues of gas exchange and work-cost of breathing are important, they are beyond the scope of this chapter.

The non–gas-exchange hemodynamic effects of ventilation can be separated into those factors associated with changes in lung volume and ITP:

I. Changes in lung volume
   A. Alter autonomic tone (respiratory sinus dysrhythmia)
   B. Alter PVR
   C. Mechanically compress the heart
II. Changes in ITP
   A. Alter the pressure gradient for venous return
   B. Alter the pressure gradient for LV ejection

Changes in Lung Volume

The lung is supplied with a large number of vagal and sympathetic afferent fibers. Normal ventilation is associated with an inspiration-induced tachycardia (respiratory sinus dysrhythmia) induced by transient withdrawal of parasympathetic tone.[11-13] Large tidal volume ventilation, on the other hand, induces cardiodepression by withdrawal of sympathetic tone.[14,15] These interactions rarely impair cardiovascular function but may complicate the interpretation of cardiovascular function in critically ill patients.

As lung volume changes, so does PVR. Under normal conditions PVR is least at end-expiration, which is the functional residual capacity (FRC). PVR increases as lung volume varies in either direction from FRC.[16-18] As lung volume increases above FRC, alveolar vessels are compressed, decreasing the pulmonary vascular cross-sectional area (increased alveolar vessel resistance).[16,19] As lung volume decreases below FRC, terminal airways collapse, and by the process of hypoxic pulmonary vasoconstriction, pulmonary vasomotor tone increases, increasing PVR (increased extra-alveolar vessel resistance).[20,21] FRC is a very dynamic volume, even in healthy humans. End-expiratory lung volume decreases with recumbency, muscle weakness, and tense ascites. In the perioperative period it decreases after abdominal surgery and thoracic surgery and in most patients with acute hypoxemic respiratory failure (i.e., adult respiratory distress syndrome [ARDS]). End-expiratory lung volume increases during acute hyperventilation associated with exercise, during acute hyperinflation associated with acute exacerbations of obstructive lung disease (e.g., chronic obstructive pulmonary disease [COPD], asthma), or if inadequate expiratory time does not allow for complete exhalation.

Positive end-expiratory pressure (PEEP) increases end-expiratory lung volume. All the gas-exchange and hemodynamic effects of PEEP therapy are related to the degree that global and regional lung volumes are increased.[22-30] To the extent that end-expiratory lung volume is below FRC and PEEP increases it to normal, PVR should decrease, terminal airways should reopen, and detrimental hemodynamic effects should be minimal.[22,23,25] If PEEP therapy over-distends lung units, either regionally or globally, PVR also will increase, impede RV ejection, and decrease CO.[23] This overdistention-induced decrease in CO is most pronounced in patients with acute hypovolemia[26] and during exacerbations of obstructive lung disease. In patients with the latter condition, the decrease in CO is due to the combined effects of increased RV ejection pressure load and RV distention-induced decreased venous return.

The heart exists in an intrathoracic fossa, the cardiac fossa, which is surrounded on two sides across the mediastinal membrane by the lungs.[31] As lung volume increases above FRC, the heart is compressed within the cardiac fossa. Since RV volume and diastolic compliance are greater than LV volume and diastolic compliance, the initial effects of increasing lung volume are to decrease RV end-diastolic volumes.[32] Eventually, biventricular diastolic compliance will decrease if lung volume increases enough.

Changes in ITP

Although all forms of ventilation phasically increase lung volume, spontaneous and positive-pressure ventilation have the exact opposite effects on ITP swings during ventilation. Spontaneous inspiration decreases ITP, lung compliance, and airway resistance. The decrease in ITP is a function of respiratory muscle effort. Positive-pressure inspiration, in contrast, increases ITP as a function of tidal volume delivered and thoracic cage compliance. Vigorous spontaneous inspiratory efforts against an inspiratory load (e.g., bronchospasm, vocal cord paralysis, upper airway obstruction, excessive resistance of inspiratory values in a continuous positive airway pressure [CPAP] system) markedly decrease ITP. Large tidal volume (≥ 15 ml/kg) positive-pressure breathing, "normal" tidal volume (≤ 12 ml/kg) positive-pressure breathing in the presence of decreased chest wall compliance, tense ascites, or the use of excessive amounts of PEEP markedly increases ITP.

Before the effects of ITP on cardiac function are addressed, the relationship between airway pressure and ITP should be examined. Increases in airway pressure may not reflect proportionally similar increases in ITP in all patients. Although approximately two thirds of the increase in airway pressure is transmitted to the pleural space in patients with healthy lungs and normal tidal volumes, a comparable degree of pressure transmission may not occur in patients with lung disease.[1,5,28,33-35] Patients with acute lung injury have reduced lung compliance and may not transmit as much of the increase in airway pressure to the pleural surface as do patients with normal lung compliance. Patients with obstructive lung disease may transmit more of the airway pressure to the pleural surface than do healthy individuals and may manifest intrinsic hyperinflation (often referred to as *auto*-PEEP) so that end-expiratory airway pressure is atmospheric (by convention referred to as *zero*), but lung volume is increased as if an external amount of PEEP were present. Clinically, it can be documented that a patient has auto-PEEP by a variety of methods. The easiest procedure is occlusion of the airway at end-expiration with immediate measurement of the airway pressure. If auto-PEEP is present, airway pressure should rapidly rise to the least auto-PEEP level. Furthermore, although it is difficult to measure the degree to which airway pressure is transmitted to the pleural surface, if a pulmonary artery catheter is present, the swings in diastolic pulmonary arterial pressure can be examined to ascertain the relative swings in ITP with ventilation. Changes in pulmonary arterial diastolic pressure should closely follow changes in ITP in most patients with conditions not associated with pulmonary hypertension.

Venous return to the heart from the body is determined by the pressure gradient between the heart (right atrial pressure) and the large venous reservoirs (mean systemic pressure).[7] Mean systemic pressure is determined by the circulating blood volume, peripheral vasomotor tone, and blood flow distribution. Any process that increases right atrial pressure will decrease this pressure gradient, decrease venous return, and ultimately lower CO. Since the right ventricle is a highly compliant structure, changes in surrounding ITP are directly transmitted to right atrial pressure. Since ITP is normally subatmospheric at end-expiration and decreases more during spontaneous inspiration, right atrial pressure usually does not rise during spontaneous ventilation. In fact, when the pressure gradient for venous return is increased (e.g., with recumbency and with fluid overload), spontaneous inspiration-induced decreases in right atrial pressure accelerate venous blood flow.[6,8,36-38] This process is referred to as the *thoracic pump.* Positive-pressure inspiration, on the other hand, by increasing ITP, increases right atrial pressure and impedes venous blood flow.[5,7,8,39,40] This ITP-induced decrease in venous return is the primary hemodynamic effect of positive-pressure ventilation on the cardiovascular system under most conditions.[28]

The left ventricle ejects its blood into an extrathoracic arterial circuit. However, the pressure required to generate this ejection pressure is the pressure across the wall of the left ventricle, transmural pressure.[41] Assuming that pericardial pressure and ITP are approximately similar and that no aortic outflow obstruction exists, transmural LV ejection pressure can be determined by the following equation:

Transmural LV ejection pressure =
Aortic pressure − ITP

For a constant aortic pressure, an increasing ITP will decrease LV ejection pressure; on the other hand, a decreasing ITP will increase LV ejection pressure. Thus both increases and decreases in ITP alter LV ejection pressure and LV afterload.[41-43] Vigorous spontaneous inspiratory efforts against an inspiratory resistance (e.g., bronchospasm, stiff lungs, airway obstruction) can induce profound decreases in ITP, which, by both markedly increasing LV ejection pressure and augmenting venous return, can precipitate acute LV failure and cardiogenic pulmonary edema.[44] Removing these exaggerated negative swings in ITP by removing the inspiratory obstruction and spontaneous respiratory efforts will decrease LV afterload. The resulting decrease in LV afterload may be the cause of the initial hemodynamic improvement seen in patients with cardiogenic pulmonary edema who are intubated and ventilated on an emergency basis.[35,45] Furthermore, in the hemody-

namically unstable patient requiring mechanical ventilatory support, removing such support may increase afterload and metabolic stress to a degree that exceeds the patient's physiologic reserve.[46] Such patients will not only "fail" their weaning trial, but they will develop worsening cardiovascular instability during the weaning process. Management of such a situation may require the temporary use of inotropic agents or adjustment of the intravascular volume status.

Superimposed positive swings in ITP, such as occur during positive-pressure inspiration, will further decrease LV afterload but also will decrease venous return.[43] Since the ability to increase ITP by mechanical means is usually associated with similar ITP-induced decreases in venous return, the beneficial effects of increasing ITP on cardiovascular function are limited.[22,25] Clearly, the overall effect of increasing ITP is dependent on the degree to which CO is responsive to changes in LV preload and afterload.[43] In patients with LV failure and volume overload, increases in ITP increase CO because ITP-induced decreases in LV ejection pressure override the ITP-induced decreases in pressure gradient for venous return.[22,25,45]

Changes in lung volume and ITP, by altering the RV end-diastolic volume, also alter LV diastolic compliance by the process of ventricular interdependence.[32,47,48] Increasing RV volume decreases LV diastolic compliance, and decreasing RV volume increases LV diastolic compliance. Thus in the setting of acute RV failure caused by pressure overload, acute cor pulmonale, the left ventricle may become oligemic despite having a "normal" LV filling pressure. LV oligemia, as a function of this mechanism, may occur after either massive pulmonary embolism or hyperinflation with fluid resuscitation. Accordingly, measures of LV filling pressure alone (i.e., wedge pressure) will not reflect actual LV volume status when ITP and RV volumes are changing. This concern is greater with spontaneous inspiration, when RV volumes normally increase, than with positive-pressure inspiration, when RV volumes normally decrease. The ventilation-induced changes in RV volume, by reciprocally changing LV diastolic compliance and, by inference, LV preload, are believed the major cause of pulsus paradoxus that occurs in patients with acute exacerbations of asthma and COPD.[32,36,49,50]

Based on the previous discussion, physiologic strategies can be predicted that will be effective in minimizing the detrimental effects of ventilation while optimizing the beneficial ones:

I. Maximize venous return (decreases venous return by increasing right atrial pressure).
   A. Keep ITP elevations small.
      1. Small tidal volumes ($\leq$10 ml/kg)
      2. Brief inspiratory time
      3. Least amount of PEEP necessary to maintain arterial oxygenation
   B. Maximize mean systemic pressure.
      1. Fluid resuscitation as necessary to maintain LV filling
      2. Military antishock trousers (MAST)
      3. Judicious use of vasopressor agents in the fluid-resuscitated patient
II. Minimize LV afterload
   A. Clinical significance relates primarily to abolishing negative swings in ITP during spontaneous ventilation: remove impediments to spontaneous inspiratory efforts
   B. In partial ventilatory assist modes (e.g., intermittent mandatory ventilation [IMV], pressure support), provide the following:
      1. Low-resistance respiratory circuits
      2. High bias flows
      3. Patient-matched inspiratory flow rates

CLINICAL APPLICATIONS OF HEART-LUNG INTERACTIONS

The effect of ventilation on a patient depends on the baseline level of cardiorespiratory function and mode of ventilation. In treatment of the spontaneously ventilating patient, concerns about ventilatory support, with or without endotracheal intubation, should be directed toward determining the primary factor or factors

that may induce cardiovascular instability. Hypovolemia, if associated with hypoperfusion, can induce acute respiratory muscle failure and death if it is prolonged.[3,26] Loss of vasomotor tone (e.g., in patients with sepsis or anaphylactic shock) can have the same effects.

Several cardiac factors appear to play major roles in determining the degree of ventilation-induced cardiovascular instability. Hyperinflation can induce a tamponade-like physiology, with pulsus paradoxus and diastolic equilibration of intracardiac pressures.[6] Globally increased ITP and, for the left ventricle, RV dilation can induce a relative hypovolemia, which may respond to fluid resuscitation.[32,48] Both hyperinflation and pulmonary embolism can induce RV-pressure overload (acute cor pulmonale), which often responds only to reversal of the primary process.[51] The RV overload will impair LV filling by the mechanism of ventricular interdependence. Finally, LV failure can occur if marked negative swings in ITP increase LV ejection pressure enough.[41,44] How then can these processes be prevented or reversed? Following two general principles can help minimize the detrimental effects of mechanical ventilation:

I. Allow the patient to breathe spontaneously.
   A. Provide assist-control ventilation.
   B. Provide partial ventilatory support.
      1. Intermittent mandatory ventilation
      2. Pressure-support ventilation
II. Avoid hyperinflation.
   A. Provide for prolonged expiratory time.
   B. Provide bronchodilator therapy.
   C. Use the lowest PEEP.

However, when such a group of patients is being treated, including those breathing spontaneously, these suggestions can be distilled into the following principles:

- Avoid large swings in ITP.
- Minimize the work-cost of breathing.
- Return end-expiratory lung volume to FRC.

Clearly, a balance must be reached to achieve adequate gas exchange while minimizing increases in lung volume and ITP. Usually a strategy for achieving adequate gas exchange without undue increases in airway pressure or lung volumes can be devised. New studies have suggested that permissive hypercarbia, if not associated with acidemia, can be well tolerated in the patient with severe reversible airflow obstruction. The benefits of permissive hypercarbia are less barotrauma and hemodynamic instability.

Although these principles seem reasonable, no controlled clinical trial has proved their effectiveness in maintaining hemodynamic stability. Given the complex nature and unpredictable course of critically ill patients, conducting such a clinical study would be extremely difficult, if at all possible. However, if these broad principles are used, the work-cost of breathing can be minimized and both the metabolic oxygen load of the respiratory muscles and patient anxiety reduced.[3] Since dynamic hyperinflation commonly occurs in patients with COPD, there is some rationale in using enough externally applied PEEP to offset the patient's own auto-PEEP during spontaneous ventilation. This is usually done by giving CPAP by a bias-flow circuit, with or without the application of positive-pressure breaths. If end-expiratory airway and alveolar pressures can be equalized by this procedure, excessive negative swings in ITP during spontaneous inspiration can be avoided. Like auto-PEEP, these large negative swings in ITP may not be appreciated from inspection of the airway pressure waveform alone.

Pressure-support ventilation is associated with the smallest fluctuations in ITP during matched tidal volume breaths of all the partial ventilatory support modes. It may be the optimal method of providing partial ventilatory support in the hemodynamically unstable patient who needs mechanical ventilatory support. It also may represent the least stressful method of weaning such patients if other methods, such as T-tube weaning and IMV withdrawal, are unsuccessful.

The practical goals of the physician caring for such patients are to define which cardiopulmonary factor or factors are determinants of the cardiovascular status of the patient and to optimize the beneficial aspects of these interactions without impairing gas exchange or venous return.

SUMMARY

- Mechanical ventilation determines work-cost of breathing, PVR, ITP, and ventricular interdependence.
- Positive pressure ventilation increases ITP and decreases CO by decreasing venous return.
- PVR increases as lung volume becomes either greater or less than FRC.
- PEEP increases end-expiratory lung volume. PVR will be minimized if PEEP brings lung volumes to normal FRC.
- Biventricular diastolic compliance will decrease if lung volume increases are of sufficient magnitude.

- The right ventricle is a compliant structure, and increases in ITP are transmitted to the right ventricle and right atrium. Venous blood flow may decrease.
- Changes in ITP modulate LV ejection pressure.
- Increasing RV volume decreases LV compliance.
- To minimize detrimental effects of mechanical ventilation, avoid large swings in ITP, minimize the work-cost of breathing, and return end-expiratory lung volume to FRC.

REFERENCES

1. Grenvik A. Respiratory, circulatory and metabolic effects of respiratory treatment. A clinical study in postoperative thoracic surgical patients. Acta Anaesth Scand 19(Suppl):1-122, 1966.
2. Vatner SF, Rutherford JD. Control of the myocardial contractile state by carotid chemo- and baroreceptor and pulmonary inflation reflexes in conscious dogs. J Clin Invest 61:1593-1601, 1978.
3. Roussos C, Macklem PT. The respiratory muscles. N Engl J Med 307:786-797, 1982.
4. Brecher GA, Hubay CA. Pulmonary blood flow and venous return during spontaneous respiration. Circ Res 3:210-214, 1955.
5. Cournaud A, Motley HL, Werko L, et al. Physiologic studies of the effect of intermittent positive pressure breathing on cardiac output in man. Am J Physiol 152:162-174, 1948.
6. Guntheroth WG, Morgan BC, Mullins GL. Effect of respiration on venous return and stroke volume in cardiac tamponade. Mechanism of pulsus paradoxus. Circ Res 20:381-390, 1967.
7. Guyton AC, Lindsey AW, Abernathy B, et al. Venous return at various right atrial pressures and the normal venous return curve. Am J Physiol 189:609-615, 1957.
8. Holt JP. The effect of positive and negative intrathoracic pressure on cardiac output and venous return in the dog. Am J Physiol 142:594-603, 1944.
9. Morgan BC, Martin WE, Hornbein TF, et al. Hemodynamic effects of intermittent positive pressure respiration. Anesthesiology 27:584-590, 1960.
10. Seely RD. Dynamic effects of inspiration on the simultaneous stroke volumes of the right and left ventricles. Am J Physiol 154:273-280, 1948.
11. Paintal AS. Vagal sensory receptors and their reflex effects. Physiol Rev 53:159-227, 1973.
12. Shepherd JT. The lungs as receptor sites for cardiovascular regulation. Circulation 63:1-10, 1981.
13. Tang PC, Marie FW, Amassain VE. Respiratory influence on the vasomotor center. Am J Physiol 191:218-224, 1957.
14. De Burgh Daly MB, Hazzledine JL, Ungar A. The reflex effects of alterations in lung volume on systemic vascular resistance in the dog. J Physiol (Lond) 188:331-351, 1967.
15. Glick G, Wechsler AS, Epstein SE. Reflex cardiovascular depression produced by stimulation of pulmonary stretch receptors in the dog. J Clin Invest 48:467-473, 1969.
16. Hakim TS, Michel RP, Chang HK. Effect of lung inflation on pulmonary vascular resistance by arterial and venous occlusion. J Appl Physiol 53:1110-1115, 1982.
17. West JB, Dollery CT, Naimark A. Distribution of blood flow in isolated lung; Relation to vascular and alveolar pressures. J Appl Physiol 19:713-724, 1964.
18. Whittenberger JL, McGregor M, Berglund E, et al. Influence of state of inflation of the lung on pulmonary vascular resistance. J Appl Physiol 15:878-882, 1960.
19. Howell JBL, Permutt S, Proctor DF, et al. Effect of inflation of the lung on different parts of the pulmonary vascular bed. J Appl Physiol 16:71-76, 1961.
20. Brower RG, Gottlieb J, Wise RA, Permutt W, Sylvester JT. Locus of hypoxic vasoconstriction in isolated ferret lungs. J Appl Physiol 63:58-65, 1987.
21. Hakim TS, Michel RP, Minami H, Chang HK. Site of pulmonary hypoxic vasoconstriction studied with arterial and venous occlusion. J Appl Physiol 54:1298-1302, 1983.
22. Calvin JE, Driedger AA, Sibbald WJ. Positive end-expiratory pressure (PEEP) does not depress left ventricular function in patients with pulmonary edema. Am Rev Resp Dis 124:121-128, 1981.
23. Canada E, Benumof JL, Tousdale FR. Pulmonary vascular resistance correlates in intact normal and abnormal canine lungs. Crit Care Med 10:719-723, 1982.
24. Cassidy SS, Robertson CH, Pierce AK, et al. Cardiovascular effects of positive end-expiratory pressure in dogs. J Appl Physiol 44:743-750, 1978.
25. Grace MP, Greenbaum DM. Cardiac performance in response to PEEP in patients with cardiac dysfunction. Crit Care Med 10:358-360, 1982.
26. Harken AH, Brennan MF, Smith B, Barsamian EM. The hemodynamic response to positive end-expiratory ventilation in hypovolemic patients. Surgery 76:786-793, 1974.
27. Jardin F, Farcot JC, Boisante L, et al. Influence of positive end-expiratory pressure on left ventricular performance. N Engl J Med 304:387-392, 1981.
28. Luce JM. The cardiovascular effects of mechanical ventilation and positive end-expiratory pressure. JAMA 252:807-811, 1984.
29. Marini JJ, Culver BH, Butler J. Mechanical effect of lung distension with positive pressure on cardiac function. Am Rev Resp Dis 124:382-386, 1981.
30. Pick RA, Handler JB, Murata GH, Friedman AS. The cardiovascular effect of positive end-expiratory pressure. Chest 82:345-350, 1982.

31. Butler J. The heart is in good hands. Circulation 67:1163-1168, 1983.

32. Janicki JS, Weber KT. The pericardium and ventricular interaction, distensibility and function. Am J Physiol 238:H494–H503, 1980.

33. Conway CM. Haemodynamic effects of pulmonary ventilation. Br J Anaesth 47:761-766, 1975.

34. Goldberg HS, Rabson J. Control of cardiac output by systemic vessels. Circulatory adjustments to acute and chronic respiratory failure and the effects of therapeutic interventions. Am J Cardiol 47:696-702, 1981.

35. Rasanen J, Vaisanen IT, Heikkila J, et al. Acute myocardial infarction complicated by left ventricular dysfunction and respiratory failure. The effect of continuous positive airway pressure. Chest 87:158-162, 1985.

36. Bromberger-Barnea B. Mechanical effects of inspiration on heart functions: A review. Fed Proc 40:2172-2177, 1981.

37. Scharf SM, Brown R, Saunders N, et al. Effects of normal and loaded spontaneous inspiration on cardiovascular function. J Appl Physiol 47:582-590, 1979.

38. Wise RA, Robotham JL, Summer WR. Effects of spontaneous ventilation on the circulation. Lung 159:175-186, 1981.

39. Braunwald E, Binion JT, Morgan WL, Sarnoff SJ. Alterations in central blood volume and cardiac output induced by positive pressure breathing and counteracted by metaraminol (Aramine). Circ Res 5:670-675, 1957.

40. Pinsky MR. Determinants of pulmonary arterial flow variation during respiration. J Appl Physiol 56:1237-1245, 1984.

41. Buda AJ, Pinsky MR, Ingels NB, et al. Effect of intrathoracic pressure on left ventricular performance. N Engl J Med 301:453-459, 1979.

42. Peters J, Kindred MK, Robotham JL. Transient analysis of cardiopulmonary interactions. II. Systolic events. J Appl Physiol 64:1518-1526, 1988.

43. Pinsky MR, Matuschak GM, Klain M. Determinants of cardiac augmentation by elevations in intrathoracic pressure. J Appl Physiol 58:1189-1198, 1985.

44. Stalcup SA, Mellins RB. Mechanical forces producing pulmonary edema in acute asthma. N Engl J Med 297:592-596, 1977.

45. Rasanen J, Nikki P, Heikkila J. Acute myocardial infarction complicated by respiratory failure. The effects of mechanical ventilation. Chest 85:21-28, 1984.

46. Beach T, Millen E, Grenvik A. Hemodynamic response to discontinuance of mechanical ventilation. Crit Care Med 1:85-90, 1973.

47. Olsen CO, Tyson GS, Maier GW, et al. Dynamic ventricular interaction in the conscious dog. Circ Res 52:85-104, 1983.

48. Taylor RR, Covell JW, Sonnenblick EH, Ross J Jr. Dependence of ventricular distensibility on filling of the opposite ventricle. Am J Physiol 213:711-718, 1967.

49. Brinker JA, Weiss JL, Lappe DL, et al. Leftward septal displacement during right ventricular loading in man. Circulation 61:626-633, 1980.

50. Ruskin J, Bache RJ, Rembert JC, Greenfield JC Jr. Pressure-flow studies in man: Effect of respiration on left ventricular stroke volume. Circulation 48:79-85, 1973.

51. Sibbald W, Driedger AA. Right ventricular function in acute disease states: Pathophysiologic considerations. Crit Care Med 11:339-345, 1983.

CHAPTER 25

Acute Lung Injury

Larry A. Woods · James P. Davison · Alan J. Cropp

Acute lung injury (ALI) is a disorder encompassing varying degrees of pulmonary cellular damage (parenchymal and vascular) that alters membrane permeability, produces an accumulation of noncardiogenic lung water, decreases compliance, and ultimately results in the clinical presentation of acute respiratory failure. This spectrum of cellular damage results in a lung injury continuum of clinical, physiologic, and roentgenographic abnormalities that in the most severe form constitutes the adult respiratory distress syndrome (ARDS).[1,2] First described by Ashbaugh et al.[3] approximately 25 years ago, ARDS has been defined as a severe form of acute respiratory failure characterized by dyspnea, refractory hypoxemia, decreased lung compliance, and diffuse radiologic changes that occur in the absence of cardiac failure or chronic lung disease.

The "classic" definition of ARDS recently has been expanded by Murray et al.[4] and Matthay[5] into the three-part definition of ALI shown in the accompanying box. The definition considers lung injury, underlying cause, and systemic nonpulmonary organ dysfunction as a basis for this expanded definition. The presence of certain "high-risk" clinical disorders and nonpulmonary systemic organ dysfunction correlates in a positive fashion with prognosis of lung

---

Factors That Define ALI*

Severity of injury

Arterial oxygenation (Pa_{O_2}/FI_{O_2})
CXR
Static lung compliance
Level of positive end-expiratory pressure

Associated clinical disorder(s)

Sepsis (microbiology, anatomic site)
Aspiration (type)
Major trauma
Drug overdose
Cardiopulmonary bypass

Systemic organ function

Acid-base status
Renal function
Hematologic abnormalities
Hepatic function
CNS function

---

*Modified from Matthay MA. The adult respiratory distress syndrome: New insights into diagnosis, pathophysiology and treatment. West J Med 150:190, 1989. Reprinted by permission of The Western Journal of Medicine.

FI_{O_2}, fraction of inspired oxygen; Pa_{O_2}, partial pressure of arterial oxygen.

injury, clinical course, and mortality. The lung injury score, as shown in Table 25-1, is a measure of the severity of lung injury and has prognostic importance. The numerical grading procedure consists of four physiologic and radiologic components. Each component is assigned a number reflecting severity. Each score, ranging from 0 to 4, is added and then divided by the number of components to yield the lung injury score. The designation of ARDS is reserved for those patients with severe lung injury (i.e., lung injury score >2.5).

INCIDENCE AND PRECIPITATING CAUSES

At present, the incidence of ALI and ARDS is unknown. The figure of 150,000 cases of ARDS per year quoted in most studies is an estimate from the early 1970s. Recent estimates place the incidence of ARDS both above and below 150,000 cases per year.[6,7] Two recent studies using the lung injury score and serum markers for predicting ARDS in septic patients report a 60% incidence of some degree of ALI.[8,9]

The conditions associated with ALI and ARDS are multiple (see box). The risk of developing ALI and progression to ARDS varies among the many clinical disorders. Three independent studies by Fowler et al.,[10] Pepe et al.,[11] and

---

Clinical Disorders Associated With ALI and ARDS	
Sepsis*	High-altitude sickness
Aspiration of gastric contents*	Disseminated intravascular coagulation
Trauma*	Postcardiopulmonary bypass
Burns	Pneumonia*
Multiple fractures	Nosocomial
Lung contusion	Viral
Massive blood transfusion	*Pneumocystis carinii*
Near-drowning	Oxygen toxicity
Drug ingestion	Eclampsia
Narcotics	Pancreatitis
Paraquat	
Smoke and toxic chemical inhalation	

*Commonly associated with ALI and ARDS.

TABLE 25-1 Components and Individual Values of Lung Injury Score*

Components	Value
CXR	
No alveolar consolidation	0
Alveolar consolidation confined to one quadrant	1
Alveolar consolidation confined to two quadrants	2
Alveolar consolidation confined to three quadrants	3
Alveolar consolidation in all four quadrants	4
Hypoxemia score (Pao_2/Fio_2)	
≥300	0
225-299	1
175-224	2
100-174	3
<100	4
PEEP score (when ventilated)	
≥5 cm H_2O	0
6-8 cm H_2O	1
9-11 cm H_2O	2
12-14 cm H_2O	3
≥15 cm H_2O	4
Respiratory system compliance score (when available)	
≥80 ml/cm H_2O	0
60-79 ml/cm H_2O	1
40-59 ml/cm H_2O	2
20-39 ml/cm H_2O	3
≤19 ml/cm H_2O	4

The final value is obtained by dividing the aggregate sum by the number of components that were used.

Lung injury	*Score*
None	0
Mild-to-moderate	0.1-2.5
Severe (ARDS)	>2.5

*Modified from Murray JF, Matthay MA, Luce J, et al. An expanded definition of the adult respiratory distress syndrome. Am Rev Respir Dis 138:721, 1988.

Pao_2/Fio_2, arterial oxygen tension to inspired oxygen concentration ratio; PEEP, positive end-expiratory pressure.

Maunder[12] show that sepsis, gastric aspiration, and trauma account for the vast majority of ARDS. These studies also show that the more clinical disorders present, the higher is the risk of developing ARDS. In the study by Pepe et al.[11] the risk for developing ARDS approximately doubles for each concurrent disorder present. In these studies time to onset of ARDS from the initial clinical insult was rapid, in most cases only 24 hours and usually less than 72 hours. In those patients developing ARDS after 72 hours, ALI was usually caused by a delayed infectious process.

Although groups at risk for developing lung injury and ARDS have been identified, it is still not possible to determine which patients within these groups will develop lung injury. Serum markers for ALI and ARDS are not clinically useful at this time. Such markers as factor VIII antigen (an indicator of endothelial injury) and an early decrease in dynamic and static compliance look promising.[8,13] However, further studies are needed to confirm the usefulness of these variables in predicting ALI.

MEDIATORS OF ACUTE LUNG INJURY

The primary mediator of ALI is unknown. Research has shown a series of cascading inflammatory events thought to be responsible for the capillary membrane breakdown and vascular changes seen in ALI (see accompanying box for a partial listing).

Bacterial endotoxin activates complement, kills endothelial cells, and causes sequestrations of neutrophils in the lung.[14] Complement activation, principally of C5 and C3, mediates neutrophil sequestration in the lung and induces the "respiratory burst" in polymorphonuclear neutrophil leukocytes (PMNs), which is probably a key event leading to endothelial destruction and increased permeability.[14] Neutrophils are thought to play a prominent role in the destruction of the endothelial-epithelial membranes. Through various chemotaxins, the PMNs become sequestered, adhere, and then emigrate from the vascular lumen into the interstitial and alveolar beds. Degranulation, secretion of various proteases, and enzymatic production of oxygen metabolites (i.e., hydrogen peroxide, superoxide anion, and the hydroxyl

radicals) have been shown experimentally to cause endothelial and epithelial cellular destruction, allowing for increased permeability of the alveolar-capillary membranes.[15]

Eicosanoid metabolites, through cyclooxygenase- and lipoxygenase-derived compounds, are secreted from various cell lines, affecting membrane permeability and causing vasoconstriction and dilation. These changes disrupt the normal vasoregulation of hypoxia in pulmonary and possibly systemic vascular beds. Eicosanoid metabolites also have been linked to modulation of cytokines.[16]

Cytokines, including tumor necrosis factor (TNF), have recently been shown to play a significant role in ALI. Chemotaxis, adherence of PMNs, induction of intravascular coagulation, and release of other cytokines have been attributed to TNF and other mediators.[17]

The inflammatory cascade is a complex mechanism of multiple feedback and amplifying pathways. Potentiators of this cascade may be triggered by an initial insult but also are activated by therapeutic interventions aimed at eliminating hypoxemia. In some studies high

---

Mediators and Modulators of ALI

Cellular components

Neutrophils
Macrophages
Platelets
? Endothelial cells

Chemical components

Endotoxin
Complement
Various neutrophil proteases
Neutrophil oxygen metabolites
Eicosanoid metabolites
    Cyclooxygenase pathway
    Lipoxygenase pathway
    Platelet-activating factor

Cytokines

Tumor necrosis factor (cachectin)
Interleukin-1
Macrophage inflammatory proteins 1 and 2
Neutrophil-activating peptide 1

oxygen concentrations and peak inspiratory pressures as low as 30 cm H_2O have been shown to cause reduction in pulmonary function as measured by partial pressure of oxygen in arterial blood (PaO_2), static lung compliance, and functional residual capacity.[18-20] Although the normal lung may be relatively resistant to the effects of high concentrations of inspired oxygen, a comparable resistance may not be true for the acutely injured lung. It is thought that high levels of inspired oxygen (fraction of inspired oxygen [FIO_2] >0.5) and possibly elevated peak airway pressures used in conventional ventilatory strategies may further compromise lung function, hinder lung repair, and induce injury in areas of the lung not involved in the neutrophil-mediated injury.[18-20]

PATHOPHYSIOLOGY

The pathologic progession of ALI and ARDS is consistent, regardless of the cause. The process follows three overlapping phases of injury and repair, with involvement of both lung parenchyma and pulmonary vasculature. The pathophysiologic changes are summarized in Table 25-2.

TABLE 25-2   Pathologic, Physiologic, and Clinical Abnormalities Associated With ALI*

Acute Phase	Proliferative Phase	Fibrotic Phase
Pathologic		
Bronchoconstriction	Granulation of edema fluid	Increased collagen formation and deposition
Endothelial and epithelial destruction	Alveolar cell type II hyperplasia	Vascular: intimal and medial hypertrophy; loss of alveoli and vasculature through remodeling
Decreased surfactant		
Microthrombi		
Hyaline membranes		
Vasoconstriction		
Vasodilation		
Physiologic		
Increased vascular permeability	Continued shunting with additional ventilation/perfusion mismatch and gas diffusion abnormalities; further decreased compliance; pulmonary hypertension	
Intrapulmonary shunting		
Decreased compliance		
Decreased functional residual capacity		
Loss of vascular regulation to hypoxia		
Pulmonary hypertension		
Clinical		
Noncardiogenic pulmonary edema	Interstitial fibrosis	
Diffuse fluffy pattern on radiograph	Ground-glass appearance on radiograph	
Hypoxemia	Continued hypoxemia	
Increased alveolar-arterial gradient		
Increased work of breathing	Tachypnea	
Decreased carbon dioxide removal		
Tachypnea	Resolution vs. progression to multiple organ system failure	

*Organ system failure may precede, be concurrent with, or follow acute lung injury. Phases overlap and may occur simultaneously in different areas of the lung.

Phase I, lasting 0 to 7 days, is the *acute* or *exudative phase*. Its hallmark is the breakdown of the pulmonary capillary-alveolar membrane, leading to an increase in vascular permeability. This injury results in interstitial-alveolar edema, often recognized on CXR as pulmonary edema. Proteins and cellular debris form hyaline membranes and result in multiple alveoli collapse. Intravascular platelet aggregation and fibrin deposition form microthrombi and perpetuate pulmonary hypertension.

During days 5 to 14 the first signs of repair appear. This interval is the *subacute* or *proliferative phase*. During this period there is a hyperplastic response of type II alveolar epithelial cells. Fibroblasts begin the transformation of the intra-alveolar fluid into granulation tissue, a process that precedes the deposition of collagen in the third phase. This *fibrotic phase* may start as early as day 10 in some areas of the lung.

The result of this fibrotic process is loss of alveoli, thickened membranes, and a less distensible lung. The lung parenchyma takes on a diffuse emphysematous-like picture as the third phase progresses. The pulmonary vasculature is not spared in the inflammatory process. The microthrombi seen in the acute phase persist and may obstruct larger arterioles. Thickening of vessel walls results from intimal and medial hypertrophy that occurs in the subacute and fibrotic phases. Finally, there is an overall loss of pulmonary vasculature concomitant with the decrease in alveolar units. All of these events result in a continuation of the pulmonary hypertension seen at the onset of the acute stage.

Underlying changes in structure foreshadow changes in function. Breakdown of the pulmonary capillary membrane increases permeability. This increased permeability is not only to fluids but to large-molecular-weight proteins. Destruction of the epithelial side of the membrane allows passage of an exudative fluid directly into alveoli. In sharp contrast, in patients with cardiogenic pulmonary edema caused by increased hydrostatic forces in the presence of an intact membrane, protein content is low and alveolar edema is less pronounced. Worsened gas exchange occurs as a result of ventilation-perfusion mismatch. Non-cardiogenic lung water, high in protein, caused by increased membrane permeability results in widespread alveolar flooding and large areas of unventilated lung still perfused. This intrapulmonary shunt causes hypoxia, which characteristically is not responsive to supplemental levels of inspired oxygen. Also seen are underperfused but well-ventilated areas of the lung, which result in increased dead space.

The decrease in compliance that occurs in the acute phase is not fully understood. It is thought to occur initially by quantitative and qualitative changes in surfactant produced by type II alveolar epithelial cells. The presence of leaking plasma proteins renders surfactant ineffective in reducing surface tension. Lung compliance is therefore decreased, and increased pressures are needed to expand the lungs.

Increased pulmonary vascular pressures without a concomitant increase in left ventricular filling pressures are thought to occur in the early phase of ARDS. Initially, pulmonary hypertension is caused by cell-injury mediators, resulting in vasoconstriction followed and perpetuated by microthrombi and vascular collapse as extravascular lung water increases.

As the process continues into the second and third phases, the underlying causes of hypoxemia, decreased compliance, and pulmonary hypertension become more complex. In the proliferative and fibrotic phases causes of hypoxemia include not only increased right-to-left intrapulmonary shunting but also newly developed ventilation/perfusion (V/Q) areas of mismatch and gas diffusion abnormalities. This condition results from loss of alveolar units, loss of pulmonary vasculature, and the widened septal membranes seen with fibrosis. Surfactant is replaced by the proliferating type II alveolar epithelial cells. Lung compliance remains low, usually further decreased by the large amount of collagen deposited in the repair phase. Obliteration of pulmonary vasculature and diffuse vessel wall hypertrophy sustain the previously increased pulmonary arterial pressures.

CLINICAL SETTING AND PROGNOSIS

Despite multiple causes, the clinical presentation of ALI is quite uniform. After the initial insult, a latent period extends from a few hours to several days. As the cell-injury mediators are released and the capillary permeability increases, tachypnea appears. ABG studies reveal hypoxemia with a widening alveolar-arterial (A-a) gradient, a reflection of intrapulmonary shunting. The shunt fraction, QS/QT (i.e., the portion of nonventilated blood flow divided by the total pulmonary blood flow), is increased and may be 30% or greater in patients with severe lung injury. Resulting hypoxemia is usually refractory to conservative measures and often requires aggressive intervention. Static lung compliance, measured by dividing the tidal volume by the plateau pressure minus the positive end-expiratory pressure (PEEP) is also decreased. The plateau pressure is obtained by occluding the exhalation circuit at end inspiration or by adding an inspiratory pause of 1 to 2 seconds. The decreased lung compliance can be <30 ml/cm H_2O in ARDS patients (normal is 80 to 100 ml/cm H_2O).

Radiographic examination early in the course of ALI is nondiagnostic and may reveal completely normal results. As the injury progresses, interstitial edema followed by bilateral fluffy infiltrates representing alveolar flooding occurs. Normal heart size and lack of pleural effusion may help distinguish noncardiogenic pulmonary edema from cardiac-induced pulmonary edema. The institution of mechanical ventilation and PEEP may initially appear to cause clearing of the CXR because of hyperinflation, but results should not be confused with injury regression. The CXR eventually takes on the "ground-glass" appearance of interstitial fibrosis and may demonstrate hyperlucent zones representing lung remodeling and emphysematous changes.

During physical examination the patient may appear tachypneic and agitated. Lung auscultation reveals coarse breath sounds followed later by scattered rhonchi. Use of respiratory accessory muscles, sternal retractions, and paradoxic abdominal movements with respirations may signal impending respiratory collapse.

The clinical course of ALI may take several paths and is dependent on a variety of factors.[21] ALI with rapid reversal is seen in patients who are otherwise healthy and young and who develop the injury secondary to a single cause (i.e., high-altitude sickness, drug ingestion, or fat embolism). Improvement may be as rapid as the onset, with little or no pulmonary sequelae. Patients who are older, have underlying disease, or develop ALI secondary to "high-risk" or multiple causes (e.g., sepsis) have a more protracted course and experience greater morbidity and mortality. Overall the mortality rate for ARDS is >50% and approaches 90% for those cases associated with sepsis.[1,22] The majority of deaths caused by ALI are not secondary to respiratory failure but to ongoing sepsis and multiple organ system failure.[23]

Pulmonary sequelae in survivors of ALI vary with severity and duration of the injury. Those patients with rapid disease reversal have little, if any, pulmonary abnormalities compared to those who progress to the chronic stages. Some patients have residual hyperactive airway disease, whereas others may develop varying degrees of restrictive lung disease and gas exchange abnormalities.[24,25]

MANAGEMENT AND INTERVENTIONS

The management of ALI and ARDS is mainly supportive. Treatment of the underlying cause is the initial step in the management of this syndrome. At this time there is no known treatment to reverse increased vascular permeability changes or fibrosis occurring with ALI.

To support arterial oxygenation, providing mechanical ventilation and PEEP is often necessary. The goal is to maintain an arterial oxygenation saturation >90% with less injurious concentrations of oxygen (FIO_2 ≤0.50). An FIO_2 of 1.0 may be required initially to adequately oxygenate the patient. PEEP is then applied starting at 5 cm H_2O and is increased in 2.5 to 5 cm H_2O increments until adequate arterial oxygenation and nontoxic concentration of inspired oxygen are achieved. Pulse oximetry is helpful in following the trend of arterial oxygen saturations and can aid in achieving a rapid and safe decrease from high concentrations of inspired oxygen to concentrations considered nontoxic. Inverse inspiration/expiration (I/E) ratio ventilation, use of inspiratory pause, and use of extracorporeal gas exchange at this time are investigational. Use of alternative modes of ventilation may require additional expertise and consultation should these modalities be necessary.

The need to assess volume status and proceed with fluid resuscitation and management is an essential basic step to managing ARDS. Intravascular volume must be adequate to maintain gas exchange, oxygen delivery, and hemodynamic stability. Pulmonary arterial catheter insertion is necessary in these assessments. Although volume-pressure relationships are variable, maintaining a pulmonary capillary wedge pressure (PCWP) between 12 and 15 mm Hg is recommended. Cardiac output may be negatively affected by the use of PEEP (see Chapter 24). Inotropic support may therefore be needed if adequate intravascular volume has already been achieved. Controversy about the preference for crystalloid or colloid solutions persists. Maintaining adequate oxygen-carrying capacity provided by hemoglobin should not be neglected, and patients should be transfused when indicated to maximize oxygen delivery and transport (see Chapter 2).

Continued vigilance for signs of infection is necessary. Fastidious care should be given to all invasive intravascular monitoring and indwelling devices in accordance with infection control policies devised by each institution in compliance with acceptable and current standards of care. In cases in which fever and leukocytosis are present without an obvious source, fungal infection, sepsis from indwelling invasive lines, and sinus infection as a result of intubation should be considered. If fever and leukocytosis occur without an obvious source before lung injury, suspicion should be focused on the lower torso as the source of infection. If this phenomenon should occur after the establishment of ALI, a pulmonary source is likewise strongly suspected.[23]

Malnutrition compromises host defense. Early and appropriate nutritional support is therefore vital and is discussed in more detail in Chapter 3.

The treating physician must be aware of and anticipate many of the general medical complications resulting from ALI, for example, aspiration, cardiac dysrhythmias, stress ulcers with GI bleeding, and pulmonary embolism. Ventilator-associated complications may include barotrauma with mediastinal and retroperitoneal dissection of air, pneumothorax, subcutaneous emphysema without pneumothorax, nosocomial pneumonias, and sinusitis. Prophylactic measures (e.g., the use of sequential leg compression devices, stress ulcer prophylaxis, and careful attention to intravenous and arterial access lines) may be beneficial in avoiding some of these complications.

Although the treatment of ALI and ARDS is mainly supportive, understanding the immunologic basis of this syndrome as it unfolds will largely shape the future of its treatment. Use of surfactant replacement and the use of antibodies to endotoxin, TNF, complement, and others are currently being investigated.[26] Use of NSAIDs that interfere with eicosanoid metabolism is also investigational and shows promise for the future.[26] Although theoretically steroid use may be beneficial, clinical trials have shown the reverse is true in most instances. Consideration of steroid administration for treating a fat embolism may be the only exception. The use of bronchodilators may be indicated for use in patients with bronchospasm. Investigational evidence also suggests attenuation of neutrophil-mediated injury by xanthine derivatives. Such agents as pentoxifylline, terbutaline, and aminophylline have been used and may be beneficial but are still considered investigational for this purpose at present.[26,27]

SUMMARY

- ARDS is severe respiratory failure with dyspnea, refractory hypoxemia, decreased lung compliance, and diffuse CXR changes in the absence of cardiac failure or chronic lung disease. Newer definitions consider lung injury, underlying cause, and systemic nonpulmonary oxygen dysfunction.
- Sepsis, gastric aspiration, and trauma are the most common causes of ARDS.
- Mediators of ALI include endotoxins, eicosanoid metabolites, and cytokines.
- ALI proceeds through an acute (exudative), subacute (proliferative), and chronic (fibrotic) phase. This process produces loss of alveoli,

thickened membranes, and decreased compliance.
- Clinical presentation of ALI is stereotypic. After a latent interval, shunt fraction increases, and hypoxemia requires aggressive support. CXR usually reveals a "ground-glass" appearance.
- Overall mortality rate of ARDS is >50%. Death usually results from organ failure syndrome.
- Treatment of ALI and ARDS usually requires mechanical ventilation with PEEP, volume resuscitation to maintain oxygen transport and hemodynamic pressure stability, inotropic support, and metabolic support.

REFERENCES

1. Bersten A, Sibbald WJ. Acute lung injury and septic shock. Crit Care Clin 5:49-79, 1989.
2. Shapiro BA, Cane RD. Acute lung injury and positive end-expiratory pressure. In Cane RD, Shapiro BA, Davison R. Case studies in Critical Care Medicine. Chicago: Year Book Medical, 1991, pp 321-346.
3. Ashbaugh DG, Bigelow DB, Petty TL, et al. Acute respiratory distress in adults. Lancet 2:319-323, 1967.
4. Murray JF, Matthay MA, Luce J, et al. An expanded definition of the adult respiratory distress syndrome. Am Rev Respir Dis 138:720-723, 1988.
5. Matthay MA. The adult respiratory distress syndrome: New insights into diagnosis, pathophysiology and treatment. West J Med 150:187-194, 1989.
6. Shoemaker WC. Pathophysiology and fluid management of post-operative and post-traumatic ARDS. In Shoemaker WC, Ayres S, Grenvik A, et al., eds. Textbook of Critical Care, 2nd ed. Philadelphia: WB Saunders, 1989, p 616.
7. Villar J, Slutsky AS. The incidence of the adult respiratory distress syndrome. Am Rev Respir Dis 140:814-816, 1989.
8. Rubin DB, Wiener-Kronish JP, Murray JE, et al. Elevated von Willebrand factor antigen is an early plasma predictor of acute lung injury in non-pulmonary sepsis syndrome. J Clin Invest 86:474-480, 1990.
9. Weinberg PF, Matthay MA, Webster RO, et al. Biologically active products of complement and acute lung injury in patients with the sepsis syndrome. Am Rev Respir Dis 130:791-796, 1984.
10. Fowler AA, Hamman RF, Good JT, et al. Adult respiratory distress syndrome: Risk with common predispositions. Ann Intern Med 98:593-597, 1983.
11. Pepe PE, Potkin RT, Holtman Reus D, et al. Clinical predictors of adult respiratory distress syndrome. Am J Surg 144:124-130, 1982.
12. Maunder RJ. Clinical prediction of the adult respiratory distress syndrome. Clin Chest Med 6:413-426, 1985.
13. Byrne K, Cooper KR, Carey PD, et al. Pulmonary compliance: Early assessment of evolving lung injury after onset of sepsis. J Appl Physiol 69:2290-2295, 1990.
14. Rinaldo JE, Christman JW. Mechanisms and mediators of the adult respiratory distress syndrome. Clin Chest Med 11:621-632, 1990.
15. Tate RM, Repine JE. Neutrophils and the adult respiratory distress syndrome. Am Rev Respir Dis 128:552-559, 1983.
16. Voelkel NF, Stenmark KR, Westcott JY, et al. Lung eicosanoid metabolism. Clin Chest Med 10:95-105, 1989.
17. Welbourn R, Goldman G, O'Riordain M, et al. Role for tumor necrosis factor as mediator of lung injury following lower torso ischemia. J Appl Physiol 70:2645-2649, 1991.

18. Jackson RM. Pulmonary oxygen toxicity. Chest 88:900-905, 1985.
19. Hickling KG. Ventilatory management of ARDS: Can it affect the outcome? Intensive Care Med 16:219-226, 1990.
20. Kolobow T. Acute respiratory failure: On how to injure healthy lungs (and prevent sick lungs from recovering). Trans ASAIO 34:31-34, 1988.
21. Hansen-Flaschen J, Fishman AP. Adult respiratory distress syndrome: Clinical features and pathogenesis. In Fishman AP. Pulmonary Diseases and Disorders, 2nd ed., vol 3. New York: McGraw-Hill, 1988, pp 2201-2213.
22. Fein AM, Lippman M, Holtzmann H, et al. The risk factors incidence and prognosis of ARDS following septicemia. Chest 83:40-42, 1983.
23. Montgomery AB, Stager MA, Carrico CJ, et al. Causes of mortality in patients with the adult respiratory distress syndrome. Am Rev Resp Dis 132:485-489, 1985.
24. Elliot CG, Morris AH, Cengiz M. Pulmonary function and exercise gas exchange in survivors of adult respiratory distress syndrome. Am Rev Respir Dis 123:492-495, 1981.
25. Elliott CG. Pulmonary sequelae in survivors of adult respiratory distress syndrome. Clin Chest Med 4:789-800, 1990.
26. Said SI, Foda HD. Pharmacologic modulation of lung injury. Am Rev Respir Dis 139:1553-1564, 1989.
27. Raffin TA. Acute lung injury and pentoxifylline. Crit Care Med 18:1485-1486, 1990.

SUGGESTED READINGS

Bone RC. Adult respiratory distress syndrome. Clin Chest Med 3:1-212, 1982.

A review of ARDS and all its aspects, containing manuscripts from leading investigators.

Wiedman HP, Matthay MA, Matthay RA. Adult respiratory distress syndrome. Clin Chest Med 11:575-800, 1990.

A collection of articles from various authors updating the earlier review from 1982 in Clinics in Chest Medicine.

Hansen-Flaschen J, Fishmann AP. Adult respiratory distress syndrome clinical features and pathogenesis (Chapter 141) and Management (Chapter 143). In Pulmonary Disease and Disorders, 2nd ed. New York: McGraw-Hill, 1988.

An excellent short review of ARDS with special attention to pathogenesis, clinical course, and management. It contains an excellent list of associated clinical causes and their references.

CHAPTER 26

Life-Threatening Bronchospasm

R. Phillip Dellinger

The surgeon may be required to participate in the intensive care management of the broncospastic patient as part of preoperative management when bronchospasm exacerbations occur following surgery and in the posttraumatic patient. Bronchospasm is defined as reversible obstructive airway disease. The hallmark of obstructive airway disease is impediment to expiration. Asthma is the prototype of bronchospasm; however, chronic obstructive pulmonary disease (COPD) patients also may have some variable degree of reversible obstruction. The pharmacologic therapy of bronchospasm is similar for asthma and COPD. Although reversibility is anticipated in asthma, in COPD it may vary from significant response to bronchodilator therapy to no response at all. Bronchospasm also predisposes to postoperative or posttraumatic pulmonary complications since the pathophysiology of bronchospasm as described below predisposes to premature airway closure in patients with atelectasis.

PATHOPHYSIOLOGY

Small airway smooth muscle contracts in patients with bronchospasm producing obstruction to airflow. The overwhelming majority of patients with bronchospasm has significant chronic inflammation that is driving the bronchospasm. This inflammation is characterized by infiltration of the bronchial wall with inflammatory cells, bronchial mucosal edema, mucous production, and smooth muscle hyperplasia. Treatment must be directed at both the bronchospasm (bronchodilator therapy) and

the inflammation (anti-inflammatory therapy). Although bronchodilators may be temporizing and lifesaving, anti-inflammatory drugs are necessary to reverse the underlying inflammation.

With acute bronchospasm, increased expiratory time is needed to allow complete emptying of the breath. With severe bronchospasm, "air trapping" occurs as the need for increased expiratory time becomes greater and greater, culminating in inspiration before total emptying of the previous breath. Air trapping is associated with higher end-expiratory lung volumes (functional residual capacity). Worsened compliance is due to an increase in functional residual capacity, resulting in an increase in the inspiratory work of breathing. Although hypoxemia occurs with acute bronchospasm from decreased ventilation relative to perfusion (low V/Q areas), ventilatory failure may progress to respiratory arrest as the work of breathing increases significantly from the combination of air trapping, mucosal edema, increased secretions, and diaphragm dysfunction. The diaphragm, which normally has optimal contractile force in its dome-shaped resting position, assumes a flattened position as air trapping increases lung volume. Compromise of diaphragmatic function results.

CLINICAL FINDINGS AND PHYSICAL EXAMINATION

All wheezing is not bronchospasm. The differential diagnosis of wheezing and clues to diagnosis are shown in the box on p. 294. The patient with severe bronchospasm is usually

---

Differential Diagnosis of Wheezing

Congestive heart failure: neck vein distention, S_3, rales on physical examination, CXR findings of failure, risk factors for heart failure

Upper airway obstruction: wheezing greatest over trachea, inspiratory stridor, risk factors

Anaphylaxis: insect sting or drug ingestion

Pulmonary embolus: rare presentation, leg findings, pleuritic chest pain, risk factors for pulmonary embolism

Toxic fume exposure: history

Endobronchial obstruction: localized wheezing, risk factors for lung cancer or foreign body

---

profoundly tachypneic and tachycardiac and may have difficulty talking.

Expiratory wheezing correlates with the degree of obstruction. Inspiratory wheezing also may be heard. The absence of wheezing in the severely bronchospastic patient may imply such low expiratory flow that wheezing cannot be heard.

Physicians are notoriously inaccurate in judging the severity of bronchospasm based on physical examination and subjective patient assessment.[1] Although routine spirometry (performed by first obtaining a full inspiration, followed by a maximal forced expiration) is the gold standard of measuring obstruction (forced expiratory volume in 1 second [FEV_1]), it is impractical in the patient in severe distress. A more practical test is peak expiratory flow rate (PEFR). This measurement can be done with a portable handheld spirometer, is reliable, and requires less patient cooperation than full spirometry since peak PEFRs occur early in the forced expiratory maneuver. Interpretation does assume the patient performed the test correctly and gave a full and cooperative effort. PEFR is higher with younger adults, males, and taller individuals.

Indications for intubation of the bronchospastic patient include the following conditions:

- Apnea or near-apnea
- Altered mental status related to bronchospasm

- Central cyanosis
- Severe distress not responding to aggressive bronchodilator therapy
- Rising partial pressure of arterial carbon dioxide ($Paco_2$) and pH falling to less than 7.25 despite aggressive bronchodilator therapy

Laboratory and Radiographic Data Base

Routine laboratory tests offer little of value for the management of acute severe bronchospasm. White blood cell count may be elevated as a consequence of stress or the adrenergic agents used for treatment. ABG values may be important for decisions concerning intubation (but only after the patient has received significant therapy) and for ongoing management of severe bronchospasm in the intubated patient. At the onset of bronchospasm, ABGs may be impressively abnormal, but the patient may still respond quickly and impressively to vigorous bronchodilator therapy.

TRADITIONAL MEDICAL THERAPY
Bronchodilator Therapy

All initial bronchodilator regimens should be built around inhaled beta-2 selective agonists since onset of effect is immediate and the therapeutic-toxicity ratio is optimal.[2] Nebulized albuterol or metaproterenol is recommended. Although there may be some difference in beta-2 selectivity between albuterol and other beta-2 selective agonists, for routine clinical practice, albuterol, metaproterenol, and terbutaline have a similar beta-2 selective agonist profile. Terbutaline is not available in solution for nebulization and is available as a metered dose inhaler only. Subcutaneous adrenergic therapy offers less of a therapeutic-toxicity ratio advantage and should be used only in selected subpopulations of acute bronchospasm. Epinephrine and terbutaline, when given subcutaneously, have similar side effect profiles.[3] The use of subcutaneous epinephrine or terbutaline for patients with asthma is indicated as follows:

- In combination with inhaled therapy for patients in extreme distress with new-onset bronchospasm
- In patients who have not responded significantly to inhaled therapy

TABLE 26-1	Adrenergic Agonists for Acute Severe Bronchospasm		
Agent	Route of Administration	Duration (hr)	Dosage
Albuterol	Aerosol, 0.5% solution	4-6	Adults: 0.5 ml with 3 ml normal saline solution
Metaproterenol	Aerosol, 5% solution	3-5	Adults: 0.5 ml with 3 ml normal saline solution
Terbutaline	Parenteral, 0.1% solution (SC)	4-6	0.01 ml/kg; maximum of 0.25 ml
Epinephrine	Parenteral, 0.2% solution (SC)	1-2	0.01 ml/kg; maximum of 0.3-0.5 ml

▪ In patients who are mechanically ventilated as a result of bronchospasm, particularly if they have been intubated and are not improving

Beta-1 cardiac toxicity (tachycardia and increased oxygen demand) is particularly important in older patients and patients with known cardiac ischemic disease, and it is significantly greater when subcutaneous and oral routes are used. There is no role for oral adrenergic agents in the management of acute severe bronchospasm. Inhaled beta-2 selective agonists can be delivered successfully in patients with acute severe bronchospasm with a metered dose inhaler and spacer,[4] with potential cost savings. The disadvantage is that this method requires patient instruction and health care professional supervision to make sure the patient is using the device properly. In general, nebulization is preferred for acute severe bronchospasm and is readily adaptable to use with mechanical ventilation. The advantages of nebulized therapy are that the patient is essentially "taken out of the loop" and maximal delivery is ensured. The handheld nebulizer is preferred but requires lip-sealing around the mouthpiece. If a lip-seal cannot be maintained by the patient, delivery of nebulized therapy by mask is needed. Dosages of therapeutic agents for bronchospasm are shown in Table 26-1.

The frequency of inhaled therapy is dependent on the severity of bronchospasm and risk for cardiac side effects. In the young, previously healthy bronchospastic patient with life-threatening asthma, inhalation therapy may be continuous. In the patient with a moderately severe attack who is not in extreme distress and with no significant risk factors for coronary artery disease, inhalation therapy is administered q 15 min × 3 or 4 and then q 1 hr.[5] In older patients and patients at risk for coronary artery disease, the frequency of therapy must be decreased. With improvement, the inhaled therapy dosing interval is broadened to q 3 hr, q 4 hr, and finally q 6 hr. Tachycardia is not an appropriate indicator for limiting aggressiveness of inhaled beta-agonist therapy in patients with life-threatening bronchospasm. Chest pain or premature ventricular contractions (PVCs) believed related to adrenergic therapy are more specific reasons to decrease inhaled beta-agonists.

The use of theophylline (intravenous aminophylline) for acute bronchospasm is controversial.[6,7] Although theophylline is a proven bronchodilator vs. placebo, when added to a full therapeutic regimen of inhaled beta-2 selective agonist, additional clinical efficacy is questionable. Although some prospective studies do demonstrate its efficacy when added to a beta-agonist in a patient with acute bronchospasm, most studies do not, and meta-analysis fails to demonstrate a statistically significant treatment effect but does reveal significant toxicity. If the use of IV aminophylline is elected, the maintenance infusion rate depends on patient age and other metabolism issues.

The dose ranges for maintenance infusion of theophylline are as follows:

- Maintenance infusion dose ranges: adult, 0.6 mg/kg/hr; youth, 0.9 mg/kg/hr; elderly, 0.4 mg/kg/hr; patient in heart failure, 0.2 to 0.3 mg/kg/hr; patient with liver disease, 0.2 to 0.3 mg/kg/hr
- Increased continuous infusion for cigarette smokers
- Decreased continuous infusion for patients receiving cimetidine or who have upper respiratory tract infection

If the patient is not currently taking theophylline, a loading dose of 6 mg/kg over 30 minutes should be administered at the start of the maintenance infusion.

Although inhaled anticholinergic therapy is not as effective as inhaled beta-agonists for acute bronchospasm, it has an adjunctive therapeutic role. The role of inhaled anticholinergic therapy as an additive to adrenergic therapy for acute bronchospasm is more strongly supported than the adding of IV aminophylline.[8,9] Although in the literature support is mixed for the addition of inhaled anticholinergic therapy to a full dosing regimen of adrenergic bronchodilator therapy, most prospective studies demonstrate additional benefit. The onset of action of anticholinergic therapy begins approximately 30 minutes after administration and peaks in approximately 2 to 3 hours. The effect lasts 4 to 6 hours. Although atropine can be used, ipratropium is preferred. Inhaled anticholinergic effect does not require serum concentrations. Atropine, when given by the inhaled route, achieves significant serum levels and may be associated with cardiac and CNS side effects and may precipitate bladder neck obstruction and acute-closure, narrow-angle glaucoma. Inhaled ipratropium is as effective as atropine and is poorly absorbed into the systemic circulation when given by the inhaled route. Side effects are minimal. If ipratropium is sprayed directly into the eyes, however, it may precipitate acute-closure, narrow-angle glaucoma. In the United States ipratropium is available only as a metered dose inhaler, and an inspiratory limb adapter with spacer must be used for the mechanically ventilated patient.

Anti-inflammatory Therapy

Steroid therapy should be administered to all patients with severe or persistent bronchospasm.[10] Methylprednisolone, 60 to 125 mg IV q 4 to 6 hr, initially is recommended. As the patient improves, the IV dose is tapered and replaced with an oral regimen. The oral therapy is then tapered and replaced with inhaled steroid therapy.

NEWER MEDICAL THERAPEUTIC APPROACHES

Patients whose condition is refractory to traditional medical therapy for life-threatening bronchospasm may receive temporary (i.e., 30 minutes) benefit from magnesium, a long-known smooth muscle relaxer, in doses of 1 to 2 grains intravenously.[11] In an anecdotal case series (without placebo controls), glucagon has also been advocated to promote bronchodilation.[12] Neither of these drugs has undergone rigorous, well-designed clinical trials to establish efficacy.

Considerations in Patient With Acute Severe Bronchospasm

There is no role for use of IV fluids to overhydrate for the purposing of liquefying or loosening secretions; however, repletion of decreased intravascular volume is clearly indicated. Antibiotics are not indicated for acute bronchospasm unless pneumonia is present. Although acetylcysteine (Mucomyst) may be helpful in some patients with cystic fibrosis, it has no role in the management of acute bronchospasm.

Considerations in Intubated and Mechanically Ventilated Patient[13]

Patients with acute bronchospasm are at risk for barotrauma caused by air trapping. This risk is increased significantly by mechanical ventilation. If hypotension occurs shortly after intubation and institution of mechanical ventilation, the possibility of tension pneumothorax (diagnosed by physical examination and treated with needle aspiration followed by chest tube insertion) should immediately come to mind. A CXR should not be required for the diagnosis of life-threatening tension pneumothorax.

If the physical examination does not support the diagnosis of tension pneumothorax, a CXR should be ordered, and the effect of positive pressure ventilation on venous return to the right side of the heart should be considered. The cause of the hypotension may be as simple as the conversion of negative intrathoracic pressure to positive intrathoracic pressure in a patient with low intravascular volume status (volume therapy required) or as complex as the presence of intrinsic PEEP[14] (see Chapter 24). Intrinsic PEEP occurs when ventilator settings dictate an inadequate inspiratory to expiratory (I:E) ratio. Expiratory time is inadequate to allow full exhalation of ventilator breath, and expiratory flow is still occurring when the next ventilator breath is delivered. This condition may be associated with a marked elevation in intrathoracic pressure and associated hypotension (decreased venous return to the heart) and barotrauma (pneumothorax). Since obstructive airway disease increases the need for expiratory time, mechanically ventilated patients with bronchospasm are at increased risk for intrinsic PEEP. Inspiratory time is determined by minute ventilation (tidal volume and rate) and peak inspiratory flow. The latter determines how rapidly the breath will be delivered. On some ventilators a choice of inspiratory waveform may also influence I:E ratio.

Since the flow at end expiration is not zero, a pressure gradient at end expiration exists. Therefore PEEP exists, even though it is not set on the ventilator. Diagnosis of intrinsic PEEP should be made clinically after institution of mechanical ventilation in patients with hypotension in whom there is no other obvious cause. Higher minute ventilations, especially in the assist-control mode in the awake bronchospastic patient in distress, predispose the patient to intrinsic PEEP. Breathing at a high ventilator breath rate or inappropriately high physician-selected minute ventilation may exacerbate intrinsic PEEP. The treatment of intrinsic PEEP is to decrease inspiratory time, usually by decreasing rate. If hypotension resolves, this maneuver is both diagnostic and therapeutic. Occasionally intrinsic PEEP may manifest itself on the water manometer dial of the ventilator as failure of the dial to return to zero at end expiration. Severe intrinsic PEEP may be present even in the absence of this finding. Severe obstruction may prevent rise of proximal airway pressure, even in the presence of high pressures in the distal alveolar area.

In the intubated patient with severe bronchospasm, inducing heavy sedation and paralysis may be necessary to ensure adequate ventilation and carbon dioxide removal. Unplanned extubation in the paralyzed patient can be catastrophic. In the mechanically ventilated bronchospastic patient with carbon dioxide retention, high peak airway pressure may occur with delivery of the selected inspired tidal volume. To minimize peak airway pressure, the clinician may use sodium bicarbonate to achieve an acceptable pH level (>7.25 to 7.3).[15] When bronchodilator therapy is administered in the intubated bronchospastic patient, the dose of aerosol medication should be doubled. Particles on the endotracheal tube may reduce delivery by 50% or more.

SUMMARY

- Bronchospasm is reversible obstructive airway disease.
- In COPD, bronchospasm is highly variable and may be a major component.
- Therapy should focus on treatment of bronchospasm (bronchodilator therapy) and inflammation (anti-inflammatory therapy).
- All wheezing is not bronchospasm (see box on p. 294).
- Use inhaled beta-2 selective agonists for initial therapy (albuterol or metaproterenol). Use subcutaneous epinephrine or terbutaline in combination with inhaled therapy in patients who are in extreme distress or those in whom inhalation therapy failed.

- Use of theophylline in acute bronchospasm is controversial.
- Inhaled anticholinergic therapy has an adjunctive role (ipratropium is preferred).
- Administer steroids to patients with severe or persistent bronchospasm.
- Intubated patients with bronchospasm who have ventilator support are at risk for barotrauma. Suspect tension pneumothorax if hypotension occurs.
- Monitor respiratory rate and I:E carefully to limit intrinsic PEEP.

REFERENCES

1. Shim CS, Williams MH. Evaluation of the severity of asthma: Patients versus physicians. Am J Med 68:11-13, 1980.
2. Stiell IG, Rivington RN. Adrenergic agents in acute asthma: Valuable new alternatives. Ann Emerg Med 12:493-500, 1983.
3. Amory DW, Burnham SC, Cheney FW. Comparison of the cardiopulmonary effects of subcutaneously administered epinephrine and terbutaline in patients with reversible airway obstruction. Chest 67:279-286, 1975.
4. Newhouse MT, Dolovich MB. Control of asthma by aerosols. N Engl J Med 315:870-874, 1986.
5. Dellinger RP. Status asthmaticus. In Civetta JM, Taylor RW, Kirby RR, eds. Critical Care. Philadelphia: JP Lippincott, 1988, pp 1115-1125.
6. Newhouse MT. Is theophylline obsolete? Chest 98:1-4, 1990.
7. Niewoehner DE. Theophylline therapy—A continued dilemma. Chest 98:5, 1990.
8. Ward MJ, Fentem PH, Smith WH, et al. Ipratropium bromide in acute asthma. Br Med J 282:598-600, 1981.
9. Bryant DH. Nebulized ipratropium bromide in the treatment of acute asthma. Chest 88:24-29, 1985.
10. Haskell RJ, Wong BM, Hansen JE. A double-blind, randomized clinical trial of methylprednisolone in status asthmaticus. Arch Intern Med 143:1324-1325, 1983.
11. Skobeloff EM, Spivey WH, McNamara RM. Intravenous sulfate for the treatment of acute asthma in the emergency department. JAMA 262:1210-1213, 1989.
12. Wilson JE, Nelson RN. Glucagon as a therapeutic agent in the treatment of asthma. J Emerg Med 8:127-130, 1990.
13. Mansel JK, Stogner SW, Petrini MR, et al. Mechanical ventilation in patients with acute severe asthma. Am J Med 89:42-48, 1990.
14. Tobin MJ, Lodato RF. PEEP, auto-PEEP, and waterfalls. Chest 96:449-451, 1989.
15. Menitove SM, Goldring RM. Combined ventilator and bicarbonate strategy in the management of status asthmaticus. Am J Med 74:898, 1983.

CHAPTER 27

Conventional Ventilator Support

Karl L. Yang · Guillermo Gutierrez

The primary goal of mechanical ventilatory support in critically ill patients is to help the lungs eliminate CO_2 produced by cellular metabolic processes while waiting for the underlying disease process to resolve. Furthermore, endotracheal intubation, a requirement for positive-pressure mechanical ventilation, allows a direct route for the administration of gases with high oxygen concentration. Therefore mechanical ventilation serves two functions, ventilation or removal of CO_2, and oxygenation, the enrichment of arterial blood with oxygen (Table 27-1).

Management of respiratory failure begins with the identification of the patient with respiratory distress. Evaluation should begin with clinical findings. One of the most easily evaluated clinical variables is the respiratory rate. Nearly all patients with respiratory distress demonstrate tachypnea. A respiratory rate of 25

TABLE 27-1 Arterial Blood Variables Affected by Ventilation and Oxygenation

	Ventilation	Oxygenation
Variables controlled by clinician	Minute ventilation	FIO_2
Variables affected	PCO_2 pH	PO_2 O_2 saturation

breaths/min or greater is a sensitive although not specific indicator of respiratory dysfunction. Another important clinical sign of respiratory distress is the use of accessory muscles of breathing. These muscles include the strap muscles, the abdominal muscles, and the intercostal muscles. Further clinical signs of worsening respiratory failure include those of increased sympathetic tone. Tachycardia, hypertension, and diaphoresis, along with an increased respiratory rate, imply impending respiratory collapse. When these signs are present, the patient should be intubated endotracheally and appropriate respiratory support provided. More commonly, the critical care physician must decide about intubation and mechanical ventilation when patients demonstrate some degree of compensation. If the patient is sufficiently stable to allow more information to be gathered, a decision concerning intubation and mechanical ventilation can be made by looking at additional variables that apply to several categories of respiratory function. These additional categories include gas exchange and mechanics of breathing.

GAS EXCHANGE

Adequate gas exchange requires saturation of the hemoglobin molecules with O_2 and elimination of CO_2 to prevent acid-base imbalance. Practically, arterial blood gas measurements are used to assess gas exchange of both O_2 and CO_2 simultaneously. A useful clinical target for adequate oxygenation is the PaO_2 that provides an arterial oxygen saturation of 90% or greater. Another helpful variable is PaO_2/FIO_2. A ratio of less than 250 suggests serious ventilation/perfusion mismatch. Hypoxemia alone should raise another question. Is loss of functional residual capacity (FRC) the cause of the hypoxemia? Is compliance decreased enough to make a patient's work of breathing excessive? Such patients may require an intervention to improve compliance. Some of these patients may be candidates for continuous positive airway pressure (CPAP). If CPAP is successful, endotracheal intubation and mechanical ventilation may be avoided. The $PaCO_2$ provides a clinical measure of CO_2 elimination and alveolar ventilation. If the $PaCO_2$ is elevated such that an acute respiratory acidosis is present, the patient almost certainly requires endotracheal intubation and mechanical ventilatory support. The pH value is the key to interpreting the $PaCO_2$. An elevated $PaCO_2$ with a normal pH may indicate that an underlying acid-base abnormality exists and that the retained CO_2 is compensatory. A pulse oximeter provides no information about $PaCO_2$. Use of the pulse oximeter alone, without the additional information of arterial blood gases, may provide insufficient information in the SICU.

RESPIRATORY MECHANICS

Patients may require ventilator support, even if arterial blood gases appear to be satisfactory. For these patients, the work of breathing may be excessive. Variables that reflect the work of breathing include respiratory rate, vital capacity, and expired minute ventilation. For example, a patient is unlikely to maintain the effort necessary to continue a respiratory rate of 30 to 35 breaths/min. Serious consideration should be given to intubating and mechanically supporting the patient with a respiratory rate of 30 to 35 breaths/min. Patients who have markedly diminished vital capacity, less than 10 to 12 ml/kg, are unlikely to maintain adequate ventilation. Finally, patients with large minute ventilations, the product of respiratory rate and tidal volume, are also unlikely to sustain the effort necessary to maintain gas exchange. Minute ventilations of greater than 10 L/min are excessive for most patients. If gas exchange is adequate, the patient does not have physical signs of respiratory collapse, and respiratory mechanics appear to be compromised, a trial of CPAP may be worthwhile. If CPAP improves lung compliance and reduces the work of breathing, the patient may be able to avoid intubation and mechanical ventilation.

Fig. 27-1 summarizes clinical guidelines for ventilator support. The clinician may need to deviate from them for specific patients.

Once the decision has been made to intubate and mechanically ventilate the patient, several additional decisions must be made, including modes of ventilation, recommended settings of respiratory rate, inspired gas concentration, the use of positive end-expiratory pressure (PEEP), and appropriate tidal volumes. Chapter 28 discusses the management of patients who fail conventional ventilator support. The usual problem in patients who fail conventional support is the inability to exchange gas in the lungs at pressures that the lungs can tolerate without further injury. Alternative therapies are available and are of current interest. Finally, Chapter 54 contains a discussion of variables that are useful in monitoring pulmonary function.

MODES OF VENTILATION

The two major modes of mechanical ventilation are negative pressure, akin to the normal physiologic function in which air moves into the lungs in response to negative pleural pressure, and positive-pressure ventilation, in which air is pushed into the lungs by increases in airway pressure. Negative-pressure ventilation was used widely during the polio epidemic of the 1940s and 1950s ("the iron lungs"), and it remains a viable alternative in patients with neuromuscular disorders and compliant lungs. However, the vast majority of critically ill patients with respiratory failure have stiff lungs, and it would be impossible to ventilate them with a negative-pressure device. Therefore positive-pressure ventilation has been the standard ventilatory method for the last 25 years. This chapter reviews the various modes of positive-pressure mechanical ventilation and the indications for their use.

The three basic modes of positive-pressure mechanical ventilation are control-mode ventilation, assist-control ventilation, and intermittent mandatory ventilation.

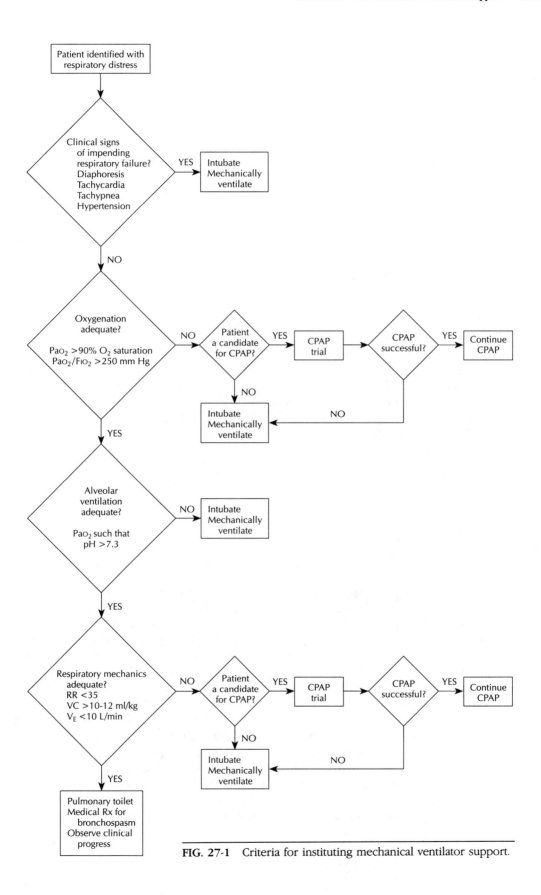

FIG. 27-1 Criteria for instituting mechanical ventilator support.

Control Mode Ventilation

The oldest mode of ventilation is control-mode ventilation (CMV), in which a preset tidal volume is delivered at specified time intervals and at a given flow rate. Total ventilation is regulated by the physician, who determines the respiratory rate and tidal volume delivered by the ventilator. With this mode of ventilation, spontaneous efforts by the patient do not trigger the ventilator to deliver a breath. Depending on the ventilator, a small spontaneous breath may still be generated if the patient uses an extraordinary degree of effort.[1] CMV is rarely used today because the patient has no control of ventilator functions, whereas the support required from the ventilator may vary according to the metabolic activity of the tissues. As a result of this lack of cooperation between patient and ventilator, struggles against the ventilator can be extremely uncomfortable or dangerous unless the patient is sedated. This mode has little use in the critical care setting. It should be used only if the patient is apneic, paralyzed, or deeply sedated and the respiratory drive depressed. By assuming control of the patient's ventilation, the physician also becomes fully responsible for the maintenance of adequate gas exchange. Therefore careful observation and frequent blood gas tests are mandatory.

Assist-Control Ventilation

Assist-control ventilation (ACV) was developed to overcome the major disadvantage of CMV, lack of patient-ventilator feedback interaction. This mode allows the patient to set the minute ventilation most adequate for a given level of CO_2 production by delivering a preset tidal volume whenever the patient produces a negative inspiratory effort. A pressure transducer detects the subatmospheric, or negative, airway pressure and triggers the ventilator, resulting in the delivery of the preset tidal volume. If the patient fails to initiate a spontaneous effort, a predetermined number of breaths (backup rate) with a set tidal volume will be delivered to the patient to ensure adequate ventilation. In other words, the patient receives a guaranteed minimum minute ventilation. Because the ventilator assists on every spontaneous breath, minute ventilation can be increased with minimal increases in the work of breathing. ACV is used frequently for full ventilatory support of critically ill patients. Although the work of breathing is usually decreased with this mode of ventilation, a decrease in the work of breathing may not always be the case. Significant muscular effort may result from improper ventilator setup.[2]

Intermittent Mandatory Ventilation

Intermittent mandatory ventilation (IMV) is possibly the most common mode of mechanical ventilation used today. With IMV, the ventilator delivers a fixed number of breaths at a predetermined tidal volume, but in between those breaths, the patient is allowed to breathe spontaneously at the tidal volume developed by his/her own efforts. To avoid air stacking of ventilator-initiated and spontaneous breaths, the ventilator-initiated breath is synchronized with the patient's own inspiratory effort. This mode is termed "synchronized intermittent mandatory ventilation" (SIMV). By initially setting a high ventilatory rate, most of the work of breathing is done by the ventilator. As the lungs improve, the ventilator-initiated breaths are gradually decreased so that the patient assumes a greater load of the work associated with breathing. The patient's minute ventilation during IMV is the sum of the ventilator-initiated breaths at the predetermined tidal volume and the patient's spontaneous breaths, with their associated tidal volumes. SIMV was originally developed as a method to wean difficult patients from mechanical ventilation. With IMV, it is possible to progressively decrease the number of ventilator-initiated breaths until the patient's own efforts provide the level of ventilation needed. Such an approach avoids the stresses imposed on the patient by a T-tube weaning procedure, in which the patient is disconnected from the ventilator and observed for a short time. During these trials, breathing occurs through the endotracheal tube attached to a T piece.[3] Well-designed prospective studies have not shown IMV to be more effective than the traditional T tube as a weaning technique.[4,5] Investigators have proposed that SIMV decreases the detrimental hemodynamic effects of positive-pressure ventilation by decreasing mean airway pressure,[6,7] but little evidence to support this theory exists.[8] Other proposed advantages of SIMV over ACV are the avoidance of respiratory alkalosis,[9] the prevention of muscle atrophy,[3] and decreased patient-ventilator dyssynchrony, resulting in a reduced need for sedation.[10] Again, little evidence supports these claims. In a recent study, investigators[11,12] found no differences in the incidence of respiratory alkalosis between patients ventilated with ACV and IMV.[13] The patient's underlying condition is more likely to be the major contributing factor to the development of respiratory alkalosis than the mode of ventilation chosen.

A major disadvantage of SIMV is the presence of a demand valve that is activated by the patient's breathing effort. The purpose of this valve is to allow spontaneous breaths. It opens when the airway pressure becomes negative as the patient initiates a breath, allowing the gas mixture to flow into the ventilator circuit and into the lungs. Because of the large negative pressure required to open this valve, and the delay of fresh gas inflow required to meet the demand of the patient, the work of breathing in a patient hungry for air may be extremely high. It must be stressed that improper selection of ventilator settings causes further distress to the already fatigued muscles of respiration by forcing them to work excessively. By carefully observing the patient and by appropriately adjusting the ventilator settings, the patient's discomfort during mechanical ventilation can be minimized, if not totally avoided.

OTHER VENTILATORY VARIABLES

In addition to the mode of ventilation, a number of other settings should be specified when writing mechanical ventilator orders. These include the respiratory rate, FIO_2, PEEP, tidal volume, trigger sensitivity, ventilator flow pattern, and inspiratory time.

Respiratory Rate

One of the goals of mechanical ventilation is to allow the respiratory muscles to rest; therefore it is important to select a respiratory rate that meets the patient's ventilatory requirement.

Generally, the backup rate may be set at 2 to 4 breaths/min fewer than the patient's spontaneous respiratory rate. This should provide adequate ventilation and prevent serious hypoventilation if the patient becomes apneic.

Oxygen Concentration in Inspired Gas

An adequate FIO_2 is important to prevent arterial hypoxemia. How much oxygen should be given to a patient depends on the level of arterial O_2 saturation. A general rule is to use the lowest possible FIO_2 capable of maintaining an arterial O_2 saturation >90%. The rationale for using low levels of FIO_2 is the avoidance of O_2 toxicity, which may occur even at relatively low levels of FIO_2. Whereas an FIO_2 of 1 can produce gas-exchange alterations in 24 to 48 hours, the use of an FIO_2 of 0.50 or less for a long time (up to several weeks) is generally considered safe.[14]

Positive End-Expiratory Pressure

If necessary, PEEP should be used to keep the FIO_2 at or below 0.50. The effects of PEEP on cardiac output and O_2 transport should be considered when using this therapeutic modality. The use of PEEP is indicated in patients with severe hypoxemia, such as those with the adult respiratory distress syndrome, since it improves oxygenation and minimizes the risk of O_2 toxicity. PEEP improves oxygenation by recruiting previously closed alveoli for gas exchange.[15] PEEP also helps redistribute the fluid in partially filled alveoli from the center to the periphery[16] to facilitate better gas exchange. The major complications of PEEP are hemodynamic compromise and barotrauma.[17] PEEP levels ≥10 cm H_2O can result in hemodynamic instability as venous return decreases and the interventricular septum is either stiffened or even pushed into the left ventricle. These changes decrease stroke volume. A flow-directed pulmonary artery catheter should be inserted to monitor the intrathoracic hemodynamics when using high levels of PEEP.

Patients with severe airway obstruction may exhibit a phenomenon termed "intrinsic PEEP." This phrase describes the presence of a positive intrathoracic pressure at the end of expiration when the expiratory time is not long enough to allow full exhalation of the tidal volume. In mechanically ventilated patients with obstructive airway disease, a significant level of intrinsic PEEP occurs 60% of the time.[18] Hemodynamic compromise also may result from high levels of intrinsic PEEP. To decrease the effect of intrinsic PEEP, intensive bronchodilation, a longer expiratory time, or PEEP ventilation at a slightly lower level than the intrinsic PEEP may be tried. (See Chapters 25 and 54.)

Tidal Volume

Tidal volume may be set at 5 to 15 ml/kg body weight. The use of smaller tidal volumes is preferable, because an excessively large tidal volume can actually increase lung injury by the stretching of lung tissue. High tidal volumes are also associated with increased intrathoracic pressure, which in some situations may cause hemodynamic instability. The advantage of using large tidal volumes is the prevention of alveolar collapse resulting from a higher mean airway pressure.[19,20] In turn, this increase in FRC improves oxygenation. On the other hand, large tidal volumes also predispose to hemodynamic compromise and barotrauma. It is important to recognize that a significant fraction of the selected tidal volume never reaches the patient, since it goes into the expansion of circuit tubing, especially in those patients with low lung compliance and elevated airway pressures. The extent of the volume loss depends on the length, size, and compliance of the ventilator tubing.

Trigger Sensitivity

Trigger sensitivity is the level of negative pressure that a patient is required to generate before the ventilator senses the effort and delivers a breath. Usually, the trigger sensitivity is set at -2 cm H_2O. The setting is important because a low trigger sensitivity can increase the work of breathing by forcing the patient to generate large negative inspiratory pressures in order to trigger the ventilator. In some cases, the patient's work of breathing with a ventilator exceeds the work with spontaneous breathing, thus causing further respiratory muscle fatigue.[21,22] Therefore trigger sensitivity should be

carefully titrated by observing the patient's breathing pattern.

Ventilator Flow Patterns

Most ventilators have two flow patterns: the square wave flow, in which flow remains constant during much of inspiration, and decelerating flow pattern, in which an initial high inspiratory flow is gradually tapered. Conflicting information exists concerning the influence of flow pattern on the work of breathing and gas exchange. One study showed no significant differences in gas exchange in patients ventilated with either flow pattern,[23] although a decelerating pattern resulted in lower mean airway pressure. Another study showed that a decelerating flow pattern resulted in better oxygenation and lower respiratory system compliance.[24] A high inspiratory flow rate also improves gas exchange and ventilation distribution[25] and reduces the work of breathing[22,26] in patients with chronic obstructive pulmonary disease. This improvement appears to relate to the prolongation of expiratory time.

Safety Features

Every ventilator has a number of alarms designed to alert the health care team when certain ventilatory measurements of function are exceeded or not met. Given the importance of ventilation to the patient's survival, these alarms should be heeded immediately. If the caregiver is unsure as to their origin, the patient should be disconnected from the ventilator and ventilated manually.

To prevent barotrauma, the peak airway pressure limit can be specified, and when it exceeds the specified pressure, an expiratory valve opens to prevent further increase in airway pressure. However, adequate ventilation may not be delivered to the patient if the high-pressure limit is exceeded frequently and significant volume is lost through the expiratory valve. Peak airway pressure can be reduced by lowering the tidal volume, decreasing the inspiratory flow rate, and lowering airway resistance. Inspiratory flow rate is also important, because an inappropriate flow rate can increase the patient's work of breathing with the venti-

TABLE 27-2   Initial Settings for Mechanical Ventilation

Factor	Setting
Mode	ACV or SIMV
Respiratory frequency	Two breaths below spontaneous
Tidal volume	5-15 ml/kg body weight
FIO_2	1 initially, then titrate to keep SaO_2 >90%
Inspiratory flow rate	60-80 L/min
Trigger sensitivity	−2 cm H_2O
PEEP	Use if required to maintain SaO_2 >90% with FIO_2 ≤0.5

lator.[2,22] For a normal lung, a respiratory flow rate of 60 L/min is adequate. For someone with increased respiratory drive, a higher flow rate (80 L/min) is more appropriate (Table 27-2).

OTHER MODES OF MECHANICAL VENTILATION
Pressure-Support Ventilation

Pressure-support ventilation (PSV) is a new and popular mode of ventilation. It can be used to provide full ventilatory support and also to wean patients from ventilatory support. During PSV, each spontaneous breath is augmented by a predetermined pressure. PSV is triggered by the patient's effort to breathe, and inspiratory flow continues while the airway pressure rapidly approaches the predetermined level. The inspiratory flow is terminated when the inspiratory flow rate has decreased to a specified rate (5 L/min in some ventilators and 25% of peak flow rate in others). PSV is not recommended in patients with a blunted respiratory drive or in those with high respiratory impedance.[27] PSV in these patients leads to a severe respiratory acidosis when the paitent is apneic.

A major advantage of PSV over other modes of ventilation is that the patient can control the respiratory rate, duration of inspiration, and inspiratory flow rate; therefore better synchronization between mechanical ventilation and spontaneous breathing can be achieved. This property may explain why PSV is better tolerated and more comfortable for the patient than other modes.[28] A number of studies have demonstrated the usefulness of PSV in ventilatory support, especially during weaning. A pressure-support level of 20 cm H_2O has been shown to decrease the work of breathing and electromyographic activity of the diaphragm in a group of patients who could not be weaned from the ventilator. Furthermore, because of the increased airway resistance from the endotracheal tube, some physicians use a small amount of pressure support (usually 5 to 10 cm H_2O) to overcome this resistance. Extubation from this level of support is usually well tolerated. However, despite the encouraging results from several studies, specific clinical indications for PSV have not been thoroughly defined.

Airway Pressure Release Ventilation

Another new mode of mechanical ventilation is airway pressure release ventilation (APRV). With APRV, the patient receives CPAP that is transiently decreased during expiration. The duration of pressure release is approximately 1.5 seconds. The theory behind APRV is that airway pressure should be kept at a positive level for as much of the respiratory cycle as possible in order to stabilize those alveoli which tend to collapse. APRV theoretically should help improve oxygenation, although its major advantage is a lower *peak* airway pressure than conventional intermittent positive-pressure ventilation. Yet *mean* airway pressure may be higher. Since APRV is relatively new, specific indications for its use are still evolving.

High-Frequency Ventilation

High-frequency ventilation (HFV) is a concept totally different from that of intermittent positive pressure. With HFV the respiratory frequency is substantially greater, and the tidal volumes are much less than those used in conventional ventilation. The three types of HFV are (1) high-frequency positive-pressure ventilation, (2) high-frequency jet ventilation (HFJV), and (3) high-frequency oscillation.

HFV is associated with lower intrathoracic pressure swings because of the relatively small tidal volume delivered, resulting in a lower peak airway pressure. On the other hand, the incidence of barotrauma with HFV has been reported to be similar to that of CMV in a number of studies.[29] HFV has been reported to be more effective than conventional positive-pressure ventilation in patients with large bronchopleural fistulae.[30] Clinical trials with HFV showed that patients with relatively normal lung compliance experienced better gas exchange than those with decreased lung compliance.[31] Another theoretic advantage of HFV is less hemodynamic compromise than that found with CMV. As discussed in Chapter 24, the reduced magnitude of intrathoracic pressure swings may improve cardiac function. However, clinical studies have not supported these claims.[32] Because HFV requires high flow rates, its operation can result in dangerous levels of air trapping and intrathoracic pressure increases. Patients with obstructive disease and those with increased lung compliance are especially at risk. In summary, HFV has no clear advantage over CMV, and its operation requires considerable expertise. Its application in clinical practice has been limited.

WEANING FROM MECHANICAL VENTILATION

The clinician should consider weaning a patient from the ventilator when the patient's underlying condition begins to improve. The decision to wean is not the same as the decision to extubate a patient. Excessive secretions or depressed mental status may require endotracheal intubation, even if positive-pressure ventilation is not necessary. Since both elevated pressures and FIO_2 have the potential of lung injury, wean the most injurious component first. For example, if a patient were managed with an FIO_2 of 0.9, a PEEP of 8 cm H_2O, a peak airway pressure of 45 cm H_2O, and a mean airway pressure of 18 cm H_2O, wean the FIO_2 first. On the other hand, if a patient were managed with an FIO_2 of 0.6, a PEEP of 18 cm H_2O, a peak airway pressure of 60 cm H_2O, and a mean airway pressure of 34 cm H_2O, reduce the airway pressures first. If the tidal volume is reasonable, reducing PEEP is a logical step.

Three methods of weaning currently employed include T-tube wean, IMV, and PSV (Table 27-3).

The selection of a weaning method is often determined by the familiarity of the physician with that method. Current literature does not support the claims made for a superior advantage of one method over the others. If the tra-

TABLE 27-3 Methods of Weaning From Mechanical Ventilator

Method	Description
T tube	T piece is placed for 30 minutes and patient carefully observed for signs of respiratory distress; if arterial blood gases remain adequate and respiratory distress does not occur, patient is extubated
IMV	IMV rate is decreased by 2-breath decrements until it reaches 4 breaths/min; if arterial blood gases remain adequate and no distress occurs, patient is extubated
PSV	Pressure-support level is gradually decreased by 3 to 6 cm H_2O decrements for as long as the patient can tolerate; patient can be extubated once pressure support reaches 5 cm H_2O

TABLE 27-4 Predictors of Weaning Outcome*

Predictor	Value
Respiratory frequency	<30 breaths/min
Tidal volume	>300 ml/breath
Maximal inspiratory pressure	<−30 cm H_2O
Minute ventilation	<10 L/min
Static compliance	>30 ml/cm H_2O
Rapid shallow breathing index (respiratory frequency/tidal volume)	<100 breaths/min/L

*All predictors should be measured during spontaneous breathing except for static compliance, which is measured during mechanical ventilation.

ditional T-tube trial is employed, weaning parameters should be obtained to assess the ability of a patient to undergo a weaning trial (Table 27-4). A new index called the rapid shallow breathing index, consisting of the ratio of respiratory frequency in breaths per minute to the tidal volume in liters, was found to be more accurate than traditional variables in predicting the weaning outcome. When the rapid shallow index is greater than 100 breaths/min/L, it is unlikely that the patient can be successfully weaned from the ventilator.[33]

Mechanical ventilation is a life-saving procedure in most circumstances, but its use is not without risks. The physician should maintain a high level of vigilance, and monitoring should be carefully matched to the patient's degree of respiratory failure. With careful attention, adjustment of ventilator settings can help reduce the patient's respiratory distress.

SUMMARY

- Mechanical ventilation is a lifesaving procedure but has inherent risks.
- The primary goal of mechanical ventilatory support is elimination of CO_2 produced by metabolism, while waiting for the underlying disease process to resolve.
- Criteria for intubating and mechanically supporting patients consider clinical correlation, gas exchange, and respiratory mechanics (see Fig. 27-1).
- ACV and IMV are generally used modes of ventilator support of critically ill patients.

- PSV, APRV, and HFV are newer modes of ventilation. Their use depends on clinical condition of patient and requires experienced users.
- In general, for acute respiratory failure, use a backup ventilator rate 2 to 4 breaths/min below the patient's spontaneous respiratory rate.
- In general, use the lowest FIO_2 that allows one arterial O_2 saturation >90%.
- PEEP is indicated for severe hypoxemia. Use PEEP to help keep FIO_2 at or below 0.50.
- In general, use tidal volume 5 to 15 mg/kg body weight.

REFERENCES

1. Bonner JT, Hall JR. Respiratory Intensive Care of the Adult Patient. St. Louis: CV Mosby, 1985, p 90.
2. Marini JJ, Capps JS, Culver BH. The inspiratory work of breathing during assisted mechanical ventilation. Chest 87:612, 1985.
3. Downs JB, Klein EF, Desautels D, et al. Intermittent mandatory ventilation: A new approach to weaning patients from mechanical ventilators. Chest 64:331, 1973.
4. Hastings PR, Bushnell LS, Skillman JJ, et al. Cardiorespiratory dynamics during weaning with IMV versus spontaneous ventilation in good-risk cardiac-surgery patients. Anesthesiology 58:429, 1980.
5. Schachter EN, Tucker D, Beck GJ. Does intermittent mandatory ventilation accelerate weaning? JAMA 246:1210, 1981.
6. Kirby RR, Downs JB, Civetta JM, et al. High level positive end-expiratory pressure (PEEP) in acute respiratory insufficiency. Chest 67:156, 1975.
7. Downs JB, Douglas ME, Sanfelippo PM, et al. Ventilatory pattern, intrapleural pressure, and cardiac output. Anesth Analg 56:88, 1977.
8. Hudson LD, Tooker J, Haisch C, et al. Comparison of assisted ventilation and PEEP with IMV and CPAP in ARDS patients [abstract]. Am Rev Respir Dis 177:129, 1978.
9. Downs JB, Block AJ, Venum KB. Intermittent mandatory ventilation in the treatment of patients with chronic obstructive pulmonary disease. Anesth Analg 55:437, 1974.
10. Petty TL. Intermittent mandatory ventilation reconsidered. Crit Care Med 9:620, 1981.
11. Christopher KL, Neff TA, Bowman JL, et al. Demand and continuous flow intermittent mandatory ventilation systems. Chest 87:625, 1985.
12. Op't Holt TB, Hall MW, Bass JB, et al. Comparison of changes in airway pressure during continuous positive airway pressure (CPAP) between demand valve and continuous flow devices. Respir Care 82:1200, 1982.
13. Culpepper JA, Rinaldo JE, Rogers RM. Effect of mechanical ventilator mode on tendency to-

wards respiratory alkalosis. Am Rev Respir Dis 120:1039, 1979.

14. Bryan CL, Jenkinson SG. Oxygen toxicity. Clin Chest Med 9:141-152, 1988.

15. Katz JA, Ozanne GM, Zinn SE, et al. Time course and mechanisms of lung volume increase with PEEP in acute pulmonary failure. Anesthesiology 54:9, 1981.

16. Malo J, Ali J, Wood LDH. How does positive end-expiratory pressure reduce intrapulmonary shunt in canine pulmonary edema? J Appl Physiol 57:1002, 1984.

17. Quist J, Ponto PP, Idan H, Wilson RS, et al. Hemodynamic response to mechanical ventilation with PEEP. The effect of hypervolemia. Anesthesiology 55:53, 1981.

18. Rossi A, Gottfried SB, Zocchi L. Measurements of static lung compliance of the total respiratory system in patients with acute respiratory failure during mechanical ventilation: The effect of intrinsic positive end-expiratory pressure. Am Rev Respir Dis 131:672, 1985.

19. Burnham SC, Martin WE, Cheney FW. The effects of various tidal volumes on gas exchange in pulmonary edema. Anesthesiology 37:27, 1972.

20. Bendixen HH, Bullwinkle B, Hedley-White J, Laver MB. Atelectasis and shunting during spontaneous ventilation in anesthetized patients. Anesthesiology 25:297, 1964.

21. Ayres SM, Kozam RL, Lukas DS. The effects of intermittent positive pressure breathing on intrathoracic pressure, pulmonary mechanics and the work of breathing. Am Rev Respir Dis 87:370, 1976.

22. Marini JJ, Rodriguez RM, Lamb V. The inspiratory workload of patient-initiated mechanical ventilation. Am Rev Respir Dis 134:902, 1986.

23. Johansson H. Effects on breathing mechanics and gas exchange of different inspiratory gas flow patterns in patients undergoing respiratory treatment. Acta Anaesthesiol Scand 19:19, 1975.

24. Al-Saady N, Bennett ED. Decelerating inspiratory flow waveform improves lung mechanics and gas exchange in patients on intermittent positive pressure ventilation. Intensive Care Med 11:68, 1985.

25. Connors AF, McCaffree DR, Gray BA. Effect of inspiratory flow rate on gas exchange during mechanical ventilation. Am Rev Respir Dis 124:537, 1981.

26. Sassoon CSH, Mahutte CK, Te T, et al. Work of breathing and airway occlusion pressure during assist-mode mechanical ventilation. Chest 93:571, 1988.

27. Marini JJ. Mechanical ventilation. In Simmons DH, ed. Current Pulmonology, vol 9. Chicago: Year Book, 1988, p 165.

28. MacIntyre NR. Respiratory function during pressure support ventilation. Chest 89:677, 1986.

29. High-frequency oscillatory ventilation compared with conventional mechanical ventilation in the treatment of respiratory failure in premature infants. N Engl J Med 320:88, 1989.

30. Carlon G, Ray C Jr, Klain M, et al. High frequency positive pressure ventilation in management of a patient with bronchopleural fistula. Anesthesiology 52:160, 1980.

31. Turnbull A, Carlton G, Howland W, et al. High frequency jet ventilation in major airway or pulmonary disruption. Ann Thorac Surg 32:468, 1981.

32. Traverse J, Korvenranta H, Adams E, et al. Cardiovascular effects of high frequency oscillatory and jet ventilation. Chest 96:1400, 1989.

33. Yang KL, Tobin MJ. A prospective study of indexes predicting the outcome of trials of weaning from mechanical ventilation. N Engl J Med 324:1445, 1991.

CHAPTER 28

Strategies for Pulmonary Support When Conventional Ventilation Methods Fail

Jerome H. Abrams

Conventional approaches to ventilator support fail in a subset of patients who have had a trial of positive-pressure ventilation. For these patients, satisfactory gas exchange at acceptable levels of fraction of inspired oxygen (FIO_2) and airway pressure is impossible. When patients reach this point in their clinical course, pulmonary compliance is usually markedly decreased, peak airway pressures are elevated, and mean airway pressures are high. The result is probable continued injury to the lung by the very means used to support pulmonary function during severe pulmonary failure.

Three features of acute lung injury deserve special mention. The first is that lung injury is frequently heterogeneous. Gattinoni et al.[1] have estimated that in severe acute lung injury, 30% to 40% of the total lung volume can participate in gas exchange. The residual functional lung must perform not simply the gas exchange necessary for an adult at rest, but the supranormal gas exchange of a patient with systemic hypermetabolism. In such patients, minute ventilation may exceed 20 L/min, rather than the normal 5 to 7 L/min. More striking specific ventilation, or ventilation per gram of tissue participating in gas exchange, may be 10 to 20 times greater than normal.[1] The situation may be worsened by another type of mismatch. The greater the lung injury, the smaller the remaining residual functional lung. However, the greater the lung injury, the greater the associated systemic hypermetabolism. When systemic oxygen delivery needs are the greatest, corresponding to the most severe lung injury, the amount of functional lung available for increased oxygen and carbon dioxide exchange is the smallest. Under these circumstances, conventional pulmonary support requires elevated inspired partial pressures of oxygen and increased airway pressures to maintain gas exchange. Each of these features has potential for worsening the lung injury.

Second, conventional ventilator support uses oscillatory breathing patterns and requires the lung to function as a bellows. Higher frequencies typically are selected as lung injury worsens. The clinician should recognize that the bellows action of the lung is necessary for carbon dioxide elimination, but is not required for oxygenation. Oxygenation can be accomplished with the method of apneic oxygenation, in which the lungs are maintained in inflation and oxygen is administered continuously.[2] Alternative strategies of pulmonary support exploit this distinction.

Third, the time course of lung injury has implications for therapy. Changing populations of cellular anatomic components, changing compliance, and varying tensile strength of tissues all contribute to time-varying constraints on support. The clinician's approach to a patient varies with the duration of acute lung injury.

TIME COURSE OF ACUTE LUNG INJURY

Acute lung injury has been divided into the acute phase, the subacute phase, and the chronic phase.[3,4] The acute phase lasts from the initial insult through approximately day 6 and is marked by edema fluid that produces thickened alveolar walls and interlobular septa. Of importance for the present discussion, type I pneumocytes are early sites of injury in the course of pulmonary failure. In the acute phase, the epithelial lining may have sloughed in certain areas, and only a bare basement membrane remains. Type II pneumocytes appear to be less susceptible to early injury. Subsequently, we shall argue that the early disappearance of type I pneumocytes results in airway pressure, rather than elevated oxygen concentration, as the source of greater injury potential to lung tissue. By the fourth or fifth day after injury, alveoli are lined by type II penumocytes. The capillary endothelium demonstrates edema, but sparing of interendothelial junctions is the rule.

The subacute phase lasts from day 4 to approximately day 10. During this phase, edema and vascular congestion are decreased. Alveoli are lined by type II pneumocytes, and mild interstitial fibrosis appears. The chronic phase continues approximately from day 8 onward. These stages overlap (Fig. 28-1). As Bachofen and Weibel[4] eloquently state: "The transition from the acute to the subacute pattern of changes is gradual and sometimes delayed. Cell proliferation starts while signs of a leaky barrier prevail, and even in far advanced stages edematous areas may be observed side by side with fibrotic regions." Meyrick[3] and Bachofen and Weibel[4] provide extensive discussions of structural changes in acute lung injury. The time course of these changes has implications for therapy, particularly in the management of airway pressure and the elevated inspired oxygen concentrations used in supporting patients with acute respiratory failure.

OXYGEN TOXICITY

Use of inspired concentrations of oxygen above that of room air is associated with a wide range of abnormalities. In one study, breathing 100% oxygen for 24 hours produced substernal distress, sore throat, paresthesias, decreased vital capacity, and symptoms related to eyes and ears.[5] Oxygen therapy may produce injury by free radical production. The damaging agent is not the oxygen molecule itself, but, rather, rad-

Days after injury		Characteristics
		Alveolar hemorrhage / Protein-rich edema fluid in alveoli
0 1 2 3 4 5	Acute phase	Edema fluid / Thickened alveolar walls and interlobular septae / Infiltration of mononuclear cells / Eosinophilic hyaline membranes / Type I pneumocyte injury / Capillary endothelial swelling
6 7	Subacute phase	Edema and vascular congestion decreased / Alveoli lined by type II cells / Mild interstitial fibrosis
8 (or 8+)	Chronic condition	Fibrosis prominent / Coordinated lung repair in survivors

FIG. 28-1 Stages of acute lung injury.

icals of peroxides generated by intracellular metabolic processes. Damage caused by oxygen radicals includes lipid perioxidation, oxidation of protein sulfhydryl groups, and oxidation of nucleic acids. The result is damage to cell membranes, enzyme inactivation, and genetic damage. All of these processes may lead to cell death. As noted previously, type I pneumocytes are among the earliest sites of injury, probably at least in part from elevated oxygen concentrations. With prolonged use of inspired oxygen fractions in current clinical use (60% to 85%), atelectasis, edema, inflammation, and hyalinization of alveolar membranes have been demonstrated. In vitro, the lung macrophage, in the presence of oxygen of 40% to 60% inspired oxygen concentration, demonstrated decreased phagocytosis and decreased chemotaxis.

The white blood cell may play a role in lung damage as a result of hyperoxia. Correlation between white blood cell recruitment and lung damage has been demonstrated in rats and rabbits. Neutropenia induced by nitrogen mustard protects the lung. Macrophages exposed to oxygen have been shown to produce white blood cell chemotactic factors.

Fig. 28-2 summarizes the events believed to

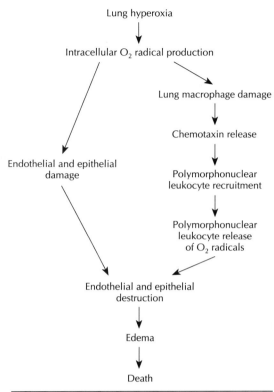

FIG. 28-2 Current mechanism of pulmonary oxygen toxicity. (From Deneke SM, Fanburg BL. Oxygen toxicity of the lung: An update. Br J Anaesth 54:737-749, 1982.)

occur with oxygen toxicity. Reviews of oxygen toxicity may be found in Lodato[6] and Deneke and Fanburg.[7]

EFFECTS OF PRESSURE

Pressure is another factor known to injure lung tissue. Intermittent positive-pressure ventilation with peak pressures of 30 to 45 cm H_2O has resulted in increased pulmonary edema.[8] Disruption of the epithelial layer and alveolar flooding have been demonstrated experimentally in animals receiving ventilation with high airway pressures and high tidal volumes.[9] Healthy sheep demonstrated pulmonary deterioration when ventilated with airway pressures used clinically to treat acute respiratory failure. The investigators concluded that peak airway pressures of 50 cm H_2O contributed to lung

injury and prevented healing processes from being effective.[10]

IMPLICATIONS FOR CARE

Consider a patient with adult respiratory distress syndrome who is receiving mechanical ventilation, usually in the volume control or intermittent mandatory ventilation mode. If the lung injury worsens, pulmonary compliance typically deteriorates. Peak inspiratory pressures, mean airway pressures, and inspired oxygen concentrations all may need to be increased. With these maneuvers, gas exchange frequently improves. However, the increased distending pressures, increased inspired oxygen concentration, and disease process may all contribute to the lung injury. Compliance may then deteriorate further and, at the volumes necessary for gas exchange, airway pressures increase. In an effort to reduce the potential of pressure injury to the lung, the tidal volume is frequently decreased, and the respiratory rate is simultaneously increased to provide comparable alveolar ventilation. With decreased tidal volumes, distribution of ventilation may be inadequate, and oxygenation may deteriorate further. At this point, the duration of lung injury is important. To reach this degree of lung stiffness, the duration of acute lung injury is generally greater than 5 days. Type I pneumocyte injury may already be at a maximum. Consequently, airway pressure injury may have greater potential for injury than elevated inspired concentrations of oxygen. At this stage in the patient's clinical course, we generally make an effort to reduce airway pressures, even at the cost of increased inspired oxygen tension. If both mean and peak airway pressures are at the maximum level that the clinician intends to use, inverse-ratio ventilation may simultaneously improve distribution of ventilation and limit airway pressures.[11,12] Although the use of smaller tidal volumes to decrease pressure may allow satisfactory oxygenation by holding the inspired breath longer, inverse-ratio ventilation may simultaneously compromise alveolar ventilation and produce hypercapnia. If the change to inverse-ratio ventilation is done in a gradual

APPROACH TO ALTERNATIVE VENTILATION STRATEGIES

Is conventional ventilation adequate?

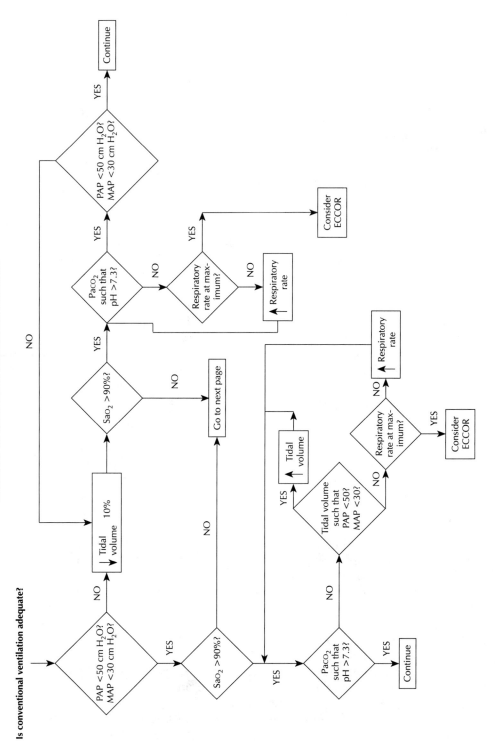

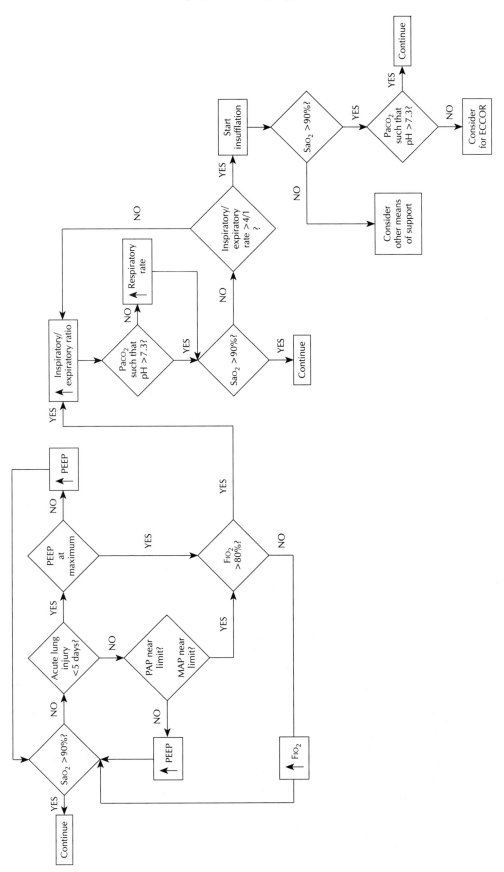

way and renal compensation is adequate, patients may tolerate a gradual increase in $Paco_2$ without clinically significant acidemia.

These ideas may be carried further. Small tidal volumes at rates of 150 or greater are used in high-frequency jet ventilation (HFJV). Currently, bronchopleural fistula is the main indication for HFJV.[13,14] If carbon dioxide elimination is inadequate with jet ventilation, the patient may require extracorporeal pulmonary support. For adults, extracorporeal carbon dioxide removal (ECCOR) is the logical extreme of the idea of reducing tidal volumes and increasing respiratory rate. Tidal volume is reduced to near zero: oxygen is insufflated into lungs that are maintained in inflation with positive end-expiratory pressure (PEEP). The respiratory rate is infinite because the oxygen is insufflated at a constant continuous rate. As Gattinoni et al.[1] have eloquently discussed, ECCOR separates lung function into two distinct components. The lung does not need to perform both oxygenation and carbon dioxide removal at the expense of increased peak airway pressures. Using extracorporeal support, peak airway pressure and specific hyperventilation can be decreased.[1,15,16] Fig. 28-3 shows the essential components of venovenous bypass. In adults, arteriovenous bypass has not been successful.[17]

Venovenous bypass has had recent success in the management of acute lung injury. Apneic oxygenation is used to oxygenate blood. Oxygen is supplied by an insufflation catheter at a constant rate. Functional residual capacity is maintained by PEEP set initially at the patient's mean airway pressure before instituting venovenous bypass. Further consolidation of the lung is prevented by occasional breaths, 2 to 4 breaths/min, that are pressure limited. Mass transport of oxygen is driven by pulmonary blood flow. Because the lungs are not serving as a bellows, elimination of carbon dioxide through the lungs is negligible. Carbon dioxide must therefore be removed extracorporeally, using either a centrifugal or roller pump and gas exchange membranes. One of the advantages of venovenous bypass is elimination of ventilation/perfusion mismatch. In the lung, the only gas exchange that occurs is uptake of

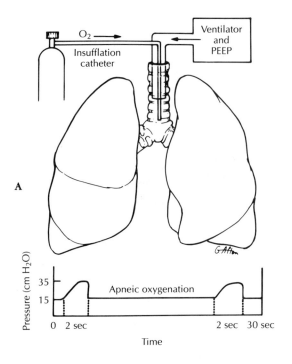

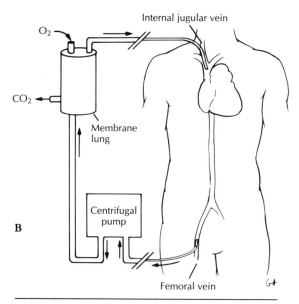

FIG. 28-3 Components of venovenous bypass. **A,** Procedure for maintenance of apneic oxygenation through use of insufflation catheter and ventilator. **B,** Venovenous bypass circuit.

oxygen. With ECCOR, all alveoli that communicate with the tracheobronchial tree ultimately achieve the same alveolar gas composition. All pulmonary blood flow to these alveoli becomes effective, and thus minimizing ventilation/perfusion mismatch.[1,15,16] Other advantages of the venovenous bypass include the following: (1) no reduction in pulmonary blood flow, (2) perfusion of the lung with more fully oxygenated blood, (3) decrease of mean airway pressure, and (4) decreased pulmonary artery pressure.[18]

The flow chart on pp. 312 and 313 outlines our current approach to the use of alternative strategies of ventilation, including venovenous bypass. The problem of adult respiratory distress syndrome that fails support with conventional approaches remains an extremely difficult problem. The increase in survival reported with the use of extracorporeal support was many times greater than that obtained with conventional support. No standard currently exists for the use of alternate ventilation strategies. Current understanding of the true cause of lung injury, the injurious potential of elevated FIO_2, and the potential for damage of increased airway pressures make the approach described on pp. 312 and 313 reasonable.

SUMMARY

- Consider alternate approaches to pulmonary support when satisfactory gas exchange at acceptable FIO_2 and airway pressure is difficult.
- Heterogeneity of lung injury, need for bellows action of lung, and time course of lung injury provide time-varying constraints on pulmonary support.
- Alternate strategies for pulmonary support recognize that bellows action of lung is necessary

for CO_2 removal only. In the extreme, apneic oxygenation is possible.
- Goals of pulmonary support include arterial oxygen saturation ≥90% at minimum FIO_2 and airway pressures. As acute lung injury progresses, pressure injury may be more significant than oxygen toxicity. The flow chart on pp. 312 and 313 demonstrates our suggested approach.

REFERENCES

1. Gattinoni L, Pesenti A, Marcolin R, Damia G. Extracorporeal support in acute respiratory failure. Intensive Care World 5:42-45, 1980.
2. Frumin MJ, Epstein RM, Cohen G. Apneic oxygenation in man. Anesthesiology 20:789, 1959.
3. Meyrick B. Pathology of the adult respiratory distress syndrome. Crit Care Clin 2:405, 1986.
4. Bachofen M, Weibel ER. Structural alterations of lung parenchyma in the adult respiratory distress syndrome. Clin Chest Med 3:35, 1982.
5. Comroe JH, Dripps RD, Dumke PR. Oxygen toxicity: The effect of inhalation of high concentrations of oxygen for 24 hours on normal men at sea level and at a simulated altitude of 18,000. JAMA 128:710, 1945.
6. Lodato RF. Oxygen toxicity. Crit Care Clin 6:749, 1990.
7. Deneke SM, Fanburg BL. Oxygen toxicity of the lung: An update. Br J Anaesth 54:737, 1982.
8. Webb H, Tierney DF. Experimental pulmonary edema due to intermittent positive pressure ventilation with high inflation pressures and protection by positive end-expiratory pressure. Am Rev Respir Dis 110:556-565, 1974.
9. Dreyfuss D, Basset G, Soler P, Saumoz G. Intermittent positive-pressure hyperventilation with high inflation pressures produces pulmonary microvascular injury in rats. Am Rev Respir Dis 132:880-884, 1985.
10. Kolobow T, Moretti MP, Fumagalli R. Severe impairment in lung function induced by high peak airway pressure during mechanical ventilation. Am Rev Respir Dis 135:312-315, 1987.
11. Gurevitch MJ, Van Dyke J, Young E, Jackson K. Improved oxygenation and lower peak airway pressure in severe adult respiratory distress syndrome: Treatment with inverse ratio ventilation. Chest 89:211-213, 1986.
12. Tharratt RS, Allen RP, Albertson TE. Pressure controlled inverse ratio ventilation in severe adult respiratory failure. Chest 94:755-762, 1988.

13. Spinale FG, Linker RW, Crawford FA. Conventional versus high frequency jet ventilation with a bronchopleural fistula. J Surg Res 46:147-151, 1989.

14. Rouby J-J, Viars P. Clinical use of high frequency ventilation. Acta Anaesthesiol Scand Suppl 90:134-139, 1989.

15. Gattinoni L, Pesenti A, Rossi GP. Treatment of acute respiratory failure with low-frequency positive pressure ventilation and extracorporeal removal of CO_2. Lancet 2:292-295, 1980.

16. Gattinoni L, Pesenti A, Pelizzola A. Reversal of terminal acute respiratory failure by low frequency positive pressure ventilation with extracorporeal removal of CO_2. Trans Am Soc Artif Organs 28:289-293, 1981.

17. Zapek WM, Snider MT, Hill JD. Extracorporeal membrane oxygenation in severe acute respiratory failure. JAMA 242:2193-2196, 1979.

18. Hickling KG. Extracorporeal CO_2 removal in severe adult respiratory distress syndrome. Anaesth Intens Care 14:46-53, 1986.

CHAPTER 29

Disturbances of Acid-Base Homeostasis

Jon F. Berlauk

ABG chemistries are among the laboratory tests most frequently ordered in the SICU, for ABG analysis provides a wealth of critical information about the SICU patient. Contained in the four variables measured (i.e., pH, partial pressure of carbon dioxide [Pco_2], partial pressure of oxygen [Po_2], and bicarbonate [HCO_3^-]) are an overall assessment of the patient's respiratory adequacy and cellular metabolic environment. Therefore an accurate interpretation of ABGs, along with clinical and electrolyte data, can provide a circumscribed differential diagnosis of some or all of a patient's medical problems. In addition, a patient's response to cardiovascular and respiratory support is monitored through ABG values. This chapter provides a simplified approach to the interpretation of ABG values and the physiology of acid-base disturbances, along with diagnostic clues available to differentiate the disturbances of acid-base homeostasis. The emphasis is on diagnosis. Treatment of the specific acid-base disturbances is not discussed.

ABG INTERPRETATION

Acid-base physiology can be reduced to simple terms in order to understand ABG analysis. Under normal, *unstressed* metabolic conditions

the human body produces excess acid. An adult produces 40 to 100 mEq of organic acids and 13,000 to 15,000 mmol of CO_2 daily (see Fig. 29-1).

To mediate the tissue pH changes that would accompany the continual organic acid production, intracellular and extracellular fluids in the body contain conjugate acid-base pairs. These conjugate pairs act as buffers within the range of normal pH:7.4. The major extracellular buffer in blood and interstitial fluid is the HCO_3^- buffer system:

$$HCO_3^- + H^+ \overset{CA}{\rightleftharpoons} H_2CO_3 \rightleftharpoons CO_2 + H_2O$$

where CA is carbonic anhydrase and H_2CO_3 is carbonic acid.

Once the organic acids are buffered (HCO_3^- is consumed), they are excreted by the kidney. New bicarbonate is regenerated through this hydrogen ion (H^+) excretion process (see Fig. 29-2). This mechanism is the body's only source of endogenous bicarbonate. Abnormalities in HCO_3^-, as measured by the ABG analysis, will reflect *metabolic* acid-base disorders or metabolic compensation for a respiratory disorder.

The continuous cellular CO_2 production would cause drastic pH changes were it not for the intracellular hemoglobin buffer system. Reduced hemoglobin will absorb approximately 0.7 mmol H^+ for each millimole of oxygen released to the tissues without a subsequent change in serum pH. Although this H^+ buffering is mediated through the action of carbonic anhydrase, HCO_3^- is not consumed in the process. The CO_2 ultimately is eliminated through pulmonary gas exchange. Therefore abnormalities in PCO_2, as measured by the ABG analysis, will reflect *respiratory* acid-base disorders or respiratory compensation for a metabolic disorder.

This interplay of renal-pulmonary regulation of acid excretion is ultimately determined through the Henderson-Hasselbalch equation for the bicarbonate buffer system:

$$pH = 6.1 + \log \frac{[HCO_3^-]}{[H_2CO_3] + [CO_2]}$$

CO_2 dissolved in the blood greatly exceeds the concentration of H_2CO_3 at equilibrium (809X); therefore the equation can be simplified to:

$$pH = 6.1 + \log \frac{[HCO_3^-]}{[CO_2]}$$

Since HCO_3^- and H_2CO_3 are not clinically measured but total CO_2 and PCO_2 are, this equation becomes:

$$pH = 6.1 + \log \frac{Total\ CO_2 - 0.03\ PCO_2}{0.03\ PCO_2}$$

Changes in PCO_2 significantly affect pH and HCO_3^-. In addition, these three variables are interdependent. A change in any one variable results in simultaneous changes in the others, as determined by the Henderson-Hasselbalch relationship. Since CO_2 causes a predictable, albeit nonlinear, change in pH through a wide physiologic range of pH, the key to interpreting ABG values is the PCO_2.

Finally, the Henderson-Hasselbalch equation has been rewritten as:

$$pH = Constant + \frac{Kidneys}{Lungs}\ or\ \frac{Metabolic}{Respiratory}$$

It is clear from this restatement that a change in either component of this equilibrium must be "compensated" by a similar change (increase or decrease) in the reciprocal component if the pH is to remain near normal.

With these concepts in mind, the SICU physician can rely on fairly simple and practical guidelines to interpret ABG data. Four steps are involved:

1. Check the pH.
2. Assume all perturbations in pH are due to an *acute* change in PCO_2.
3. Confirm or refute this assumption (diagnose the primary acid-base disorder).
4. Check for normal physiologic compensation (diagnose the secondary acid-base disorder, if present).

Step 1

Note the measured pH. (Analysis of PO_2 in conjunction with acid-base changes is discussed in Chapter 54.) By convention, a pH of 7.4 is considered neutral or "normal" (normal pH is actually within a range of values from 7.38 to 7.42). Likewise, a PCO_2 of 40 torr (mm Hg) is normal. *Acidosis* refers to any serum pH below 7.4 and *alkalosis* refers to pH values above 7.4. Yet quite often a patient with a normal serum pH is mistakenly believed to have an acidosis simply because the HCO_3^- reported on the ABG analysis is low.

ABG analysis should begin with pH because there are only four primary acid-base disorders: metabolic acidosis, metabolic alkalosis, respiratory acidosis, and respiratory alkalosis. Of these four, only one, chronic respiratory alkalosis, ultimately compensates enough to result in a normal serum pH. The primary disorder will never "overcompensate." Therefore the pH reveals if the patient has acidosis (metabolic vs. respiratory) or alkalosis (metabolic vs. respiratory). With this information, half of the analysis is done.

Step 2

After the measured pH has been checked, the PCO_2 should be addressed. It should be assumed that *the pH measured from the ABG was the result of an acute change in PCO_2*. Acute changes in the PCO_2 result in predictable changes in serum pH (the converse is not true, however). For an acute 10 torr increase in PCO_2 above 40 torr, the pH will decrease by approximately 0.05 units. However, for an identical acute 10 torr decrease in PCO_2, the pH will increase approximately 0.1 unit (see accompanying box). An equivalent change in P_{CO_2} results in different changes in pH. (As a memory aid: *alkalosis* [9 letters] is greater than *acidosis* [8 letters]). By using these two rules, a pH predicted by the assumption can be calculated from the measured P_{CO_2}, resulting in both measured pH and predicted pH.

Step 3

By comparing the predicted pH with the measured pH, a primary acid-base diagnosis can be made.

- If the predicted pH and measured pH correlate very well, an acute respiratory disorder is present.
- If the predicted pH and measured pH lie in opposite directions of a pH of 7.4, a primary metabolic disorder exists. A secondary respiratory disorder is also possible (see step 4).
- If the predicted pH and measured pH lie on the same side of a pH of 7.4 but otherwise do not correlate, several possibilities exist:

   A primary (chronic) respiratory disorder exists, and renal compensation has occurred. The combination of a low P_{CO_2} and normal pH (7.38 to 7.42) almost always indicates chronic respiratory alkalosis.

   A combined disorder exists (i.e., metabolic and respiratory acidosis). A combined disorder is easy to diagnose because the measured pH is more acidotic or alkalotic than the predicted pH.

   A mixed disorder exists.

Step 4

The first three steps determine whether an acid-base disorder exists and, if so, whether the primary disorder is respiratory or metabolic. If the primary disorder is respiratory (ΔP_{CO_2}), physiologic compensation would be expected to occur through renal (ΔHCO_3^-) mechanisms and vice-versa. This physiologic compensation has been well defined and does have limits (rules 3 to 8 in the accompanying box). Two principles apply: (1) only chronic respiratory alkalosis will completely compensate to a normal pH, and (2) without iatrogenic intervention, no primary disorder will overcompensate. *Establishing whether the physiologic compensation*

for a primary acid-base disorder falls within expected limits or not can determine if a second acid-base disorder exists.

The metabolic (ΔHCO_3^-) compensation for a primary respiratory disorder (ΔP_{CO_2}) occurs in two steps. First, there is a rapid re-equilibration of HCO_3^- as described by the Henderson-Hasselbalch equation. This occurs within minutes (acute). The subsequent loss or regeneration of HCO_3^- is much slower and occurs through renal mechanisms over 12 to 36 hours (chronic). Rules 3 to 6 in the box below describe this compensation and the expected lim-

---

Rules for ABG Analysis

1. Each acute 10 torr increase in P_{CO_2} above 40 torr will decrease blood pH approximately 0.05 unit.
2. Each acute 10 torr decrease in P_{CO_2} below 40 torr will increase blood pH approximately 0.1 units.
3. An acute 10 torr increase in P_{CO_2} will be buffered by an increase in HCO_3^- of approximately 1 mEq/L (upper limit, HCO_3^- of 30 mEq/L).
4. A chronic 10 torr increase in P_{CO_2} will be compensated by an increase in HCO_3^- of approximately 3.5 mEq/L (upper limit, HCO_3^- of 45 mEq/L).
5. An acute 10 torr decrease in P_{CO_2} will be buffered by a decrease in HCO_3^- of approximately 2.5 mEq/L (lower limit, HCO_3^- of 18 mEq/L).
6. A chronic 10 torr decrease in P_{CO_2} will be compensated by a decrease in HCO_3^- of approximately 5 mEq/L (lower limit, HCO_3^- of 12 mEq/L).
7. For metabolic acidosis only:
   Expected P_{CO_2} = 1.5 [HCO_3^-] + 8 ± 2 (lower limit, P_{CO_2} of 10 torr) (modified Winter's formula)
   Expected P_{CO_2} approximates last two digits of the pH
   Expected P_{CO_2} is approximately 15 + [HCO_3^-]
8. For metabolic alkalosis only:
   Each 10 mEq/L increase in HCO_3^- will be compensated by an increase in P_{CO_2} of approximately 6 torr (upper limit, P_{CO_2} of 55 torr).
9. Between 6-7 mEq of HCO_3^- per liter of HCO_3^- distribution space will change the pH approximately 0.1 unit.

its of normal compensation. If the compensation for a primary respiratory disorder is more or less than expected, a secondary acid-base disorder should be diagnosed. Again, compensation for alkalosis is greater than for acidosis.

The respiratory (ΔPco_2) compensation for a primary metabolic (ΔHCO_3^-) disorder can occur rapidly. However, the rules (see box on p. 319, rules 7 and 8) defining this compensation are unique and cannot be extrapolated from the previous rules. If the compensation for a primary metabolic disorder is more than or less than expected, a secondary acid-base disorder is present.

These are the basics. Once ABG has been analyzed, it should be recalled that acid-base changes are dynamic. Especially in an SICU setting, the interplay of patient pathophysiology and physician intervention can create interesting ABG results. It is helpful and sometimes essential to review previous ABG values if they are available, interpret them accurately and completely, and then obtain additional information to define a specific diagnosis further.

METABOLIC ACID-BASE DISORDERS
Metabolic Acidosis

Metabolic acidosis is arguably the most interesting of the four primary acid-base disorders. By combining clinical information with ABG and serum electrolyte data, a precise diagnosis is very often possible.

Physiology

An unstressed adult produces 40 to 100 mEq of acid daily as a by-product of intermediary metabolism. This acid is in the form of sulfuric, phosphoric, and additional hydrogen phosphate, and other minor organic acids. Extracellular buffers are required to ameliorate the pH changes imposed by this continual acid production. These buffers are predominantly HCO_3^-, proteins, and the skeletal system (Fig. 29-1). Eventually the kidneys must excrete the acid load and, additionally, resynthesize HCO_3^- lost in the buffering process. Overproduction of acids, loss of buffer stores, or underexcretion of acid can disrupt this delicately balanced system and induce metabolic acidosis. Regardless of the mechanism of systemic acidosis, even-

tually the pH in the CSF also declines. Medullary chemoreceptors respond to the elevated H^+ by stimulating respiration. Hyperventilation will cause hypocapnia, which will return the systemic pH toward normal, but compensation is never complete.[1,2]

Winter's formula[3] is a sophisticated calculation for determining the expected Pco_2 compensation for any degree of acidosis (as reflected in HCO_3^-). A simplified version of Winter's formula is given in the box on p. 319. The lower limit of normal compensation is Pco_2 of approximately 10 torr.[4] If the actual Pco_2 deviates significantly from the expected Pco_2, secondary disorder is possible.

When the acid load reaches the kidney, excretion depends on the ability of the renal tubule to excrete H^+ and ammonia (NH_3) normally. H^+ secretion occurs in both proximal and distal renal tubular cells. The amount secreted depends on intracellular production of H^+, cellular carbonic anhydrase concentration, and Pco_2. In the proximal tubule H^+ secretion is most dependent on Pco_2. In the distal tubule H^+ secretion is independent of Pco_2 and is primarily dependent on carbonic anhydrase concentration. In the renal tubular cell, carbon dioxide combines with water under the influence of carbonic anhydrase. H^+ is secreted into the tubular fluid (urine) in exchange for sodium. The HCO_3^- is reabsorbed into the blood (Fig. 29-2). To prevent secreted H^+ from recombining with tubular HCO_3^- to reverse the previous reactions, H^+ must be chemically "trapped" and excreted. This is accomplished through phosphate and ammonia secretion into the *distal* tubular lumen. For each H^+ that is trapped and excreted, one HCO_3^- is regenerated. This process is the only mechanism available for new HCO_3^- generation. Potassium-for-sodium exchange also occurs in the distal tubule, but will not generate new HCO_3^-.

Differential diagnosis

The upper box on p. 321 lists a broad classification of metabolic acidoses. These conditions are divided by their effect on the serum electrolytes, calculated by the anion gap.[5,6] Acidoses are categorized as producing a normal anion gap or an elevated anion gap. The term "anion gap," however, is a misnomer since it implies there is a disequilibrium (gap) between the concentration of serum anions and serum cations. In reality, only frequently measured serum anions and cations are used to calculate the anion gap (AG):

$$AG = (Na^+) - [Cl^-] + [HCO_3^-]$$

The normal anion gap is approximately 12 mEq/L if potassium is omitted. The true anion gap, however, reflects the unmeasured anions (UA) and unmeasured cations (UC) in blood:

$$AG = UA - UC$$

The lower box on p. 321 lists most of the common unmeasured anions and cations.

Based on these observations, if chloride is ultimately the anion that accumulates during an acidosis, the resulting anion gap will be normal

Metabolic Acidoses

	Normal anion gap acidoses (10-12 mEq/L)	*Elevated anion gap acidoses (>12 mEq/L)*
Hypokalemia	*Normal to hyperkalemia*	*Hyperkalemia*
Renal tubular acidosis	Early renal failure	Chronic renal failure
Proximal	Hydronephrosis	Lactic acidosis
Distal	Hypoaldosteronism	Ketoacidoses
Buffer deficiency (phosphate	Acidifying agents	Diabetes mellitus
or ammonia)	Hydrochloric acid	Alcohol induced
Diarrhea	Ammonium chloride	Starvation
Posthypocapnic acidosis	Arginine chloride	Toxins
Carbonic anhydrase inhibitors	Lysine chloride	Methanol
Acetazolamide (Diamox)	Sulfur toxicity	Ethylene glycol
Mefenamide (Sulfamylon)		Paraldehyde
Ureteral diversions		Salicylates
Ureterosigmoidostomy		
Ileal bladder		
Ileal ureter		

Anion Gap

Increased anion gap (>12 mEq/L)
Increased unmeasured anions

Organic anions (lactate, ketoacids)
Exogenous anions (salicylate, formate, penicillin)
Inorganic anions (phosphate, sulfate)
Hyperalbuminemia (transient)
Incompletely identified anion (paraldehyde poisoning)

Laboratory error

High sodium measured
Low chloride or bicarbonate measured

Decreased unmeasured cation

Hypokalemia, hypocalcemia, hypomagnesemia

Decreased anion gap (<10 mEq/L)
Decreased unmeasured anion

Hypoalbuminemia

Laboratory error

Falsely low sodium secondary to viscous serum (hyperglycemia, hyperlipidemia)
Bromide intoxication
Low sodium measured
High chloride or bicarbonate measured

Increased unmeasured cation

Normal cation (hyperkalemia, hypercalcemia, hypermagnesemia)
Abnormal cation (IgG, lithium, TRIS buffer)

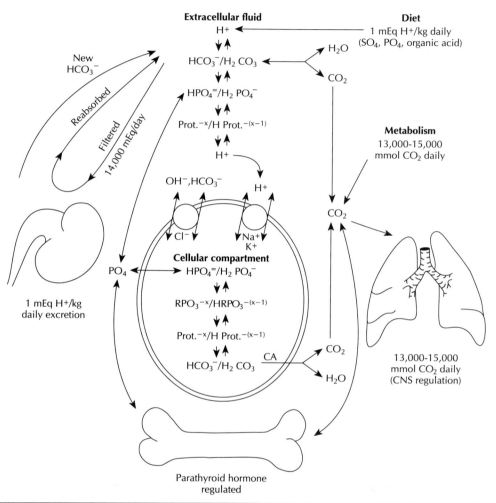

FIG. 29-1 Interactions that occur between body fluid compartments with respect to buffering and major organ systems involved in maintenance of acid-base balance. Major buffers are shown in compartments in which they occur. Buffers within either intracellular or extracellular compartments are in equilibrium by isohydric principle; intracellular and extracellular compartments are linked by ion exchange systems indicated and by Pco_2. Carbonic anhydrase (CA) occurs only intracellularly. Not illustrated are renal and gut handling of phosphate and hormonal control of these processes. When normal balance is being maintained, daily production of "new" bicarbonate (HCO_3^-) by the kidney equals amount of HCO_3^- consumed during acute buffering of acid loads ingested. (From Laski ME. Normal regulation of acid-base balance. Renal and pulmonary response and other extrarenal buffering mechanisms. Med Clin North Am 67:771, 1983.)

(or approximately 12 mEq/L), producing the hyperchloremic metabolic acidoses. Although potassium does not play an important role in determining the anion gap, it provides valuable information to differentiate further the hyperchloremic metabolic acidoses. In contrast, elevated anion gap acidoses are characterized by the accumulation of an anion other than chloride (see lower box on p. 321). Historically, these are the disorders most frequently associated with metabolic acidosis.

Metabolic Alkalosis

Metabolic alkalosis is the most common acid-base disorder in the general hospital patient population.[7] The metabolic alkaloses are characterized by a sustained hyperbicarbonatemia. This condition can result from loss of acid, loss of volume (extracellular fluid), exogenously administered alkali, or imbalances in the renal-adrenal axis.

Physiology

Alkalinization of the serum by any of the above mechanisms eventually will lead to alkalinization of the CSF. Medullary chemoreceptors will respond by depressing respiration. Hypoventilation will cause hypercapnia, which will return the elevated serum pH toward normal, but pH compensation will never be complete. The P_{CO_2} will rise approximately 6 torr for each 10 mEq/L rise in HCO_3^-.[8] The maximum CO_2 compensation occurs at approximately 55 torr.[9-12] If the measured P_{CO_2} falls outside these limits, a secondary disorder should be suspected.

In patients with metabolic acidosis renal tubular cell function is essential to eliminate the acid load. In contrast, the renal mechanism to

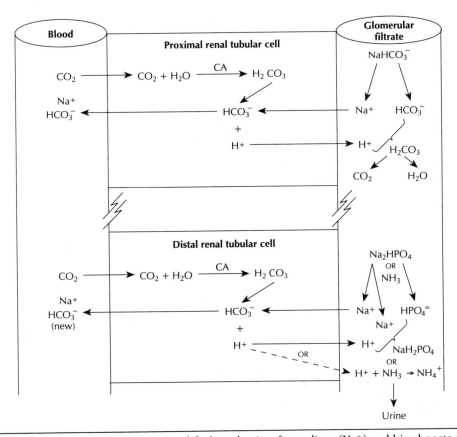

FIG. 29-2 Proximal renal tubular cell: simplified mechanism for sodium (Na^+) and bicarbonate (HCO_3^-) reabsorption. Distal renal tubule cell: simplified mechanism for acidification of urine and new HCO_3^- regeneration. CA, carbonic anhydrase.

eliminate excess bicarbonate is determined primarily through changes in glomerular filtration rate (GFR). Under normal conditions, bicarbonate reabsorption, like sodium reabsorption, changes directly with the GFR, and very little filtered bicarbonate is excreted. This bicarbonate reabsorption is probably mediated through a combination of H^+ secretion by tubular cells and alteration in tubular size. The most common mechanism for the development of metabolic alkalosis involves loss of chloride-rich fluid.[13] When the kidney detects volume depletion, it attempts to protect renal blood flow through sodium (hence volume) reabsorption. The accompanying anion reabsorbed is the relatively more abundant HCO_3^-. Eventually mild hyperbicarbonatremia occurs. If the volume deficit is not restored, this protective mechanism would initiate a vicious cycle, leading to increasingly severe alkalosis, were it not for the renal tubular maximum for HCO_3^-. The normal renal tubular maximum for HCO_3^- is 27 to 29 mEq/L. If a higher concentration of HCO_3^- is filtered, it is promptly excreted. Although the elevated Pco_2 (respiratory compensation) will enhance H^+ secretion and HCO_3^- reabsorption in the proximal tubule (see Fig. 29-2), this addition to serum HCO_3^- is minor. Therefore if the GFR remains constant, large amounts of HCO_3^- are excreted after the tubular maximum for HCO_3^- is reached. Severe systemic alkalosis is prevented, but once alkalosis is initiated, the kidney will perpetuate it.[14] Mineralocortical hormones, serum calcium, and serum chloride also influence HCO_3^- homeostasis through poorly understood mechanisms. Under pathologic conditions, they are the factors that elevate the renal tubular for maximum HCO_3^-. The result is sustained hyperbicarbonatemia and serious alkalosis.

Differential diagnosis

The differential diagnosis for metabolic alkalosis involves extracellular fluid volume and mineralocortical hormones. The anion gap is not helpful since it is slightly elevated (5 to 9

Classification of Metabolic Alkaloses

Saline responsive (urinary chloride <15 mEq/L)	*Saline unresponsive (urinary chloride >15 mEq/L)*
Normotensive	*Normotensive*
Renal	Renal
Diuretic induced	Bartter's syndrome
Poorly reabsorbable anion therapy (carbenicillin, sulfate, phosphate)	Magnesium deficiency
Posthypercapnic alkalosis	Severe potassium depletion
Gastrointestinal	Refeeding alkalosis
Vomiting	Hypercalcemia
Nasogastric drainage	Hyperparathyroidism
Villous adenoma	
Congenital chloride diarrhea	*Hypertensive*
Exogenous alkali	Renal or adrenal
Baking soda ($NaHCO_3^-$)	Primary aldosteronism (Conn's syndrome)
Antacids	Hyperreninism
Salts of strong acids (citrate, lactate, acetate)	Cushing's syndrome
Blood product transfusion	Liddle's syndrome
"Overshoot" alkalosis	Adrenal 11-beta or 17-alpha hydroxylase deficiency
Contraction alkalosis	Glycyrrhizinic acid (licorice, chewing tobacco)
	Carbenoxolone

mEq/L) in all metabolic alkaloses.[15] Rather, classification of metabolic alkaloses includes a saline-responsive group and a saline-resistant group (see box on p. 324). These groups are separated by urinary chloride excretion. The majority of alkaloses in the SICU are saline responsive and are mediated through a chloride deficiency (Fig. 29-3). Avid chloride retention (with sodium) by the kidney results in little chloride excretion, hence low urinary chloride concentration. The majority of the saline-resistant alkaloses are mediated by imbalances in the renal-adrenal axis. Volume state and hypertension provide additional clinical clues to these disorders.

RESPIRATORY ACID-BASE DISORDERS

Respiratory acid-base disorders result from alteration in normal CO_2 excretion. Therefore the physiology of CO_2 transport and elimination is common to both respiratory acidosis and alkalosis.

As stated previously, hemoglobin is the primary buffer against the pH changes imposed by continual CO_2 production.[16] HCO_3^- is not the best buffer in blood because the pK of the HCO_3^- buffer system (see Henderson-Hasselbalch equation) is remote from the physiologic pH of 7.4. The hemoglobin molecule serves as an important buffer because it is rich in the amino acid histidine. The imidazole group of histidine has a pK of 7, which is in the physiologic pH range of blood. It is the imidazole group on reduced hemoglobin that absorbs as much as 50% of the H^+ generated by cellular CO_2 production. The total CO_2 produced is finally carried in one of four forms: (1) HCO_3^- (70%), (2) carbamino compounds (20%), (3) dissolved CO_2 (<10%), and (4) H_2CO_3 (a small fraction) (Fig. 29-4). Once the venous blood reaches the lungs, the concentration gradients for oxygen and CO_2 are reversed from those present at the tissue level. Reactions that occurred at the tissue level are also reversed (Fig. 29-5). Yet in contrast to tissue reactions, in the lung these reactions proceed against an unfavorable thermodynamic gradient. The primary driving force is continual depletion of CO_2.

The healthy lung has an enormous capacity to excrete CO_2. Saturation of this excretion mechanism through overproduction of CO_2 is unknown. In addition, medullary chemoreceptors that control ventilation are exquisitely sensitive to changes in Pco_2. The result is a finely balanced feedback system to regulate CO_2 excretion through CO_2 production, thereby maintaining a stable Pco_2. Imbalances in the regulation of ventilation or the excretion of CO_2 result in respiratory acid-base disorders.

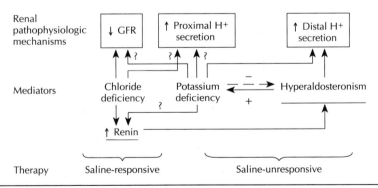

FIG. 29-3 Factors contributing to maintenance of metabolic alkalosis. Renal retention of bicarbonate can be affected by a decrease in glomerular filtration rate and/or an increase in proximal or distal bicarbonate reabsorption. These mechanisms in turn can be activated by combinations of chloride deficiency, potassium deficiency, and hyperaldosteronism. Saline therapy corrects only those pathophysiologic factors attributable to chloride deficiency. (From Cogan MG, Liu F, Berger BE, et al. Metabolic alkalosis. Med Clin North Am 67:903, 1983.)

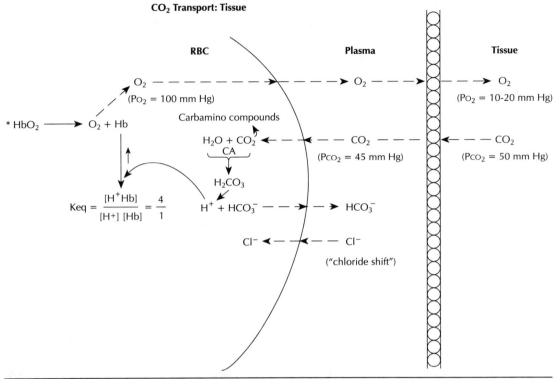

FIG. 29-4   Reaction (*) favors dissociation to oxygen and reduced hemoglobin. However, main driving force is continual depletion of both end products. CA, carbonic anhydrase.

Respiratory Acidosis

If central respiratory centers are depressed or CO_2 is underexcreted relative to production, the Pco_2 becomes elevated. Since renal compensation (increased HCO_3^-) for an acute rise in Pco_2 requires 36 hours or more, buffering the acidemia produced by an abrupt and sustained elevation in Pco_2 is dependent on plasma and intracellular buffers described in previous sections. An acute 10 torr rise in Pco_2 is accompanied by approximately a 1 mEq/L rise in HCO_3^-, described by the Henderson-Hasselbalch relationship.[8] The maximal compensation through this mechanism occurs at a HCO_3^- level of approximately 30 mEq/L. Over the subsequent hours to days, the kidney compensates for a sustained Pco_2 elevation by reabsorbing all filtered HCO_3^- and secreting H^+ into the distal tubule.[17,18] The secreted H^+ is "trapped" by ammonia and excreted; one new HCO_3^- is

generated and absorbed into the blood (see Fig. 29-2). This sustained HCO_3^- reabsorption is accompanied by a chronic loss of chloride. This mechanism provides adequate, but never complete, pH compensation for chronic CO_2 retention. In addition, severe CO_2 elevation (Pco_2 >60 torr) begins to impair renal tubular ammonia production, which reduces HCO_3^- regeneration and results in severe systemic acidosis. Overall, chronic renal compensation can be expected to raise the HCO_3^- approximately 3.5 mEq/L for each sustained 10 torr rise in Pco_2.[8,19,20] The limit of compensation is HCO_3^- level of approximately 45 mEq/L.[17,21] If the actual HCO_3^- deviates from these expectations, a secondary disorder may exist.

Differential diagnosis

The causes of acute and chronic respiratory acidosis are given in the box on p. 328.

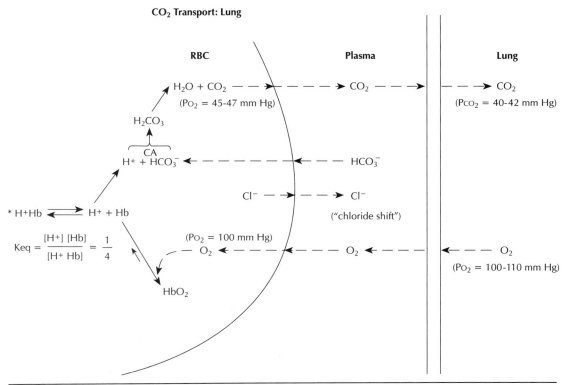

CO$_2$ Transport: Lung

FIG. 29-5 Reaction (*) does not favor dissociation to H$^+$ and reduced hemoglobin. Main driving force is continual depletion of both end products to form stable compounds.

Respiratory Alkalosis

Simple respiratory alkalosis is characterized by low P_{CO_2} induced by sustained hyperventilation. As in respiratory acidosis, compensation occurs in two phases. Intracellular and extracellular buffering are complete within 5 to 15 minutes, and renal compensation follows. An acute 10 torr fall in P_{CO_2} will be buffered by a decrease in HCO_3^- of approximately 2.5 mEq/L.[8,22] The limit for acute compensation is approximately 18 mEq/L.[23] Over the next 12 to 36 hours, up to 5 mEq/L of HCO_3^- are lost for a sustained 10 torr drop in P_{CO_2}.[23] The renal mechanism involves the decreased serum H$^+$ and CO$_2$ concentrations presented to the renal tubular cells as a result of hypocapnia. The alteration in H$^+$ and CO$_2$ concentrations tends to decrease proximal tubular absorption of the filtered HCO_3^- and inhibit distal tubular regeneration of HCO_3^- (urinary acid excretion stops).

Potassium (and sodium) is lost with HCO_3^-, whereas chloride is retained. The resultant electrolyte pattern of hyperchloremia and hypokalemia can mimic some patterns seen with normal anion gap metabolic acidoses.[24] Significant amounts of HCO_3^- are lost to a maximum of HCO_3^- of approximately 12 to 15 mEq/L.[23] This acid-base disorder can compensate to a normal pH through this mechanism. It should be noted that respiratory alkalosis is the most frequently seen ABG abnormality in the SICU patient population.[25]

Differential diagnosis

Hypocapnia does not result from abnormal CO$_2$ excretion; therefore all causes of respiratory alkalosis involve disturbances in respiratory control. The causes of respiratory alkalosis involve central mechanisms, pulmonary mechanisms, and complex mechanisms (see box on p. 329).

Causes of Respiratory Acidosis

Acute
Secondary to respiratory control failure

Central nervous system
    Cerebrovascular accident
    Drug overdose (sedatives, narcotics)
    Anesthesia
    Central sleep apnea
    Trauma

Secondary to carbon dioxide excretory failure

Spinal cord
    Cervical cord trauma
    Guillain-Barré syndrome
Neuromuscular
    Neurotoxins (botulism, tetanus, organophosphates)
    Neuromuscular blocking drugs (e.g., succinylcholine, curare, pancuronium)
    Neuromuscular blocking antibiotics (e.g., streptomycin, kanamycin, polymyxin)
    Myasthenic crisis
    Hypokalemic paralysis
    Hypophosphatemia
    Hypermagnesemia
Thoracic
    Flail chest
    Pneumothorax
    Hemothorax
Upper airway
    Obstructive sleep apnea
    Epiglottitis, laryngotracheitis
    Vocal cord paralysis
    Postintubation laryngeal edema
    Laryngospasm
    Foreign body aspiration
Cardiovascular
    Massive pulmonary embolism
    Fat embolism

Snake bite
Cardiac arrest
Lower airway or alveolar
    Gastric aspiration (particulate)
    Severe pulmonary edema
    Adult respiratory distress syndrome
    Severe pneumonia
    Severe bronchospasm (asthma)

Chronic
Secondary to respiratory control failure

Central nervous system
    Obesity and hypoventilation (Pickwickian syndrome)
    Brainstem infarcts
    Tumor
    Chronic sedative or tranquilizer overdose
    Myxedema
    Metabolic alkalosis
    Bulbar poliomyelitis

Secondary to carbon dioxide excretory failure

Spinal cord
    Poliomyelitis
    Amyotrophic lateral sclerosis
    Cervical cord trauma
Neuromuscular
    Myasthenia gravis
    Multiple sclerosis
    Myxedema
Thoracic
    Muscular dystrophy
    Kyphoscoliosis
    Spondylitis
Lower airway or alveolar
    Chronic obstructive lung disease
    Severe interstitial lung disease
    Bronchiectasis

Causes of Respiratory Alkalosis

Central mechanisms

Central nervous system disorders
  Cerebrovascular accident
  Trauma
  Infection
  Tumor
Hypoxemia
  Altitude
  Ventilation-perfusion abnormalities
  Pulmonary shunts
  Pulmonary diffusion abnormalities
  Hypotension, low cardiac output
Drugs or hormones
  Salicylates
  Nicotine
  Progesterone (pregnancy)
  Xanthines
  Thyroid hormone

Anxiety, hysteria
Fever
Pain

Pulmonary mechanisms

Pneumonia
Asthma
Pulmonary embolus
Congestive heart failure
Interstitial lung disease

Complex mechanisms

Cirrhosis
Gram-negative sepsis
Hyponatremia
Heat exposure
Mechanical ventilation

SUMMARY

- Abnormalities in P_{CO_2} reflect a respiratory acid-base disorder or respiratory compensation for a metabolic disorder.
- The key to interpreting ABG values is the P_{CO_2}.
- Guidelines for interpreting ABG values include checking the pH (assuming all perturbations in pH are due to acute changes in P_{CO_2}), confirming or refuting the assumption of acute changes, and checking for normal physiologic compensation.
- Primary acid-base disorders are metabolic acidosis, metabolic alkalosis, respiratory acidosis, and respiratory alkalosis.
- Only chronic respiratory alkalosis can compensate enough to produce a normal pH. No primary disorder will overcompensate without iatrogenic interventions.
- By determining whether physiologic compensation for a primary acid-base disturbance falls within expected limits, the clinician can identify the presence or absence of a second acid-base disorder.

REFERENCES

1. Pierce NF, Fedson DS, Brigham KL, et al. The ventilatory response to acute base deficit in humans: Time course during development and correction of metabolic acidosis. Ann Intern Med 72:633, 1970.
2. Lennon EJ, Lemann J. Defense of hydrogen ion concentration in chronic metabolic acidosis: A new evaluation of an old approach. Ann Intern Med 65:265, 1966.
3. Albert MD, Dell RB, Winters RW. Quantitative displacement of acid-base equilibrium in metabolic acidosis. Ann Intern Med 66:312, 1967.
4. Relman AS. Metabolic acidosis. Med Times 96:1094, 1968.
5. Emmett M, Narins RG. Clinical use of the anion gap. Medicine (Baltimore) 56:38, 1977.
6. Oh MS, Carroll HJ. The anion gap. N Engl J Med 297:814, 1977.
7. Hodgkin JE, Soeprono FF, Chan DM. Incidence of metabolic alkalemia in hospitalized patients. Crit Care Med 8:725, 1980.
8. Narins RG, Emmett M. Simple and mixed acid-base disorders: A practical approach. Medicine (Baltimore) 59:161, 1980.

9. Goldring RM, Cannon PJ, Heinemann HO, et al. Respiratory adjustment to chronic metabolic alkalosis in man. J Clin Invest 47:188, 1968.
10. Bone JM, Cowie J, Lambie A, et al. The relationship between arterial Pco_2 and hydrogen ion concentration in chronic metabolic acidosis and alkalosis. Clin Sci Mol Med 46:113, 1974.
11. Elkington JR. Clinical disorders of acid-base regulation. A survey of seventeen years' diagnostic experience. Med Clin North Am 50:1325, 1966.
12. Fulop M. Hypercapnia in metabolic alkalosis. NY State J Med 76:19, 1976.
13. Garella S, Chang BS, Kahn SI. Dilution acidosis and contraction alkalosis. Review of a concept. Kidney Int 8:279, 1975.
14. Seldin DW, Rector FC Jr. The generation and maintenance of metabolic alkalosis. Kidney Int 1:306, 1972.
15. Madias NE, Ayus JC, Androgué HJ. Increased anion gap in metabolic alkalosis: The role of plasma protein equivalency. N Engl J Med 300:1421, 1979.
16. Giebisch G, Berger L, Pitts RF. The extrarenal response to acute acid-base disturbances of respiratory origin. J Clin Invest 34:231, 1955.
17. Schwartz WB, Brackett NC Jr, Cohen JJ. The response of extracellular hydrogen ion concentration to graded degrees of chronic hypercapnia. The physiologic limits of the defense of pH. J Clin Invest 44:291, 1965.
18. VanYpersele de Strihou C, Brasseur CL, De-Coninck J. The "carbon dioxide response curve" for chronic hypercapnia in man. N Engl J Med 275:117, 1966.
19. Brackett NC Jr, Cohen JJ, Schwartz WB. Carbon dioxide titration curve of normal man: Effect of increasing degrees of acute hypercapnia on acid-base balance. N Engl J Med 272:6, 1965.
20. Schwartz WB, Cohen JJ. The nature of the renal response to chronic disorders of acid-base equilibrium. Am J Med 64:417, 1978.
21. Robin ED. Abnormalities of acid-base regulation in chronic pulmonary diseases with special reference to hypercapnia and extracellular alkalosis. N Engl J Med 268:917, 1963.
22. Arbus GS, Hebert LA, Levesque PR, et al. Characterization and clinical application of the "significance band" for acute respiratory alkalosis. N Engl J Med 280:117, 1969.
23. Gennari FJ, Goldstein MB, Schwartz WB. The nature of the renal adaption to chronic hypocapnia. J Clin Invest 51:1722, 1972.
24. Brown EB. Electrolyte changes with chronic passive hyperventilation in man. J Appl Physiol 1:848, 1949.
25. Mazzara JT, Ayres SM, Grace WJ. Extreme hypocapnia in the critically ill patient. Am J Med 56:450, 1974.

CHAPTER 30

Acute Renal Failure

Mark E. Rosenberg

Acute renal failure (ARF) is a clinical syndrome characterized by rapid deterioration of renal function that results in the accumulation of nitrogenous wastes. This syndrome complicates the hospital course of 5% of patients. As an isolated organ system failure, ARF carries a low mortality of approximately 8%. However, ARF that accompanies multiorgan system failure, as is usually the case in the critically ill surgical patient, involves a much poorer prognosis. For instance, ARF that is part of two-organ system failure has a mortality of 75%. The mortality increases to 90% to 100% with involvement of more than two organs. The outcome of ARF is most often linked to the resolution of the patient's underlying problems. However, prompt recognition and management of renal failure is critical to improving patient survival.

Since the terminology regarding ARF is confusing, selected terms are defined here:

Acute renal failure—a syndrome characterized by rapid deterioration of kidney function resulting in the accumulation of nitrogenous wastes.

Acute tubular necrosis—the most common form of ARF caused by ischemic or nephrotoxic injury to the kidney leading to necrosis of tubules

Acute cortical necrosis—a rare form of ARF due to necrosis of all elements of the renal cortex resulting in irreversible renal failure

Oliguric renal failure—ARF from any cause associated with a urine output <400 ml/day

Nonoliguric renal failure—ARF from any cause associated with a urine output >400 ml/day

DIFFERENTIAL DIAGNOSIS

ARF is first recognized by a decrease in urine output, rising BUN and creatinine (Cr), or both. The differential diagnosis of ARF is best approached by dividing the possible etiologies into prerenal, intrinsic renal, and postrenal causes. This approach not only obviates the need to memorize long lists of possible causes but also provides a useful starting point for the diagnostic evaluation and management of the patient with failing kidneys. The common causes of ARF are listed in the differential diagnosis shown in the left box on p. 332, and the clinical evaluation of the patient with ARF is summarized in the right box on p. 332.

Prerenal Acute Renal Failure
Causes

A prerenal etiologic condition for ARF is the most common cause of renal failure in the hospitalized patient. It is critical to recognize prerenal causes since they are potentially reversible yet can lead to acute tubular necrosis if left untreated. In addition, a prerenal factor often contributes to other forms of ARF. The fundamental abnormality is a decrease in renal perfusion, which results in a fall in the glomerular filtration rate (GFR). Some of the causes of prerenal ARF are listed in the left box on p. 332.

Differential Diagnosis of ARF

Prerenal

Decreased cardiac output
  Decreased circulating blood volume
    Decreased input
    External fluid losses (bleeding, gastrointestinal, renal, skin)
    Redistribution (peritonitis, pancreatitis, hypoalbuminemia)
    Peripheral vasodilation (sepsis, liver disease, antihypertensives)
  Renal artery occlusion

Renal

Glomerular
  Glomerulonephritis
Vascular
  Vasculitis
  Hemolytic uremic syndrome
  Malignant hypertension
  Cholesterol emboli
Interstitial
  Allergic (methicillin, sulfonamide, allopurinol)
  Infiltration (leukemia, lymphoma)
  Infections (staphylococcus, Gram-negative, tuberculosis)
Tubular (ATN)
  Ischemic (shock, cardiac failure)
  Nephrotoxic (drugs, pigment)

Postrenal

Urethra (stricture)
Bladder (prostatic disease, carcinoma, neurogenic, stones, clot)
Ureter and pelvis
  Intrinsic (stones, blood clot, papillary necrosis, fungus)
  Extrinsic (retroperitoneal fibrosis, tumor, abscess, ligation)

Evaluation of Patient With ARF

History

Predisposing medical conditions
Preexisting renal function
Input, output, and weights
Hypotensive episodes
Anesthesia report
Medications
Toxin exposure
Crush injury

Physical

Postural blood pressure and pulse
Temperature
Weight
Fundi (exudates, hemorrhages, Roth's spots)
Skin (rash, jaundice)
Jugular venous pressure (volume status, atrial fibrillation, tamponade)
Lungs (rales, pneumonia)
Heart (gallop, rub, new murmur)
Abdomen (mass, ascites, enlarged kidneys)
Edema

Central venous pressure monitoring

Central venous catheter
Swan-Ganz catheter

Laboratory studies

Serial BUN/creatinine
Urinalysis
CBC and smear
Electrolytes (anion gap)
Arterial blood gas

X-ray examination

Renal ultrasound (excluding obstruction)

Renal hypoperfusion can be caused by a decrease in cardiac output (CO), effective circulating blood volume depletion, or renal artery occlusion. Although in some cases volume loss is obvious, such as with diarrhea, blood loss, or overdiuresis, in other cases the loss of fluid can be internal, for example, as with third-space losses in the patient with peritonitis. "Effective circulating blood volume" is a term that takes into account the amount of circulating blood, how well the blood is being pumped throughout the body, and, most important, how well the tissues are being perfused. For instance, in the patient with sepsis, effective circulating blood volume depletion may occur as a result of peripheral vasodilation and shunting of blood despite a high CO and no loss of extracellular fluid.

Diagnosis

The patient history should focus on the possible sources and quantity of fluid loss, the symptoms of volume depletion (including orthostatic dizziness or weight loss), and the existence of underlying cardiac or liver disease. In the hospitalized patient the chart should be reviewed; particular attention should be given to input, output, and daily weight (the weight of the patient with third-space losses actually may increase despite the presence of intravascular volume depletion). On physical examination, the volume status of the patient can be estimated by careful attention to postural blood pressure and pulse, height of the neck veins, and presence or absence of signs of congestive heart failure (pulmonary rales, S_3, edema). Often the volume status is difficult to define, particularly in the patient with sepsis, who may have vascular leak with peripheral edema, or in the patient with cardiac decompensation. When there is doubt, central venous pressures should be measured, preferably the pulmonary capillary wedge pressure (PCWP), in an attempt to optimize circulating volume.

Laboratory evaluation of prerenal ARF is based on the ability of the functioning kidney to avidly conserve sodium and water when it senses a decrease in renal perfusion. Thus measurement of blood and urinary parameters not only provide an index of volume status but also help to differentiate prerenal ARF from acute tubular necrosis (ATN), in which the kidney loses its ability to reabsorb sodium. Table 30-1 lists some useful variables to measure and the expected results in differentiating prerenal ARF from ATN. These measurements need to be performed prior to volume replacement or administration of mannitol or diuretics.

Treatment

The treatment of prerenal ARF focuses on restoring the circulating volume to normal. If true volume depletion is present, normal saline or

TABLE 30-1 Prerenal Acute Renal Failure vs. Acute Tubular Necrosis

Variable	Prerenal	ATN
BUN/creatinine	>20	10-20
Urine specific gravity	>1.02	<1.01
Urine osmolality (mOsm/kg)	>500	<350
Urinary sodium (mEq/L)	<20	>40
FENa* (%)	<1	>1
Renal failure index† (%)	<1	>1

*FENa = $(U_{Na} \times P_{Cr}/U_{Cr} \times P_{Na}) \times 100$.
†Renal failure index = $(U_{Na} \times P_{Cr}/U_{Cr}) \times 100$.

colloid should be infused, with the physical examination, central venous pressures, urine output, and improvement in BUN and creatinine used as clinical markers. Most important, therapy should be directed at the underlying disease, for example, vasodilator therapy for heart failure or antibiotics for sepsis.

Intrinsic Acute Renal Failure
Causes

The major structures in the kidney are the glomeruli, tubules, vasculature, and interstitium. Disease of any of these structures can lead to ARF. Although glomerular disease is rare in the surgical patient, it can occur. For instance, postinfectious glomerulonephritis can complicate chronic infections or bacterial endocarditis. Occlusion of the renal microvasculature can occur as part of a vasculitic process, in hemolytic uremic syndrome, in malignant hypertension, or following cholesterol embolization from an atheroma. Acute interstitial nephritis is characterized by an inflammatory infiltrate and edema in the interstitium accompanied by varying degrees of tubular injury.

The most common cause of ARF is ATN, a diagnosis made after prerenal and postrenal causes have been excluded and glomerulonephritis, interstitial nephritis, and intrarenal vascular disease have been ruled out. ATN is caused by ischemic or nephrotoxic injury to the kidney. Prolonged renal hypoperfusion from any prerenal cause can lead to ATN (see left box, p. 332). The most common nephrotoxins that cause ATN are drugs—particularly aminoglycosides, amphotericin B, cis-platinum, NSAIDs, and radiocontrast agents.

Diagnosis

Prerenal ARF must be differentiated from ATN (see discussion of diagnosis of prerenal ARF). Volume infusion is crucial in the prerenal patient, but it is potentially hazardous in the oliguric patient with ATN. Comparison of the onset of renal failure with the start of a new medication may provide some clues to the cause of the renal disease. Nephrotoxic agents such as aminoglycosides need to be administered for a long period for nephrotoxicity to occur, whereas radiocontrast agents may result in more immediate nephrotoxicity. The analysis of a fresh urine specimen can be quite helpful in differentiating the causes of intrinsic renal ARF. The presence of proteinuria, hematuria, and RBC casts is characteristic of glomerulonephritis and renal vasculitis. In acute interstitial nephritis, urinary abnormalities may be minimal, or they can include the presence of small amounts of protein, WBCs, WBC casts, eosinophils (in only 30% to 50% of cases), and renal tubular epithelial (RTE) cells and casts. In ATN the urine is classically a muddy-brown color and contains RBCs, WBCs, RTE cells, and pigmented granular and RTE casts. In some circumstances, particularly if the diagnosis of ARF is unclear, a renal biopsy should be considered.

Renal failure secondary to rhabdomyolysis can occur in patients with crush injury. Other conditions associated with rhabdomyolysis include ethanol abuse, seizures, metabolic derangements, and infections. In damaged muscle, intracellular calcium concentrations increase as a result of impaired ionic pumping of calcium from the cell. Increased intracellular calcium concentration leads to increased protease activity and subsequent myofibril disruption. Stretching of muscle fiber increases cellular membrane permeability to calcium, a phenomenon that may help explain the sensitivity of skeletal muscle to mechanical pressure. In an injured muscle, intramuscular pressure may exceed arterial blood pressure within minutes of injury. The resulting swelling may lead to the development of compartmental syndrome.

Within hours of crush injury, while serum BUN and creatinine remain within normal limits, dangerous hyperkalemia, hypocalcemia, hyperphosphatemia, and metabolic acidosis may occur. Hyperuricemia is also noted. If replacement of intravenous fluid is delayed by 6 hours or more, ARF is likely to develop. In experimental models of crush injury, systemic hypovolemia, casts obstructing tubules, and renal vasoconstriction as a consequence of endothelial relaxing factor inhibition all have been implicated in producing renal failure. The catalysis of oxygen free radical formation by ferrous compounds, hyperphosphatemia, hyperuricemia, and disseminated intravascular coagulation also may be a contributing factor to renal failure.

Treatment

If glomerulonephritis or vasculitis is suspected, a renal biopsy should be performed to help guide therapy. In drug-induced acute interstitial nephritis, the offending agent (or any suspected drug) should be discontinued. The use of steroids to treat interstitial nephritis is controversial. Approaches to the management of ATN and rhabdomyolysis-induced renal failure are discussed in the following sections.

Postrenal Acute Renal Failure
Causes

Obstruction of the urinary tract is an uncommon cause of ARF but one that is easily treatable and therefore crucial to recognize. The common causes of obstruction are listed in the left box on p. 332.

Diagnosis

Complete anuria suggests urinary tract obstruction. On abdominal examination, careful palpation for abdominal masses, enlarged kidneys, and an enlarged bladder (requires >500 ml to be palpable) should be performed. The first diagnostic test is bladder catheterization, which yields a large volume of relatively normal urine (by urinalysis) in patients with urethral or bladder neck obstruction. Renal ultrasound is a safe, noninvasive, and sensitive method for diagnosing obstruction. The diagnosis is based on demonstration of dilation of the collecting system. Therefore false negatives may occur when obstruction is present but dilation is not, such as with early obstruction (first 24 to 36 hours) or encasement of the collecting system by tumor, which prevents dilation from occurring. Dilation of the collecting system in the absence of obstruction (false positive) is found in 15% to 20% of cases and may be caused by vesicoureteral reflux, previous high urine flow states, pregnancy, adynamic ureter, pelvic cysts, or previously treated obstruction. Radiocontrast studies, particularly intravenous pyelography, should be avoided in patients in whom obstruction is suspected. Once obstruction has been diagnosed, the site of the obstruction needs to be localized, which may involve antegrade or retrograde pyelograms.

Treatment

Therapy must be directed at relieving the obstruction. This therapy may be as simple as inserting a urinary catheter, or it may involve more complex procedures such as percutaneous nephrostomy or internal ureteral stenting. Return of renal function can occur after 1 to 2 weeks of obstruction, but there have been some reports of return of function after much longer periods. The thinner the renal cortex appears on ultrasound, the less chance for recovery of function. In general, attempts should be made to salvage as much renal function as possible, which may involve decompression of both kidneys in patients with bilateral obstruction.

After relief of the obstruction, diuresis may occur as a result of sodium, urea, and water retention during the period of obstruction. Such diuresis is therefore appropriate and does not require fluid replacement above maintenance requirements. Matching of the urine output will maintain volume expansion and the diuresis will continue.

PREVENTION

Prompt correction of prerenal factors is the most critical preventive measure for ARF. In the case of volume depletion, fluid should be administered. Time should be taken to optimize volume status prior to surgery. Sepsis should be treated promptly with volume expanders and antibiotics. In cardiac failure, therapy with inotropes (dopamine or dobutamine), vasodilators (nitroprusside), or an intra-aortic balloon pump should be instituted as necessary. Aminoglycoside drug levels should be monitored closely and drug dosages adjusted accordingly. Prophylaxis against radiocontrast-induced ARF (see Chapter 9) should include hydration and the administration of mannitol and/or loop diuretics. In the setting of intravascular hemolysis or rhabdomyolysis, hydration and urine alkalinization comprise the treatment of choice.

Mannitol and Loop Diuretics

These agents have been used for (1) prophylaxis in circumstances associated with a high incidence of ARF (e.g., administration of radiocontrast agents, major cardiovascular surgery, massive trauma); (2) treatment of the oliguric patient whose urine volume remains low despite correction of prerenal factors such as volume depletion ("incipient ATN"); and (3) hastening the recovery of renal function in patients with established ATN. However, the efficacy of these agents is still unproven. Mannitol and loop diuretics are capable of increasing urine flow in some patients, but increased urine volume does not necessarily translate into improved GFR or reduced mortality. Furthermore, a beneficial response to these agents may simply indicate those patients with less severe renal dysfunction. Mannitol and/or loop diuretics have some proven value as prophylaxis against radiocontrast nephrotoxicity, and a trial of these agents seems warranted in patients with "incipient ATN" after optimization of prerenal factors. However, these agents are not warranted for therapy of established ATN. Table 30-2 lists the doses and side effects of these and other agents. If no beneficial effect is seen, these therapies should be discontinued.

Dopamine

Low-dose dopamine (1 to 3 μg/kg/min), administered alone or with mannitol and/or diuretics, has been used to increase renal blood flow in states of renal vasoconstriction such as sepsis or liver failure. No consistent beneficial effect has been found with dopamine therapy;

TABLE 30-2 Prophylaxis of Acute Renal Failure		
Agent	Dose	Side Effects
Mannitol	12.5-25 g IV	Volume overload
Furosemide	40-320 mg IV in divided doses	Deafness, allergic interstitial nephritis
Bumetanide	1-8 mg IV in divided doses	Allergic interstitial nephritis (rare)
Dopamine	1-3 μg/kg/min	Minimal at low dose

if an increase in urine output or a fall in creatinine is observed, it occurs shortly after the initiation of therapy. Therefore, if low-dose dopamine is used and no response occurs within the first few hours, therapy can be discontinued.

MANAGEMENT

Complications of ARF appear in almost any organ system and are often the major determinant of prognosis. The most common complications of ARF are listed in Table 30-3. General principles of management include careful monitoring of input and output, changes in the physical examination, serum electrolytes, and drug dosages and levels. Because of the high incidence of infection associated with invasive catheters, their use should be kept to a minimum. For example, a chronic indwelling urinary catheter is often not needed in the patient with ARF.

Fluid Balance

In the absence of fluid overload, the volume of maintenance fluids should equal measured fluid losses (urine, gastrointestinal fluids, surgical drains) plus insensible losses, which can be estimated at 600 ml/day. Higher insensible losses occur with fever. Often a higher fluid intake is needed to deliver medications or perform hyperalimentation. In such cases dialysis therapy is often necessary to manage volume. Whenever possible, excess fluid intake should be kept to a minimum. The electrolyte composition of infused fluid is dictated by the type of loss (which can be measured) and the serum electrolytes.

Hyperkalemia

Potassium should almost never be administered, particularly in the oliguric patient. Be-

TABLE 30-3 Complications of Acute Renal Failure	
System/ Function	Complication
Metabolic	Retention of nitrogenous wastes, hyperkalemia, hyponatremia, metabolic acidosis, hyperphosphatemia, hypocalcemia, hyperuricemia, muscle catabolism
Cardiovascular	Fluid overload, pericarditis, dysrythmias, hypertension, myocardial infarction
Infectious	Urine, bacteremia, catheter, pneumonia, surgical sites
Neurologic	Disorientation, confusion, coma, seizures
Hematologic	Anemia, coagulopathy, disseminated intravascular coagulation, platelet dysfunction
Gastrointestinal	Hemorrhage, nausea, vomiting, gastritis
Pulmonary	Pulmonary edema, pneumonia, emboli, acute respiratory distress syndrome

cause of the potential for serious dysrythmias, hyperkalemia should be treated promptly. Emergency therapy for hyperkalemia is outlined in Table 30-4.

Hyponatremia

Hyponatremia implies a disorder of osmolarity and not an abnormality of sodium metabolism. The patient with oliguric ARF has impaired

TABLE 30-4   Therapy of Hyperkalemia*

Treatment	Dosage	Time of Onset	Mechanism
Calcium gluconate (10%)	5-10 ml IV over 2 min; second dose may be repeated in 5 min	Immediate	Antagonize cardiac and neuro-muscular effects of potassium
Glucose (50%) and insulin	50 ml of glucose and 5-10 U of regular insulin IV over 5 min	30 to 60 min	Shifts potassium into cells
Sodium bicarbonate (7.5%)	50 ml IV over 5 min	30 to 60 min	Shifts potassium into cells; particularly effective in acidotic patients
Cation-exchange resin	15-30 g of resin in 50-100 ml of 20% sorbitol po (or by rectal catheter); may repeat q 4 hr	Hours	Removes 1 mEq of potassium/g of resin by exchange for 1.5 mEq of sodium
Dialysis	As needed	Hours	Diffusive loss

*Cardiac monitoring done at all times.

free water excretion and is therefore suscep-tible to hyponatremia, particularly if large amounts of dilute solutions are administered. The therapy is free water restriction, which means limiting not only intake by mouth but also intravenous fluids (including hyperalimen-tation). Hypertonic sodium infusion can lead to pulmonary edema in the oliguric patient. Dialysis is often needed to correct hypona-tremia.

Hypocalcemia and Hyperphosphatemia

Failure of urinary excretion of phosphate leads to hyperphosphatemia with a reciprocal de-crease in calcium levels. Higher levels of phos-phate are found in patients in a catabolic state or those with rhabdomyolysis. Phosphate intake should be minimized, and phosphate binders, such as aluminum-containing antacids or cal-cium carbonate, should be administered. Mag-nesium-containing antacids should be avoided because renal excretion of magnesium is im-paired in ARF. The calcium-phosphate product should be kept at <70. If symptoms of hypo-calcemia, such as carpopedal spasm (Trous-seau's sign), a positive Chvostek's sign, or dys-rythmias are present, calcium needs to be ad-ministered.

Acidosis

Sodium bicarbonate should be administered if severe metabolic acidosis (serum bicarbonate concentration <15) is present.

Nutrition

Although early studies demonstrated that nu-tritional therapy improved survival and has-tened recovery of renal function in patients with ARF, these studies have not been confirmed. Still, one of the goals of therapy is to maintain good general health since the course of ARF is likely to last several weeks. The nutritional re-quirements of patients with ARF vary greatly and are largely dependent on the nature of the un-derlying disease and the integrity of other organ systems. For specifics of the nutrition prescrip-tion, the reader is referred to recent reviews (see Chapter 3 and Bibliography at end of this chapter).

Dialysis

Dialytic therapy for ARF is discussed in detail in Chapter 31. The timing of dialysis is impor-tant because early dialysis improves survival. Indications for initiation of dialysis are listed in the box on p. 338. The absolute levels of BUN and creatinine are not as important a factor in the decision to initiate dialysis as the patient's overall condition. Dialysis should be instituted when the BUN is >150, particularly if other metabolic abnormalities are present (e.g., acidosis or hyperkalemia). Many complications of uremia, such as neurologic manifestations, nausea and vomiting, and bleeding disorders, are improved with dialysis.

Bleeding

A clotting defect due to abnormal platelet function is present in ARF, and this defect may contribute to a bleeding tendency. Also, in the hemodialyzed patient, heparin is used to prevent dialyzer clotting. Treatment of the uremic platelet defect is discussed in Chapters 9 and 44. No-heparin dialysis can be performed if necessary.

Drug Dosing

Dosage adjustments need to be made for many drugs according to the level of renal function and the degree of drug removal resulting from dialysis. (See Bibliography and Chapters 9 and 15 for further information.)

Treatment of Rhabdomyolysis

Isotonic saline should be infused. If a patient has a crush injury, for example, after being caught under the rubble of a collapsed building, isotonic saline should be infused at 1.5 L/hr as soon as the trapped person's limbs are freed. Once the patient achieves hemodynamic stability and the urine flow is confirmed, intravenous hydration should be continued. Mannitol should be added. Administration of sodium bicarbonate will alkalinize the urine and reduce the nephrotoxic effects of myoglobin.

Indications for Dialysis

Volume overload
Uremia
Pericarditis
Hyperkalemia
Hyponatremia
Acid-base disturbance
Coma or seizures
Uremic bleeding

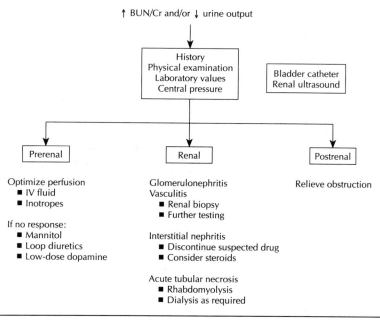

FIG. 30-1 Diagnostic and treatment approach to acute renal failure.

COURSE AND PROGNOSIS

For the hospitalized patient with ARF, the prognosis is highly dependent on resolution of the underlying disease since no patient, if properly managed, should die of uremia or its associated metabolic disturbances. In the surgical patient with ARF, the prognosis is often poor, with a mortality of 30% to 60%. Predictors of poor prognosis are listed in the accompanying box. As shown in the box, the number and type of complications are often the most important determinants of a poor prognosis.

In the oliguric patient with ARF whose underlying disease resolves, renal function begins to return after an average of 10 to 21 days. However, the course may be much shorter or prolonged for several months. Recovery is heralded by an increase in urine volume that is followed by a delayed fall in BUN and creatinine. In the nonoliguric patient, recovery often occurs earlier. In 10% of patients, no recovery of renal function occurs; in approximately 30%, only incomplete recovery is found, with a small percentage (5%) developing late deterioration of renal function.

Predictors of Poor Prognosis in Course of ARF

Dialysis requirement
Increment in serum creatinine >3 mg/dl
Oliguria
Abnormal urine sediment
Second episode of ARF
Number of complications
Multiorgan system failure
Respiratory failure
Cardiac failure
Sepsis
Coma

SUMMARY

- Determine whether ARF is prerenal, renal, or postrenal.
- Prerenal causes are suggested by postural blood pressure changes, acute weight loss, low central venous pressures, BUN/Cr >20, FENa <1, urine specific gravity >1.02, or urine osmolality >350.
- ATN is the most common cause of intrinsic ARF in the SICU.
- Normal to elevated central venous pressures, BUN/Cr of 10-20, FENa >1, urine specific gravity <1.01, and urine osmolality <350 suggest ATN.
- Examination of fresh urine specimen for protein, blood, WBCs, eosinophils, and RTE casts is important for diagnosis of intrinsic renal failure.
- Complete anuria suggests obstruction. Perform bladder catheterization as first diagnostic test. Renal ultrasound provides useful diagnostic information at minimal risk.

- Prompt correction of prerenal cause is the most effective approach to prevention.
- Mannitol and loop diuretics have value as prophylactic agents against radiocontrast nephrotoxicity but are not intended for treatment of established ATN.
- In euvolemic patients, maintenance fluid replacement should equal measured fluid losses plus estimated insensible loss.
- Do not routinely administer potassium in the oliguric patient. Use serum concentration to guide potassium replacement.
- Hyponatremia usually implies free water excess. Restrict free water.
- Minimize phosphate intake.
- Dialyze early if indications are present (see box, p. 338).
- Diagnosis and treatment are summarized in Fig. 30-1.

BIBLIOGRAPHY

Anderson RJ, Linas SL, Berns AS, et al. Nonoliguric acute renal failure. N Engl J Med 296:1134-1138, 1977.

Bennett WM. Practical guidelines for drug dosing in renal failure. In Brenner BM, Stein JH. Pharmacotherapy of Renal Disease and Hypertension. New York: Churchill Livingstone, 1987, p 349.

Better OS, Stein JH. Early management of shock and prophylaxis of acute renal failure in traumatic rhabdomyolysis. N Engl J Med 322:825-829, 1990.

Bonventre JV. Mediators of ischemic renal injury. Ann Rev Med 39:531-544, 1988.

Conger JD. Management of acute renal failure. In Jacobson HR, Striker GE, Klahr S, eds. The Principles and Practice of Nephrology. Philadelphia: BC Decker, 1991, p 667.

Gabow PA, Kaehny WD, Kelleher SP. The spectrum of rhabdomyolysis. Medicine 61:141-152, 1982.

Hou SH, Bushinsky DA, Wish JB, Cohen JJ, Harrington JT. Hospital acquired renal insufficiency: A prospective study. Am J Med 74:243-248, 1983.

Lange HW, Aappli DM, Brown DC. Survival of patients with acute renal failure requiring dialysis after open heart surgery: Early prognostic indicators. Am Heart J 113:1138-1143, 1987.

Miller TR, Anderson SRJ, Linas SL, Hendrich WL, Berns A, Gabow PA, Schrier RW. Urinary diagnostic indices in acute renal failure. A prospective study. Ann Intern Med 89:47-50, 1978.

Mitch WE, Wilmore DW. Nutritional considerations in the treatment of acute renal failure. In Brenner BM, Lazarus JM. Acute Renal Failure. New York: Churchill Livingstone, 1988, p 743.

Myers BD, Moran SM. Hemodynamically mediated acute renal failure. N Engl J Med 314:97-105, 1986.

Rudnick MR, Bastl CP, Elfinbein IB, Narins RG. The differential diagnosis of acute renal failure. In Brenner BM, Lazarus JM. Acute Renal Failure. New York: Churchill Livingstone, 1988, p 177.

Wheeler DC, Feehally J, Walls J. High risk acute renal failure. Q J Med 61:977-984, 1986.

CHAPTER 31

Support of Renal Function

Connie L. Manske

HEMODIALYSIS

In healthy individuals, the kidney serves the dual function of eliminating waste products and controlling fluid balance. Critically ill patients frequently sustain a loss of one or both of these renal functions and require support with dialysis. Dialysis therapy is initiated when the level of waste products in the blood is toxic, or when fluid balance cannot be maintained with the aggressive use of diuretics. The major indications for emergency dialysis include fluid overload that compromises oxygenation, hyperkalemia that cannot be managed with ion-exchange resins or diuretics, uncontrollable bleeding not attributable to a cause other than uremia, or anuria. Additional indications are summarized in Chapter 30.

The dialysis process alters the solute composition of blood by exposing it to a dialysis solution through a semipermeable membrane (Fig. 31-1). Water molecules and small-molecular-weight solutes in the blood can pass through the membrane pores into the dialysate, but large solutes, such as proteins, cannot pass through the membrane and remain in the plasma.

The factors listed in Table 31-1 affect solute and water transport across the dialysis membrane.

The ability of dialysis to remove many solutes depends on the area of the dialysis membrane and the rate of blood flow through the dialyzer (Fig. 31-2). However, large or highly protein-bound solutes cannot be removed well with dialysis. The ability of dialysis to remove fluid depends on the area of the dialysis membrane and the amount of pressure applied

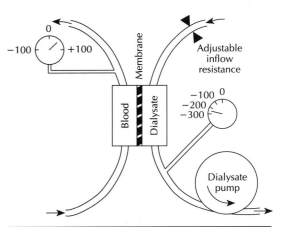

FIG. 31-1 Dialyzer with blood flowing in one direction and dialysis solution flowing in opposite direction. Hydrostatic pressure across membrane (and ultrafiltration) is adjusted by varying resistance to inflow of dialysis solution. Position of gauges monitoring pressure at blood and dialysate outflow ports also is shown, along with typical operating pressures. In this case transmembrane pressure is 300 mg Hg (+50 at the blood outlet − [−250] at dialysate outlet). (Redrawn from Daugirdas JT, Ing TS, eds. Handbook of Dialysis. Boston: Little, Brown, 1988, p 14.)

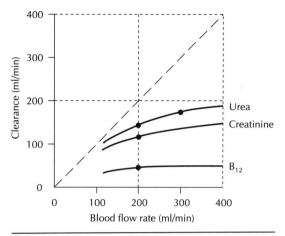

FIG. 31-2 Relationship between blood flow rate and dialyzer whole blood clearance rates for urea, creatinine, and vitamin B_{12} (for a low-efficiency dialyzer). (Redrawn from Daugirdas JT, Ing TS, eds. Handbook of Dialysis. Boston: Little, Brown, 1988, p 16.)

TABLE 31-1	The Dialysis Process

Dialysis Function	Factors Affecting Dialysis
Solute removal	Molecular size of solute
	Concentration gradient between blood and dialysate for solute
Fluid removal	Ultrafiltration capacity of dialysis membrane (K_{uf})
	Transmembrane pressure

across the membrane. For both solute and water removal, increasing the amount of time a patient receives dialysis can be used to increase efficiency. Because solute removal depends on the initial solute concentration, dialysis becomes progressively less efficient as the solute concentration is lowered. For this reason, dialysis is performed intermittently, when toxic levels of waste products have accumulated in the bloodstream.

Successful dialysis depends on access to the bloodstream. Temporary access can be estab-lished using a double-lumen dialysis catheter, in which the catheter contains both the venous and arterial ports, or a Scribner shunt, which is created surgically by inserting external tubing between the radial artery and cephalic vein. Access characteristics are summarized in Table 31-2.

The dialysis procedure is performed by a trained hemodialysis nurse as specified by written orders from a nephrologist. Before dialysis, the nephrologist assesses the patient and determines an appropriate "dry" weight. Table 31-3 lists the variables that must be specified for dialysis. During the dialysis run, the nurse records the blood pressure every 15 minutes and sends laboratory tests as ordered.

The expected fluid removal with dialysis is determined by the transmembrane pressure and is calculated as shown in Table 31-3. Newer dialysis machines can measure the actual quantity of fluid removed. A single dialysis procedure can remove up to 4 L of fluid, but many critically ill patients cannot tolerate this amount of fluid removal.

Removal of toxic waste products is less straightforward than removal of fluid. Although lower molecular weight substances such as potassium and magnesium can be easily removed, higher molecular weight compounds may be dialyzed less easily. The blood urea nitrogen (BUN) and creatinine concentrations are often used as indicators of dialysis adequacy. However, these values are often unreliable in critically ill patients (Table 31-4).

Regular dialysis, done thrice weekly for 4 hours at a time and at a blood flow rate of at least 200 ml/min, gives the patient the equivalent of an average weekly glomerular filtration rate (GFR) of 10 to 15 ml/min. No large prospective studies compare daily dialysis with thrice-weekly dialysis, but the limited data available suggest no benefit from intensive dialysis. This finding is consistent with the accepted approach to patients with chronic renal failure, in whom dialysis is not begun until the GFR drops to 5 to 10 ml/min.

A number of complications can occur while the patient is undergoing dialysis. The most common one is hypotension (see box, p. 344).

TABLE 31-2 Access for Hemodialysis

Access Mode	Advantages	Disadvantages	Relative Contraindications
Subclavian catheter	Usable for many weeks	Potentially life-threatening complications: pneumothorax, air embolism, arterial puncture, superior cava puncture, tamponade; high incidence of subclavian vein stenosis	Patient cannot lie flat; coagulopathy; severe pulmonary compromise; lack of skilled operator to insert; bacteremic patient (risk of catheter seeding)
Femoral catheter	Low rate of catheter-associated bacteremia: easy to insert	Temporary (<72 hours)	Agitated patient, previous lower extremity bypass procedure with prosthetic or vein graft
Scribner shunt	Low risk of insertion	High incidence of infection, thrombosis; permanent loss of artery	Future need for permanent dialysis; poor ulnar circulation, bacteremic patient

TABLE 31-3 Dialysis Orders

Variable	Options Available	Usual Choice
Dialyzer K_{uf} (ml/hr/mm Hg)	1.4-7.8	4-6
Dialyzer surface area (m^2)	0.5-1.9	1.4-1.8
Blood flow rate (ml/min)	100-350	250
Transmembrane pressure (TMP) (mm Hg)	0-500	Calculate from desired fluid loss (F): $TMP = F/(K_{uf} \times hr$ of dialysis)
Dialysate composition		
Potassium (mEq/L)	0-4	2 (varies with patient)
Base	Acetate or bicarbonate (35 mEq/l)	Bicarbonate
Dextrose (g/dl)	0-200	200
Anticoagulation	Administer to patient or dialyzer only	Administer heparin
Length of dialysis (hr)	2.5-5	4

TABLE 31-4 Factors Other Than Renal Function That Affect Creatinine and BUN Values

	Increase	Decrease
Creatinine	Muscle catabolism Diabetic ketoacidosis	Decreased muscle mass (immobilization, amputation, advanced age)
BUN	Gastrointestinal bleeding Catabolic state Steroid therapy Volume depletion Excessive protein intake Diuretics Acidosis	Hepatic failure

Causes of Hypotension During Dialysis

Common causes

Excessive decrease in blood volume because of high ultrafiltration rate, low target dry weight
Lack of vasoconstriction because of antihypertensives, acetate in dialysate
Poor cardiac function

Uncommon causes

Tamponade
Myocardial infarction
Hemorrhage
Septicemia
Dysrhythmias
Anaphylaxis
Hemodialysis
Air embolism

Possible solutions

Evaluate patient for blood loss
Increase target dry weight
Reduce transmembrane pressure or decrease dialyzer size
Increase pressor medications
Stop antihypertensives
Transfuse any required blood products during dialysis
Consider uncommon causes listed above

Less common complications include cramps, nausea, vomiting, headache, dialysis disequilibrium, anaphylactic reaction to the dialyzer, and air embolus. Dialysis also can be associated with hypoxemia. The P_{O_2} may fall 5 to 30 mm Hg, a decrease that may be dangerous in a critically ill patient who is not receiving mechanical ventilation. This hypoxemia is nearly always a result of hypoventilation induced by metabolic alkalosis caused by bicarbonate transfer from the dialyzer or by loss of carbon dioxide into the dialysate. Complement activation by the dialysis membrane may also disturb ventilation/perfusion matching when Cuprophane membranes are used.

Medication and hyperalimentation require special attention in dialysis patients. Because the major waste products removed by dialysis are derived from protein catabolism and because many critically ill patients are catabolic, excessively high protein loads should be avoided. (See Chapter 3 for metabolic support guidelines.) Drug metabolism is altered in patients with renal failure, and many unmeasured metabolites accumulate in the bloodstream. In addition, highly protein bound drugs such as warfarin and phenytoin are displaced from albumin by organic acids. High levels of free drug then result. The number of medications should be minimized in dialysis patients. Specific guidelines for common drugs are summarized in the upper box on p. 345 and in Chapter 15. Clinical pharmacologists and nephrologists can help determine appropriate medication regimens. The *Physicians' Desk Reference* also includes information on drug use in renal failure.

Fluid removal with dialysis is limited by the patient's hemodynamic status and the time spent receiving dialysis. Because removal of more than 4 L of fluid at a time is generally not possible, the patient's total fluid intake, including blood products, should be limited to no more than 2 L plus replacement of urine and nasogastric drainage. Urine output can frequently be increased by diuretic use. An effective strategy is to combine a loop diuretic such as furosemide or bumetanide with a thiazide diuretic such as metolazone or hydrochlorothiazide. The use of bolus doses of loop diuretics should be avoided because of the high risk of ototoxicity. Intravenous furosemide in doses greater than 100 mg should be given as a controlled infusion of 4 mg/min. Alternatively, a recent study suggests that a continuous low-dose intravenous infusion of bumetanide may be effective in patients with chronic renal failure. The need for fluid removal with dialysis should be minimized by concentrating all medications and alimentation solutions in the smallest possible volume of fluid.

CONTINUOUS ARTERIOVENOUS HEMOFILTRATION

Continuous arteriovenous hemofiltration, or CAVH, is a method of renal replacement therapy developed to facilitate fluid removal. In this procedure, a large catheter similar to a hemodialysis catheter is used to deliver blood to a hemofilter (Fig. 31-3). The patient's blood pressure maintains blood flow, and no external pump is needed. The ultrafiltrate passes through the membrane into the ultrafiltration space and drains into a collection bag. Gravity drainage creates subatmospheric pressure in the filter, which increases the ultrafiltration rate. The blood cells and proteins remaining in the blood chamber are then returned to the patient. The process is continued 24 hours per day. Large volumes of fluid (up to 900 ml/hr) can be removed with this therapy, and replacement fluid must be infused into the patient (Fig. 31-3). Because of this fluid exchange, a limited clearance of waste products also occurs.

CAVH can be modified to slow continuous ultrafiltration if solute clearance is not necessary. Ultrafiltration rate is limited to <5 ml/min and replacement fluid is not given. With either procedure, volume status and medication dosages must be monitored carefully.

Continuous Arteriovenous Hemofiltration With Dialysis

Patients with severe renal failure cannot achieve adequate solute clearance with CAVH. In this situation, intermittent hemodialysis can be instituted or CAVH can be modified to include dialysis (CAVHD) (Fig. 31-4). Dialysate is infused into the dialyzer, countercurrent to blood flow. Solute removal is effected as in hemodialysis (see earlier discussion). The ultrafiltration rate can be decreased to <5 ml/min, diminishing the need for replacement fluid.

CHOOSING A METHOD OF RENAL REPLACEMENT THERAPY

Advantages and disadvantages of CAVH compared to hemodialysis are summarized in the lower box. Unfortunately, randomized prospective studies are not available comparing the

---

Use of Medications in Dialysis Patients

Medications to avoid

Meperidine (Demerol): Metabolite causes seizures

Magnesium-containing compounds

Medications requiring altered administration

Antibiotics: Many require reduction in maintenance dose; penicillin in high levels can cause seizures

Cimetidine: Dosage decreased to 300 mg bid should be given after dialysis

Digoxin: Loading dose is decreased 50% because of reduction in volume of distribution; maintenance dose also decreased

Procainamide: Active drug and active metabolite accumulate at different rates; use only if levels are available for both and only in inpatient setting

Ranitidine: Dose decreased to 50 mg q 18-24 hr

Sedatives and pain medications: Efficacy achieved with low doses in many patients; may accumulate and cause excessive sedation

---

CAVH Compared to Hemodialysis

Advantages

Well tolerated in hypotension

Allows greater volume of fluid removal

Does not require continuous presence of dialysis nurse

Disadvantages

Requires anticoagulation

Requires continuous bedrest

Requires high volume of fluid replacement

Has low efficiency in removing urea and other metabolic end products

Medication dosage adjustment can be problematic

Expensive

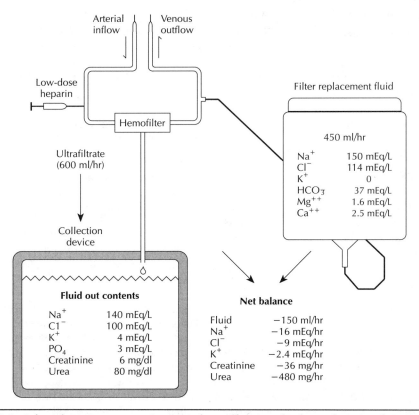

FIG. 31-3 Principles of continuous arteriovenous hemofiltration. (Redrawn from Mault JR, Dirkes SM, Swartz RD, Bartlett RH. Continuous Hemofiltration: A Reference Guide for SCUF, CAVH, and CAVHD. Copyright © 1988, James R. Mault. Used by permission.)

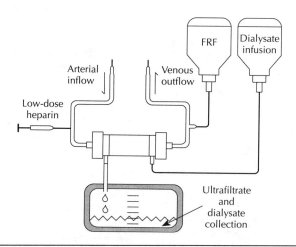

FIG. 31-4 Continuous arteriovenous hemodialysis. *FRF,* filtration replacement fluid. (Redrawn from Mault JR, Dirkes SM, Swartz RD, Bartlett RH. Continuous Hemofiltration: A Reference Guide for SCUF, CAVH, and CAVHD. Copyright © 1988, James R. Mault. Used by permission.)

morbidity and mortality of these dialysis methods. Hemodialysis has the advantage of being widely available. CAVH and CAVHD require skilled nursing staff, specifically trained in their use, as well as clinical pharmacologists, to aid in the modification of medication doses. CAVH may be useful in patients who do not tolerate hemodialysis or who require large amounts of alimentation solutions or blood products. In addition, intriguing evidence exists that CAVH may remove endotoxin-triggered mediators, such as thromboxane A_2 and leukotrienes, and may possibly increase survival rates in persons with multiorgan system failure. For the purpose of mediator removal, even larger volumes of fluid removal may be required, necessitating continuous use of a blood pump.

SUMMARY

- Monitor variables of fluid balance, including daily weights, blood pressure in lying and standing positions, pulse, and hemodynamic measurements if available.
- Monitor variables of uremia, including creatinine and BUN values, pericardial rub, and anorexia and nausea.
- Be alert for serious complications of dialysis, including hypoxemia, hypotension, and anaphylactic reaction to dialyzer membrane.
- Monitor patient for evidence of bleeding.
- Limit intravenous fluid administration.
- Limit hyperalimentation to less than 1.5 g/kg/day of protein, if appropriate for level of metabolic stress.
- Check all medication dosages for necessary adjustments, including the need for a supplemental dose after hemodialysis.
- Consider use of CAVH in patients with refractory volume overload or need for large quantities of blood products.

BIBLIOGRAPHY

Bartlett RH, Mault JR, Dechert RE, et al. Continuous arteriovenous hemofiltration: Improved survival in surgical acute renal failure? Surgery 100:400-408, 1986.

Barzilay E, Kessler D, Berlot G, et al. Use of extracorporeal supportive techniques as additional treatment for septic-induced multiple organ failure patients. Crit Care Med 17:634-637, 1989.

Brater C. Handbook of Drug Use in Patients with Renal Disease. Lancaster, Tex.: Improved Therapeutics, 1989.

Cogan MG, Garovoy MR, eds. Introduction to Dialysis. New York: Churchill Livingstone, 1985.

Daugirdas JT, Ing TS, eds. Handbook of Dialysis. Boston: Little, Brown, 1988.

Golper TA. Continuous arteriovenous hemofiltration in acute renal failure. Am J Kidney Dis 6:373-386, 1985.

Mault JR, Dirkes SM, Swartz RD, Bartlett RH. Continuous hemofiltration: A reference guide for SCUF, CAVH, and CAVHD, 1988.

Rudy DW, Voelker JR, Greene PK, et al. Loop diuretics for chronic renal insufficiency: A continuous infusion is more efficacious than bolus therapy. Ann Intern Med 115:360-366, 1991.

Schneider NS, Geronemus RP. Continuous arteriovenous hemodialysis. Kidney Int 24(Suppl):S159-S162, 1988.

Storck M, Hartl WH, Zimmerer E, Inthorn D. Comparison of pump-driven and spontaneous continuous hemofiltration in postoperative acute renal failure. Lancet 337:452-455, 1991.

CHAPTER 32

Physiologic Alterations of the Gut Mucosal Barrier

David C. Evans • Oren K. Steinmetz • Jonathan L. Meakins

NORMAL GUT BARRIOR FUNCTION

The gut mucosal barrier (GMB) is a multitiered defense against systemic invasion by intestinally contained microorganisms, which are potentially lethal to the host. Whereas the stomach and upper tract normally are sparsely inhabited by *Lactobacillus* and Gram-positive species, the colon harbors hundreds of bacterial strains, including Enterobacteriaceae, *Proteus,* enterococcus, *Pseudomonas, Lactobacillus,* and a greater than 1000-fold predominance of anaerobic species. The consequences of failure to contain these strains and the toxins they elaborate are well appreciated in the critically ill patient.[1,2] To the end that supportive therapy can be directed appropriately, it is essential that all components of the GMB be understood (see box, p. 349).

Physical Barrier
Mechanical barrier

The enterocyte's lipid membrane, bound to adjacent cells by tight junctions, is a physical barrier to bacterial invasion. The orderly turnover of healthy cells is crucial to maintenance of this barrier. Malnutrition, hypoxia, and the reduced trophic stimulation of gut hormones characteristic of the catabolic state impair cell migration and regeneration, thereby compromising this barrier. Coordinated intestinal motility, also commonly disrupted in the SICU patient, is not only an essential stimulus to cellular turnover but also maintains the flow of bacterial toxins through the digestive tract.

Chemical and enzymatic barriers

A gastric pH <4.5 is antibacterial. Pepsinogen is activated to pepsin at this pH level and helps to counter further the action of microbes and their toxins. Like bile salts, mucin secreted throughout the GI tract nonspecifically binds bacteria and endotoxins within the bowel lumen. Substances such as lactoferrin and salivary lysozyme also serve in part to inhibit the growth of sensitive organisms. Mucin also protects the enterocyte from gastric acidity by maintaining an alkaline gradient of bicarbonate against the cell surface. SICU patients, particularly those who are intubated, often fail to maintain normal gastric sterility. Their upper GI tracts can become colonized by enteric and extrinsic nosocomial organisms, a threat exacerbated by antacid antiulcer therapy.[3]

Elements of Gut Mucosal Barrier

Physical

Mechanical

Healthy enterocyte
Tight junction
Cell turnover
Normal motility

Chemical

Gastric acidity
Salivary lysozyme
Lactoferrin
Mucous secretion
Bile salts

Immunologic

Local

Gut-associated lymphoid tissue (GALT):
Intraepithelial lymphocytes
Submucosal aggregates
Peyer's patches
Mesenteric nodes' secretory IgA

Systemic

Kupffer cell bed
Circulating lymphocytes

Bacteriologic

Balanced enteric microflora

Immunologic Barrier
Local barrier

The intestinal mucosa and submucosa are richly inhabited by macrophages, lymphocytes, neutrophils, eosinophils, and mast cells. Peyer's patches are strategically located to sample the antigenic load of the gut contents. Along with the lymphoid tissue of the lamina propria, they give rise to activated B lymphocytes, which mature in mesenteric lymph nodes and reach the systemic circulation by way of the thoracic duct. These B cells differentiate predominantly into secretory IgA-producing plasmocytes, which selectively relocate along mucosal surfaces to secrete antibodies into saliva, bile, and succus. Secretory IgA binds bowel bacteria, inducing bacteriolysis, and prevents their adherence to mucosal surfaces. A population of T lymphocytes also resides alongside the enterocytes of the gut mucosa to provide a cytotoxic line of defense.

Systemic barrier

Bacteria and toxins translocating across the GMB enter the portal circulation and filter through the Kupffer-cell macrophage bed of the liver. After sampling portal antigens, these cells are involved in the mediation of systemic immune responses.[4] Gram-negative bacteria, which either colonize the small bowel or are injected into the portal circulation, depress the delayed-type hypersensitivity response to subcutaneously injected antigens.[5] Kupffer cells appear to produce immunologic mediators in response to antigenic stimulation by the gut. These cells also prompt increased interleukin-1 and prostaglandin E_2 production when exposed to endotoxin. Unregulated antigenic stimulation possibly prompts an exaggerated immune response that culminates in the syndrome of multiple system organ failure (MSOF).[6]

Bacteriologic Barrier

The maintenance of normal gut microbial ecology is critical in the prevention of enteric autoinfection. Not only do intestinal microflora stimulate and nourish the mucosal cells, preserving barrier integrity and enhancing mechanical function, they also act to prevent overgrowth or colonization by potentially harmful organisms. Enteric bacteria translocate across gut mucosa when antibiotic use has altered normal microbial populations.[7] Furthermore, common SICU-acquired infections relate to overgrowth of certain gut commensals, including enterococcus, *Staphylococcus epidermidis, Pseudomonas,* and *Candida.* Alterations of gut microflora also impair local host immunity and increase the potential for GMB failure. Translocation of *Candida* across gut mucosa in debilitated surgical patients has been demonstrated.[8]

TRANSLOCATION

Translocation refers to the extraintestinal migration of gut bacteria and bacterial toxins under conditions of compromised intestinal mucosal barrier function. This phenomenon has been demonstrated convincingly under experimental conditions that mimic those present in the critically ill.[9,10] Gut bacteria have been isolated in homogenates of liver, spleen, and mesenteric lymph nodes in amounts proportional to the degree of imposed hypovolemic shock in laboratory animals.[11] Bacteremia of enteric origin is also described as a fatal complication of chemotherapy in neutropenic patients. Other stress factors thought to enhance translocation are peritonitis, bowel obstruction, inflammatory bowel disease, thermal injury, bacterial overgrowth, immunosuppression, splanchnic low-flow states, and endotoxemia. Bacteremic organisms in patients with these conditions are often the predominant aerobic fecal strains.

Enteric microflora enhance gut function by facilitating digestion, nutritionally supporting the mucosal epithelium, and maintaining a crucial balance of commensal organisms; in addition, they represent a threat to the host should the gut fail to contain them adequately. The lipopolysaccharide component of the gram-negative bacterial cell wall known as endotoxin is a well-recognized trigger of the septic clinical state marked by fever, confusion, tachycardia, hyperdynamic circulation, water retention, hyperbilirubinemia, compromised renal function, and impaired respiratory function. Because endotoxin is a product of both viable and nonviable bacteria, the gut comprises the body's largest reservoir of potentially harmful bacterial products. "Autointoxication" by these microbial substances is regarded by many as the first step in a cascade of systemic events culminating in the highly fatal syndrome of MSOF.[12]

MULTIPLE SYSTEM ORGAN FAILURE AS SEQUELA OF ENDOTOXEMIA

Although the syndrome of MSOF is familiar to the critical care physician, its causes and mechanisms are elusive, and its management disappointing. Triple organ failure persisting longer than 3 days is almost uniformly fatal. Whereas advanced age and severity of illness are commonly associated, clinical sepsis is almost always present. Untreated infection has largely been held responsible, but the frequent failure to identify an infectious focus by routine cultures, postmortem studies, and blind laparotomy has resulted in the concept of nonbacterial clinical sepsis.[2]

The septic state can arise in the absence of infection by systemic exposure to endotoxin, an obvious source of which is the compromised gut. Tumor necrosis factor (TNF), interleukin-1, interleukin-2, and prostaglandins are host-derived mediators in this process and are capable of invoking the "septic response" independent of endotoxin, implicating endotoxin as an activator. A recent controlled prospective clinical trial using HA-1A human IgM antibody against the lipid A domain of endotoxin showed that monoclonal immunotherapy can reduce mortality effectively in patients with Gram-negative bacteremia.[13] In all other clinical settings this protection was not observed, a finding that questions the true role of endotoxin as a trigger for MSOF. Therapeutic intervention directed at the mediators of the septic response offers a promising and focused approach to this complex physiologic problem.

The unhealthy gut thus must be recognized as a potential instigator of MSOF.[9] As long as the management of MSOF remains generalized, attempted prevention through intestinal support is paramount in the SICU setting. Although numerous prophylactic automatisms have become well established, current thinking challenges common protocols, particularly the value of "bowel rest" and a pH-neutral stomach, and calls for a rational updated approach.

SUPPORTING GUT BARRIER FUNCTION

Assessment of intestinal function traditionally has been a clinical exercise based on the presence of ileus, diarrhea, gastritis, and stress ulceration. Maintenance of the gut mucosal barrier per se previously has been a nonissue that now must assume critical significance. Although providing support of intestinal physiology as described in the following material is important, the key to preserving mucosal function is control of the process initiating or contributing to its compromise. Be it infection, ischemia, or rejection, rapid resolution of the inciting process is pivotal to the effective management of sepsis. Sepsis, and ultimately MSOF, is a late-stage manifestation of the biologic response to some initial physiologic derangement, and effective therapy must integrate the following concept: *Infection is a process—sepsis is a response.*

To control the response, the process first must be controlled. This concept, however, addresses squarely the need for diligence in the clinical approach to the prevention and treatment of MSOF in which gut mucosal barrier dysfunction is but one of many components that may comprise either the primary inciting event or some secondary sequelae.

Because reliable variables to monitor the health of the GMB do not currently exist, the most appropriate approach aims at bolstering GMB's three constituents: mucosal integrity, the balance of commensal microflora, and immunocompetency. Optimum support is achieved by careful attention to the following objectives.

Oxygenation

Breakdown of the GMB and bacterial translocation occur in splanchnic low-flow states such as hypovolemic shock or cardiac arrest. Hypoxia, enterocyte-protease activation, and superoxide free radical generation are postulated mechanisms. Experimental evidence supports a role for therapy with antiprostaglandins and free radical scavengers. In practice, therapy is limited to maintaining adequately oxygenated circulation to the splanchnic bed. Volume therapy, appropriate oxygen-carrying capacity (hemoglobin), and adequate resuscitation incorporating an oxygen saturation >90% are essential. Hemodynamic monitoring and support and assisted ventilation should be used as required. Some investigators advocate pharmacologic dilation of the splanchnic vascular bed with low-dose dopamine. In the experimental setting beta-adrenergic agonists (isoproterenol),[2] cholinergic agents, and peptide hormones have all shown promise.[14]

Nutritional Support

Providing adequate nutrition is essential to bolster the immune machinery and reverse the catabolic state. Controversy exists about the appropriate role for parenteral vs. enteral nutrition. Barring obvious contraindications, enteral nutrition should be begun as soon as possible in the critically ill. If total gastric output is <600 ml per day, the risk of aspiration is negligible. Intrajejunal feeding with gastrostomy decompression of the stomach provides the safest access because the esophageal sphincters remain competent and aspiration-inducing reflux is limited. Tolerance to such feeding is assessed over a 24-hour trial period and is deemed adequate when the 4-hour gastric residuum is

<50 ml, vomiting and cramps are absent, and no worsening of abdominal distention or diarrhea occurs. Passage of flatus and presence of bowel sounds are unreliable indicators of tolerance to enteral feeding.

Parenteral nutrition

The beneficial role of total parenteral nutrition (TPN) for the support of the catabolic patient is undisputed. However, experimental studies document mucosal villus atrophy and impaired intestinal motility with fasting and TPN use.[15] The nonessential amino acid glutamine, supplied by release from skeletal muscle in the stressed state, constitutes the major oxidizable fuel source for the small bowel. TPN supplementation with 2% glutamine attenuates mucosal wasting and increases enterocyte turnover.[16] Furthermore, bile S-IgA levels are increased, and bacterial translocation reportedly is reduced. TPN should be used only when thorough clinical assessment of gut function determines enteral feeding inappropriate or impossible. TPN is costly and assumes a definite risk of complication, which may contribute to patient morbidity.

Enteral nutrition

Experimental evidence suggests that enteral feedings stimulate the gut and strengthen mucosal barrier function.[17] Motility is enhanced; consequently, the contact time of gut toxins with the mucosa is reduced. Villus height is maintained, and absorptive capacity is protected. The colonocyte specifically requires butyrate for sodium and water resorption. Butyrate normally is made available by bacterial fermentation. Pectin added to enteral feeds provides a fermentable polysaccharide that enhances this function and promotes colonic epithelial growth.

Stress Ulcer Prophylaxis

Superficial gastric erosions causing serious hemorrhage are well recognized in the SICU patient population. Intragastric administration of antacids to maintain a pH of 5 or higher is the most effective mode of gastric alkalinization, but IV histamine type-2 (H_2) blockers are also commonly used. Although both antacids and H_2 blockers provide effective ulcer prophylaxis, the overall effect on morbidity and mortality remains unclear. Although antacids and H_2 blockers are routinely used in North America, they are rarely used in Europe, with no apparent cost in important GI hemorrhage. The catastrophic bleeding episodes seen in SICU patients in the 1970s now rarely occur. It has been hypothesized that improved methods of resuscitation and supportive care are more responsible for their prevention than the use of routine gastric alkalinization. A significant adverse effect of alkalinization is colonization of the stomach with Gram-negative bacteria. These organisms can gain access to the upper airways and cause pneumonia.[18]

Recent work by Driks et al.[3] suggests that when intubated patients are treated with cytoprotective agents such as sucralfate, gastric acidity and relative gastric sterility are preserved. Compared to antacids, use of these agents in a randomized controlled trial was associated with half the rate of pneumonia and a lower overall mortality rate.

Antibiotic Prophylaxis

The appropriate use of antibiotics in the SICU for the prophylaxis of infection of enteric origin is a contentious issue. Selective decontamination of the digestive tract (SDD) was introduced by Stoutenbeck et al.[19] as a means to control enteric sepsis by (1) eliminating aerobic Gram-negative gut bacteria, (2) preventing fungal overgrowth, and (3) preserving commensal anaerobic microflora of the oropharynx and GI tract. The usual regimen is as follows:

Topical oral paste (tid):
  Polymyxin E, 2%, wt/wt
  Tobramycin, 2%, wt/wt
  Amphotericin B, 2%, wt/wt

Intragastric antibiotics (tid):
  Polymyxin E, 100 mg
  Tobramycin, 80 mg
  Amphotericin B, 500 mg

Systemic antibiotic:
  Cefotaxime, 50 mg/kg/day IV for 4 days

Microbiologic monitoring in the form of thrice-weekly cultures from the nasopharynx,

tracheobronchial aspirate, gastric aspirate, urine, blood, and rectum is required to assess the efficacy of sterilization and the emergence of resistant bacterial strains. As concluded by numerous investigators, this intervention appears to sterilize the nasopharynx successfully and to reduce bacterial counts variably in the stomach and rectum.[6,19,20] It is also useful in the elimination of resistant nosocomial strains of gut-colonizing bacteria in an SICU patient.[21] When compared to control results, SDD prophylaxis is associated with a lower overall incidence of nosocomial infection in SICU patients.[20] Pneumonia, the most common infectious complication, can be reduced significantly, and patients appear to suffer fewer septic episodes associated with Gram-negative bacteremia.

Theoretically, SDD should diminish the risk of exposure to circulating endotoxin and attendant MSOF. However, the mortality rate is reduced only in certain subgroups, namely, patients with trauma, long-stay patients, and those with midrange APACHE II scores.[22] The effect on MSOF specifically is unclear.

The use of a systemic cephalosporin to prevent infection before the triple-antibiotic regimen can attain a sterilizing effect may promote colonization with resistant organisms.[23] Studies show that aminoglycoside-resistant strains can emerge in SDD-treated patients and early colonization with staphylococcus may be enhanced. Presumably the decreased rate of nosocomial infection in SDD patients is due primarily to sterilization of the upper oropharynx and digestive tract. In this way the results of SDD compare to similar findings in patients receiving cytoprotective sucralfate therapy, which preserves bacteriostatic gastric acidity.[3]

The precise role of SDD and the elucidation of effective regimens need further clarification. It appears that hemodynamic and nutritional measures to support both the intestine and the immune system constitute the more rational approach to prophylaxis against sepsis of enteric origin and endotoxin-mediated MSOF (Fig. 32-1).

■   ■   ■

Like the so-called "vital organs," the intestine must be regarded by the SICU physician as a target organ requiring aggressive support to ensure patient survival. Evidence exists to implicate the debilitated gut as an instigator of MSOF.

Currently therapeutic measures aimed at maintaining gut homeostasis fall into the realm of generalized supportive care, but promising new approaches based on focused research are beginning to evolve.

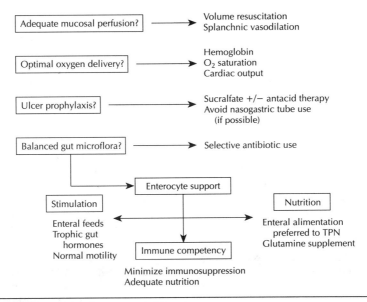

FIG. 32-1 Approach to support of gut mucosal barrier.

SUMMARY

- GMB protects the host against potentially lethal microorganisms contained in the gut.
- GMB consists of mechanical, chemical, enzymatic, immunologic, and bacteriologic components.
- Translocation is the extraintestinal migration of gut bacteria and bacterial toxins and is regarded as a first step in the path to MSOF.
- Source control includes maintenance of GMB. Support of GMB includes nutritional support, especially with enteral nutrition; stress ulcer prophylaxis with cytoprotective agents, which may preserve gastric sterility; and antibiotic prophylaxis (use of SDD remains controversial).

REFERENCES

1. Saadia R, Schein M, MacFarlane C, Boffard KD. Gut barrier function and the surgeon. Br J Surg 77:487-492, 1990.
2. Steinmetz OK, Meakins JL. Care of the gut in the surgical intensive care unit: Fact or fiction? Can J Surg 34:207-215, 1991.
3. Driks MR, Craven DE, Celli BR, et al. Nosocomial pneumonia in intubated patients given sucralfate as compared with antacids or histamine type-2 blockers. N Engl J Med 317:1376-1381, 1987.
4. Marshall J, Lee C, Meakins JL. Kupffer cell modulation of the systemic immune response. Arch Surg 122:191-196, 1987.
5. Marshall J, Christou NJ, Meakins JL. Immunomodulation by altered gastrointestinal tract flora. Arch Surg 123:1465-1469, 1988.
6. Billiar TR, Maddaus MA, West MA, et al. Intestinal

gram-negative overgrowth in vivo augments the in vitro response of Kupffer cells to endotoxin. Ann Surg 208:532-540, 1988.

7. Berg RD. Promotion of the translocation of enteric bacilli from the gastrointestinal tracts of mice by oral treatment with penicillin, clindamycin or metronidazole. Infect Immun 33:854-861, 1981.

8. Stone HH, Kolb LD, Currie CA, et al. *Candida* sepsis: Pathogenesis and principles of treatment. Ann Surg 179:697-711, 1974.

9. Deitch EA. The role of intestinal barrier failure and bacterial translocation in the development of systemic infection and multiple organ failure. Arch Surg 125:403-404, 1990.

10. Schweinburg FR, Seligman AM, Fine J. Transmural migration of intestinal bacteria—A study based on the use of radioactive *Escherichia coli.* N Engl J Med 242:747-752, 1950.

11. Baker JW, Deitch EA, Berg RD, Specian RD. Hemodynamic shock induces bacterial translocation from the gut. J Trauma 28:896-906, 1988.

12. Fry DE. Multiple system organ failure. Surg Clin North Am 68:107-122, 1988.

13. Ziegler EJ, Fisher CJ, Sprung CL, et al. Treatment of gram-negative bacteremia and septic shock with HA-1A human monoclonal antibody against endotoxin. N Engl J Med 324:429-436, 1991.

14. Richardson PDI. Pharmacology of intestinal blood flow and oxygen uptake. In Shepherd AP, Granger DN. Physiology of the Intestinal Circulation. New York: Raven Press, 1984.

15. Eastwood GL. Small bowel morphology and epithelial proliferation in intravenously alimented rats. Surgery 82:613-620, 1977.

16. Hwanu TL, O'Dwyer ST, Smith RJ, et al. Preservation of the small bowel mucosa using glutamine enriched parenteral nutrition. Surg Forum 37:56-58, 1986.

17. Alverdy JC, Chi HS, Sheldon GF. The effect of parenteral nutrition on gastrointestinal immunity: The importance of enteral stimulation. Ann Surg 202:681-684, 1985.

18. DuMoulin GC, Patterson DG, Hedley-Whyte J, et al. Aspiration of gastric bacteria in antacid-treated patients: A frequent cause of postoperative colonization of the airway. Lancet 1:242-245, 1982.

19. Stoutenbeck CP, Van Saene HKF, Miranda DR, Zandstra DF. The effect of selective decontamination of the digestive tract on colonisation and infection rate in multiple trauma patients. Intensive Care Med 10:185-192, 1984.

20. Blair P, Rowlands BJ, Lowry K, et al. Selective decontamination of the digestive tract: A stratified, randomized, prospective study in a mixed intensive care unit. Surgery 110:303-310, 1991.

21. Brun-Buisson C, Legrand P, Rauss A. Intestinal decontamination for control of nosocomial multiresistant gram-negative bacilli—Study of an outbreak in an intensive care unit. Ann Intern Med 110:873-881, 1989.

22. Ledingham IM, Alcock SR, Eastaway AT, McDonald JL, McKay IC, Ramsay G. Triple regimen of selective decontamination of the digestive tract, systemic cefotaxime, and microbiological surveillance for prevention of acquired infection in intensive care. Lancet 2:785-790, 1988.

23. Sanderson PJ. Selective decontamination of the digestive tract. Br Med J 299:1413-1414, 1989.

CHAPTER 33

Acute Gastrointestinal Hemorrhage

Jerome H. Abrams

Acute gastrointestinal hemorrhage is a frequent reason for admission to the SICU. Upper gastrointestinal (UGI) causes are more common (85%) than lower gastrointestinal (LGI) causes (15%). The likelihood that emergency surgery will be necessary is 40% for UGI sources and 30% for LGI bleeding.[1] Clinically, the distinction between UGI and LGI sources is important. Practically, LGI bleeding is hemorrhage that occurs beyond the range of the UGI endoscope. Fortunately, bleeding ceases in 85% of patients without intervention. The remaining 15% of patients require early and accurate diagnosis and urgent therapy.[2]

UPPER GASTROINTESTINAL HEMORRHAGE

The estimated rate of hospitalization for UGI bleeding is approximately 150 per 100,000 population per year, or approximately 300,000 hospitalizations per year, in the United States. Typically, patients are elderly, usually more than 70 years of age, and have one or more major chronic organ system diseases.[3] Patients hospitalized for another reason before massive bleeding begins have a mortality of 70%.[4] In the hospitalized patient, tachycardia, hypotension, or anemia should suggest the possibility of GI hemorrhage.

The most common causes of UGI hemorrhage are esophageal varices, gastric ulcer, and duodenal ulcers. In two large series these entities accounted for ≥20% of UGI bleeding sources.[4,5] Other causes included esophageal ulcers, malignant ulcers, bleeding from hiatal hernias, and diverticuli. Each of these entities had an association with UGI hemorrhage of <5%. In the series of Chalmers et al.,[5] esophageal varices were demonstrated in 33 of 44 patients with cirrhosis. In 16 of these 33 patients, no point of rupture of the varices was found. Yet, in only one of these patients was another possible source of bleeding seen, a chronic duodenal ulcer. When faced with the unusual situation of a patient with apparent GI bleeding, known varices, no evidence of bleeding from the varices, and no other identifiable source, the clinician should continue to suspect variceal bleeding until another source can be identified.

UGI endoscopy can be an aid in the management of UGI hemorrhage to locate the lesion, to assess the risk of rebleeding, and, with increasing frequency, to control bleeding. With respect to locating the lesion, diagnostic accuracy of approximately 90% is typical.[6,7] A series of 500 consecutive emergency UGI endoscopic procedures reported successful location of bleeding sites in 449 of 500 patients (89%).[6]

With respect to the risk of rebleeding, several observations have special importance. Active arterial bleeding with streaming of blood, clot adherence to a lesion, an exposed vessel that protrudes from the lesion, and staining of the ulcer base within a lesion have become known as stigmata of recent hemorrhage (SRH).[8] Presence of SRH is associated with increased rebleeding risk and increased mortality. For ulcers actively bleeding at the time of endoscopy, the rebleeding rate has been reported to range from 53% to 100%. For collected series, the mean rate is 66%.[9] For patients with visible vessels in ulcers, the rebleeding rate is approximately 50%, and the emergency surgery rate has been reported at 52%.[9,10] Other SRH have a lower incidence of rebleeding.[10] In one large series, mortality for patients with SRH was 12% and 0% for patients without SRH.[11]

The timing of endoscopy in the management of UGI bleeding is controversial. Early endoscopy in acutely bleeding patients presumably would have several advantages. First, surgery, when indicated, would be performed earlier. With more rapid definitive therapy, the patient would receive fewer transfusions. Second, the operation could be directed at the specific lesion and site. Accurate preoperative diagnosis would reduce operating time and eliminate inappropriate surgical procedures. Accurate diagnosis also should eliminate the need for blind gastrectomy. Third, accurate preoperative diagnosis would eliminate surgical exploration to detect the bleeding source. Fourth, surgical risk could be predicted better, especially for treatments with an expected high morbidity, for example, total gastrectomy for hemorrhagic gastritis. Iced lavage, which precedes endoscopy, may slow or stop bleeding. In addition, endoscopy can suggest long-term therapy, such as abstention from aspirin or alcohol.[12] Despite these advantages, no clear evidence exists that morbidity of UGI bleeding is reduced by emergency endoscopy in patients in whom bleeding has ceased. For patients with continued active bleeding, early and specific diagnosis with UGI endoscopy remains vital for selecting appropriate therapy.[13]

Common Causes
Mallory-Weiss syndrome

Endoscopic diagnosis of a Mallory-Weiss lesion has a 94% accuracy. The Mallory-Weiss syndrome consists of a linear mucosal tear, usually found on the lesser curvature of the stomach, either at or below the gastroesophageal junction. Seventy percent of cases of Mallory-Weiss syndrome can be treated effectively with blood transfusion, antacid, and saline irrigation. A Sengstaken-Blakemore tube may be a useful temporary treatment. If surgery is necessary, a gastrotomy is made high on the stomach to allow oversewing of the bleeding points. Endoscopic coagulation also has been used successfully.[14]

Esophageal varices

Treatment of esophageal varices is varied. Balloon tamponade can provide temporary control of bleeding. For combined series, a 78% rate of bleeding control has been achieved, with a rebleeding rate of 42%. For optimum control of bleeding with minimum complications, the clinician should follow a careful protocol (Table 33-1). Vasoconstrictor therapy has been useful in controlling acute variceal bleeding. Vasopressin is commonly used and achieves control of variceal bleeding in approximately 55% of patients. Vasopressin and nitroglycerin used together have achieved comparable control with fewer side effects.[15]

In controlled trials with follow-up of 2 to 5 years, sclerotherapy resulted in a decreased rebleeding rate or decreased transfusion requirements, when compared to medical therapy. Despite improved control of bleeding, studies do not demonstrate a clear increase in survival.[16-20] When compared to portacaval shunt, sclerotherapy has a significantly higher rebleeding rate. Despite better control of bleeding, portacaval shunt does not improve either encephalopathy or mortality.[21] Three controlled trials have compared sclerotherapy with distal splenorenal shunt (DSRS). In all three trials DSRS significantly decreased the rebleeding rate but did not change survival.[22-24] Current management of variceal bleeding employs sclerotherapy, different types of portacaval shunts, and pharmacotherapy. A comprehensive current review can be found in the reference list.[25]

Gastritis

Association of ulceration of the gastric mucosa and subsequent stress bleeding with critical illness has a long history. Cushing reported acute duodenal ulceration in patients with major burn injury in 1842. Cushing's ulcer refers to the association of peptic ulcers with traumatic brain injury. With advances in resuscitation,

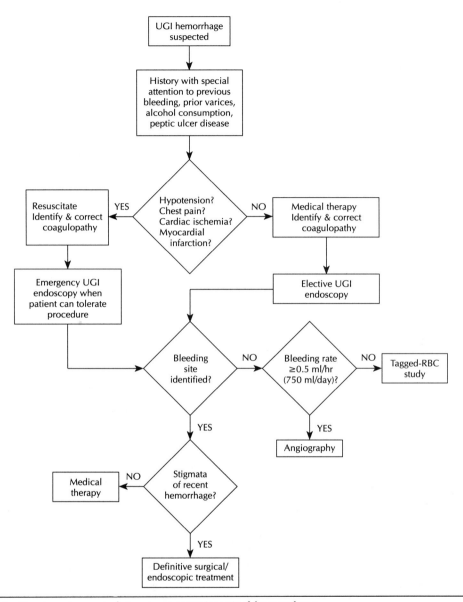

FIG. 33-1 Treatment approach to upper gastrointestinal hemorrhage.

metabolic support, and prophylaxis, the incidence of stress bleeding and stress bleeding requiring surgical intervention has decreased. The mortality for patients who require intervention for stress-related bleeding remains high, up to 50%.[1,26]

Prophylaxis against stress bleeding is effective. Antacids, H_2-receptor antagonists, and sucralfate are commonly used agents. Several studies demonstrate that antacids decrease stress bleeding when compared to placebo or control groups. For collected series, a bleeding rate of 18.9% in the placebo or control groups was reduced to 7.1% in the antacid group. To achieve this degree of success, enough antacid (30 to 60 ml) should be administered frequently, hourly if necessary, to maintain a pH $\geq$ 4. H_2-receptor antagonists can provide a similar degree of bleeding prophylaxis. Again, from collected series, bleeding in control groups was 17.1%. In patients treated with H_2 blockers, the bleeding rates in collected series

TABLE 33-1 Protocol for Use of Sengstaken-Blakemore Tube*

Before insertion

1. Consider nasotracheal intubation.
2. Use new tube and check balloon for leaks.
3. Attach no. 18 Salem sump tube above esophageal balloon.
4. Evacuate blood from stomach with a large tube.
5. Insert tube through nose using ring forceps if necessary.

After insertion

1. Apply low, intermittent suction to stomach tube.
2. Apply constant suction to Salem sump.
3. Inflate gastric balloon with 25-ml increments of air to 100 ml, observing patient for pain.
4. Snug gastric balloon to gastroesophageal junction and affix to nose, under slight tension, with soft rubber pad.
5. Add 150 ml of air to gastric balloon.
6. Place two clamps (one taped close) on tube to gastric balloon.
7. Inflate esophageal balloon to 24 to 45 mm Hg, clamp, and check every hour.
8. Perform heavily penetrated upper abdomen–lower chest roentgenography (portable) to confirm balloon positions.
9. Determine serial hematocrit levels every 4 to 6 hours (gastric tube may occlude and fail to detect recurrent hemorrhage).
10. Tape scissors to head of bed so tube can be transected and rapidly removed if respiratory distress develops.
11. Deflate esophageal and gastric balloons after 24 hours.
12. Remove tube in an additional 24 hours if there is no recurrent hemorrhage.

*From Rikkers LF, ed. Non-operative emergency treatment of variceal hemorrhage. Surg Clin North Am 70:297, 1990.

ranged from 6% to 7%. Sucralfate also has provided satisfactory prophylaxis. Several series confirm the efficacy of sucralfate. Prophylaxis is comparable to that of antacids and H_2 blockers. From pooled data, the bleeding incidence in the sucralfate group was noted as 3.8%; in the antacids/H_2 blocker groups, it was 8%.

Although effective prophylaxis can be achieved by alkalinizing stomach secretions to a pH ≥4, an increased incidence of nosocomial pneumonia with increasing pH has been demonstrated. The risk of gastric colorization and consequent nosocomial pneumonia may be comparable to the risk of stress bleeding. Gut decontamination is effective in reducing nosocomial pneumonia and other infections. For critically ill patients, who are expected to remain in the SICU for at least 5 days, gut decontamination is effective in reducing nosocomial infection. The use of a gut decontamination regimen should be considered for patients receiving gastric stress bleeding prophylaxis with antacids or H_2 blockers, especially if these patients are simultaneously receiving broad-spectrum antibiotic therapy. An excellent summary of current therapy and assessment of risk may be found in the reference list.[26]

Peptic ulcer disease

The mainstay of peptic ulcer disease treatment is use of antacids or H_2-blockers. In the case of ulcers that are acutely bleeding at the time of endoscopy, further therapy, including emergency surgery, is frequently necessary. The rebleeding rate is approximately 65%. Other stigmata of recent hemorrhage are associated with an increased risk of rebleeding. For selected patients, endoscopic therapy is successful. Epinephrine-saline solution and absolute ethanol injection of ulcers have been used successfully.[27,28] Endoscopic thermal methods include monopolar electrodes, bipolar elec-

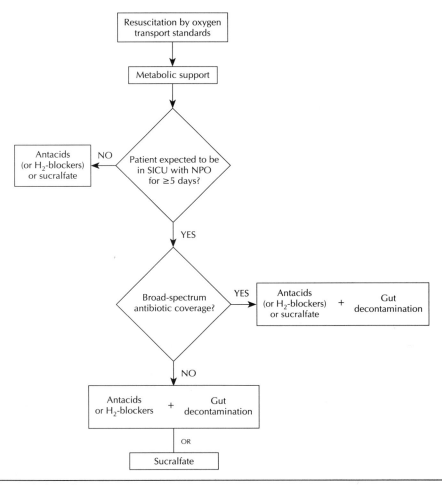

FIG. 33-2 Prophylaxis for gastritis.

trodes, and laser photocoagulation. In principle, the bipolar electrode can deliver more heat locally. Of seven randomized, prospective, controlled trials of endoscopic electrocoagulation, three demonstrated a significant decrease in rebleeding rate when compared to medical therapy. These demonstrated a reduced requirement for surgical control of bleeding. Of six prospective controlled trials of nd:YAG laser coagulation, four have shown a decreased rebleeding rate. Two indicated a decreased need for surgical intervention.[9]

Surgery for peptic ulcer disease is indicated for treatment of severe or unrelenting bleeding. A definitive ulcer procedure can be performed; the choice of procedure depends on the condition of the patient and the severity of bleed-

ing. In a series of more than 1000 patients with bleeding duodenal ulcers, 250 patients had emergency surgery. Truncal vagotomy and anterectomy were performed in all. In the emergency surgery group, the mortality was 5.5%.[29] A discussion of specific surgical considerations is beyond the scope of this chapter but may be found in the reference list.[29]

LOWER GASTROINTESTINAL HEMORRHAGE

The most likely causes of LGI bleeding are related to age. In children, Meckel's diverticulum is common, whereas in adults over 60 years of age, vascular ectasias are frequently associated with severe LGI hemorrhage.[30] In one large series, the most common causes of LGI bleeding were diverticular disease, colon cancer, inflammatory bowel disease, and colonic polyps[31] (Table 33-2). Vascular ectasias, ischemic colitis, rectal cancer, and hemorrhoids all had an incidence of 10% or less. Although vascular ectasias had a 6% incidence, they accounted for one third of patients requiring emergency surgery and 50% of patients requiring more than four units of blood in the first 24 hours.

Vascular ectasias are usually multiple and almost always occur in the cecum or proximal ascending colon. Two thirds of affected patients are over 70 years old. The lesions are thought to be acquired.[30]

A transfusion requirement of three to four units or more of blood in the first 24 hours is a risk factor for emergency surgery. Approximately 20% of patients overall can be expected to have a transfusion requirement of three or more units. In one large series, all patients who required emergency surgery needed four or more units of blood in the first 24 hours.

TABLE 33-2 Causes of Acute Lower Gastrointestinal Hemorrhage in a Series of Patients During a 4-Year Period*

Diagnosis	No. of Patients
Diverticular disease	30
Carcinoma of colon	28
Inflammatory bowel disease	17
Colonic polyps	10
Vascular ectasia	6
Ischaemic colitis	3
Rectal ulcer	3
Hemorrhoids	2
Anticoagulant treatment	1
Thrombocytopenia	1
Aortosigmoid fistula	1
Malignant histiocytosis	1
Anastomotic bleeding	1
Undetermined	1
TOTAL	105

*From Farrands PA, Taylor I. Management of acute lower gastrointestinal haemorrhage in a surgical unit over a 4-year period. J Royal Soc Med 80:79-82, 1987.

Patient Evaluation

Evaluation of patients with LGI hemorrhage should begin with a thorough physical examination, including a careful rectal examination. Coagulation studies and platelet counts should be obtained. A BUN/creatinine >25 distinguishes UGI bleeding from LGI bleeding in 90% of patients.[32] Nasogastric aspiration is the next study. In 10% to 15% of patients, the source of presumed LGI bleeding is actually the UGI tract. Absence of blood and presence of bile in the aspirate virtually excludes a GI bleeding source proximal to the ligament of Treitz.[30]

If the patient's condition is stable or cessation of bleeding is not certain, sigmoidoscopy, followed by a radionuclide tagged-RBC study (if no diagnosis is made by sigmoidoscopy) should be done. Although not as precise as angiography in identifying the site of bleeding, the tagged-RBC study may be more sensitive in detecting bleeding. The nuclear medicine study is amplified because it can be integrated over hours and does not depend on active bleeding during the brief period of colonoscopy or injection of radiocontrast material. With the labeled RBCs, bleeding rates of 0.1 ml/min have been detected. Furthermore, several studies can be obtained for up to 36 hours after injection of the radionuclide.[33] If the radionuclide study suggests a site of bleeding and the patient's condition is stable, colonoscopy is next performed. The examination should be abandoned if technical problems are encountered. If the patient continues to bleed actively, superior mesenteric artery angiography should be done next. Bleeding rates of 0.5 ml/min can be detected. Angiography is successful in locating the source of bleeding in one half to two thirds of patients.[30,34]

In most patients, bleeding will spontaneously stop. Colonoscopy should be performed in the patient when nasogastric aspirates and sigmoidoscopy are nondiagnostic and bleeding has ceased. If colonscopy fails to reveal a diagnosis, double-contrast barium studies of the UGI tract, small bowel, and colon should be done. Finally, in the small group of patients in whom a diagnosis cannot be made, angiography should be done.[30]

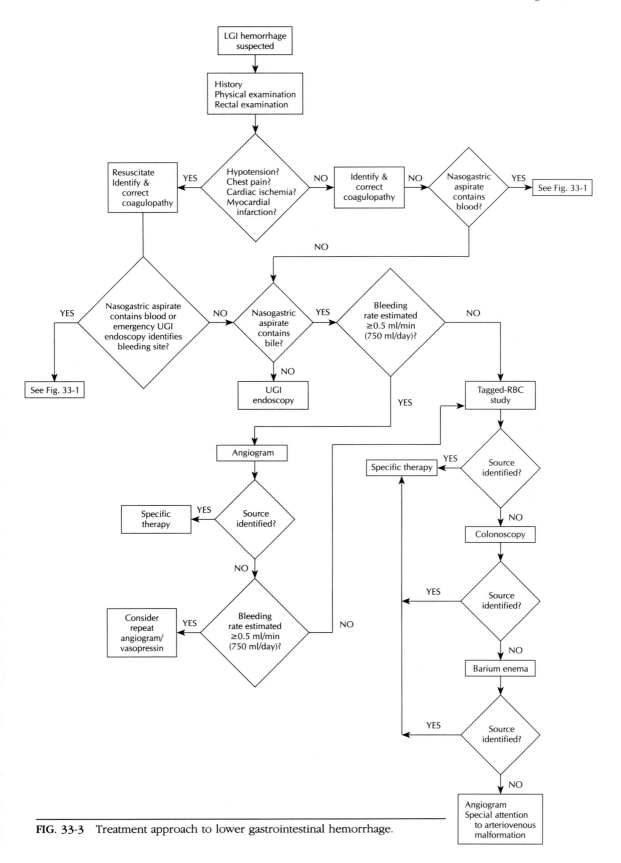

FIG. 33-3   Treatment approach to lower gastrointestinal hemorrhage.

Treatment of Severe Bleeding

Conservative management of LGI hemorrhage is indicated initially. Approximately 90% of bleeding will stop before transfusion requirements exceed two units. If more than four units are required in 24 hours, the chance that surgery will be necessary approaches 50%. An aggressive search for the source should be undertaken. If a bleeding source is clearly identified, segmental resection is recommended. If a bleeding source is not clearly identified, subtotal colectomy with or without ileorectal anastomosis should be done.[31]

SUMMARY

- Acute GI hemorrhage can complicate critical illness. When GI bleeding occurs in hospitalized patients, mortality is high.
- Prophylaxis of acute GI bleeding is effective. Antacids, H_2-receptor antagonists, and sucralfate can reduce GI bleeding.
- Nosocomial infection increases with rising gastric pH. Selective gut decontamination has been shown to decrease the nosocomial infection rate and should be considered in critically ill patients receiving antacids or H_2 blockers.
- Stigmata of recent hemorrhage (SRH), especially bleeding at the time of endoscopy and a visible vessel, have a high rebleeding rate. Consideration should be given to definitive therapy, either surgically or endoscopically, when SRH is identified.
- LGI bleeding requiring transfusion of three or more units of blood in 24 hours has a probability of requiring emergency surgery that approaches 50%. Efforts at establishing a diagnosis rapidly are essential for therapy. Angiography in patients with a large transfusion requirement can establish the bleeding site in up to two thirds of patients, especially when performed early in the patient's hospital course.

REFERENCES

1. Greenburg AG, Saik RP, Bell RH. Changing patterns of gastrointestinal bleeding. Arch Surg 120:341-344, 1985.
2. Gostout CS. Acute gastrointestinal bleeding—A common problem revisited. Mayo Clin Proc 63:596-604, 1988.
3. Cutler JA, Mendeloff AI. Upper gastrointestinal bleeding: Nature and magnitude of the problem in the U.S. Dig Dis Sci (Suppl 7) 26:90S-96S, 1981.
4. Chojkier M, Laine L, Conn HO. Predictors of outcome in massive upper gastrointestinal hemorrhage. J Clin Gastroenterol 8:16-22, 1986.
5. Chalmers TC, Zamcheck N, Curtins GW. Fatal gastrointestinal hemorrhage: Clinicopathologic correlations in 101 patients. Am J Clin Pathol 22:633-645, 1952.
6. Dagradi AE, Arguello JF, Weingasten ZG. Failure of endoscopy to establish a source for upper gastrointestinal bleeding. Am J Gastroenterol 72:395-402, 1979.
7. Cotton PB, Rosenberg MT, Walram RPL. Early endoscopy of oesophagus, stomach, and duodenal bulb in patients with haematemesis and melaena. Br Med J (Clin Res) 2:505-509, 1973.
8. Foster DN, Miloszewski KJA, Losowsky MS. Stigmata of recent haemorrhage in diagnosis and prognosis of upper gastrointestinal bleeding. Br Med J 1:1173-1177, 1978.
9. Pescovitz MD, Satterberg TL, Shearen JG. Endoscopic control of bleeding ulcers: The Minnesota experience with several methods. In Najarian JS, Delaney JP, eds. Progress in Gastrointestinal Surgery. Chicago: Year Book, 1989, pp 247-254.
10. Swain CP, Storey DW, Bown SG. Nature of the bleeding vessel in recurrently bleeding gastric ulcers. Gastroenterology 90:595-608, 1986.
11. Brearley S, Morris DL, Hawker PC. Prediction of mortality at endoscopy in bleeding peptic ulcer disease. Endoscopy 17:173-174, 1985.
12. Dagradi AE, Ruiz RA, Weingarten ZG. Influence of emergency endoscopy on the management and outcome of patients with upper gastrointes-

tinal hemorrhage. Am J Gastroenterol 72:403-415, 1979.

13. Domschke W, Lederer P, Lux G. The value of emergency endoscopy in upper gastrointestinal bleeding: Review and analysis of 2014 cases. Endoscopy 15:126-131, 1983.

14. Todd GJ, Zikria BA. Mallory-Weiss Syndrome. Ann Surg 186:146-148, 1977.

15. Burnett DA, Rikkers LF. Nonoperative emergency treatment of variceal hemorrhage. Surg Clin North Am 70:291-306, 1990.

16. Terblanche J, Borrunaln PC, Kahn D. Failure of repeated injection sclerotherapy to improve long-term survival after oesophageal variceal bleeding. A five-year prospective controlled trial. Lancet 2:1328-1332, 1983.

17. Copenhagen Esophageal Varices and Sclerotherapy Project. Sclerotherapy after first variceal hemorrhage in cirrhosis: A randomized multicenter trial. N Engl J Med 311:1594-1600, 1984.

18. Westaby D, MacDargall BRD, Williams R. Improved survival following injection sclerotherapy for esophageal varices: Final analysis of a controlled trial. Hepatology 5:827-930, 1985.

19. Korula J, Balast LA, Radvan G. A prospective, randomized controlled trial of chronic esophageal variceal schlerotherapy. Hepatology 5:584-589, 1985.

20. Soderlund C, Ihre T. Endoscopic sclerotherapy v. conservative management of bleeding oesophageal varices. A 5-year prospective controlled trial of emergency and long-term treatment. Acta Chir Scand 151:449-456, 1985.

21. Cello JP, Grendell JH, Crass RA. Endoscopic sclerotherapy versus portacaval shunt in patients with severe cirrhosis and acute variceal hemorrhage: Long-term follow-up. N Engl J Med 316:11-15, 1987.

22. Warren WD, Henderson JM, Millikas WJ. Distal splenorenal shunt versus endoscopic sclerotherapy for long-term management of variceal bleeding. Ann Surg 203:454-462, 1986.

23. Rikkers LF, Burnett DA, Volentine GD. Shunt surgery versus endoscopic sclerotherapy for long-term treatment of variceal bleeding. Early results of a randomized trial. Ann Surg 206:261-271, 1987.

24. Teres J, Bordas JM, Bravo D. Sclerotherapy vs. distal splenorenal shunt in the elective treatment of variceal hemorrhage: A randomized controlled trial. Hepatology 7:430-436, 1987.

25. Rikkers LF, ed. Management of variceal hemorrhage. Surg Clin North Am 70:251-493, 1990.

26. Gourdin TG, Smith BF, Craven DE. Prevention of stress bleeding in critical care patients: Current concepts on risk and benefit. Perspect Crit Care 2(2):44-73, 1989.

27. Chen P-C, Wu C-S, Liaw Y-F. Hemostatic effect of endoscopic local injection with hypertonic saline-epinephrine solution and pure ethanol for digestive tract bleeding. Gastrointest Endosc 32:319-323, 1986.

28. Nakagawa K, Asaki S, Sato T. Endoscopic treatment of bleeding peptic ulcers. World J Surg 13:154, 1989.

29. Herrington JL, Davidson J III. Bleeding gastroduodenal ulcers: Choice of operations. World J Surg 11:304-314, 1987.

30. Dickstein G, Boley SJ. Severe lower intestinal bleeding in the elderly. In Najarian JS, Delaney JP, eds. Progress in Gastrointestinal Surgery. Chicago: Year Book, 1989, pp 525-542.

31. Farrands PA, Taylor I. Management of acute lower gastrointestinal haemorrhage in a surgical unit over a 4-year period. J Royal Soc Med 80:79-82, 1987.

32. Snook JA, Holdstock GE, Banforth J. Value of a simple biochemical ratio in distinguishing upper and lower sites of gastrointestinal hemorrhage. Lancet 1:1064-1065, 1986.

33. Winzelberg GG, Froelich JW, McKusick KA. Scintigraphic detection of gastrointestinal bleeding: A review of current methods. Am J Gastroenterol 78:324-327, 1983.

34. Nusbaum M, Baum S. Radiographic demonstration of unknown sites of gastrointestinal bleeding. Surg Forum 14:374-375, 1963.

CHAPTER 34

Pancreatitis

Barry W. Feig

Despite a wealth of investigation and debate, pancreatitis remains a poorly understood disease. In three fourths of the patients who develop pancreatitis, the disease runs a self-limited course. The factors that determine whether the disease process will be self-limited or life-threatening remain a mystery. Those patients who develop severe complicated pancreatitis can be the greatest challenge to the diagnostic and technical skills of the surgical critical care team. Similarly, the complications of severe acute pancreatitis present challenging diagnostic and therapeutic dilemmas for which clear answers are not always evident. The metabolic response evoked by the disease process is manifest in almost all the organ systems of the body. The earlier in the course of the disease that patients with severe pancreatitis can be identified, the better will be the chance of optimizing management, restoring oxygen transport, and preventing the later complications of the disease.

Patients with acute pancreatitis have the potential for the most severe metabolic and physiologic derangements. Each of the four sections of this chapter will address both the well-established principles and the controversial, unresolved issues that make pancreatitis such a fascinating disease process.

CLASSIFICATION

The term "pancreatitis" has been used to describe a wide spectrum of clinical and pathologic conditions that affect the pancreas. Clinically, the disease can vary from a mild, local inflammatory process to a severe necrotizing process complicated by extreme hypermetabolism and multisystem organ failure. Pathologically, acute pancreatitis can range from simple interstitial edema to gross necrosis of gland parenchyma. This variety of clinical and pathologic findings and the inability to obtain a histologic diagnosis early in the disease process make it difficult to arrive at a uniform classification of pancreatitis, especially one that can be used to predict the severity and course of the disease process.

Two international workshops were held in an attempt to address this issue (in Cambridge, England, in 1983, and in Marseilles, France, in 1984). Despite this worldwide cooperation, disagreement about the classification of the disease persists. Certainly, both an acute and a chronic form of pancreatitis do exist. The Cambridge group made the following clinical definitions[1]:

1. *Acute pancreatitis* was defined as an acute condition typically presenting with abdominal pain and usually associated with raised pancreatic enzymes in the blood or urine owing to inflammatory disease of the pancreas.

2. *Chronic pancreatitis* was defined as a continuing inflammatory disease of the pancreas, characterized by irreversible morphologic change and typically causing pain and/or permanent loss of function.

The Cambridge group further subdivided acute pancreatitis into a mild form, in which there was no evidence of multisystem failure, and a severe form, in which multisystem failure was present along with local or systemic complications. The complications defined were phlegmon, pseudocyst, and abscess.

The Marseille group used similar definitions for acute and chronic pancreatitis, but they added pathologic as well as functional criteria to their definitions. They pointed out that the mild form of acute pancreatitis is usually characterized by interstitial edema, with pancreatic necrosis being a rare finding. However, the mild form can progress to a severe type characterized by necrosis of gland parenchyma and peripancreatic fat. They also stated that both exocrine and endocrine functions of the pancreas are impaired to a variable extent.[1a] Even with this addition of morphologic criteria, these classifications are not always reproducible with respect to estimating severity and outcome of disease.

PATHOGENESIS

Although a variety of causes have been linked to the onset of acute pancreatitis, little is known about the initiation of the disease process at the cellular level or the factors that control the severity and course of the disease. In most cases the cause of the disease process can be identified. In the United States alcohol and biliary tract disease are the two most common causes of acute pancreatitis, and they account for 80% to 90% of all patients with the disease. The actual leading cause of pancreatitis (alcohol vs. biliary tract disease) has depended on the population sampled. In those series performed at inner-city hospitals that treat indigent patients, alcohol is the number one cause, whereas studies done in private hospitals have shown gallstones to be more common.[2] The accompanying box lists the etiologic factors known to be associated with acute pancreatitis.

Many clinical and experimental theories have been postulated about the mechanism by which the inflammatory process is initiated. Despite this extensive investigation, the connection between the cause and the pathologic events inciting the pancreatic inflammation have not been clearly elucidated. Certainly, the release and activation of pancreatic digestive enzymes is part of the cycle of the pathogenesis of acute pancreatitis. The proteolytic and lipolytic enzymes that are synthesized in the pancreas are capable of causing significant tissue destruction. Many authors attribute the early inflammatory process in the pancreas to the intrapancreatic activation of these enzymes. In patients with acute pancreatitis, the presence of activated forms of these enzymes in pancreatic parenchyma, pancreatic juice, ascitic fluid, and blood has been taken as evidence that these enzymes play an important role in pathogenesis. Experimental evidence for this process has been based on the ability to induce pancreatitis in animal models by injection of these enzymes into the pancreatic duct or the parenchyma.[3] The key question, which remains unanswered, is whether the release and activation of these enzymes is a result of or a cause of acute pancreatic inflammation and cellular destruction. Edema, vascular injury, ruptured pancreatic ducts, and acinar damage are all pathologic features present in the pancreatic glands at an early stage in both experimental and clinically observed pancreatitis. The combination of these features can lead to cellular hypoxia and cell death, further fueling the cycle of pancreatic autodigestion (Fig. 34-1).

Three main theories that are current expla-

Etiologic Factors of Pancreatitis
Biliary tract disease
Alcohol
Tumor
Infection
Bacterial
Viral
Drugs
Prednisone
Azathioprine
Estrogen
Pentamidine
Thiazides
Cimetidine
Tetracycline
Hyperparathyroidism
Hypertriglyceridemia
Postoperative trauma

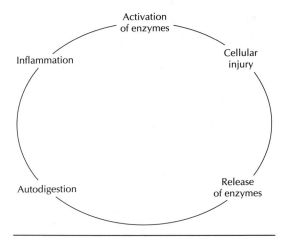

FIG. 34-1 Cycle of pancreatic autodigestion.

nations for the gross and microscopic changes seen with pancreatitis are[4]:

1. Reflux of duodenal contents into the pancreatic duct could cause premature activation of pancreatic enzymes. Normally, these enzymes are stored and secreted in an inactive form with activation occurring in the duodenum. Presence of duodenal contents in the pancreatic duct would cause premature activation of these digestive enzymes and thus damage the pancreas.

2. Bile, ethanol, and aspirin have been shown experimentally to increase the permeability of the pancreatic duct mucosa, thereby allowing pancreatic enzymes to leak into the gland parenchyma.

3. Hypersecretion by the pancreatic gland against a completely or partially obstructed duct may result in acute pancreatitis secondary to rupture of small ductules with release of digestive enzymes into the gland proper. Obstruction may be mechanical (i.e., secondary to a gallstone) or physiologic (i.e., spasm of the sphincter of Oddi secondary to alcohol use).

DIAGNOSIS

The diagnosis of acute pancreatitis has been predicated on the patient's history and the physical examination along with determination of the serum amylase concentration. The classic presentation of acute pancreatitis is readily diagnosed by these criteria. However, the term "pancreatitis" has been applied to such a wide spectrum of inflammatory conditions of the pancreas that the diagnosis often can be difficult. The second problem in diagnosis lies in the early identification of those cases that are complicated by destruction of glandular tissue necessitating more aggressive monitoring and resuscitation and invasive procedures to control the inflammatory process.

Almost all patients with pancreatitis complain of abdominal pain. Typically, the pain is located in the epigastrium and radiates to the back. The majority of patients also experience nausea and emesis. Other symptoms include jaundice, altered mental status, and shortness of breath. On physical examination, there is usually tenderness on palpation of the epigastric region with abdominal distention and fever (usually low-grade). It is not unusual to see tachypnea, tachycardia, and arterial hypotension. Occasionally, an abdominal mass may be palpated.

The accepted standard laboratory test for acute pancreatitis is the serum amylase concentration. A patient with abdominal pain and an elevated serum amylase concentration should be considered as having pancreatitis until proven otherwise. Unfortunately, a significant incidence of false positive and false negative diagnoses occurs if the diagnosis is based on the serum amylase concentration. The two most common causes for a false negative diagnosis are the timing of the venipuncture for the serum amylase concentration in relation to the onset of pancreatitis and the presence of an acute exacerbation of chronic pancreatitis. In more than 50% of patients, the serum amylase returns to normal within 3 days of the onset of pancreatitis.[5] Therefore a normal serum amylase concentration is obtained in a patient who presents for evaluation several days after the onset of the attack. In patients with a chronically inflamed pancreas, the pancreas may be unable to continue producing amylase. Therefore the amylase concentration will remain normal even during an acute exacerbation of the pancreatitis.[6] Another reason for a normal amylase concentration in a patient with pancreatitis has been described by Warshaw et al.[7] These authors found that 10% of patients with acute pancreatitis who were studied prospectively had lipemic serum on gross inspection. A significant number of these patients had normal amylase concentrations. Warshaw et al. postulate that an amylase inhibitor present in the serum of these patients interferes with the amylase determination. Therefore in patients with abdominal pain and lipemic serum, pancreatitis should be strongly considered in the differential diagnosis, even if the amylase concentration is normal.

An extensive list of disease processes other than pancreatitis can cause hyperamylasemia. A false positive diagnosis of pancreatitis most commonly is caused by perforation of the gastrointestinal tract. The intestine is normally impermeable to the large amount of amylase within its lumen. Perforation of the gastrointestinal tract allows amylase-rich fluid to leak into the peritoneal cavity, from which it is absorbed into the systemic circulation via the abdominal lymphatics. Similarly, mesenteric infarction can violate the integrity of the bowel wall and allow leakage of amylase into the peritoneal cavity. These possibilities must be evaluated in patients with abdominal pain, tenderness, and an elevated serum amylase concentration. Renal failure is a common cause of hyperamylasemia in critically ill patients. Normally, the kidney will catabolize amylase and excrete it in the urine. An amylase >2.5 times normal, however, should arouse suspicion of a diagnosis other than renal failure. The salivary glands are a source of a large quantity of amylase. Increased concentrations of salivary amylase in the blood are seen with salivary gland infection, trauma, and tumors. Serum isoamylase determination can distinguish amylase produced in the salivary glands from that produced in the pancreas. Electrophoresis and ion-exchange chromatography can be used to separate and quantify pancreatic and salivary amylase and help clarify the diagnosis.[8]

Since serum amylase is not a totally reliable indicator of pancreatitis, numerous other laboratory studies have been investigated as possible replacements for this test. Amylase is normally excreted in the urine. The kidney's ability to reabsorb amylase from the urine is exceeded at fairly low concentrations of amylase in the glomerular filtrate. This finding has led to the suggestion that urinary amylase might be a more sensitive indicator of pancreatic inflammation than serum amylase. However, clinical trials have not proven this hypothesis. It also has been suggested that the amylase clearance be determined to compensate for abnormal renal function. This determination also has been found to be no more sensitive or more specific than serum amylase.

The serum lipase concentration has been postulated as potentially more specific for pancreatic disease than serum amylase since no known extra pancreatic source for the enzyme exists. However, false positive elevations of serum lipase have been reported with intra-abdominal conditions such as cholecystitis, appendicitis, bowel obstruction, bowel perforation, and mesenteric infarction.[9,10] Although several studies claim that lipase is more sensitive and more specific for pancreatic disease,[11,12] some authors have noted no difference between the two determinations.[9,13,14]

In the effort to find the definitive test for acute pancreatitis, several assays for other enzymes produced in the pancreas have been developed. These include trypsin, chymotrypsin, elastase, ribonuclease, and phospholipase A_2. In general, none of these tests has been shown to be consistently more sensitive or more specific than serum amylase in predicting the presence of pancreatitis or the severity or outcome of a specific episode of the disease.

Currently, the diagnosis of acute pancreatitis is most often based on clinical criteria and serum amylase determination. No radiologic test that is specific for pancreatitis exists, and radiologic evaluation serves to confirm the clinical diagnosis and to exclude other causes of abdominal pain. Initial evaluation in patients with acute pancreatitis generally includes plain films of the abdomen. Although such films have no classic diagnostic findings in acute pancreatitis, the most commonly associated abnormality is a focal ileus, which is manifest as a distended loop of small bowel in the left upper quadrant of the abdomen ("sentinel loop"). Other less frequently observed signs are noted

TABLE 34-1   Radiographic Signs of Acute Pancreatitis on Plain Films of Abdomen*

Sign	Disruption	Mechanism
Sentinel loop	Distended loop of small bowel in LUQ	Focal ileus from pancreatic inflammation
Colon cutoff	Dilation of right and transverse colon with abrupt termination of gas pattern at splenic flexure	Colonic spasm from leaking pancreatic enzymes
Renal halo	Area of decreased density around kidney	Fluid collection in perirenal space accentuates perirenal fat
Diffuse mottling	Diffuse mottling	Abdominal fat necrosis

*From Freeny PC. Radiology of actue pancreatitis: Diagnosis, detection of complications and interventional therapy. In Glazer G, Ranson JHC, eds. Acute Pancreatitis. London: Baillière Tindall, 1988, pp 275-302.

in Table 34-1. Radiology also plays an important role in the diagnosis of structural and morphologic abnormalities (i.e., obstruction by a pancreatic duct stone or areas of focal stricture of the pancreatic duct secondary to chronic pancreatitis or pancreas divisum) and in the identification and treatment of the complications of acute pancreatitis (i.e., identifying pancreatic necrosis, phlegmon, or pseudocyst formation with CT scanning or ultrasound-guided fine-needle aspiration used to identify the presence of infection).

Until the general availability of high-resolution CT scanners, ultrasonography was considered the best modality for visualizing the pancreas. Ultrasonography is frequently unsatisfactory for two reasons: (1) visualization of the pancreas may be obscured by bowel gas, and (2) loss of tissue planes from fat necrosis reduces resolution. These difficulties have been documented in up to 70% of cases of acute pancreatitis.[15,16] The findings of acute pancreatitis on ultrasonography include an enlarged gland, loss of normal intraparenchymal echogenicity, and peripancreatic fluid collections.

Currently, CT scanning is considered the most accurate means of imaging the pancreatic gland. In acute pancreatitis, the CT scan shows an irregular, enlarged gland with areas of inhomogeneity, peripancreatic edema, and peripancreatic inflammatory changes in the pararenal space and the mesenteric fat. The severity of pancreatitis correlates with the degree of changes seen on CT scan. Areas of pancreatic gland necrosis, hemorrhage, and peripancreatic fluid collections, such as abscesses and pseudocysts, will be seen. Balthazar et al.[17] were able to classify the degree of severity of the pancreatitis based on the presence and degree of lack of enhancement on the initial CT scan. This information was then correlated with initial patient management and prognosis.

Concerns that acute pancreatitis will be worsened make acute pancreatitis a relative contraindication to endoscopic retrograde cholangiopancreatography (ERCP). Early ERCP is being performed by some investigators for pancreatitis secondary to an impacted common bile duct stone. The procedure is performed without cannulation or complete filling of the pancreatic duct with contrast material.[18] ERCP should not be used to make the diagnosis of acute pancreatitis.

At present, the role of MRI in pancreatitis is not well established.

Despite the wealth of clinical, laboratory, and radiologic information that can be obtained during an attack of acute pancreatitis, a definitive diagnosis of this condition may be difficult to confirm. Rarely, an exploratory laparotomy may be necessary to distinguish acute pancreatitis from another intra-abdominal catastrophe.

TREATMENT

The initial treatment of acute pancreatitis is based on clinical assessment of the severity of the attack. The classic report by Ranson et al.[19] in 1974 identified 11 prognostic signs in acute

| Prognostic Indicators of Severe
| Pancreatitis*

On admission

Age >55 years
WBC >16,000/mm³
Glucose >200 mg/dl
LDH >350 IU/L
SGOT >120 IU/L

During first 48 hours

Hematocrit decrease >10%
BUN increase >5 mg/dl
Serum calcium <8 mg/dl
Arterial P_{O_2} <60 mm Hg
Base deficit >4 mEq/L
Fluid sequestration >6 L

*From Ranson JHC, Rifkind KM, Roses DF, et al. Prognostic signs and the role of operative management in acute pancreatitis. Surg Gynecol Obstet 139:69, 1974. By permission.

pancreatitis (see box). The number of signs present correlated with mortality. Although these signs give an indication of the severity and prognosis of the condition, it is usually difficult to collect all these data early enough to be helpful in the initial management of the patient. Many clinical indicators of severity have been advocated. These include hypotension, tachycardia, fever, increased respiratory rate, severity of abdominal pain, Cullen's sign (periumbilical bluish discoloration) and Grey Turner's sign (bluish flank discoloration). Laboratory values, such as hypocalcemia (serum calcium <7.5 mg/dl), hemoconcentration (hematocrit >45%), and degree of elevation of the serum amylase concentration, also have been tested as possible individual indicators of the severity of disease. Most authors feel that these signs alone are poorly predictive of the severity of an attack of pancreatitis. Mortality is higher with the first attack of pancreatitis than it is with subsequent attacks.[20,21] Therefore patients who have had multiple attacks of acute pancreatitis in the past are less likely to have a severe attack. Many British physicians have advocated early peritoneal lavage for determination of the severity of pancreatitis. However, this procedure has not achieved widespread popularity in the United States.

Once a patient presents with an attack of acute pancreatitis, the main therapeutic objectives are to remove the inciting process if possible, limit the degree of inflammation, support the patient physiologically, and treat complications as they occur. Once the diagnosis of pancreatitis has been made, the clinician must first decide if it is a mild or a severe case. Although such a determination presumably is a minor task, even the most experienced clinician will have difficulty categorizing those cases that are of intermediate severity on initial presentation. The clinician must take into account all the previously mentioned laboratory, radiologic, and clinical data to assess the severity of an attack and attempt to predict each individual patient's course. Patients with mild pancreatitis generally can be treated on the ward with routine vital signs taken, blood tests performed, and urine output monitored. Patients with severe pancreatitis must be admitted to the SICU for closer monitoring of vital signs, invasive hemodynamic monitoring (via pulmonary artery catheter), restoration of oxygen transport, and support of multisystem organ failure (Fig. 34-2). Although only 25% of patients develop this severe form of pancreatitis, 10% of all patients with pancreatitis will die from the disease or its complications. Previously, patients died as a result of fluid sequestration and multisystem organ failure during the first week of the disease process. Despite better understanding and treatment of the pathophysiology of severe acute pancreatitis and multisystem organ failure, the 10% mortality associated with pancreatitis has persisted. Patients now die of complications occurring later in the course of the disease.[22]

To prevent early death in severe acute pancreatitis, the principles of managing multisystem organ failure and the altered metabolic response must be implemented (see Chapters 1 to 3). The predominant pathophysiologic response in such patients is massive fluid sequestration. The patients will lose liters of intravascular volume into the nonfunctional "third space." Part of a patient's adaptive response is an increase in cardiac output. Both pulse rate and stroke volume are greatly increased initially with severe disease. Cardiac output may be insufficient to meet the tissue oxygen demands,

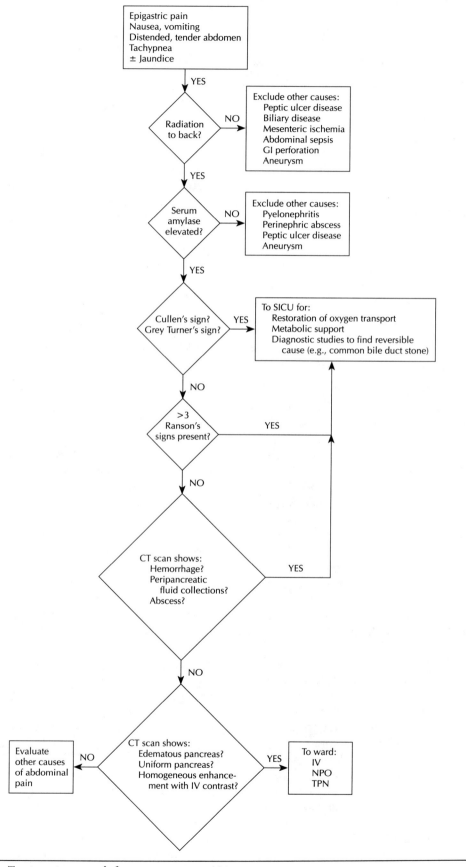

FIG. 34-2 Treatment approach for severe pancreatitis.

a result of myocardial dysfunction and increased tissue oxygen demands. Respiratory insufficiency, a frequent complication of severe pancreatitis, is usually manifest initially as arterial hypoxemia. Significant ventilation/perfusion mismatch is common (see Chapters 27 and 28).

Acute renal failure is another complication of severe pancreatitis, the presence of which is associated with increased mortality. In acute pancreatitis, oliguria is most commonly a result of poor renal perfusion. This problem may be compounded by the presence of hypotension and sepsis. Ileus, nausea, and emesis are the most common gastrointestinal complications. Several studies have shown no benefit to nasogastric suction in acute pancreatitis.[23,24] However, these studies were conducted mainly in small groups of patients with mild pancreatitis. Most authors consider nasogastric aspiration to be beneficial in cases of severe pancreatitis to both treat the ileus present and prevent gastric dilation. Whether nasogastric suction actually puts the pancreas "at rest" by diverting gastric acid and decreases stimulation of the pancreas through decreased release of secretin and cholecystokinin remains a debatable issue. No prospective randomized controlled study has demonstrated a benefit in using prophylactic antibiotics. Electrolyte abnormalities, particularly hypokalemia, hypocalcemia, and hypomagnesemia, are common during an attack of acute pancreatitis. Hypocalcemia is one of the prognostic indicators, as identified by Ranson et al.,[19] that predicts mortality. It is important to remember that total serum calcium determination may be low as a result of hypoalbuminemia, whereas the ionized calcium concentration (the physiologically active form) may be normal. Overcorrection of calcium may be detrimental to the patient since hypercalcemia has been implicated as a possible cause of pancreatitis. All patients should have some form of gastric acid neutralization to prevent stress ulceration. The use of morphine is usually not advisable for pain control because of potential spasm of the sphincter of Oddi. Meperidine, one of the semisynthetic narcotics, or an NSAID should be used. Patients with pancreatitis are often malnourished as a result of their disease

process. Intravenous hyperalimentation should be begun as soon as possible. Intravenous lipid infusion does not exacerbate the pancreatitis and should be used appropriately.[25] Hyperamylasemia is not a specific contraindication to enteral feedings. Timing of enteral feedings depends on overall patient response to acute pancreatitis. Maintenance of enteral feedings depends on the clinical response to a trial of jejunal feedings.

The majority of patients will show some signs of clinical improvement within 4 to 5 days of the onset of the medical treatment described here. The role of surgery in the treatment of acute pancreatitis and the timing and type of intervention remain subjects of controversy. Laparotomy may be necessary to make the diagnosis of pancreatitis. Four basic procedures have been advocated as a means of limiting the severity of pancreatic inflammation early in the disease process: (1) pancreatic drainage, (2) pancreatic debridement, (3) peritoneal lavage, and (4) biliary procedures. The proponents of early surgical intervention believe that interruption of the inflammatory process early in the course of the disease will decrease systemic manifestations and later infectious complications. Although this seems logical, clinical trials have not provided convincing proof. In some cases (i.e., gallstone pancreatitis) early operative intervention actually has been shown to be detrimental.[26]

Those patients who do not respond to conservative medical management and continue to show signs of systemic manifestations of pancreatitis 1 week after the initiation of treatment should be considered as possible candidates for operative intervention. If it has not already been performed, CT scanning should be done to evaluate the presence of pancreatic necrosis and/or peripancreatic fluid collections. Often these collections may show infection, and CT-guided aspiration can provide diagnosis and identification of infecting organisms. The presence of infected pancreatic necrosis or peripancreatic fluid mandates some form of intervention. Whether this should be performed via the percutaneous route or operatively remains an area of debate in the literature at this time.[27,28]

SUMMARY

- Pancreatitis can vary from mild to life-threatening, with associated multiple organ failure. Acute and chronic forms exist.
- Current classifications do not always correlate with severity and outcome.
- Alcohol consumption and biliary disease are the two most common causes of acute pancreatitis.
- A patient with abdominal pain and an elevated serum amylase level is considered as having pancreatitis until proven otherwise. Note that GI perforation can produce hyperamylasemia.

- Radiologic evaluation identifies standard abnormalities, pancreatic necrosis, phlegmon or pseudocyst formation. CT scan is currently the most accurate method for imaging the pancreas.
- Initial treatment of acute pancreatitis is matched to the severity. Ranson's criteria correlate with severity of the condition.
- Manage severe cases with source control, restoration of oxygen transport, and metabolic support.

REFERENCES

1. Sarner M, Cotton PB. Definitions of acute and chronic pancreatitis. Clin Gastroenterol 13:865, 1984.
1a. Banks PA, Bradley EL, Dreiling DA, et al. Classification of pancreatitis—Cambridge and Marseille. Gastroenterology 89:928, 1985.
2. Howard JM. Pancreatitis in the United States of America. In Howard JM, Jordan GL, Reber HA, eds. Surgical Diseases of the Pancreas. Philadelphia: Lea & Febiger, 1987, pp 231-233.
3. Sarner M. Etiology and pathophysiology of acute pancreatitis. In Go VLW, Gardner JD, Brooks FP, Lebenthal E, Dimagno EP, Scheele GA, eds. The Exocrine Pancreas: Biology, Pathobiology, and Diseases. New York: Raven Press, 1986, pp 465-474.
4. Wedgwood K, Reber HA. Pathogenesis of acute pancreatitis. In Howard JM, Jordan GL, Reber HA, eds. Surgical Diseases of the Pancreas. Philadelphia: Lea & Febiger, 1987, pp 371-376.
5. Kolars JC, Ellis CJ, Levitt MD. Comparison of serum amylase, pancreatic isoamylase, and lipase in patients with hyperamylasemia. Dig Dis Sci 29:289, 1984.
6. Spechler SJ, Dalton JW, Robbins AH, et al. Prevalence of normal serum amylase levels in patients with acute alcoholic pancreatitis. Dig Dis Sci 28:865, 1983.
7. Warshaw AL, Bellini CA, Lesser PB. Inhibition of serum and urine amylase activity in pancreatitis with hyperlipidemia. Ann Surg 182:72, 1975.
8. Warshaw AL, Nath BJ. Laboratory diagnosis of acute pancreatitis. In Howard JM, Jordan GL, Reber HA, eds. Surgical Disease of the Pancreas. Philadelphia: Lea & Febiger, 1987, pp 386-411.
9. Banks PA. Pancreatitis. New York: Plenum Medical, 1979, pp 75-76.
10. Patt HH, Kramer SP, Woel G. Serum lipase determination in acute pancreatitis. Clinical appraisal of a new method. Arch Surg 92:718, 1966.
11. Kolars JC, Ellis CJ, Levitt MD. Sensitivity of serum total amylase, pancreatic isoamylase and lipase measurements in the diagnosis of acute pancreatitis. Gastroenterology 82:1104, 1982.
12. Berk JE. Serum amylase and lipase. JAMA 199:134, 1967.
13. Lifton JL, Slickers KA, Pragay DA, et al. Pancreatitis and lipase. A reevaluation with a five-minute turbidimetric lipase determination. JAMA 229:47, 1974.
14. Ticktin HE, Trujillo NP, Evans PF, et al. Diagnostic value of a new serum lipase method. Gastroenterology 48:12, 1965.
15. Pistolesi GF, Fuggazola C, Procacci C, et al. Radiologic approach to acute and chronic pancreatitis. In Scuro LA, Dagradi A. Topics in Acute and Chronic Pancreatitis. New York: Springer-Verlag, 1981, pp 63-83.
16. Silverstein W, Isikoff MB, Hill MC, et al. Diagnostic imaging of acute pancreatitis: Prospective study using CT and sonography. Am J Roentgenol 137:497, 1981.
17. Balthazar EJ, Robinson DL, Megibow AJ, et al. Acute pancreatitis: Value of CT in establishing prognosis. Radiology 174:331, 1990.
18. Safrany L, Cotton PB. A preliminary report: Urgent duodenoscopic sphincterotomy for acute gallstone pancreatitis. Surgery 89:424, 1981.

19. Ranson JHC, Rifkind KM, Roses DF, et al. Prognostic signs and the role of operative management in acute pancreatitis. Surg Gynecol Obstet 139:69, 1974.

20. Trapnell JE, Duncan EHL. Patterns of incidence of acute pancreatitis. Br Med J 2:179, 1975.

21. Ranson JHC. Prognostication in acute pancreatitis. In Glazer G, Ranson JHC, eds. Acute Pancreatitis. London: Balliere Tindall, 1988, pp 303-330.

22. Frey CF, Bradley EL, Beger HG. Progress in acute pancreatitis. Surg Gynecol Obstet 167:282, 1988.

23. Naeiji R, Salingret E, Clumeck N, et al. Is nasogastric suction necessary in acute pancreatitis? Brit Med J 2:659, 1978.

24. Sarr MG, Sanfey H, Cameron JL. Prospective, randomized trial of nasogastric suction in patients with acute pancreatitis. Surgery 100:500, 1986.

25. Havala T, Shrants E, Cerra F. Nutritional support in acute pancreatitis. Gastroenterol Clin North Am 18:525, 1989.

26. Ranson JHC. The role of surgery in the management of acute pancreatitis. Ann Surg 311:392, 1990.

27. Bradley EL, Allen K. A prospective longitudinal study of observation versus surgical intervention in the management of necrotizing pancreatitis. Am J Surg 161:19, 1991.

28. Adams DB, Harvey TS, Anderson MC. Percutaneous catheter drainage of infected pancreatic and peripancreatic fluid collections. Arch Surg 125:1554, 1990.

CHAPTER 35

Acute Abdomen

Michael D. Pasquale · Roderick A. Barke

Diagnosis and management of the acute abdomen are fundamental in general surgery. Few other conditions provide an equal challenge to the clinician's knowledge and judgment. This challenge becomes even more formidable when the patient is critically ill. The diagnosis of acute abdomen in the critically ill is made under two circumstances. The first is the patient for whom acute abdomen is the original medical indication for admission to the SICU, whereas the second is in the setting of the postoperative surgical patient whose recovery is interrupted by an acute abdominal event. Although the diagnostic regimen for each is similar, the information available at the time of presentation to the surgical intensivist may be considerably different.

In a study done by the Department of Veterans Affairs, a typical presentation of potentially treatable abdominal pathologic conditions was revealed as a common cause of class I error (major unexpected findings at autopsy that would have led to a change in therapy and an improved survival rate had they been diagnosed before death) in veterans who received mechanical ventilation. The diagnoses were missed in two thirds of patients because the clinicians failed to consider and pursue the diagnoses, not because they were misled by inconclusive or incorrect information from diagnostic procedures. This observation further reinforces the idea that identification of patients with an acute abdomen is of great importance for the surgical intensivist. A recommended approach to the patient with acute abdominal pain is shown in Fig. 35-1.

HISTORY AND PHYSICAL EXAMINATION

Despite the technologic advances in medicine, a detailed history and physical examination remain the most important tools in the initial evaluation of the patient. The history, obtained either from the patient or individuals close to the patient, directs further investigation. A complete medical history with attention to major illnesses, previous surgical procedures, and current medications is essential. In the subset of patients seen in the recovery room after a surgical procedure, historical details include the history of present illness leading to the surgical procedure, operative notes, and anesthesia record. In addition, the classic historical details such as the time course of the illness and associated constitutional symptoms (e.g., nausea, vomiting, diarrhea, chills, character of pain) provide the clues necessary for rapid definitive diagnosis and treatment.

Pain is often the presenting complaint of patients with acute abdomens, and knowing its location at onset and at the time of examination, its duration, quality, and aggravating factors is of substantial importance in the diagnostic process. Abdominal pain is mediated through both the autonomic and somatic sensory nervous systems.

Visceral pain is elicited from abdominal organs that are innervated by the autonomic sys-

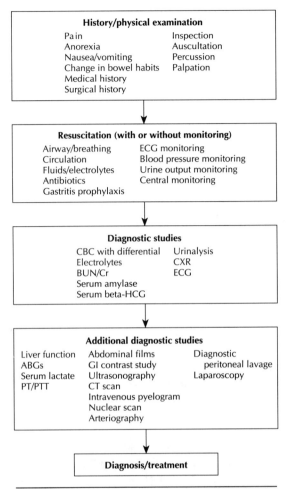

FIG. 35-1 Approach to the patient with acute abdominal pain.

---

tem. This type of pain is usually crampy, poorly localized, and often associated with nausea and vomiting. Stimuli that produce visceral pain are increased hollow viscus wall tension, solid viscus capsule stretching, ischemia, and certain chemicals. Visceral pain usually is transmitted according to developmental patterns—foregut (stomach, duodenum, liver, biliary tract, pancreas, spleen) radiating to the epigastrium, midgut (small bowel, appendix, right side of the colon) radiating to the periumbilical region, and hindgut (left side of the colon, rectum) radiating to the hypogastrium. This pattern is seen because the autonomic nerves follow the distribution of the blood supply from the major splanchnic arteries (celiac, superior mesen-

teric, and inferior mesenteric). Severe visceral pain also results in autonomic reflexes such as sweating, tachycardia or bradycardia, hypotension, cutaneous hyperalgesia, hyperesthesia, and involuntary spastic contractions of the abdominal musculature.

Somatic pain arises from irritation of parietal peritoneum, mesentery, or respiratory diaphragm. It is transmitted through somatic sensory nerves and is sharper, more distinct, and well localized to the site of stimulation. This pain is often associated with the classic "peritoneal" signs of rigidity: spasm of overlying muscles and rebound tenderness from inflammation of the parietal peritoneum. Referred pain arises at a distance from the pathologic site and follows neural pathways, often dermatome distributions. It is important to document when pain began, where it originated, what was its character, what precipitated it, what was associated with it, and whether it has varied.

Anorexia, nausea, and vomiting often occur in the setting of intra-abdominal pathology. Paralytic ileus accompanies most intraperitoneal inflammatory processes. Anorexia may be caused by a variety of organic and psychologic disturbances that are poorly understood. Nausea and vomiting may occur separately but usually are closely related. Nausea generally precedes vomiting. The act of vomiting is controlled by the vomiting center and the chemoreceptor trigger zone (CTZ) in the medulla. The CTZ receives afferent stimulation from the GI tract and sends impulses to the vomiting center. In some cases afferent impulses from the GI tract bypass the CTZ. Emesis without antecedent nausea suggests a CNS lesion with increased intracranial pressure. Emesis that relieves epigastric pain usually is associated with intragastric lesions or pyloric spasm associated with pyloric channel ulcer. Immediate postprandial vomiting may represent a toxic or psychogenic cause, hyperemesis gravidarum, gastritis, high intestinal obstruction, or a gastric neoplasm. Vomiting larger amounts of undigested food at 12- to 24-hour intervals suggests chronic pyloric obstruction. Vomiting 1 or more hours after meals is consistent with gastric outlet obstruction, diabetic gastropathy, and postvagotomy disorders. Feculent emesis often indicates either a gastrocolic fistula or a complete low intestinal obstruction.

Change in bowel habits, typically constipation or obstipation, occurs in a patient with obstruction or ileus. Diarrhea also may occur in a patient with intra-abdominal inflammation, although diarrhea is more common with enterocolitis syndromes.

In females the menstrual history is important. Amenorrhea, hypogastric pain, or uterine bleeding suggests ectopic pregnancy.

When the patient is unable to communicate (sedation, paralysis, intubation, previous cerebrovascular accident), the history may prove inconclusive. Physical examination in this situation achieves greater importance in directing further diagnostic procedures. The initial physical examination of the critically ill patient must be complete and provides the basis for further comparisons. Ideally, the patient should be reassured and a good rapport established before the examination is begun. A sense of trust in the examiner serves to relax the patient and allow the evaluation to proceed without undue discomfort. Routine vital signs should be taken and evaluated. Both fever and hypothermia are significant signs of intra-abdominal sepsis. The rate and quality of the pulse should be noted, as should the character of respirations. Tachycardia and tachypnea with shallow inspirations suggest the possibility of impending instability and/or abdominal catastrophe. Blood pressure should be documented and compared to the patient's pre-illness value. The abdominal examination should be conducted in a systematic manner with attention to the fundamentals of inspection, auscultation, percussion, and palpation.

The first step in a thorough examination is careful inspection of the anterior and posterior abdominal wall, perineum, and flank areas. Defects (e.g., hernias, scars), ecchymoses (e.g., retroperitoneal bleeding), abnormal pulsations (e.g., abdominal aneurysm), engorged subcutaneous veins (e.g., from portal hypertension), jaundice (e.g., from hepatobiliary disease), and umbilical deformities (e.g., Sister Joseph's nodule [metastatic intra-abdominal carcinoma], eversion, ascites, fistula [either patent urachal or enterocutaneous]) should be sought. Surgical wounds should be inspected to evaluate them for bleeding, purulent drainage, crepitus, and/or dehiscence.

Auscultation should be performed next. The character of the bowel sounds and presence of bruits should be noted. Hypoactive or absent bowel sounds may indicate an ileus associated with an intra-abdominal infection, whereas hyperactive sounds with rushes are characteristic of intestinal obstruction. Bruits may signify the presence of aneurysms or significant hemangiomas, especially hepatic hemangiomas.

Percussion, which is performed next, is useful as a means to assess organ size, determine the presence of ascites (shifting dullness), and evaluate bladder fullness. Tympany over the midabdomen suggests obstruction, whereas tympany over the lateral liver is a clue to bowel perforation. Percussion is also useful in demonstrating peritoneal irritation.

Palpation of the abdomen is last and should be performed in a systematic fashion. If possible, the area of most discomfort should be evaluated last. Attempts to localize pain should be made, as should assessing the presence of rigidity and rebound tenderness. The presence of any masses should also be noted. A rectal examination, pelvic examination in females, and genital examination should be considered a part of the abdominal examination. The presence of blood, mass, or tenderness in these areas provides invaluable clues about the cause of acute abdominal pain.

After completion of a thorough history and physical examination, the intensive care physician should be able to formulate a working differential diagnosis for the patient.

At this point several questions must be addressed. (1) Is the patient adequately resuscitated? (2) Does the patient require invasive monitoring? (3) What further diagnostic studies are required? (4) Should the patient be taken to the operating room, and if so, when?

RESUSCITATION AND MONITORING

Resuscitation first involves attention to airway, breathing, and circulation. The patient with an acute abdomen may have altered pulmonary function with increased atelectasis, hypoxia, and increased work of breathing. Patients with preexisting pulmonary disease may not tolerate this pulmonary compromise, and early respiratory support may be needed. In general, most patients with an acute abdomen have had limited oral intake and associated GI losses via diarrhea, emesis, bleeding, or "third space" fluid shifts. They usually are dehydrated and demonstrate alterations in electrolyte balance. Early IV fluid and electrolyte replacement is mandatory. When the possibility of intra-abdominal sepsis exists, empiric antibiotic administration becomes an important early treatment. Before administering antibiotics, a definitive plan of action should be made. Antibiotics may mask the signs and symptoms of the intra-abdominal disease and delay appropriate therapy. Prophylaxis against stress gastritis is warranted in all critically ill patients.

All patients in the SICU with an acute abdomen should have ECG, blood pressure, and urinary output monitoring. Invasive monitoring generally is not required to resuscitate the patient with an acute abdomen. Selected patients (i.e., those with underlying cardiac, pulmonary, or renal disease) may require more sophisticated monitoring both to ensure adequate restoration of oxygen transport and to determine when the patient's condition is optimal for surgery. The guidelines for invasive monitoring set forth in Chapter 2 of this text also apply to the patient with an acute abdomen.

DIAGNOSTIC EVALUATION

The availability of a laboratory or radiologic test does not mandate its use. Cope's classic treatise on the diagnosis of the acute abdomen states that "overreliance on laboratory tests and radiologic evaluations will very often mislead the clinician, especially if the history and physical examination are less than complete." This observation applies equally well to the critically ill patient.

Laboratory Tests

A complete blood count with differential should be done on all patients to detect anemia, chronic blood loss, and hemoconcentration. El-

evation or depression of the WBC count with a shift to more immature forms may suggest an inflammatory process. This leukocytic response can be masked by dehydration. Platelet counts frequently are elevated by chronic infection and usually are depressed with overwhelming sepsis or disseminated intravascular coagulopathy (DIC).

Electrolyte values are useful in evaluating all patients with a potentially acute abdomen. Electrolyte concentrations may be abnormal with GI losses and dehydration. A low serum bicarbonate value suggests metabolic acidosis. Hypokalemia and hypochloremia, with metabolic alkalosis, suggest upper intestinal obstruction. Hyperglycemia can be the first sign of uncontrolled sepsis. Blood urea nitrogen and serum creatinine levels are often determined along with serum electrolyte values and are helpful in determining whether a patient has prerenal azotemia or renal failure.

Urinalysis is useful in differentiating genitourinary causes of abdominal pain. The urinalysis should reveal the presence or absence of WBC, RBC, bacteria, bilirubin, and ketone bodies, the specific gravity, and pH of the urine. Pyuria may also be associated with intra-abdominal inflammatory conditions.

Serum analyase evaluation usually is obtained because elevations are common with acute pancreatitis. Hyperamylasemia, however, also may occur with cholecystitis, intestinal obstruction with strangulation, perforated viscus, ectopic pregnancy, and renal failure.

Serum beta-human chorionic gonadotropin (beta-HCG) levels should be obtained in all women of childbearing age. The complications of pregnancy associated with the acute abdomen include ectopic gestation and concurrent intra-abdominal pathology (e.g., appendicitis, cholecystitis).

Liver function studies (bilirubin, alanine and aspartate transaminases, lactate dehydrogenase, alkaline phosphatase) can be deranged by any hepatobiliary disorder. Marked elevations of the transaminases usually are associated with hepatitis, whereas increases in alkaline phosphatase and bilirubin are more commonly associated with biliary tract obstruction. Milder elevations of these test results are seen with cholecystitis and other nonobstructive causes.

Arterial blood gas values are useful when an acid-base abnormality is suspected. Metabolic acidosis, particularly lactic acidosis, often occurs in the patient with intra-abdominal sepsis. A serum lactate value is also helpful in this setting. It not only provides a clue to diagnosis but also helps to evaluate resuscitation efforts. Ongoing lactic acidosis despite resuscitative efforts is associated with a poorer prognosis. Diabetic ketoacidosis may also be seen. Glucose metabolism is dysregulated in the setting of sepsis. Unexplained metabolic acidosis is characteristic of intestinal ischemia.

Assessment of coagulation by determination of the prothrombin time (PT) and partial tissue thromboplastin time (PTT) is useful in patients with advanced liver disease or DIC. Correction of coagulopathy should be done before any invasive therapy.

Stool studies for WBCs and *Clostridium difficile* toxin should be done in all critically ill patients with unexplained diarrhea and abdominal pain. The use of broad-spectrum antibiotics has led to a dramatic increase in pseudomembranous colitis, which, if untreated, can progress to toxic megacolon and even colonic perforation.

Radiologic Tests

The single most valuable film for the evaluation of an abdominal process is an upright chest film. This film allows inspection of abnormalities above the diaphragm (e.g., pneumonia, atelectasis, effusion) and below the diaphragm (e.g., free intraperitoneal air). Abdominal films (supine and upright) are useful in evaluating bowel gas patterns and in assessing ascites, blurring of psoas shadows, stones, vascular calcification, or foreign bodies. Despite the potential for providing significant clinical information, the use of plain abdominal radiographs in assessing the acute abdomen influences management in only 4% of cases; thus abdominal films should be used selectively.

GI contrast studies are useful when evaluating patients with suspected obstruction or perforation. In the critically ill patient water-soluble contrast agents should be used when perforation of the GI tract is suspected. These contrast studies have been of great value in ruling out perforated gastric or duodenal ulcers and in differentiating mechanical large bowel obstruction from so-called pseudo-obstruction. Enteroclysis, on the other hand, better delineates pathologic conditions of the jejunum and ileum.

Intravenous pyelograms are used to rule out ureteral obstruction as the cause of abdominal pain and to define genitourinary involvement of intra-abdominal infections. Genitourinary disease is an important diagnostic possibility in the differential diagnosis of the acute abdomen. In the critically ill patient genitourinary disease presenting as an acute abdomen is usually associated with pyonephrosis or hydronephrosis from obstruction of the renal pelvis or ureter. Abdominal pain may also be associated with severe cystitis or bladder outlet obstruction.

Ultrasonography has been used increasingly to investigate both acute and chronic abdominal conditions. It can identify gallstones, biliary dilation, pancreatic pseudocysts, hydronephrosis, aortic aneurysms, intraperitoneal fluid collections, and pelvic pathology. It is also useful for directing percutaneous drainage of fluid collections for both diagnosis and treatment. Ultrasonography should be used selectively and not as a screening study.

CT scans may be of value in patients with acute abdominal pain but generally only when routine radiographic studies are not diagnostic and the patient's condition allows the time to complete the study. An important use of the CT scan in critically ill patients is to search for intra-abdominal abscesses. Additional information about the urinary and GI tracts is obtained when IV and luminal contrast agents are used. Percutaneous drainage of fluid collections can be guided by CT imaging.

Nuclear medicine studies (technetium-99 radionuclide scan) have been used to aid in the diagnosis of acute cholecystitis and postoperative biliary leaks (HIDA scan), to evaluate pulmonary embolism as a cause of abdominal pain (V/Q scan), and to diagnose possible Meckel's diverticulum (Meckel scan). Aside from these specific conditions, nuclear studies are of limited use in the diagnosis of the acute abdomen.

Angiography, although not routinely used in the evaluation of the acute abdomen, is invaluable for assessing the cause of mesenteric ischemia (e.g., embolism, thrombosis, nonthrombotic occlusion).

Miscellaneous Tests

An ECG, although not routinely required when evaluating abdominal pain, is probably warranted in all critically ill patients. Associated disease processes in this group of patients, along with the possibility of underlying heart disease, place increased stress on the myocardium. A patient with myocardial infarction may initially present with epigastric pain; thus it should be ruled out.

Fine-needle aspiration or diagnostic peritoneal lavage (DPL) in patients with a suspected acute abdomen is useful. Alverdy et al.[1] demonstrated a sensitivity of 100% and specificity of 88% in a study of 68 patients who underwent DPL in the evaluation of these critically ill patients with a possible acute abdomen. Criteria for a positive tap were >50,000 RBC/ml, >500 WBC/ml, the presence of bile in lavage fluid, and the presence of bacteria by Gram stain. This group concluded that a negative DPL made intra-abdominal disease requiring surgical treatment highly unlikely; however, a positive lavage result may require further diagnostic evaluation. Similar results have been reported with fine-needle aspiration.

The use of preoperative laparoscopy for acute abdominal pain is not new. Use of laparoscopy in diagnostic decision-making in the patient with an acute abdomen has been strongly suggested by a number of studies. Most of these studies found laparoscopy particularly useful in differentiating the cause of acute right iliac fossa or pelvic pain. There also has been some evidence that a selective policy of using laparoscopy in patients with acute abdominal pain for whom the decision to operate is in doubt significantly decreases management errors. Laparoscopy and DPL are invasive diagnostic techniques and are not suited to all patients.

DIAGNOSIS AND TREATMENT

The management of the critically ill patient with a suspected acute abdomen depends on the diagnosis that has been formulated at the conclusion of the diagnostic evaluation. The question that must be answered at this point is whether or not a surgically treatable cause of the abdominal pain is present (Fig. 35-2). In general, patients fall into one of four categories (Fig. 35-3):

1. Diagnosis known—immediate operation. Patients with peritonitis and patients with an abdominal catastrophe (i.e., ruptured or dissecting aneurysms, mesenteric infarction, strangulated intestinal obstruction, volvulus, GI perforation, testicular or adnexal torsion, ectopic pregnancy, splenic rupture) fall into this class. After the initial stabilization of the patient, urgent operative intervention is required to prevent excessive morbidity and mortality.

2. Diagnosis known—initial management nonsurgical. Patients with cholecystitis, diverticulitis, small bowel obstruction, and continuous abdominal peritoneal dialysis catheter–related peritonitis fall into this category. These patients undergo initial resuscitation and are followed closely to either resolution of their problem or deterioration requiring urgent intervention. The majority of these patients will require an elective operation at some time after their acute condition resolves.

3. Diagnosis unknown—presence of peritonitis. In this group of patients a definitive diagnosis has not been made; however, presence of peritonitis mandates an urgent operation. A classic example is the patient that is taken to the operating room to rule out acute appendicitis. In the critically ill patient, once a diagnosis of peritonitis is made, the patient should be prepared for operation, and time should not be wasted on further diagnostic studies.

4. Diagnosis unknown—absence of peritonitis. In this group of patients the physician is able to observe or perform further diagnostic studies. If peritonitis develops or a diagnosis mandating surgery is made, the pa-

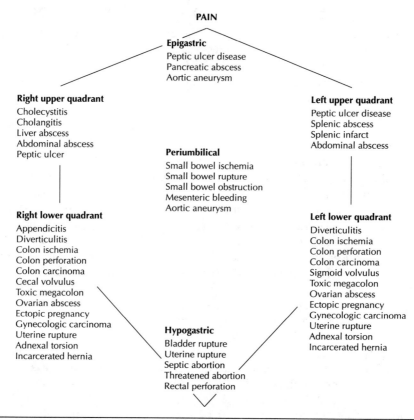

FIG. 35-2 Surgically treatable causes of abdominal pain.

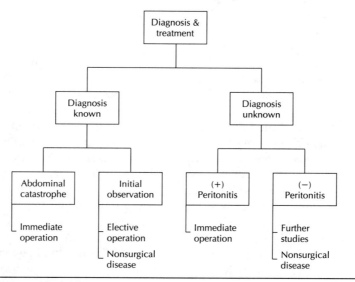

FIG. 35-3 Determination of whether surgery is necessary.

tient should be treated expeditiously. A nonsurgical cause of the abdominal pain (see box), once identified, should dictate appropriate therapy.

DIAGNOSTIC DIFFICULTIES IN THE CRITICALLY ILL PATIENT

Despite the advances that have been made in medical technology and the improved diagnostic tools currently available to the surgical

intensivist, several entities pose particular diagnostic problems.

Acalculous Cholecystitis

Acalculous cholecystitis is an acute inflammation of the gallbladder in the absence of gallstones. Its incidence as a cause of cholecystitis is estimated at 4% to 8%; however, recent evidence suggests that its incidence is rising. It occurs in patients with burns or major trauma

---

| Nonsurgical Causes of Abdominal Pain

Pulmonary

Pneumonia or pleurisy
Pulmonary embolus
Pneumothorax

Cardiac

Angina or myocardial infarct
CHF (on right side)
Pericarditis or myocarditis

Gastrointestinal

Mesenteric adenitis
Gastritis or enteritis
Inflammatory bowel disease
Hepatitis
Pancreatitis
Ileus
Pseudo-obstruction

Genitourinary

Pyelonephritis
Renal infarct
Urolithiasis
Cystitis
Prostatitis
Testicular torsion
Epididymitis or orchitis

Obstetric

Mittelschmerz
Ovarian cyst
Salpingitis
Endometritis or endometriosis
Dysmenorrhea
Threatened abortion

Musculoskeletal

Rectus sheath hematoma
Osteomyelitis
Arthritis

Neurologic

Multiple sclerosis
Tabes dorsalis
Herpes zoster
Abdominal epilepsy

Miscellaneous

Porphyria
Familial Mediterranean fever
Hemochromatosis
Diabetic ketoacidosis
Addison's disease
Thyroid disease
Hyperparathyroidism
Sickle cell anemia
Leukemia
Pernicious anemia
Measles or mumps
Malaria
Rocky Mountain spotted fever
Rheumatic fever
Connective tissue disorders
Poisons
 Lead
 Mercury
 Arsenic
 Mushroom
 Spider bite
Narcotic withdrawal
Psychosis

and after major operative procedures. Although not a constant association, a low-flow state is often an antecedent event. Other causative factors include biliary stasis and sepsis. Although the pathology is similar to acute calculous cholecystitis, the incidence of gangrene and perforation is higher. The diagnosis is notoriously difficult to make, and a high degree of suspicion based on clinical history is necessary for successful treatment. Nuclear scans have a higher incidence of false positive studies. The reduced diagnostic value of nuclear scans is due to the inadequate oral intake of these patients. Their bile usually is viscid and stagnant because the gallbladder does not contract. Ultrasonographic evidence for acalculous disease includes thickening of the gallbladder wall and the presence of pericholecystic fluid. Again, these imaging tests may be helpful, but the diagnosis rests largely on clinical suspicion. Acalculous disease mandates urgent intervention; accurate and early diagnosis is important.

Acute Mesenteric Ischemia

The bête noire of acute abdominal conditions is acute mesenteric ischemia. Diagnosing this entity is difficult, not only because laboratory and noninvasive tests tend to be inconclusive, but also because the patient's history usually is vague and a paucity of physical findings is present. Three causes of acute mesenteric ischemia are common: embolism, thrombosis, and nonocclusive mesenteric insufficiency. Emboli to the superior mesenteric artery arise from the heart (90%) or atherosclerotic plaques. The emboli generally lodge in the proximal superior mesenteric artery, a few centimeters from their origin, thus sparing the middle colic artery and the proximal jejunal branches of the superior mesenteric artery. Thrombosis of the superior mesenteric artery usually is associated with generalized atherosclerotic disease and occurs at the origin of the vessel. Thus the gut is ischemic from duodenum to midtransverse colon. Nonocclusive mesenteric insufficiency occurs in a patient with cardiac failure or dysrhythmia, digitalis intoxication, hemoconcentration, and other conditions that lead to a decrease in cardiac output and mesenteric flow.

Because of its insidious onset and the lack of obvious findings, early diagnosis of acute mesenteric ischemia is difficult. The classic findings of pain out of proportion to the examination and a "doughy" abdomen are difficult to identify in the SICU patient. Several observations that lead to early diagnosis are a markedly increased WBC count, unexplained metabolic acidosis, and elevated serum phosphate level. Based on these findings and clinical suspicion, the surgeon should decide whether or not a visceral angiogram is indicated. Treatment is based on the angiographic findings.

Pancreatitis

Although patients may come to the SICU with a diagnosis of severe pancreatitis, occult acute pancreatitis complicates any major surgical procedure. A high degree of suspicion is necessary to suggest the diagnosis since classic historical details and physical signs may be absent in the critically ill patient. Clinical clues include unexplained tachycardia, abdominal tenderness, and pleural effusion on the left side. Laboratory evidence of hyperamylasemia and elevated lipase may be helpful but are nonspecific. In patients with pancreatitis who do not appear to improve with conservative management, the possibility of evolution to necrotizing pancreatitis with abscess formation must be considered. This possibility can be confirmed with dynamic CT and needle aspiration under CT guidance. Unexplained decreases in the hemoglobin concentration in a patient with severe pancreatitis suggest the development of hemorrhagic pancreatitis. Classic diagnostic clues such as Grey Turner's sign (flank ecchymosis from retroperitoneal hemorrhage) are extremely rare.

Immunosuppression

Acute abdominal catastrophes can complicate immunosuppression associated with cancer chemotherapy, transplantation, and AIDS. In every instance the diagnostic possibilities must be placed in the context of the overall disease. For example, certain historical details are important, including the temporal relationship of the nadir of blood counts with the onset of neutropenic colitis. Although the physical examination is always important, physical signs usually associated with acute abdominal catastrophes are often confusing or absent. Similarly, typical defense responses (e.g., increased WBC count) may also be absent. Disease in critically ill patients who are immunosuppressed may be complicated by a number of unusual entities. Reported infectious complications include acalculous cholecystitis secondary to *Cryptosporidium* or *Candida,* toxic colitis with perforation caused by cytomegalovirus, or GI metastases from Kaposi's sarcoma. Although unusual infectious complications may occur, immunosuppressed patients should be treated with the thought that common causes of acute abdominal pain are more frequent.

SUMMARY

- Accurate and timely diagnosis of the acute abdomen can be very difficult in critically ill patients, especially those receiving mechanical ventilation.
- History and physical examination remain important diagnostic tools, and details of the onset of pain, character of pain, associated nausea and vomiting, location of pain, and radiation of pain are valuable diagnostic clues.
- Nausea that precedes emesis suggests abdominal pathology, whereas emesis without preceding nausea should raise the possibility of increased intracranial pressure.
- The availability of a laboratory or radiologic test does not mandate its use. Findings of the history and physical examination should guide further testing.
- Serum beta-HCG should be measured in women of childbearing age.
- In critically ill patients CT scans may be useful in identifying and percutaneously draining intra-abdominal abscesses when an abscess is suspected.
- Acalculous cholecystitis, acute mesenteric ischemia, and pancreatitis may complicate the clinical cause of SICU patients. These entities are difficult to diagnose and should be part of the differential diagnosis of abdominal pain in the critically ill patient.
- Acute abdominal crises can complicate immunosuppression. Unusual problems in the immunosuppressed patient include acalculous cholecystitis from *Cryptosporidium* or *Candida,* cytomegalovirus colitis with perforation, or GI metastases from Kaposi's sarcoma.

REFERENCE

1. Alverdy JC, Saunders J, Chamberlin WH, et al. Diagnostic peritoneal lavage in intra-abdominal sepsis. Am Surg 54:456, 1988.

SUGGESTED READINGS

Davies AH, Mastorakou I, Cobb R, et al. Ultrasonography in the acute abdomen. Br J Surg 78:1178, 1991.

Diethelm AG. The acute abdomen. In Sabiston's Textbook of Surgery, 13th ed. Philadelphia: WB Saunders, 1986.

Gregor P, Prodger JD. Symposium on mesenteric ischemia—Abdominal crisis in the intensive care unit. Can J Surg 31:331, 1988.

Hiatt JR. Management of the acute abdomen—A test of judgement. Postgrad Med 87:38, 1990.

Hiatt JR, Calabria RP, Passaro E Jr, et al. The amylase profile—A discriminant in biliary and pancreatic disease. Am J Surg 154:490, 1987.

Hickey MS, Kiernan GJ, Weaver KE. Evaluation of abdominal pain. Emerg Med Clin North Am 7:437, 1989.

Hoffman J, Lanng C, Shokouh-Amiri H. Peritoneal lavage in the diagnosis of acute peritonitis. Am J Surg 155:359, 1988.

Jamieson WG. Symposium on mesenteric ischemia—Acute intestinal ischemia. Can J Surg 31:200, 1988.

Papadakis MA, Mangione CM, Lee KK, et al. Treatable abdominal pathologic conditions and unsuspected malignant neoplasms at autopsy in veterans who received mechanical ventilation. JAMA 265:885, 1991.

Paterson-Brown S, Vipond MN. Modern aids to clinical decision-making in the acute abdomen. Br J Surg 77:13, 1990.

Rosemurgy AS, McAllister E, Karl RL. The acute surgical abdomen after cardiac surgery involving extracorporeal circulation. Ann Surg 207:323, 1988.

Schroeder T, Christoffersen JK, Andersen J, et al. Ischemic colitis complicating reconstruction of the abdominal aorta. Surg Gynecol Obstet 160:299, 1985.

Silen W. Cope's Early Diagnosis of the Acute Abdomen, 18th ed. New York: Oxford University Press, 1991.

Stower MJ, Amar SS, Mikulin T, et al. Evaluation of the plain abdominal x-ray in the acute abdomen. J R Soc Med 78:630, 1985.

Vipond MN, Paterson-Brown S, Tyrrell MR, et al. Evaluation of fine catheter aspiration cytology of the peritoneum as an adjunct to decision making in the acute abdomen. Br J Surg 77:86, 1990.

Vogt DP. The acute abdomen in the geriatric patient. Cleve Clin J Med 57:125, 1990.

Wilson SE, Robinson G, Williams RA, et al. Acquired immune deficiency syndrome (AIDS): Indications for abdominal surgery, pathology, and outcome. Ann Surg 210:428, 1989.

Young GP. Abdominal catastrophes. Emerg Med Clin North Am 7:699, 1989.

CHAPTER 36

Fractures in Blunt Multiple Trauma

James Hassett • John R. Border

FRACTURE MANAGEMENT IN THE SICU

Operative stabilization within the first 24 hours of fractures whose conservative management would otherwise produce prolonged enforced supine position in patients with two or more major injuries (Index-Injury Severity Score [ISS] >18) has been shown conclusively in retrospective and prospectively randomized studies to reduce complications and the length of SICU stage drastically.[1-9] The time on ventilator therapy, multiple organ failure, and late deaths from sepsis correlate highly in patients with blunt multiple trauma with the duration of the prolonged enforced supine position, produced by conservative management of fractures of the femur, spine, and weight-bearing pelvis.

Since the key to this relationship is the prolonged enforced supine position, the complications observed can be extrapolated to other clinical situations that produce the supine position. Such situations include protection of the many lines used for monitoring and support, use of mind-obtunding drugs, an abdomen open for prolonged periods, and, above all, the expectation of the SICU care team that severely ill patients should be flat on their backs in the horizontal crucifixion position. The link between the prolonged enforced supine position, multiple organ failure, and late septic deaths apparently is lack of oral intake and the gut-origin septic states.

PATHOPHYSIOLOGY

One of the key intellectual changes that characterizes modern medicine began in the 1940s. Physicians then recognized that the prolonged bedrest then used did not help cure most diseases. Indeed, it added a number of its own disease mechanisms, which both increased the mortality rate and greatly increased the period of disability. This change in perspective, applied to successively broader fields of medicine, has led to both decreased periods of hospital care and improved results of care. Only recently has the concept of mobilizing patients been applied in the SICU.[10]

The most important advance in medicine is the recognition that filth and disease are associated. That poor hygiene, and its associated bacteria, fungi, and probably viruses, leads to disease is a concept most aptly termed the "Florence Nightingale concept."

However, to this basic concept must be added the concept of endogenous sources of sepsis. Of special importance is the gut lumen's contents—bacteria and bacterial toxins. Gut bacteria and associated toxins have access to the systemic body through a previously unknown gut wound. Initially systemic access results from the original physiologic crisis and continues from several standard SICU support modalities, resulting in the concept of "gut-origin septic states." The SICU is a harsh environment for survival with respect to the failure to include appropriate, positive gut-support regimens and to modify regimens that have a negative effect on entry of gut-origin bacteria and their toxins.[11-17]

Another new concept must be added. The organ failures are products not of bacteria and bacterial toxins per se but of the leukocyte system activation these agents produce. The leukocyte system is activated not only by bacteria and bacterial toxins, but also by devitalized tissue. More commonly, some combination of the three mechanisms is at work. The leukocyte system includes at least monocytes and macrophages, the polymorphonuclear cells, the various lymphocyte lines, the endothelium, and some tissue cells such as the mast cell. These different cell lines function as an integrated whole under the influence of various eicosanoic acid derivatives, platelet activating factor, and cytokines. In response to activation they release these coordinating agents locally and systemically (systemically producing the septic response) and, in addition, release locally a variety of destructive products such as oxidants, lysosomal enzymes, split-complement products, and various coagulating factors. These destructive products in their extracellular function normally prepare devitalized tissue and bacteria for phagocytosis. In their intracellular function they kill bacteria and digest dead bacteria and devitalized tissue in the phagolysosome. These products are highly destructive and expand the local wound by killing the marginally viable tissue present. The result is both reduced destructive product egress and compromised antibiotic ingress.[18] Of primary importance, severe organ failures from bacteria and bacterial toxin activation of the leukocyte system occur without producing positive bacterial cultures or measurable bacterial toxins.

Failure of pulmonary oxygen transport brings about most blunt multiple trauma SICU admissions. Such inadequate gas exchange is a

product first of direct chest trauma, second of the enforced supine position, third of gut-origin bacteria and bacterial toxins, and fourth of activation of the gut's hepatic-leukocyte system, with output of leukocyte destructive products. The damage done to the lung by these multiple insults produces a bacterial nutrient–rich environment. The oral endotracheal tube provides access for oropharyngeal bacteria. The use of systemic broad-spectrum antibiotics, stomach alkalinization, and nasogastric tubes and the enforced supine position convert the normal gut commensal bacteria to more antibiotic-resistant pathogenic aerobic forms and aid their access to the oropharynx and the lung. Within a few days of intubation, bacterial pneumonia may be an additional insult to the lung. A complicating secondary pneumonia increases the duration of oral endotracheal intubation and increases the possibility of changing bacterial flora in the basic pneumonia process.[17-19]

Oral endotracheal intubation and its constraints eliminate the possibility of spontaneous eating and greatly reduce defecation. Abnormal GI function greatly reduces biliary secretion of secretory IgA and bile salts. Enterocyte replication, mucous secretion, and gut mucosa thickness are all reduced. Secretory IgA, gut mucous secretions, and enterocyte shedding as a result of cell replication are of major importance in reducing bacteria and bacterial toxin penetration of the gut mucosa. Bile salts are of major importance in detoxifying gut lumen endotoxin and probably other bacterial toxins. In the colon, defecation is of major importance in reducing bacteria and bacterial toxin penetration pressure.[17-19]

The essential point is that any therapy that prolongs oral endotracheal intubation and carries with it the standard associated therapy that produces the prolonged enforced supine position contributes greatly to the gut wound with its leukocyte system activation. This mechanism results in continued pulmonary oxygen transport failure that lengthens the need for endotracheal ventilatory support. The conservative management of femur fractures, disruption of the weight-bearing pelvis, and spinal fractures are the prototype fractures that demonstrate the path to oxygen failure. Traditional conservative management of such patients requires prolonged ventilatory support, leads to multiple organ failure, and results in a high late septic death rate. These outcomes are not a product of the magnitude of the original injury, but of the treatment of the original injury.[17]

TREATMENT

The objective of therapy is to achieve rapidly a largely pain-free mobile patient who can sit up, eat, and defecate and who requires no special gut mucosa support. In most blunt multiple trauma patients, oxygen transport and resuscitation that preserve blood clotting are easily obtained and maintained. Supra-normal oxygen transport in this initial care period is clearly of importance in preventing a variety of subsequent complications. Our treatment protocol during surgery for all patients with two or more major injuries includes maintaining the arterial oxygen level at or above 100 mm Hg and urinary output around 100 ml/hr and leaving the patients intubated after surgery and receiving ventilator support until they clearly prove in the SICU that ventilatory support is not required. Oxygen transport is maximized during this period by hypervolemia, and any pulmonary limitations are compensated by use of ventilatory support with positive end-expiratory pressure. The patient is extubated as early as possible in the SICU under carefully controlled conditions (24 to 72 hours).

In such a patient the question becomes how to organize preoperative care to include x-ray studies that define the fractures adequately for operative stabilization and how to organize the operative session to stabilize those fractures efficiently. Although standard x-ray studies provide adequate definition of most fractures, some such as those of the face, weight-bearing pelvis, or spine require CT scans. Since many of these patients have head or facial injuries that also require CT scans, most of the risks of transport to the CT scanner already are being taken. The additional CT scan work requires little additional time. However, the need to define the fractures sufficiently well by x-ray study requires additional emergency room time. We see no harm in providing additional time for evaluation if good oxygen transport can be measured and maintained. Our goal is to define all injuries in the emergency room so that the sur-

gical endeavor in those patients who respond well to resuscitation is well organized. The need for and a plan for resuscitative operations in which oxygen transport resuscitation cannot be quickly obtained are discussed subsequently.

In the patient with good oxygen transport resuscitation, the organizing principle is positioning the patient and arranging operative procedures so that as many operative teams as possible can work at one time. The first position is almost always the supine position. In this position operative teams can work on the abdomen, the legs below the knees, the forearms, and the head and neck. If a femur or tibia fracture is present, the initial abdominal operation can proceed on the fracture table. Using the fracture table saves considerable time; either the tibial fracture can be treated simultaneously with the abdominal injury or the femur fracture can undergo closed reduction in preparation for closed nailing after the laparotomy. In the supine position open tibial fractures, forearm fractures, facial fractures, and vascular repairs of the lower or upper extremity can be done concurrently with the laparotomy. The facial fractures must be stabilized operatively since the objective is to produce a mobile patient who can eat.

After the laparotomy, femur fractures or disruption of the sacroiliac joint can also be treated with the patient in the supine position. Disruption of the sacroiliac joint in patients without massive bleeding can be performed easily in the supine position. Using an ilioinguinal approach, an anterior plate can be placed over the sacroiliac joint. A number of the more stable cervical spine fractures can be treated in the same position by application of a halo-vest arrangement that allows nearly immediate mobility. A number of spinal fractures and vertical sacral fractures require the prone position for surgery. Although the patient can be placed in the prone position only after all supine surgery has been completed, treatment of these fractures should be done in the first 24 hours.

Although such a planned operative session may take several hours, we see no disadvantage if oxygen transport and blood clotting are maintained. In well-supported patients, a long operation may present problems, not with the patient, but with the surgeon. Tired surgeons make more mistakes. Surgery that is poorly done has bad consequences for both the surgeon and the patient. Our plan is organized around multiple operating teams to limit surgeon fatigue and make fatigue much less of a problem. When properly done, a multiple team organization not only reduces the problems of SICU care but also decreases the local wound and surgical complications.

Patients who require immediate resuscitative surgery to help restore oxygen transport and blood clotting present different problems. These patients necessarily go rapidly to the operating room for their laparotomy, thoracotomy, craniostomy, or control of vascular injury. The consequence is minimal diagnostic information about all other injuries. Such patients must be treated during their resuscitative surgery as though they have spinal fractures or intracranial injuries. In patients with liver injuries blood loss beyond 5 to 10 units leads to major problems with blood clotting. The use of packing to control blood loss temporarily and a second operation at 24 to 48 hours for a definitive repair seems to have proven value. With laparotomies, severe intra-abdominal edema can occur. If the abdomen is forcibly closed, the diaphragm is elevated and creates failures of pulmonary oxygen transport. The same pressure applied to the vena cava can also reduce venous return and cardiac output. The use of mesh in the abdominal closure until the intra-abdominal edema subsides has great value in supporting systemic oxygen transport. Anything that supports oxygen transport at its required supranormal levels is of great value in these patients.

After resuscitative surgery, oxygen transport and blood clotting resuscitation must be maintained and monitored closely. The resuscitative operation cannot be assumed to have produced continued restoration of oxygen transport. When good resuscitation has been achieved, these patients again enter the diagnostic phase. At this time all injuries are determined, and a second comprehensive operative session is planned. The second operative session should be done within 24 hours, when possible, and not later than 48 hours. No excuse exists for

postponing this session 7 to 10 days. Again multiple operative teams are used to eliminate using a tired surgeon.

Patients with massive pelvic bleeding from disruption of the weight-bearing pelvis require different priorities in care. The basic diagnosis is easy since they have a mobile hemipelvis, confirmatory x-ray findings, and minimal response to standard resuscitation. The major diagnostic problem is eliminating massive intra-abdominal bleeding, intrathoracic bleeding, and pericardial tamponade. Diagnostic peritoneal lavage, chest tubes, and pericardial windows in the emergency room provide these distinctions. In patients with massive pelvic bleeding most have venous bleeding that is easily tamponaded with medical anti-shock trousers (MAST). Many also have femur fractures whose bleeding is also tamponaded with MAST. Use of the MAST for the treatment of venous bleeding requires pressures of only 20 to 40 mm Hg. The use of MAST at this pressure is entirely different from its tourniquet use at 100 mm Hg. When MAST is applied to treat venous bleeding in the pelvis or femur, the patients usually are easily resuscitated unless overwhelming blood loss has damaged their myocardium. The patients who have MAST applied and do not rapidly resuscitate require interventional radiology to define and treat pelvic arterial bleeding.

If these maneuvers are successful in obtaining a resuscitated patient, the question arises as to when to proceed with their needed surgery. The tradition has been a 7- to 10-day delay. This delay is long enough to get the patient frankly into the gut-origin septic states and has no apparent surgical merits. Surgically the hematoma and the bleeding vessels must be well clotted off, a condition that probably is achieved in 24 to 48 hours. If the lesion to be treated can be reached from the ilioinguinal approach, this approach takes the surgeon directly through the clot and to the vessels that were formerly bleeding. Under these conditions blood loss control with the use of pressure and hemostats is relatively simple. If, in addition to the pelvic bleeding, a rectal injury exists or the pelvic injury is open, the hematoma must be evacuated before uncontrollable infection occurs.

SUMMARY

- Operative stabilization of fractures within 24 hours in patients with multiple injuries reduces mortality, pulmonary complications, late fracture morbidity, and life-style compromise.
- Carefully evaluate changes in mental status or vital signs in any patient with long bone or pelvic fracture.
- Fractures of the pelvic ring and acetabulum are severe injuries.
- Obtain anterior/posterior x-rays of the pelvis in all patients injured in high-energy accidents.
- Perform a careful neurologic, perineal, rectal, and vaginal examination in patients with pelvic fracture.

- Open pelvic fractures require an emergency colostomy.
- For the patient in shock, stabilizing the pelvic ring can be a lifesaving procedure. Pelvic stabilization helps tamponade bleeding.
- Fractures of the acetabulum are rarely life-threatening.
- Consider prophylaxis for deep venous thrombosis in patients with pelvic fractures.
- Surgical stabilization of femoral fractures permits early mobilization of patients.
- Fractures of the humeral shaft can be managed with both operative and nonoperative therapy.
- Radial nerve injuries are complications of humeral shaft fractures.

REFERENCES

1. Riska E, Bonsdorff H, Hakkinen S. Primary operative fixation of long bone fractures in patients with multiple injuries. Injury 6:110-116, 1976.
2. Riska E, Myllynen P. Fat embolism in patients with multiple injuries. J Trauma 22:894-895, 1982.
3. Ruedi T, Wolff G. Vemeidung posttraumatischer komplikationen duch fräke difinitive versorgung von polytraumatisiertes mit frakturen des kewegungapparats. Helv Chir Acta 42:507-512, 1975.
4. Wolff G, Dittman M, Ruedi T, Buchman B, Allgower M. Koordination von chirurgie und intensivmedizin zur vermeidgung der posttraumatischen respiratorischen insuffizienz. Unfallheilkunde 81:425-442, 1978.
5. Meek R, Vivoda E, Pirani S. Comparison of mortality of patients with multiple injuries according to type of fracture treatment. Injury 17:2-4, 1986.
6. Goris R, Gimbrere J, Van Niekerk J. Early osteosynthesis and prophylactic mechanical ventilation in the multiple trauma patient. J Trauma 22:895-903, 1982.
7. Johnson K, Cadambi A, Siebert G. Incidence of adult respiratory distress syndrome in patients with multiple musculoskeletal injuries; Effect of early operative stabilization of fractures. J Trauma 25:375-384f, 1985.
8. Seibel R, LaDuca J, Hassett J, Babikian G, Mills B, Border D, Border J. Blunt multiple trauma (ISS-36), femur traction, and the pulmonary failure septic state. Ann Surg 202:283-295, 1985.

9. Bone L, Johnson K, Weigelt J, Scheinberg R. Early versus delayed stabilization of femoral fractures. J Bone Joint Surg 71A:336-340, 1989.
10. Border J, Bone L, Babikian G, Rodriquez J. A history of the care of trauma. In Border J, Allgower M, Hansen S, Ruedi T, eds. Blunt Multiple Trauma. New York: Marcel Dekker, 1990.
11. Border J. Trauma and sepsis. In Worth M, ed. Principles and Practice of Trauma Care. Baltimore: Williams & Wilkins, 1982, pp 330-388.
12. Alexander J, MacMillan B, Stinnet J, Ogle C, Bogian R, Fischer J, Oakes J, Morriss M, Krummel R. Beneficial effect of aggressive protein feeding in severely burned children. Ann Surg 192:505-518, 1980.
13. Antonacci A, Cowles S, Reaves L. The role of nutrition in immunologic function. Infect Surg 3:590-597, 1984.
14. Alexander JW. Mechanism of immunologic suppression in burn injury. J Trauma 30:S70-S75, 1990.
15. Deitch E. Bacterial translocation of the gut flora. J Trauma 30:S184-S189, 1990.
16. van Saene H, Stoutenbeck C, Lawin P, Ledingham I. Infection control by selective decontamination. In Vincent JL. Update in Intensive Care and Emergency Medicine, 7th ed. Berlin: Springer-Verlag, 1988.
17. Border J, Hassett J, LaDuca J, Seibel R, Steinberg S, Mills B, Losi P, Border D. The gut origin septic states in blunt multiple trauma (ISS-40) in the ICU. Ann Surg 206:427-448, 1987.

18. Border J, Hassett J, Bone L, Steinberg S, Lentenegger A, Rodriquez J. Metabolic response to trauma and sepsis. In Border J, Allgower M, Hansen S, Ruedi T, eds. Blunt Multiple Trauma. New York: Marcel Dekker, 1990.

19. Border J, Steinberg S, Bone L, Hansen S, Ruedi T, Allgower M. Bacterial growth and infection: Antibiotics and other effective measures. In Border J, Allgower M, Hansen S, Ruedi T, eds. Blunt Multiple Trauma. New York: Marcel Dekker, 1990.

CHAPTER 37

Emergency Considerations for Specific Fractures

David C. Templeman

The appropriate orthopedic care of patients with multiple injuries reduces mortality rates, pulmonary complications, and late morbidity from fractures and returns patients to active and productive life-styles. The orthopedist's goal in the care of multiply injured patients is to immobilize unstable fractures. Immobilization of long-bone fractures benefits pulmonary care by removing traction, which allows patients to sit upright, and reducing fracture site pain, which reduces the need for narcotic doses that suppress pulmonary function, and assists nursing care because patients are easier to move.[1] Thus the bedside care of these patients is an extension of the operations done to stabilize their fractures and is an integral part of the philosophy of fracture care.

In general, surgical stabilization of fractures uses screw-plate combinations, intramedullary nails, or external fixation to achieve fixation. Conversely, when skeletal traction is used or when the fractures are poorly immobilized by splints, moving patients to different positions is impossible or limited by motion and pain at the fracture site. After surgical procedures to stabilize fractures, the orthopedic team should outline any restrictions in sitting and the mobilization of adjacent joints. Because patients with long-bone and pelvic fractures are at risk for fat embolism syndrome and adult respiratory distress syndrome, any changes in mental status and vital signs should be evaluated by a clinical examination that includes a search for petechiae, arterial blood gas evaluation, and chest x-ray films.

FRACTURES OF PELVIC RING AND ACETABULUM

Fractures of the pelvic ring and acetabulum are severe injuries, usually caused by high-energy accidents. These fractures often are associated with other life-threatening injuries that complicate the management of these patients. The treatment goals are to resuscitate the patient and to manage the pelvic ring disruption to provide bony union in satisfactory position. Pelvic deformities lead to leg-length inequalities, sitting problems, nonunion of the fracture site, or late sacroiliac joint pain from arthritis, all of which can cause lifelong impairment. Fractures of acetabulum must be distinguished from pelvic ring disruptions. Acetabular fractures involve disruption of the articular surface of the hip joint and, if displaced, can lead to posttraumatic arthritis. In most instances fractures of the acetabulum are not associated with the life-threatening hemorrhage that can complicate pelvic ring disruptions.

The purpose of the pelvic ring is to (1) transfer the weight of the upper body to the lower extremities; (2) provide attachment sites for lower extremity muscles used in walking; and (3) shield the pelvic viscera. The pelvic ring can be envisioned as having two arches. The posterior arch transmits weight from the femoral heads through the iliac wings to the sacrum for weight bearing. The anterior arch of the pelvis, composed of the pubic rami and the symphysis pubis, contributes little to pelvic stability. Other than performing a protective role and providing sites for muscle insertion, fractures or congenital absence of the pubic rami rarely compromises function.

Several different systems exist for the classification of pelvic ring injuries. Tile's classification[2] is based on the type of pelvic instability that exists after the injury. This system groups fractures into three categories:

I. Injuries that are rotationally and vertically stable. The pelvic ring is intact, and supportive care is required until the patient can walk comfortably.

II. Injuries that are rotationally unstable but vertically stable. The so-called "open book" injuries include disruptions of the symphysis pubis, with widening of the symphysis. Lateral compression injuries are also a subset of rotationally unstable but vertically stable pelvic ring fractures. Most lateral compression injuries do not require surgery.

III. Pelvic injuries that are rotationally and vertically unstable, frequently termed *vertical shear injuries,* or *Malgaigne fractures.* They are severe injuries. Of the three subsets of pelvic ring disruptions, vertical shear injuries have the highest incidence of neurologic injury, urologic injury, and life-threatening hemorrhage. Vertical shear injuries are also more likely to cause deformities of the pelvis that lead to permanent impairment. New techniques in the operative management of pelvic fractures are directed at restoring the pelvic anatomy to reduce the morbidity and mortality associated with vertical shear injuries.

The advantage of Tile's classification system is that it includes both ligamentous and bony injuries and describes the resultant mechanical instability, a description that is helpful in determining the ultimate functional prognosis and the indications for operative treatment.

Pelvic Ring Injuries
Assessment

Physical examination of the pelvis is difficult. Although manual stressing of the pelvis can detect relative motion between the two anterior superior iliac spines, the diagnosis of pelvic fractures is made with roentgenograms. The standard anteroposterior view of the pelvis is recommended to complement routine films of the cervical spine and chest for all patients injured in high-energy accidents (e.g., motor vehicle accidents, pedestrian vs. motor vehicle accidents, falls from heights). The clinical examination of the patient with a pelvic fracture requires a detailed neurologic examination of the lower extremity, with grading of motor function (motor grades 0 to 5), to detect injuries of the lumbosacral plexus. Foot dorsiflexion and foot eversion are the functions usually lost after a pelvic fracture with a neurologic injury. A meticulous examination of the perineum, rectum, and vaginal vault should reveal open wounds that communicate with fracture sites. A careful examination requires that patients are gently rolled onto their side to detect any posterior wounds. Any soft tissue injury in proximity to a pelvic fracture or dislocation is considered an open pelvic fracture until proved otherwise.

Patients with open pelvic fractures require an emergency colostomy to prevent death from intrapelvic sepsis, for historically mortality rates as high as 90% have been reported in association with such fractures. If any possibility exists that fecal contamination of the fracture site might occur, a colostomy must be performed; therefore any open fracture wounds in or near the perineum are clear indications for a colostomy. The orthopedic service should be consulted before performing a colostomy to ensure that the ostomy site does not interfere with the placement of an external fixator or any future surgical incisions. In addition to an anteroposterior roentgenogram of the pelvis, additional views are required. Oblique inlet and outlet views taken at 45-degree angles to the anteroposterior view (angled 45 degrees toward the feet and 45 degrees toward the head) are necessary to identify horizontal and vertical displacements of the pelvis. It is difficult to use plain films to assess the injury pattern of the posterior aspect of the pelvic ring, which includes the sacroiliac joints and the sacrum. Adequate assessment of the posterior aspect of the pelvic ring requires CT scans to define the anatomy of sacral fractures, sacroiliac dislocations, or posterior iliac wing fractures.[3,4]

Management

The orthopedic care of pelvic ring injuries should complement and proceed with the resuscitation of the patient. For patients in shock, the orthopedist plays a vital role in their resuscitation. Life-threatening hemorrhage after a pelvic ring disruption is caused by (1) injury to abdominal or pelvic viscera; (2) disruption of major vessels; and (3) bony surfaces. The superior gluteal artery and the internal iliac vessels are the vascular structures most often injured in vertical shear injuries. Angiographic studies indicate that nearly 95% of hemodynamically unstable patients with pelvic fractures do not have an identifiable vascular lesion. Therefore, when other sources of hemorrhage have been excluded, bleeding most likely comes from the highly vascular bony surfaces of the pelvis.

When horizontal or vertical instability of the pelvic ring exists, the spherical cage of the bony pelvis is disrupted, which allows unchecked swelling from hemorrhage. Since the volume of a sphere is a function of the cube of the radius (volume equals ($\frac{4}{3}$) πr^3), even small disruptions of the symphysis pubis allow for an exponential increase in pelvic volume. In this setting the pelvic disruption accommodates the expanding hematoma. Tamponade can be assisted by restoring the stability of the pelvic ring, particularly by reducing the diastasis of the pubic symphysis.[5]

Emergency application of an anterior pelvic external fixator can reapproximate the shape of the pelvic ring and, in combination with volume replacement, correct hypovolemic shock from exsanguination. Military anti-shock trousers (MAST) have also been used to control pelvic volume. However, the pressure generated by MAST is transmitted to the lower extremities, and in the presence of lower extremity fractures, compartment syndromes and limb loss are reported. Therefore a wise use of MAST is during transportation to the trauma center, followed by rapid removal of the MAST and application of an external fixator.

The external fixator is applied by inserting pins into the iliac crest through percutaneous incisions. This can be done in a matter of minutes in conjunction with any required intra-abdominal surgery. After the application of the external fixator, the patients are carefully monitored for continued blood loss. A continued fall in hemoglobin level indicates ongoing pelvic bleeding. Frequently, a falling hemoglobin level is accompanied by marked swelling in the perineum, lower abdomen, or buttock. If volume replacement and the application of an external fixator will not stop blood loss, an emergency angiogram is obtained to look for sources of intrapelvic bleeding that can be embolized. In this setting angiographic embolization of intrapelvic bleeding is lifesaving.

Permanent disability after pelvic ring injuries usually is associated with vertical shear injuries rather than type I or type II pelvic ring disruptions. A number of procedures have been developed for the treatment of vertical displacement. The principles of treating vertical disruptions of the pelvis are as follows:

- Ligamentous disruptions are unlikely to heal (sacroiliac joint dislocations).
- Leg-length inequality secondary to vertical displacement of the pelvis may lead to disabling low back pain and sitting imbalance.
- After reduction of vertical shear injuries, internal fixation of the posterior structures of the pelvis is required to resist recurrent vertical displacement.

The operative management of pelvic ring disruptions by open reduction and internal fixation is usually delayed for approximately 48 hours. This delay allows tamponade of bleeding fracture surfaces and reduces operative blood loss. It also avoids retroperitoneal dissections in the presence of an expanding intrapelvic hematoma. Before surgery, skeletal traction usually is applied to prevent or reduce vertical displacement of the hemipelvis. After the application of traction, x-ray films are taken to confirm reduction of the vertical displacement, and a repeat examination is necessary to ensure that traction has not led to a neurologic injury.

Pelvic disruptions and their associated injuries are frequently life-threatening. The patient with such injuries is best managed in a level I trauma center. Advances in trauma care, incorporating the specialties of general surgery, urology, and orthopedics, have dramatically reduced the morbidity and mortality associated with fractures of the pelvic ring.

Acetabular Injury

Fractures of the acetabulum are rarely life-threatening. However, the patient may have other associated injuries that are responsible for shock. Selected acetabular fractures are managed with open reduction and internal fixation to restore the congruity of the joint and to prevent posttraumatic arthritis. Unless rapid mobilization of a multiply injured patient is required, acetabular fracture surgery can be considered as a reconstructive procedure to prevent late morbidity of the hip. Surgery, when performed, is frequently done after 48 hours to prevent excessive intraoperative bleeding. During this period, skeletal traction is used to reduce displacement of the fracture fragments. Anteroposterior dislocations of the femoral head in association with acetabular fractures require emergency reduction to avoid avascular necrosis of the femoral head. In rare instances closed reduction is unsuccessful, and an emergency open reduction of the dislocated hip is required. Hip dislocations are associated with a significant incidence of neurologic injury, and careful evaluation of the neurovascular status and motor grading is necessary. After open reduction and internal fixation of acetabular fractures, the orthopedic team should outline carefully the restrictions on the range of motion of the hip, log rolling the patient, and care needed in sitting or bed-to-chair transfers.

DEEP VENOUS THROMBOSIS AFTER PELVIC FRACTURE

The incidence of deep venous thrombosis after fracture of the pelvis is unknown. However, by using duplex ultrasound screening, at least a 15% incidence of proximal thrombosis has been detected.[6] No prospective studies conclusively prove the value of single or combined therapies for the prevention of deep venous thrombosis after pelvic trauma. Two different subsets of patients sustain pelvic fractures—the elderly who have minimally displaced fractures that are immobilized for a period of time and younger patients who suffer high-energy injuries with associated multisystem injuries. Because of the potential for deep venous thrombosis and pulmonary embolism in these patients, the use of some form of prophylaxis seems prudent. When use of pharmacologic agents might be risky because of associated visceral injuries, at least some form of mechanical compression can be used. Intermittent compression devices can be used, with some care, even in the presence of lower extremity skeletal traction. However, the presence of lower extremity fractures contraindicates their use if there is concern about compartment syndromes. Although information about deep venous thrombosis and pulmonary embolism is incomplete, the prophylactic treatment of these disorders should be considered in all patients with pelvic fracture (see Chapter 12).

FRACTURES OF FEMUR

Femoral fractures can be divided into three anatomic groups: proximal fractures, which are fractures of the femoral neck and intertrochanteric region; femoral shaft fractures, or fractures of the femoral diaphysis; and distal one third femoral fractures, which are fractures of the distal femoral metaphysis or intra-articular fractures of the distal femur. All three types are immobilized best by internal fixation.

Femoral neck fractures, common in the elderly, usually are fixed with multiple screws or a proximal femoral endoprosthesis in cases of severe fracture site displacement. Femoral shaft fractures are fixed routinely with intramedullary nails. Frequently, interlocking bolts placed through the ends of the intramedullary nail are used to prevent shortening and rotation of comminuted fractures. Distal one third femoral fractures can cause displacement of the articular surfaces of the knee joint and lead to posttraumatic arthritis. Open reduction and internal fixation using plates and screws are done to restore joint surfaces and immobilize the fracture.

In most instances the surgical stabilization of femoral fractures permits early mobilization of patients. Postoperative splinting and range of motion are determined by the stability of the fracture fixation achieved at surgery. Continuous passive motion machines are often used after fixation of intra-articular fractures of the knee.

FRACTURES OF HUMERUS AND SUPRACONDYLAR HUMERUS

The treatment of humeral shaft fractures is controversial. Nonoperative treatment achieves high union rates and good functional results, and although they are successful, the different surgical procedures that are used have their inherent complications. Although the need for stabilization of other long-bone fractures in the multiply injured patient is established, it is still possible to splint an isolated humeral shaft fracture and mobilize the patient. Indications used for surgical stabilization of humeral fractures include bilateral fractures, unacceptable position with nonoperative management, open fractures, closed head injury, and when surgical stabilization will improve nursing care and the ability to move the patient. Internal fixation with plates and screws and the use of intramedullary nails are the commonly used techniques. The preference of the surgeon usually determines which form of surgical stabilization is used.

Radial nerve palsies are complications of humeral shaft fractures and surgical procedures. Both after surgery and during the nonoperative treatment of humeral fractures, the status of the radial nerve is assessed by grading the strength of wrist dorsiflexion. In the absence of functional extension of the wrist, wrist extension splints must be prescribed. The management of a patient with a humeral shaft fracture and an associated radial nerve injury is controversial. However, most authors recommend a 3-month period of observation before surgical exploration of the nerve. In approximately 85% of cases, spontaneous recovery of radial nerve function occurs after a closed humeral fracture.

Supracondylar humeral fractures involve the distal one third of the humerus and may be intra-articular. Displaced intra-articular fractures require open reduction and internal fixation for an accurate restoration of joint surfaces. To enhance surgical exposure, an olecranon osteotomy frequently is done. Extra-articular supracondylar fractures, which are difficult to align with nonoperative methods, are also treated with open reduction and internal fixation. Severely displaced distal humeral fractures are associated with injuries to the brachial artery, radial nerve, medial nerve, and ulnar nerve. The integrity of these structures must be carefully documented and observed during the care of this injury.

SUMMARY

- Orthopedic care of patients with multiple injuries reduces mortality, pulmonary complications, late fracture morbidity, and life-style compromise.
- Changes in mental status or vital signs should be evaluated carefully in any patient with long-bone or pelvic fracture.
- Fractures of pelvic ring and acetabulum are severe injuries, but fractures of the acetabulum are rarely life-threatening.
- Anteroposterior x-ray films of pelvis should be obtained in all patients injured in high-energy accidents.
- A careful neurologic, perineal, rectal, and vaginal examination should be performed in patients with pelvic fracture.

- Open pelvic fractures require an emergency colostomy.
- For the patient in shock, stabilizing the pelvic ring can be a lifesaving procedure. Pelvic stabilization helps tamponade bleeding.
- Use of prophylaxis for deep venous thrombosis should be considered for patients with pelvic fractures.
- Surgical stabilization of femoral fractures permits early mobilization of patients.
- Fractures of the humeral shaft can be managed with both operative and nonoperative therapy.
- Radial nerve injuries are complications of humeral shaft fractures.

REFERENCES

1. Phillips TF, Conteras DM. Current concepts review: Timing of operative treatment of fracture in patients who have multiple injuries. J Bone Joint Surg 72A:784, 1990.
2. Tile M. Fractures of the Acetabulum. Baltimore: Williams & Wilkins, 1984.
3. Bucholz RW. The pathological anatomy of Malgaigne fracture—Dislocation of the pelvis. J Bone Joint Surg 63A:400, 1981.
4. Gill K, Bucholz RW. The role of computerized tomographic scanning in the evaluation of major pelvic fractures. J Bone Joint Surg 66A:34, 1984.
5. Lange RH, Hansen ST Jr. Pelvic ring disruption with symphysis pubis diastasis: Indications, techniques and limitations of anterior internal fixation. Clin Orthop 201:130, 1985.
6. White RH, Goulet JA, Bray TJ, Daschbach MM, McGahan JP, Hartling RP. Deep vein thrombosis after fracture of the pelvis. Assessment with serial duplex ultrasound screening. J Bone Joint Surg 72A:495, 1990.

SUGGESTED READINGS

Chapman MW, ed. Operative Orthopaedics. Philadelphia: JB Lippincott, 1988.

A major orthopedic textbook, describing treatment considerations for all orthopedic injuries.

Mears DC, Rubash H. Pelvic and Acetabular Fractures. Thorofare, N.J.: Slack, 1986.

An extensive treatise describing the evaluation and surgical management of pelvic and acetabular fractures.

Schatzker J, Tile M. The Rationale of Operative Fracture Care. New York: Springer-Verlag, 1987.

A detailed description of the technical aspects of operative fracture care.

CHAPTER **38**

Endocrine Disorders

Carol H. Wysham

ADRENAL INSUFFICIENCY

Increased cortisol secretion is necessary for the normal physiologic adaptation to surgery, trauma, burns, and medical illness. If unrecognized, the body's inability to increase cortisol in response to severe stress is associated with a high mortality. Impaired cortisol secretion occurs from adrenal destruction (primary adrenal insufficiency), chronic adrenal suppression from exogenous steroids, and hypothalamic and pituitary disease (secondary adrenal insufficiency).

The clinical manifestations of acute adrenal insufficiency are listed in the accompanying box. Hypotension, often poorly responsive to pressors, is the cardinal feature of adrenal crisis; however, nausea, vomiting, and confusion are common. The typical laboratory findings of hyponatremia, hyperkalemia, and hypoglycemia may be obscured by careful fluid and electrolyte management, or they may be attributed to other medical complications (e.g., renal failure). Hyperpigmentation, common in longstanding primary adrenal insufficiency, is not present in patients with secondary adrenal insufficiency or those with primary adrenal insufficiency of recent onset.

Although primary adrenal insufficiency is uncommon, impaired cortisol reserve as a consequence of chronic glucocorticoid therapy affects an estimated 6 million Americans.[1] Any patient who has undergone more than 1 month of glucocorticoid therapy (>20 mg of prednisone or its equivalent each day) within the previous 12 months should receive stress doses of hydrocortisone when critically ill or undergoing surgery. Hypopituitarism as a cause of hypocortisolemia is less common. The causes of

---

Clinical Manifestations of Acute Adrenal Insufficiency	
Physical signs	*Laboratory abnormalities*
Hypotension and shock*	Hyponatremia*
Fever	Hyperkalemia*
Hyperpigmentation*	Uremia
Vitiligo*	Acidosis
Loss of body hair	Anemia
Abdominal pain	Eosinophilia*
Nausea and vomiting	Hypoglycemia*
Psychiatric disturbance	Hypercalcemia
Other autoimmune disorders*	

*Adrenal insufficiency should be routinely considered in patients with these signs.

397

adrenal insufficiency are listed in the upper box. In an older series, autoimmune adrenalitis accounted for 80% of the cases of primary adrenal insufficiency. However, in the SICU, infectious involvement of the adrenal glands in patients with HIV or hemorrhagic destruction of the adrenal glands is now encountered more frequently.

Adrenal hemorrhage usually occurs as a complication of critical illness and is most frequently reported in postoperative patients with underlying bleeding diathesis, such as anticoagulation, thrombocytopenia, hypoprothrombinemia, or lupus anticoagulant. The most common clinical features of acute adrenal hemorrhage (Table 38-1) are easily overlooked in the critically ill patient. Typically, an episode of abdominal or chest pain occurs, followed within 48 hours by a more than 2 g drop in the hemoglobin concentration. The serum sodium concentration falls, and the potassium concentration rises progressively over the next 5 to 7 days. Finally, if unrecognized, circulatory collapse occurs 5 to 14 days after the initial event. Failure to diagnose and treat hypocortisolemia caused by adrenal hemorrhage before the onset of hypotension is associated with a poor outcome.[2] Adrenal hemorrhage should therefore be included in the differential diagnosis of abdominal or chest pain in the patient in the SICU. If adrenal hemorrhage is suspected, an abdominal CT scan with adrenal cuts can confirm the diagnosis. The scan will show the characteristic changes of hemorrhage involving both adrenal glands.

Once the diagnosis of adrenal insufficiency is suspected, a cosyntropin stimulation test should be performed and treatment initiated promptly. In the critically ill patient, however, a basal cortisol concentration of >20 μg/dl is often sufficient to rule out acute adrenal insufficiency.[3] In this setting, a cortisol concentration <15 μg/dl confirms the diagnosis.[4] A cosyntropin stimulation test (see lower box) is the diagnostic test of choice and can be performed concomitantly with the administration of 4 mg of dexamethasone in the unstable patient. If stimulated cortisol concentrations fail to rise to >20 μg/dl, the diagnosis of adrenal insufficiency is made. The baseline adrenocorticotropic hormone (ACTH) level helps locate the defect: if the ACTH concentration is high, the defect is in the adrenal gland. A low ACTH concentration suggests a pituitary or hypothalamic process. After laboratory tests return, directed radiologic imaging is helpful in determining the cause of hypocortisolemia.

Etiology of Adrenal Insufficiency

Primary cause	Trauma
Autoimmune	Adrenal surgery
Hemorrhage	Drug reaction
HIV	
Tuberculosis	*Secondary cause*
Histoplasmosis	Hypopituitarism
Malignancy	Hypothalamic
Amyloidosis	destruction
Sarcoidosis	Exogenous
Hemochromatosis	glucocorticoid
	withdrawal

Cosyntropin Stimulation Test

- Obtain baseline ACTH and cortisol measurements.
- Administer 0.25 mg cosyntropin IV or IM.
- After 60 minutes, obtain stimulated cortisol measurement.

TABLE 38-1   Clinical Features of Adrenal Hemorrhage

Symptoms	No. of Patients (%)
Abdominal, flank, back, or chest pain	86
Fever	66
Anorexia, nausea, or vomiting	47
Psychiatric symptoms	42
Abdominal rigidity or rebound	22

Treatment of patients with a suspected adrenal crisis should not be delayed until the results of laboratory testing are received. Blood pressure should be stabilized with fluids and vasopressors. After blood has been drawn to determine the cortisol concentration, hydrocortisone, 100 mg IV, should be given immediately and repeated every 8 hours until the patient's condition is stable. Improvement is usually seen within 6 hours of initiation of therapy.[3] Once the patient's condition is stable, the hydrocortisone dosage can be decreased by 50% each day until the daily maintenance dose of 30 mg (20 mg in morning, 10 mg in evening) is reached. Mineralocorticoid therapy, in the form of fludrocortisone, 0.1 to 0.2 mg/day, may be necessary to control hyperkalemia once the daily hydrocortisone dose drops below 75 mg.

THYROID DISORDERS

Although thyroid emergencies are uncommon, thyroid dysfunction affects between 2% to 14% of hospitalized patients.[5] If unrecognized, such emergencies can have profound effects on the clinical course of the critically ill patient. Unfortunately, the diagnosis may be difficult because the symptoms of thyroid diseases are nonspecific and are often masked by the underlying illness. Furthermore, critical illness has significant effects on the results of thyroid tests, thus complicating their interpretation.

Thyroid Function Tests in Nonthyroidal Illness

An isolated low triiodothyronine (T_3) level, caused by the impaired conversion of thyroxine (T_4) to T_3, occurs in over 70% of hospitalized patients. T_3 levels begin to decline within hours of surgery, trauma, acute illness, and fasting. In more severe illness, T_4 levels are low in 30% to 50% of patients, the level of which correlates inversely with the severity of illness.[6] Patients with a T_4 concentration <3 µg/dl have a reported mortality of 50% to 84%.[7,8] Treatment with thyroid hormone has failed to improve survival in these patients. Decreased T_4 concentrations are most commonly explained by the presence of an inhibitor of T_4 binding to its

carrier proteins. Measurements of unoccupied thyroid hormone–binding sites, such as thyroid hormone–binding ratio (THBR) or T_3 resin uptake (T_3RU), are elevated. The estimated free thyroxine index (FTI) is the mathematical product of T_4 and THBR. FTI concentrations usually are normal, making this the most reliable method to determine thyroid status in critical illness. When measured by equilibrium dialysis, free T_4 concentrations are normal, except in the most severely ill patients.[9] Thyroid-stimulating hormone (TSH) concentrations are generally normal in patients with nonthyroidal illness; however, 7% to 10% of hospitalized patients may have TSH measurements outside of the normal limits of the assay.[10]

Drugs have diverse effects on thyroid function tests.[11] Elevated FTI concentrations are occasionally seen in patients receiving propranolol (>320 mg/day) and amiodarone. Anticonvulsant therapy is frequently associated with a 30% to 40% reduction in FTI concentrations through alterations in the cellular metabolism of T_4. Pituitary secretion of TSH is suppressed by dopamine and glucocorticoids. Several drugs affect the binding of T_4 to its binding proteins, affecting T_4 concentrations and THBR, but FTI concentrations are usually normal.

Thyroid function test results should be interpreted with regard to the likelihood of disease and possible interference of drugs and nonthyroidal illness (Table 38-2). In the presence of a normal TSH, an FTI concentration within or just below the normal limits suggests normal thyroid function. Endocrinologic consultation is warranted when the FTI falls below 4 µg/dl or rises above 12 µg/dl.

Hyperthyroidism and Thyroid Storm

The signs and symptoms of hyperthyroidism are the result of increased metabolic rate and energy requirements: tachycardia, atrial dysrhythmias, heat intolerance, and weight loss. Thyroid storm represents a decompensated form of preexisting hyperthyroidism with the cardinal symptoms of fever, severe tachycardia, congestive heart failure, hypotension, and mental status changes. Precipitating causes include

TABLE 38-2 Thyroid Function Tests in Critical Illness

Measurement*	Nonthyroidal Illness	Hypothyroidism	Hyperthyroidism
FTI	↔	↓	↑
TSH	↑,↔,↓	↑ †	↓
T$_3$	↓	↓	↔,↓

*FTI, free thyroxine index; TSH, thyroid-stimulating hormone.
†May be normal in patients receiving dopamine or glucocorticoids or in patients with hypopituitarism.

infection, surgery, trauma, cerebrovascular accident, and iodine administration (radiologic dyes, surgical scrubs, amiodarone). Prompt recognition and treatment of hyperthyroidism in the critically ill patient is essential to prevent decompensation or the development of thyroid storm.[12]

Any of the physical or laboratory findings listed in the upper box on p. 401 should raise suspicion of hyperthyroidism. Atrial fibrillation with a rapid ventricular rate poorly responsive to usual treatment is especially suggestive. With hyperthyroidism, characteristic changes on hemodynamic monitoring are increased heart rate, increased stroke volume, and decreased peripheral vascular resistance.

In the critically ill patient with hyperthyroidism, thyroid function testing (see Table 38-2) reveals an elevated T$_4$ and suppressed TSH concentrations. THBR may not show the characteristic elevation because of the superimposed effects of nonthyroid illness. Similarly, the T$_3$RIA concentration is often normal, reflecting the opposing effects of hyperthyroidism and nonthyroidal illness. A measurement of 24-hour radioiodine uptake may be necessary to confirm the diagnosis of hyperthyroidism; however, any iodine administration within the preceding month will invalidate the results.

When symptoms suggest thyroid storm, treatment should be instituted even if the results of thyroid function testing are not available. The following approach should be used for treatment of hyperthyroidism and thyroid storm:

1. Supportive measures
   a. Hydration
   b. External cooling and/or administration of acetaminophen
   c. Management of congestive heart failure and dysrhythmias
2. Propylthiouracil 300 to 900 mg po, as a loading dose, followed by 100 to 200 mg q 8 hr; a solution for rectal administration can be prepared
3. Propranolol 20 to 80 mg po (or 1 to 2 mg IV q 5 min up to 10 mg) q 6 hr; or esmolol 500 µg/kg loading dose, followed by 50 to 200 µg/kg/min by infusion

In life-threatening situations, these drugs should be administered:

- Iodine (give at least 1 hour after propylthiouracil): sodium iodide 1 g slow IV push; or saturated solution of potassium iodide (SSKI) 5 drops po q 8 hr (inhibits secretion of preformed T$_4$)
- Dexamethasone 2 mg IV q 6 hr (inhibits T$_4$ release and T$_4$-to-T$_3$ conversion)

Patients with less severe manifestations can be presumptively treated with beta-adrenergic receptor blockers while awaiting the results of thyroid function testing and measurement of radioiodine uptake.

HYPOTHYROIDISM AND MYXEDEMA COMA

Hypothyroidism is a common disorder, affecting up to 10% of elderly women.[13] Because of the nonspecific nature of the signs and symptoms (see lower box, p. 401), this disorder is easily overlooked, especially in the face of critical illness. Hypothyroidism is most commonly

Clinical Features of Hyperthyroidism

Physical signs	Laboratory abnormalities
Goiter*	Hyperbilirubinemia
Thyroid bruit*	Abnormal liver function
Proptosis*	Hypercalcemia
Lid retraction	Hyperglycemia
Tremor	Leukopenia
Agitation	
Tachycardia	
Atrial fibrillation*	

*Hyperthyroidism should be routinely considered in patients with these signs.

Clinical Features of Hypothyroidism

Physical signs	Laboratory abnormalities
Goiter*	Anemia
Thyroidectomy scar*	Hypercholesterolemia
Periorbital edema	Hyponatremia*
Nonpitting edema	Coagulopathy
Bradycardia*	Increased creatine
Hypothermia*	phosphokinase
Serous effusions	concentration
Hypoventilation*	Hypercapnia
Delayed reflexes*	Hypoxemia
Decreased mentation	
Psychiatric disturbances	
Ileus	
Macroglossia	

*Hypothyroidism should be routinely considered in patients with these signs.

caused by autoimmune thyroid destruction (Hashimoto's thyroiditis), previous radioiodine treatment, or surgery in patients with Graves' disease. Hypopituitarism accounts for less than 5% of all cases of hypothyroidism. In the SICU, prolonged administration of dopamine may cause hypothyroidism as a result of chronic TSH suppression.[14]

Myxedema coma, characterized by severely depressed mental status, hypothermia, bradycardia, hypoventilation, and hyponatremia, occurs in patients with long-standing untreated hypothyroidism. More than 50% develop depressed mental status after admission to the hospital. Factors that precipitate or exacerbate myxedema coma are cold exposure, trauma, infection, or the administration of CNS depressants.[15]

Management of hypothyroidism is dictated by the clinical situation. In uncomplicated hypothyroidism, levothyroxine (1.2 to 1.6 µg/kg/day) is given orally or intravenously. Lower doses (12.5 to 25 µg/day) are recommended in elderly patients or in patients with significant ischemic heart disease. Because of the high mortality (50% to 84%), patients with suspected myxedema coma should be treated more aggressively. The following approach should be used for the management of patients with myxedema coma:

1. Supportive measures
   a. Ventilatory support
   b. Passive rewarming
   c. Volume expansion
2. Thyroid hormone replacement: 300 to 500 µg levothyroxine IV push, followed by 100 µg/day; *or* 200 µg levothyroxine IV push and 25 µg triiodothyronine po q 12 hr, followed by levothyroxine, 100 µg/day; continue triiodothyronine for 2 to 4 days or until the patient is conscious
3. Anticipate possible adrenal insufficiency
   a. Draw serum cortisol
   b. Hydrocortisone 100 mg IV q 8 hr until adrenal function is confirmed to be normal

DIABETES MELLITUS

Surgery, trauma, and medical illness induce a rapid secretion of growth hormone, cortisol, epinephrine, and glucagon. The net effect of these hormonal changes is to stimulate ketogenesis, gluconeogenesis, and glycogenolysis and to impair glucose uptake.[16] Additionally, insulin secretion is decreased through alpha-adrenergic inhibition of the pancreatic B cell. Uncomplicated abdominal surgery results in a 70% increase in glucose levels in nondiabetic patients.[17] Further increases are seen with the addition of TPN.

Proper management of hyperglycemia in the critically ill patient is essential to prevent severe

Protocols for IV Infusion of Insulin*

Glucose/insulin/potassium	*Variable insulin*
32 U of human regular insulin + 20 mEq potassium chloride in 1000 ml 10% dextrose at 125 ml/hr†	50 U of human regular insulin + 20 mEq potassium chloride in 1000 ml normal saline at 1.5 U/hr†

Check blood glucose concentration by fingerstick test every 2 hours, adjusting infusion as follows:

Blood glucose	*Insulin dose*	*Insulin infusion rate*
<80	Reduce by 8 U/L	Decrease by 0.5 U/hr + 25 ml 10% dextrose
80-119	Reduce by 4 U/L	Decrease by 0.5 U/hr
120-179	Leave unchanged	No change
180-240	Add 4 U/L	Increase by 0.5 U/hr
>240	Add 8 U/L	Increase by 0.5 U/hr + 8 U IV bolus

*From Hirsch IB, McGill JB, Cryer PE, White PF. Perioperative management of surgical patients with diabetes mellitus. Anesthesiology 74:346, 1991.
†Initial infusion rate should be doubled in patients with severe infections and in those receiving steroids or TPN.

catabolism, to promote wound healing, and to normalize leukocyte function. Constant intravenous infusion is the safest method for insulin delivery because continuous infusion allows for adjustment as insulin requirements change during recovery. Intravenous infusion is more effective than subcutaneous administration of insulin at controlling hyperglycemia and is associated with a lower risk of hypoglycemia.[16] In the SICU, the subcutaneous administration of insulin is not recommended since the absorption of this hormone is unpredictable, and individual insulin requirements are difficult to determine. The proper management of ketoacidosis and hyperosmolar coma requires insulin infusion and careful attention to fluid and electrolyte replacement.[18]

Several different protocols for intravenous administration of insulin have been described in the literature. Those listed in the box are the most widely used. The protocol chosen should be standardized throughout the institution to prevent potential errors. Since the half-life of intravenous insulin is 4 to 5 minutes, the administration of intravenous bolus insulin without an insulin infusion is not a sound practice, especially in the patient with insulin-dependent diabetes mellitus. Similarly, intravenous infusions of insulin should not be disrupted for longer than 30 minutes.

The insulin infusion should be continued until the patient's condition is stable and he/she is able to tolerate oral feedings. When the plan is to switch to subcutaneous administration of insulin, at least 50% of the insulin dose should be given as intermediate-acting insulin (NPH or lente) and the remainder as regular insulin, either as an established dose or as a sliding scale. The use of sliding-scale regular insulin without intermediate-acting insulin is not recommended because such administration is often associated with wide fluctuations in glucose concentrations and even diabetic ketoacidosis. The choice of the appropriate subcutaneous regimen depends on the type of nutrition (Table 38-3). The insulin infusion should be continued for at least 1 hour after the subcutaneous dose has been given.

TABLE 38-3 Protocols for Changing From Intravenous to Subcutaneous Administration of Insulin

Source of Nutrition	Usual Insulin Regimen	
	Morning	Evening
Normal meals	2/3 TDD: 2/3 NPH, 1/3 regular	1/3 TDD: 1/2 NPH, 1/2 regular
Continuous enteral feedings	1/3 TDD of NPH q 8 hr	

TDD, total daily dose, usually 50% of hourly insulin infusion rate × 24.

For optimal nutritional support, total parenteral nutrition (TPN) may be needed in critically ill patients with diabetes. However, to prevent marked hyperglycemia, aggressive insulin therapy is mandatory. Optimally, intravenous infusion of insulin should be used to keep the blood sugar under 200 mg/dl. In the patient for whom long-term TPN is indicated, insulin can be added to the TPN solution, keeping the glucose-to-insulin ratio constant. For example, in a patient receiving TPN at a rate of 100 ml/hr and insulin at a rate of 2 U/hr, 20 units of regular insulin is added to each liter of TPN solution. When changing to enteral feedings, the daily insulin dose should be reduced by 50% and given as indicated in Table 38-3.

SUMMARY

Adrenal insufficiency

- Hypotension, poorly responsive to pressors, is the cardinal feature of adrenal crisis.
- Typical findings of hyponatremia, hyperkalemia, and hypoglycemia in the SICU may be masked by fluid administration or attributed to renal failure.
- Consider adrenal hemorrhage in patients with abdominal or chest pain, especially if decrease in hemoglobin concentration occurs and patient has underlying coagulopathy.
- A cosyntropin stimulation test confirms presence of adrenal insufficiency.

Thyroid disorders

- T_3 concentrations decline with surgery, trauma, acute illness, and fasting.
- Low T_4 concentrations are associated with high mortality.
- TSH concentrations are usually normal in patients with nonthyroidal illness.

- Treatment of thyroid storm should begin before laboratory confirmation of diagnosis is complete.
- Elevated T_4 and suppressed TSH concentration are characteristic of hyperthyroidism in critically ill patient.
- Hypothyroidism is easily identified in the SICU. Low T_3, low T_4, high reverse T_3, and elevated TSH concentrations are characteristic.

Diabetes mellitus

- Preferred treatment of hyperglycemia in the SICU is continuous intravenous infusion of insulin.
- Subcutaneously administered insulin may be unpredictably absorbed in the SICU patient.
- When patient's condition is stable and oral feedings can be tolerated, consider use of sliding scale.
- Sliding scale regular insulin always should be given as a supplement to intermediate-acting insulin.

REFERENCES

1. Rusnak RA. Adrenal and pituitary emergencies. Emerg Med Clin North Am 7:903, 1989.
2. Knowlton AI. Adrenal insufficiency in the intensive care setting. J Intensive Care Med 4:35, 1989.
3. Chin R. Adrenal crisis. Crit Care Clin 7:23, 1991.
4. Bagdade JD. Endocrine emergencies. Med Clin North Am 70:1111, 1986.
5. Simmons RJ, Simon JM, Demers LM, et al. Thyroid dysfunction in elderly hospitalized patients. Arch Intern Med 150:1249, 1990.
6. Cavalieri RR. The effects of nonthyroid disease and drugs on thyroid function tests. Med Clin North Am 75:27, 1991.
7. Slag MF, Morley JE, Elson MK, et al. Hypothyroxinemia in critically ill patients as a predictor of high mortality. JAMA 245:43, 1981.
8. Silberman H, Eisenberg D, Ryan J, et al. The relation of thyroid indices in the critically ill patient to prognosis and nutritional factors. Surg Gynecol Obstet 166:223, 1988.
9. Zaloga GP, Smallridge RC. Thyroidal alterations in acute illness. Semin Respir Med 7:95, 1985.
10. Spencer CA, Nicoloff JT. Serum TSH measurement: A 1990 status report. Thyroid Today 13:1, 1990.
11. Kaplan MN. Interactions between drugs and thyroid hormones. Thyroid Today 4:1, 1981.
12. Reasner CA, Isley WL. Thyrotoxicosis in the critically ill. Crit Care Clin 7:57, 1991.
13. Levy EG. Thyroid disease in the elderly. Med Clin North Am 75:151, 1991.
14. Kaptein EM, Kletzky OA, Spencer CA, et al. Effects of prolonged dopamine infusion on anterior pituitary function in normal males. J Clin Endocrinol Metab 51:488, 1980.
15. Myers L, Hays J. Myxedema coma. Crit Care Clin 7:43, 1991.
16. Hirsch IB, McGill JB, Cryer PE, White PF. Perioperative management of surgical patients with diabetes mellitus. Anesthesiology 74:346, 1991.
17. Brandi LS, Frediani M, Oleggini M, et al. Insulin resistance after surgery: Normalization by insulin treatment. Clin Sci 79:443, 1990.
18. Foster DW, McCarry JD. The metabolic derangements and treatment of diabetic ketoacidosis. N Engl J Med 309:159, 1983.

SUGGESTED READINGS

Alberti KG, Thomas DJ. The management of diabetes mellitus during surgery. Br J Anaesth 51:693, 1979.

Brunette DD, Rothong C. Emergency department management of thyrotoxic crisis with esmolol. Am J Emerg Med 9:232, 1991.

Davidson JK, Galloway JA, Chance RE. Insulin therapy. In Davidson JK, ed. Clinical Diabetes Mellitus. A Problem-Oriented Approach, 2nd ed. New York: Thieme Medical, 1991, p 266.

McMahon M, Manji N, Driscoll DF, et al. Parenteral nutrition in patients with diabetes mellitus: Theoretical and practical considerations. J Parenter Enteral Nutr 13:545, 1989.

Walter RM, Bartle WR. Rectal administration of propylthiouracil in the treatment of Graves' disease. Am J Med 88:69, 1990.

Watts NB, Gebhart SS, Clark RV, et al. Postoperative management of diabetes mellitus: Steady-state glucose control with bedside algorithm for insulin adjustment. Diabetes Care 10:722, 1987.

CHAPTER 39

Divalent Ions

John E. Mazuski

Disorders of divalent ions—calcium, magnesium, and phosphate—are frequently seen in the SICU. Although divalent ion abnormalities are usually asymptomatic, they have the potential to impair cardiovascular and neuromuscular function. Because of the potential consequences to the patient, a high index of suspicion for these disorders should be maintained. Thus routine monitoring of serum calcium, magnesium, and phosphorus levels is probably warranted for most critically ill patients.

CALCIUM

Calcium is the most abundant electrolyte in the body, with a total content of approximately 1300 g in the average-sized person. However, over 99% of the body's calcium is deposited in the skeleton, and, with the exception of a small pool of calcium that can be readily mobilized, this skeletal calcium does not enter into routine homeostasis.[1]

The normal total serum calcium concentration is 8.5 to 10.5 mg/dl. However, only 0.03% of the body's calcium is present in the plasma. Approximately 50% of this calcium is present as the free ionized form; approximately 40% of the calcium is bound to prcteins, primarily albumin; and approximately 10% of the plasma calcium is complexed with other ions, including bicarbonate, citrate, phosphate, carbonate, and lactate. Only the free ionized form actively participates in physiologic reactions involving calcium.[2]

A number of factors can affect the relationship between the ionized calcium level and the total serum calcium concentration. A reduction in the serum albumin concentration usually decreases the total serum calcium without affecting the ionized calcium concentration. Changes in plasma pH can alter the binding of calcium to protein. Acidosis decreases the binding of calcium to albumin, whereas alkalosis promotes increased binding of calcium to the protein. The ionized calcium concentration also may be depressed by increased concentrations of chelating ions, such as phosphate or citrate. This latter ion is especially important in patients who have received massive blood transfusions.[2]

A number of algorithms have been developed to estimate the serum ionized calcium concentration from the total serum concentration and the total protein or albumin concentration. These algorithms, do not appear to adequately estimate the ionized calcium concentration in critically ill patients.[3,4] Therefore, in most cases, the serum ionized calcium concentration should be directly measured rather than relying on one of these estimates.[2]

Calcium homeostasis is normally regulated tightly by the actions of parathyroid hormone (PTH) and calcitriol (1,25-dihydroxy vitamin D). Gastrointestinal absorption of calcium is promoted by calcitriol, and both PTH and calcitriol interact with the skeleton to maintain normal extracellular calcium concentrations. PTH acts on the kidney both to increase calcium reabsorption and to stimulate hydroxylation of 25-hydroxy vitamin D, an action that produces the hormonally active compound, calcitriol.[1,2,5,6] Thus disorders of both the parathyroid glands and of vitamin D metabolism may profoundly affect serum calcium concentrations.

Hypocalcemia

In the SICU, hypocalcemia is most often seen in patients with acute disease processes, such as trauma, pancreatitis, sepsis, and burns. Decreases in total and ionized calcium occur frequently after massive blood transfusion,[7,8] especially in patients who have had a significant period of hypovolemic shock. These changes may be partially due to the complexing of calcium with unmetabolized citrate, but the shock process itself also promotes the uptake of ionized calcium into the intracellular compartment. In most of these patients, ionized calcium concentrations return to normal within 48 hours, although total serum calcium concentrations may remain low because of hypoalbuminemia.

The association of hypocalcemia with pancreatitis is well known. Defects in the hormonal regulation of calcium concentrations and intracellular uptake of calcium probably account for the hypocalcemia, even though in the past hypocalcemia was attributed to the deposition of calcium in areas of fat necrosis. Similar defects also contribute to the decreases in total and ionized calcium concentrations observed with sepsis and burns.[2,5]

Hypocalcemia occurs in the presence of metabolic disorders such as hypomagnesemia and hyperphosphatemia. In addition, hypermagnesemia, through its impact on PTH secretion, may also produce hypocalcemia. Hypocalcemia is relatively common in patients with chronic renal failure and is related to decreased hydroxylation of 25-hydroxy vitamin D and to concomitant hyperphosphatemia and hypermagnesemia. Hypoparathyroidism as a cause of hypocalcemia is rare in the SICU, except for the reactive hypocalcemia seen after surgery for hyperparathyroidism. Chronic diseases associated with vitamin D deficiency, such as alcoholism and malnutrition, also may produce hypocalcemia.[2,5]

Symptoms and signs of acute hypocalcemia are most often seen in the neuromuscular and cardiovascular systems. Neuromuscular manifestations include tetany, muscle spasms, weakness, and paresthesias, as well as nonspecific mental status changes. Chvostek's sign and Trousseau's sign may be elicited, but these responses are not necessarily reliable, particularly in the SICU. Cardiovascular manifestations include ECG changes, such as prolongation of the QT and ST intervals, nonspecific T-wave changes, bradycardia, and ventricular dysrhythmias. Severe hypocalcemia may lead to hypotension, cardiac insufficiency unresponsive to catecholamines and digoxin, and eventually circulatory collapse.[2,5,6]

If clinical findings of hypocalcemia are present or if the clinical setting is appropriate, total and ionized serum calcium concentrations should be obtained (Fig. 39-1). If hypocalcemia is diagnosed, serum phosphorus and magnesium concentrations also should be checked since concomitant disorders of these ions are common. If no obvious cause for the hypocalcemia can be found, an endocrinologic evaluation should be initiated and may include determinations of PTH and vitamin D concentrations.

Patients with symptomatic or severe hypocalcemia should be treated urgently. In the critical care setting, intravenous calcium is the preferred treatment, with the administration of 100 to 200 mg of elemental calcium given as 10 to 20 ml of 10% calcium gluconate or 4 to 8 ml of 10% calcium chloride. Maintenance therapy will be needed for patients with severe hypocalcemia. This can be given as an intravenous infusion of 1 to 2 mg/kg/hr of elemental calcium.[2,6] Patients receiving total parenteral nutrition (TPN) should receive maintenance dosages of calcium: generally, 250 to 450 mg (6 to 11 mmol) of elemental calcium per day.[9]

Along with calcium administration, adjunctive treatment of acute hypocalcemia includes discontinuation of drugs that contribute to calcium loss, such as furosemide. Hypomagnesemia should also be treated, since the hypocalcemia will otherwise be relatively refractory to therapy. In patients with hyperphosphatemia, intravenous calcium should be given with great caution, since metastatic calcification may be provoked when the product of the serum cal-

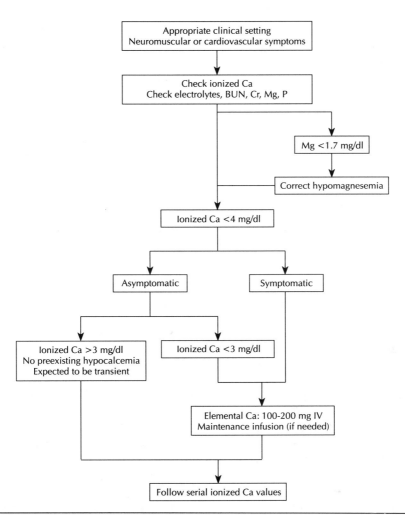

FIG. 39-1 Treatment approach to hypocalcemia.

cium and phosphorus concentrations is >75. Calcium also should be given with caution to patients receiving digoxin since dysrhythmias may be precipitated by intravenous calcium.[2,6]

Asymptomatic hypocalcemia produced by a massive blood transfusion does not necessarily require treatment. In the absence of ongoing hypovolemic shock, the ionized calcium concentrations usually return to normal within 48 hours. Under these circumstances, even very low ionized calcium concentrations do not appear to impair cardiac performance.[7,8] Thus it is probably safe to observe the patient who has an ionized calcium concentration ≥3 mg/dl.[6] Also, patients with reactive hypocalcemia after parathyroid surgery usually do not require cal-

cium supplementation unless all parathyroid tissue has been removed. Ordinarily, these patients can be monitored without treatment until the calcium concentration reaches its nadir and stabilizes. In patients with permanent hypoparathyroidism or another cause of chronic hypocalcemia, therapy with oral calcium salts, with or without vitamin D supplementation, may be needed.

Hypercalcemia

Although not as common as hypocalcemia, hypercalcemia is occasionally seen in the SICU. Most often it is associated with malignancy or immobilization, or it is produced iatrogenically by the administration of calcium salts or drugs such as thiazides that promote hypercalcemia. Hypovolemia also contributes to hypercalcemia. Hyperparathyroidism rarely warrants placing the patient in the SICU unless it is associated with severe symptomatic hypercalcemia. Other causes of hypercalcemia include familial hypercalcemia, granulomatous diseases such as sarcoidosis, and endocrine disorders such as hyperthyroidism, pheochromocytoma, and acromegaly. Patients with renal failure occasionally develop hypercalcemia, although hypocalcemia is more typically seen.[2,5]

The clinical manifestations of hypercalcemia are protean. Acute hypercalcemia is more likely to be symptomatic than is chronic hypercalcemia. With acute hypercalcemia, cardiovascular and neuromuscular symptoms predominate. The QT interval is shortened, but this may not be a reliable sign of hypercalcemia. Dysrhythmias and increased sensitivity to digitalis preparations may be seen. In addition, calcium exerts an inotropic effect on the heart and may lead to vascular smooth muscle contraction, giving rise to an increased systemic vascular resistance and hypertension. Neuromuscular symptoms include weakness and hyporeflexia. CNS problems, such as personality changes, depression, and disorientation, progressing into obtundation and frank coma, are frequently observed. Chronic hypercalcemia may produce only vague complaints such as anorexia, constipation, nausea and vomiting, or skeletal pain. In patients with long-standing hypercalcemia, nephrolithiasis and nephrocalcinosis may occur along with renal osteodystrophy.[2,5]

Diagnosis of hypercalcemia is determined by the serum calcium concentration (Fig. 39-2). Generally, an elevated total serum calcium concentration indicates an elevated ionized calcium concentration. In patients with depressed serum protein concentrations, an elevated ionized calcium concentration may be present in the face of a normal total serum calcium concentration. In these patients, then, an ionized calcium concentration should be obtained. Magnesium and phosphorus concentrations also should be checked since the incidence of concomitant disorders is relatively high. If the cause of the hypercalcemia is not immediately obvious, a diagnostic evaluation, including a PTH determination, should be initiated.

Acute symptomatic hypercalcemia should be treated as a medical emergency. General measures include restoration of any volume deficits present, stopping the administration of calcium or medications contributing to hypercalcemia, and treating the underlying disorder if at all possible. The mainstay of therapy for acute symptomatic hypercalcemia is forced diuresis, using 1 to 2 L of saline administered over a few hours, supplemented by furosemide as needed to promote diuresis. Serum potassium and magnesium concentrations must be monitored along with calcium concentrations during this intervention. In patients with significant renal dysfunction, dialysis may be the only method with which to acutely lower serum calcium concentrations.[2,5]

A number of other agents that treat hypercalcemia by inhibiting bone reabsorption are available for use. These agents include mithramycin, salmon calcitonin, glucocorticoids, and diphosphonates. Generally, these agents require several hours to days to have an effect, but their use may be initiated, if needed, in conjunction with forced diuresis. Infrequently, calcium chelators such as EDTA and phosphates have been used for acute hypercalcemia, but they are not generally recommended. Calcium channel blockers such as verapamil may be of value for the treatment of life-threatening cardiovascular manifestations of hypercalcemia.[2,5]

MAGNESIUM

Magnesium is distributed throughout the body, but approximately two thirds of the body's magnesium is present in the skeleton. One third of this magnesium is potentially available for exchange with the extracellular fluid. Most of the remaining magnesium is found intracellularly, where it represents the second most common intracellular cation after potassium. Again, only a portion of this intracellular magnesium is actually available for exchange with the extracellular fluid since much of the intracellular magnesium is complexed with proteins or phosphates. Approximately 1.3% of the body's magnesium is found in the extracellular fluid.[2,10]

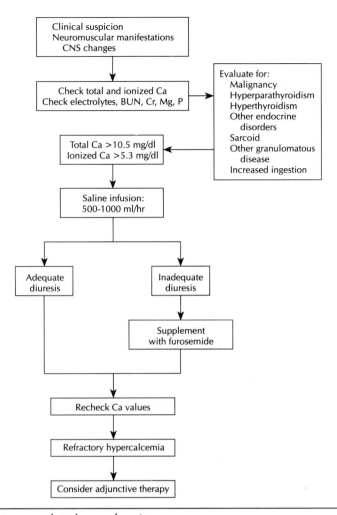

FIG. 39-2   Treatment approach to hypercalcemia.

In the plasma, free magnesium makes up approximately 50% of the total magnesium concentration, with the remainder being complexed with proteins and smaller organic and inorganic ions.[10] The normal total serum magnesium concentration is 1.7 to 2.4 mg/dl. No technique for measuring ionized magnesium concentrations is readily available at present. Therefore it must be assumed that the total serum magnesium concentration represents the physiologically active ionized plasma magnesium.[2] Of greater importance is the fact that serum concentrations of magnesium may not reflect total body magnesium content since so much of the ion is present intracellularly. A normal serum magnesium concentration may mask a significant magnesium deficiency or excess.

Plasma magnesium concentrations are regulated by some of the same factors, including PTH and vitamin D, that regulate calcium concentrations. In general, magnesium concentrations are not as tightly regulated as are calcium concentrations. Magnesium is absorbed from the intestine by both vitamin D–dependent and vitamin D–independent transport systems.[11] In addition, the amount of magnesium in the diet and the overall body stores of magnesium regulate the amount absorbed from the intestine.[12] Plasma magnesium concentrations are primarily regulated by the kidney. Although both PTH and calcitriol promote tubular reabsorption of magnesium, the majority of magnesium reabsorption depends on intrinsic renal mechanisms, which are in turn regulated by the serum magnesium concentration. The glomerular filtration rate also affects renal magnesium excretion and may account in part for the hypermagnesemia seen with renal failure.[11]

Hypomagnesemia

Hypomagnesemia is a relatively common disorder and has been found in 9% to 12% of hospitalized patients. The incidence of this disorder in the SICU may be substantially higher.[2,13] Hypomagnesemia is usually due to inadequate uptake of magnesium from the gastrointestinal tract or increased losses of the ion from the kidneys or intestines. Malabsorption caused by bowel or pancreatic disease; gastrointestinal losses from fistulas, diarrhea, or prolonged nasogastric suction; and reduced intake from prolonged bowel rest without magnesium replacement may all lead to a magnesium deficiency. Increased renal losses are common with the use of diuretics and other drugs such as aminoglycosides and amphotericin B. Hypomagnesemia is also seen in alcoholics, in whom both gastrointestinal and renal causes may play a role in the development of the deficiency. Nutritional repletion causes magnesium to shift intracellularly; thus an occult magnesium deficiency may become manifest in many patients when such repletion is undertaken.[2,10,13,14]

The primary manifestations of magnesium deficiency are in the neuromuscular and cardiovascular systems. Hyperreflexia, tetany, and muscle spasms may be seen. Neurologic disturbances, such as disorientation, obtundation, and seizures also occur. Of greater importance, however, are the cardiovascular manifestations. The ECG changes mimic those of hypokalemia and include QT prolongation, ST segment abnormalities, broadening of T waves, and occasionally the development of U waves. Myocardial irritability is increased, and frequent premature ventricular contractions are commonly seen. More severe dysrhythmias such as ventricular tachycardia and ventricular fibrillation may occur; these latter dysrhythmias may be unresponsive to conventional antiarrhythmic therapy. Hypomagnesemia is also associated with other electrolyte abnormalities, such as hypocalcemia and hypokalemia, and with an anemia of unexplained origin.[2,13]

Diagnosis is based on the serum magnesium level. However, magnesium deficiency is still possible even with a normal serum magnesium concentration, since the serum concentration may not accurately reflect intracellular stores. Serum calcium and phosphorus concentrations and standard electrolyte and renal function tests should also be checked once the diagnosis of hypomagnesemia has been entertained (Fig. 39-3).

Asymptomatic mild hypomagnesemia may be treated with parenteral administration of 1 g (8 mEq) of magnesium sulfate every 4 to 6 hours or with oral supplements such as magnesium oxide, if the patient can tolerate them. Since magnesium equilibrates relatively slowly with the intracellular compartment, therapy may have to be continued for several days to adequately replace a significant deficiency.[2] For maintenance purposes, patients receiving only parenteral fluids should receive 8 to 10 mEq of magnesium daily,[9] and supplemental amounts should be given to patients with significant gastrointestinal or renal losses of the ion.[2] Dysrhythmias and other manifestations of symptomatic magnesium deficiency may require more aggressive parenteral magnesium therapy. For severe hypomagnesemia, up to 6 g of magnesium sulfate or 5 g of magnesium chloride can be given intravenously over a 3-hour period.[2] For acute life-threatening dysrhythmias, 2 to 4 g of magnesium sulfate can be given over a 15-minute period.[13] In patients with normal serum magnesium concentrations, prophylactic treatment of dysrhythmias with 1 g of magnesium sulfate every 6 hours has been used. This therapy has been recommended specifically for dysrhythmias associated with digitalis toxicity, those related to long QT intervals, and in patients with acute myocardial infarction.[15,16]

Hypermagnesemia

Hypermagnesemia produces significant clinical problems much less commonly than does hy-

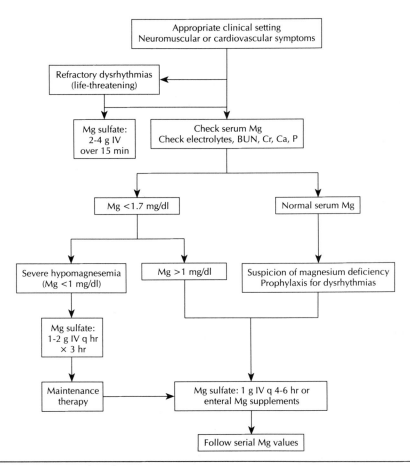

FIG. 39-3 Treatment approach to hypomagnesemia.

pomagnesemia. Most often, hypermagnesemia is caused by renal failure, and occasionally it is the result of iatrogenic administration. For instance, elevated serum magnesium concentrations are expected as part of the treatment of preeclampsia and eclampsia.

Symptoms of hypermagnesemia are not usually seen until serum magnesium concentrations approach 5 mg/dl. Above that point, muscle weakness becomes evident; with concentrations of 13 mg/dl, frank paralysis may be seen. CNS changes, including somnolence, are associated with magnesium concentrations of 9 mg/dl. ECG changes, such as prolonged PR, QRS, and ST intervals, may be seen at serum concentrations of 5 to 8 mg/dl, and bradycardia and hypotension become apparent as the serum magnesium concentration increases fur-

ther. Heart block and cardiac arrest may occur when serum magnesium concentrations approach 20 mg/dl. Because of its effect on PTH release, hypermagnesemia may produce hypocalcemia. Nonspecific gastrointestinal symptoms (e.g., nausea, vomiting) also are associated with elevated magnesium concentrations.

For asymptomatic patients, treatment consists of restriction of magnesium-containing solutions and medications. For symptomatic patients, 100 to 200 mg of elemental calcium may be given to transiently block some of the effects of hypermagnesemia. Forced diuresis helps remove excessive magnesium in patients with functioning kidneys. However, for patients with renal failure, hemodialysis may be the only method with which to treat acute hypermagnesemia.

PHOSPHORUS

Phosphorus is present in the body primarily as organic and inorganic phosphate. At physiologic pH, inorganic phosphate consists of a 4:1 mixture of the dibasic (HPO_4^{-2}) and monobasic ($H_2PO_4^-$) forms of the ion. Approximately 80% of the body's phosphate is found in the skeleton, and most of the remaining phosphate is present intracellularly, where it represents the most common intracellular anion. A small fraction of the body's phosphate is present in the extracellular compartment. In the plasma, 85% of the inorganic phosphate is present as the free ion; 5% is complexed with other cations, primarily magnesium and calcium; and 10% is bound to protein.[17] The serum phosphorus concentration is used to measure the concentration of inorganic phosphate in the plasma (normal range, 2.7 to 4.5 mg/dl or 0.8 to 1.5 mmol/L).[2]

The serum phosphorus concentration is regulated by both the absorption of phosphate from the intestines and by the excretion of phosphate by the kidneys. Although intestinal absorption of phosphate is enhanced by vitamin D, adequate amounts of phosphate can usually be absorbed even in the presence of vitamin D deficiency. The kidneys play the primary role in the regulation of plasma phosphate. PTH sets the tubular maximum for phosphate reabsorption, but intrinsic renal mechanisms also play a role in phosphate regulation. Serum phosphorus concentrations also are altered by intracellular shifting of the ion, which can be induced directly by insulin or produced indirectly by carbohydrate loading.[2,17]

Hypophosphatemia

Hypophosphatemia is another common disorder in the SICU, but many times it does not represent a true phosphorus deficiency. Hypophosphatemia is frequently seen in the postoperative patient. In one study the disorder was observed in 29% of these patients.[18] Hypophosphatemia occurs as part of the treatment or recovery from a number of conditions, including burns, sepsis, malnutrition, ketoacidosis, and hypothermia. With many of these conditions, hypophosphatemia reflects a transcellular shift of phosphates rather than a true phosphate deficiency. Hypophosphatemia is also common among alcoholics, occurring both with acute alcohol intoxication[19] and chronic alcoholism.[20] Other causes of hypophosphatemia include hyperparathyroidism, hypomagnesemia, and the administration of certain drugs that bind phosphates, such as antacids and sucralfate.[2,21]

Hypophosphatemia rarely causes symptoms unless the serum phosphorus concentration is <2 mg/dl. Below this concentration, weakness, malaise, and anorexia may be observed. As the concentration approaches 1 mg/dl, muscle weakness becomes more pronounced and clinical impairment in respiratory and cardiac function may be exhibited. With severe hypophosphatemia (<1 mg/dl), actual muscle cell injury and rhabdomyolysis may occur. Blood components are also affected by severe hypophosphatemia, which may result in platelet dysfunction, leukocyte dysfunction, and hemolysis. Because of the importance of phosphates in intermediary metabolism, hypophosphatemia also produces a host of metabolic abnormalities. The most common manifestations of this are insulin resistance and impaired glucose tolerance. Hypercalcemia and hypermagnesemia are both cause and consequence of hypophosphatemia.[2,21]

Therapy of hypophosphatemia is based on the degree of the disorder (Fig. 39-4). With severe hypophosphatemia, intravenous phosphate preparations are the treatment of choice. Consensus has not yet been reached as to how much phosphate should be replaced initially. Zaloga and Chernow[2] recommend an infusion of intravenous sodium or potassium phosphate at a rate of 0.6 mg (0.02 mmol)/kg/hr for relatively acute hypophosphatemia and an infusion of 0.9 mg (0.03 mmol)/kg/hr in cases of chronic phosphorus depletion. Others have used infusions of as much as 0.25 to 0.5 mmol/kg of phosphate given over a 4-hour period.[22] In addition to phosphate replacement, agents contributing to hypophosphatemia, such as antacids and diuretics, should be stopped, and, if possible, glucose and insulin infusions should be curtailed. Serum phosphorus concentrations

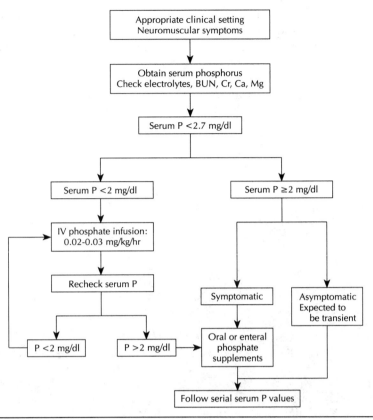

FIG. 39-4 Treatment approach to hypophosphatemia.

should be monitored frequently during phosphate replacement. Once a serum phosphorus concentration of 2 mg/dl or greater has been achieved, phosphorus supplementation should be continued by the enteral route if possible. In cases of severe phosphorus deficiency, phosphate supplements should be continued for several days to adequately replete intracellular stores.[2] In patients receiving TPN, approximately 30 mmol of phosphorus should be supplied per day for maintenance and more if needed for repletion.[2,9]

Hyperphosphatemia

Renal failure is the most common cause of hyperphosphatemia, but it is occasionally observed with overvigorous administration of phosphate supplements, particularly to patients with borderline renal insufficiency. Hyperphosphatemia is also seen with disorders in which cell destruction occurs, such as rhabdomyolysis, hemolysis, malignant hyperthermia, and severe hypothermia, as well as with metabolic problems such as lactic acidosis. Rare causes of hyperphosphatemia include hypoparathyroidism, pseudohypoparathyroidism, and vitamin D excess.[2,21]

Hyperphosphatemia usually produces relatively few symptoms. When symptoms do occur, they are a result of metastatic calcifications, which may occur when the calcium-phosphorus product exceeds 75. Other acute symptoms are related to concomitant hypocalcemia. The latter symptoms represent the strongest indication for therapy.[2,21]

Chronic treatment of hyperphosphatemia consists of controlling the absorption of phosphates from the gastrointestinal tract, usually by dietary phosphate restriction, and the use of oral phosphate binders. With acute hyperphosphatemia, treatment of the associated hypocalcemia is the first priority. However, the high phosphorus concentrations may make it difficult to provide adequate calcium supplementation. Under these circumstances, phosphate excretion can be promoted by saline diuresis and by acetazolamide in patients with normally functioning kidneys. In patients with renal failure, hemodialysis may be needed to assist in phosphate removal. The effect of dialysis is usually transient, however, since serum phosphorus concentrations typically rebound within a few hours, a consequence of phosphate release from intracellular stores.[2,21]

SUMMARY

- Divalent ion abnormalities can cause cardiovascular and neuromuscular dysfunction.
- Routinely measure calcium, magnesium, and phosphorus serum concentrations.

Hypocalcemia

- Neuromuscular irritability, tetany, muscle spasms, paresthesias, Chvostek's signs, and Trouseau's sign suggest hypocalcemia.
- ECG changes include prolonged QT and ST intervals, T-wave changes, and ventricular dysrhythmias.
- Symptomatic hypocalcemia requires urgent treatment with intravenous calcium.
- Hypomagnesemia should be treated concomitantly.
- Asymptomatic, transient hypocalcemia may not require treatment.

Hypercalcemia

- Malignancy and immobilization are common causes of hypercalcemia.
- Weakness, hyporeflexia, and a shortened QT interval suggest hypercalcemia.
- Acute symptomatic hypercalcemia is a medical emergency treated by forced diuresis.

Hypomagnesemia

- Hypomagnesemia is common in the SICU. Many factors promote urinary and gastrointestinal losses of magnesium.

- Ventricular dysrhythmias are common and may include ventricular tachycardia and ventricular fibrillation.
- Magnesium deficiency may exist despite a normal serum magnesium concentration.
- Hypomagnesemia always should be treated.
- Many cardiac dysrhythmias respond to magnesium treatment.

Hypermagnesemia

- Renal failure is most common cause.
- Very high magnesium concentrations may produce muscle weakness and ECG changes.
- Magnesium restriction and dialysis are the mainstays of therapy.

Hypophosphatemia

- Phosphorus concentrations ≥2 mg/dl rarely produce symptoms.
- Severe hypophosphatemia (<1 mg/dl) may result in rhabdomyolysis and respiratory or cardiac insufficiency.
- Use intravenous phosphorus replacement for severe hypophosphatemia; enteral phosphorus replacement may be used once serum phosphorus concentration is ≥2 mg/dl.

Hyperphosphatemia

- Renal failure is most common cause.
- Restriction of phosphate intake and oral phosphate binders is usual therapy.
- Associated hypocalcemia may require treatment.

REFERENCES

1. Marx SJ, Bourdeau JE. Calcium metabolism. In Maxwell MH, Kleeman ER, Narin RG. Clinical Disorders of Fluid and Electrolyte Metabolism, 4th ed. New York: McGraw-Hill, 1987, pp 207-244.

2. Zaloga GP, Chernow B. Divalent ions: Calcium, magnesium, and phosphorus. In Chernow B, Holaday JW, Zaloga GP, et al. The Pharmacologic Approach to the Critically Ill Patient. Baltimore: Williams & Wilkins, 1988, pp 603-636.

3. Ladenson JH, Lewis JW, Boyd JC. Failure of total calcium corrected per protein, albumin, and pH to correctly assess free calcium status. J Clin Endocrinol Metab 46:986-993, 1978.

4. Zaloga GP, Chernow B, Snyder R, Clapper M, O'Brian JC. Assessment of calcium homeostasis in the critically ill surgical patient. The diagnostic pitfalls of the McLean-Hastings nomogram. Ann Surg 202:587-594, 1985.

5. Zenabe JE, Martinez-Maldonado M. Disorders of calcium metabolism. In Maxwell MH, Kleeman ER, Narins RG, eds. Clinical Disorders of Fluid and Electrolyte Metabolism, 4th ed. New York: McGraw-Hill, 1987, pp 759-788.

6. Zaloga GP, Chernow D. Hypocalcemia in critical illness. JAMA 256:1924-1929, 1986.

7. Howland WS, Schweizer O, Carlon GC, Goldiner PL. The cardiovascular effect of low levels of ionized calcium during massive transfusion. Surg Gynecol Obstet 145:581-586, 1977.

8. Harrigan C, Lucas CE, Ledgerwood AM. Significance of hypocalcemia following hypovolemic shock. J Trauma 23:488-493, 1983.

9. Inadomi BW, Kopple JD. Fluid and electrolyte disorders in total parenteral nutrition. In Maxwell MH, Kleeman ER, Narins RG, eds. Clinical Disorders of Fluid and Electrolyte Metabolism, 4th ed. New York: McGraw-Hill, 1987, pp 945-966.

10. Quanme GA, Dirks JH. Magnesium metabolism. In Maxwell MH, Kleeman ER, Narins RG, eds. Clinical Disorders of Fluid and Electrolyte Metabolism, 4th ed. New York: McGraw-Hill, 1987, pp 297-316.

11. Lee C, Zaloga GP. Magnesium metabolism. Semin Respir Med 7:70-80, 1985.

12. Gums JG. Clinical significance of magnesium: A review. Drug Intell Clin Pharm 21:240-246, 1987.

13. Brautbar N, Massry SG. Disorders of magnesium metabolism. In Maxwell MH, Kleeman ER, Narins RG, eds. Clinical Disorders of Fluid and Electrolyte metabolism, 4th ed. New York: McGraw-Hill, 1987, pp 831-849.

14. Rude RK, Singer FR. Magnesium deficiency and excess. Ann Rev Med 32:245-259, 1981.

15. Roden DM. Magnesium treatment of ventricular arrhythmias. Am J Cardiol 53:43G-46G, 1989.

16. Sheehan J. Importance of magnesium chloride repletion after myocardial infarction. Am J Cardiol 63:35G-38G, 1989.

17. Lee DVN, Kurokawa K. Physiology of phosphorus metabolism. In Maxwell MH, Kleeman ER, Narins RG, eds. Clinical Disorders of Fluid and Electrolyte metabolism, 4th ed. New York: McGraw-Hill, 1987, pp 245-295.

18. Swaminathan R, Bradley P, Morgan DB, Hill GL. Hypophosphatemia in surgical patients. Surg Gynecol Obstet 148:448-454, 1979.

19. Stein JH, Smith WO, Ginn HE. Hypophosphatemia in acute alcoholism. Am J Med Sci 252:78-83, 1966.

20. Territo MC, Tanaka KR. Hypophosphatemia in chronic alcoholism. Arch Intern Med 134:445-447, 1974.

21. Brautbar N, Kleeman CR. Hypophosphatemia and hyperphosphatemia: Clinical and pathophysiologic aspects. In Maxwell MH, Kleeman ER, Narins RG, eds. Clinical Disorders of Fluid and Electrolyte Metabolism, 4th ed. New York: McGraw-Hill, 1987, pp 789-830.

22. Kingston M, Al-Siba'r MB. Treatment of severe hypophosphatemia. Crit Care Med 13:16-18, 1985.

PART FOUR

SYSTEMIC DYSFUNCTION

CHAPTER 40

Intra-abdominal Infection

Ori D. Rotstein • Richard L. Simmons

The principles of management of the patient initially seen with an intra-abdominal infection include providing (1) resuscitation, (2) nutritional and metabolic support, (3) broad-spectrum antibiotic therapy directed against a polymicrobial bacterial flora, and (4) surgical or radiologic intervention to treat the underlying pathology. This chapter reviews the host response to infection in the peritoneal cavity and describes an approach to the management of both bacterial peritonitis and intra-abdominal abscesses.

ANATOMY AND PHYSIOLOGY OF ABDOMINAL CAVITY

The peritoneum is a smooth, translucent membrane lining the abdominal cavity. Its surface consists of a single layer of flat mesothelial cells that reside on a basement membrane, which in turn overlies a bed of connective tissue. The overall surface area of the peritoneum approximates that of the total cutaneous surface area (approximately 1.7 m^2). The peritoneal cavity is normally sterile and contains <50 ml of fluid. The fluid has a specific gravity <1.016 and a protein concentration <3 g/dl. It contains fewer than 3000 cells/mm^3, predominantly macrophages and lymphocytes. The peritoneal membrane permits bidirectional diffusion of water and most solutes. In addition, particulate matter can be cleared through stomata between specialized peritoneal mesothelial cells that overlie lymphatic channels on the diaphragmatic surface of the peritoneal cavity. These intercellular stomata correspond with fenestrations in the basement membrane, and together they serve as channels from the peritoneal cavity to underlying specialized diaphragmatic lymphatics, called lacunae.[1] In concert with the one-way valves in the thoracic lymphatics, this unit serves as an important clearance mechanism of bacteria from the peritoneal cavity. Bacteria pass easily through the large stomata and can be recovered from the thoracic lymph duct within 6 minutes and from the blood within 12 minutes of intraperitoneal inoculation.[2] This mechanism is facilitated by an intraperitoneal flow of fluid and particles toward the diaphragm, an effect presumably produced by suction caused by the pull of gravity on the upper abdominal viscera away from the diaphragmatic surface.

DEFENSE AGAINST PERITONEAL INFECTION
Local Response

Three local defense mechanisms contribute to the ultimate clearance of bacteria from the peritoneal cavity.[3] They are (1) mechanical clearance of bacteria through the diaphragmatic lymphatics; (2) phagocytosis and destruction of suspended or adherent bacteria by phagocytic cells; and (3) sequestration and walling off of bacteria, coupled with delayed clearance by phagocytic cells. The first mechanism involves the physical removal of bacteria. Microorganisms are carried cephalad by the intraperitoneal circulation, are absorbed into the diaphragmatic lymphatics, and then are carried to the bloodstream. The interaction of bacteria and their products with macrophage populations distant from the peritoneal cavity is presumably responsible for the development of the systemic response to intraperitoneal infection.

The peritoneal response is otherwise typified by the development of local inflammation, including hyperemia of the vasculature underlying the peritoneum, exudation of fluid into the peritoneal cavity, and a marked influx of phagocytic cells. Within the first 2 to 4 hours, bacteria not cleared by the peritoneal lymphatics are mostly cell associated, presumably attached to or ingested by resident peritoneal macrophages.[4] After 4 hours, neutrophils become the predominant phagocytic cell in the peritoneal cavity.[5] The precise events surrounding the development of the peritoneal response have not been well studied but can be surmised from a combination of in vitro and in vivo studies of inflammation. For example, inflammatory exudates derived from subcutaneously implanted sponges contain measurable levels of interleukin-1, interleukin-6, tumor necrosis factor, and macrophage colony-stimulating factor.[6] The combined effects of these cytokines clearly contribute to the inflammatory response observed during peritonitis (Table 40-1). Other inflammatory mediator molecules such as leukotriene B_4, platelet-activating factor, and components of a complement cascade augment these effects by virtue of their ability to attract, prime, and activate cells in the peritoneal cavity.

Finally, a procoagulant response, manifested

TABLE 40-1 Role of Cytokines in Peritoneal Response to Infection*

Cytokine	Action
Tumor necrosis factor	Causes vascular leak
	Increases influx of neutrophils into the peritoneal cavity by augmenting neutrophil-endothelial interactions and transendothelial migration of neutrophils
	Stimulates and primes neutrophil functions
	Stimulates release of other cytokines
	Slight stimulation of macrophage procoagulant activity
Interleukin-1	Increases influx of neutrophils to peritoneum by augmenting neutrophil-endothelial interactions and transendothelial migration of neutrophils
	Chemotactic for neutrophils
	Primes neutrophil function
	Stimulates macrophage procoagulant activity
	Stimulates release of other cytokines
Cellular procoagulants	Induce intraperitoneal fibrin deposition
Interleukin-8	Strong neutrophil chemotactic activity
Colony-stimulating factor 1	Primes neutrophil function

*Modified from Rotstein OD. Peritonitis and intraabdominal abscesses. In Wilmore DW, Brennan MF, Harken AH, et al., eds. Care of the Surgical Patient. New York: Scientific American Publications, 1992. All rights reserved.

by the deposition of fibrinous exudates, is observed during peritoneal infection. Fibrin deposition apparently is important in sequestering infection, not only by incorporating large numbers of bacteria within the fibrin matrix,[7] but also by causing loops of intestine and omentum to create a physical barrier against dissemination. Fibrin deposition is promoted by the procoagulant actions of mesothelial cells and peritoneal macrophages[8] on the fibrinogen-rich peritoneal exudate and by the loss of the intrinsic fibrinolytic activity of the peritoneal surface.[9] Although under some circumstances sequestration of bacteria within these fibrinous exudates predisposes to residual infection, more commonly appropriate antibiotic therapy and surgery plus local mechanisms are able to effect clearance of bacteria with complete resolution of the infection.

Systemic Response

Several factors contribute to the systemic response to intra-abdominal infection. Dehydration caused by third-space fluid loss may cause altered hemodynamics if it is of sufficient magnitude. In addition, particularly in the resuscitated patient, the synthesis and release of various mediator molecules in response to systemic endotoxemia and bacteremia cause marked hemodynamic and metabolic alterations. They are discussed in Chapter 1 in greater detail.

DIAGNOSIS AND MANAGEMENT OF INTRA-ABDOMINAL INFECTION

Intra-abdominal infection is most commonly manifested by the development of secondary peritonitis. Secondary bacterial peritonitis is defined as peritoneal infection caused by perforation of a hollow viscus or transmural necrosis of the GI tract. Under most circumstances, the combination of appropriate antibiotic therapy and timely surgical intervention results in complete resolution of the intraperitoneal infection. When infection persists or recurs, the ability of the host to localize the infection results in the formation of discrete abscesses within the peritoneal cavity. Recently it has been recognized that a small proportion of patients with secondary peritonitis are unable either to clear or to contain infection and go

on to develop persistent diffuse peritonitis, that is, *tertiary peritonitis*. The approach to diagnosis and management for each of these three entities is discussed.

Secondary Peritonitis
Diagnosis

The most common causes of secondary bacterial peritonitis are perforated appendix; perforated duodenal ulcer; perforated sigmoid colon as a result of diverticulitis, volvulus, or cancer; strangulation obstruction of the small bowel; and postoperative peritonitis from anastomotic disruption. The diagnosis of peritonitis is almost always clinical. The symptom complex of anorexia, nausea, and abdominal pain, associated with the physical findings of fever, tachycardia, and abdominal tenderness, are diagnostic of peritonitis. The hemodynamic and metabolic responses to intra-abdominal infection varies, depending on the severity of the infectious process and the magnitude of the patient's response to the infection.

Laboratory and radiologic tests may support the diagnosis of peritonitis. Specifically, the leukocyte count characteristically is elevated with a left shift. Plain abdominal x-ray films may show evidence of ileus, with distended loops of large and small bowel, air fluid levels, and free fluid in the peritoneal cavity. Upright films demonstrate free air under the diaphragm in 80% of patients with perforated duodenal ulcer, but free air is evident in a smaller percentage of patients after perforation of other intra-abdominal organs.

Management

The principles of therapy in patients with secondary peritonitis are (1) resuscitation, (2) appropriate antimicrobial therapy, and (3) surgical intervention. All patients with peritonitis have some degree of hypovolemia related to third-space fluid loss into the peritoneal cavity. Patients should be resuscitated with crystalloid solution before surgery. The microbiology of secondary peritonitis is invariably polymicrobial[10] and consists of a mixture of Gram-negative enteric bacteria plus anaerobes (see box, p. 422). Both experimental and clinical studies suggest that antimicrobial therapy should be directed against both the aerobic and anaerobic

| Bacteria Causing Secondary Peritonitis* |

Aerobic bacteria	Anaerobic bacteria
Escherichia coli	*Bacteroides*
Streptococci	*B. fragilis*
Enterobacter, Klebsiella	Eubacteria
Enterococci	*Clostridium*
Proteus	Anaerobic streptococci

*Modified from Rotstein OD. Peritonitis and intraabdominal abscesses. In Wilmore DW, Brennan MF, Harken AH, et al., eds. Care of the Surgical Patient. New York: Scientific American Publications, 1992.

TABLE 40-2 Antibiotic Therapy for Secondary Peritonitis and Intra-Abdominal Abscesses*

Agent	Comment
Single agents	
Cefoxitin	For community-acquired infection of mild to moderate severity
Cefotetan	Same as for cefoxitin
Cefmetazole	Same as for cefoxitin
Ticarcillin-clavulinic acid	Same as for cefoxitin
Imipenem-cilastatin	For severe infection
Combination therapy†	
Antianaerobe	
Clindamycin	
Metronidazole	
Antiaerobe	
Aminoglycoside‡	Contraindicated for patient with renal compromise or shock
Cefotaxime or ceftizoxime	
Aztreonam	

*Modified from Bohnen JMA, Solomkin JS, Dellinger EP, et al. Guidelines for clinical care: Antiinfective agents for intra-abdominal infection: A Surgical Infection Society policy statement. Arch Surg 127:83, 1992. Copyright 1992, American Medical Association.
†One agent should be selected from the antianaerobe group and one from the antiaerobe group.
‡Choices include gentamicin, tobramycin, amikacin, and netilmicin.

components of these infections, typified by *Escherichia coli* and *Bacteroides fragilis*.[11,12] Single agents or combination therapy that fulfills this requirement is effective for treating secondary peritonitis. Table 40-2 summarizes the guidelines proposed by the Surgical Infection Society for the use of anti-infective agents during intra-abdominal infection.[13] The need to treat enterococci specifically remains controversial. Although experimental studies suggest that this microorganism can act as a significant copathogen with *E. coli*,[14] clinical studies demonstrate that antibiotic coverage directed against coliforms and anaerobes is sufficient treatment for intra-abdominal infection and usually does not result in treatment failure or relapse from enterococci. In contrast, enterococcal bacteremia or the recovery of enterococci from residual or recurrent intra-abdominal infection represents an indication for treatment with the appropriate antienterococcal therapy.[15] Similarly, *Candida* species may be recovered as part of the polymicrobial flora from the peritoneal exudate of patients with secondary peritonitis. As for enterococci, there is no indication for specific therapy directed against *Candida* species in patients with otherwise uncomplicated secondary peritonitis.

The duration of antibiotic therapy following operative management of secondary peritonitis should be based on the clinical status of the patient. If the patient is afebrile, has a normal leukocyte count, and a band count <3%, the chance of recurrent sepsis after discontinuation of antibiotic therapy is virtually zero.[16,17] In contrast, if the patient demonstrates a fever or leukocytosis, the probability of recurrent or residual infection ranges from 33% to 50%. With this approach, antibiotics may be discontinued as early as postoperative day 4. However, if leukocytosis or fever persists after postoperative days 7 to 10, the clinician should consider investigating the patient for the presence of residual infection. Several clinical circumstances exist in which the duration of antibiotic therapy may be as short as 1 day. They include simple acute and suppurative appendicitis, small bowel infarction without perforation, and traumatic enteric perforations operated on within 12 hours of injury.[13] The common feature of these diagnoses is the minimal degree of peritoneal soiling and inflammatory response present at the time of laparotomy. A preoperative dose of antibiotics, followed by two doses within 24 hours of surgery, is appropriate therapy for these conditions.

The goals of the surgical management of peritonitis are to eliminate the source of contamination, to reduce the bacterial inoculum, and to prevent recurrent or persistent infection. The technique used to control contamination depends on the location and the nature of the pathologic condition. In general, continued peritoneal soiling is controlled by closing, excluding, or resecting the perforated viscus. Colonic pathology is handled most effectively by resection of the diseased segment, with exteriorization of the proximal end as an end colostomy, and by creating a mucous fistula or oversewing the distal end. A primary anastomosis in a patient with diffuse peritonitis is associated with an increased rate of dehiscence and should be avoided.[18] Small intestinal pathology should be dealt with similarly by resection of the diseased segment. Since the risk of anastomotic dehiscence is reduced, a primary anastomosis may be considered in this circumstance. However, if peritoneal soiling is particularly extensive or the viability of the intestine is uncertain, the creation of stomas is preferable. A perforated duodenal ulcer caused by peptic ulcer disease is either patched with a piece of omentum or included in the creation of pyloroplasty. In the latter situation, simultaneous vagotomy should be performed. A perforated gastric ulcer is either included in a distal gastric resection with subsequent gastroduodenal or gastrojejunal anastomosis or is excised locally with primary closure. Appendicitis is treated by appendectomy.

In addition to treating the underlying pathology, gross purulent exudates are aspirated, and loculations in the pelvis, paracolic gutters, and subphrenic regions are gently opened and debrided. Adjuvant materials, including fecal matter, barium, necrotic tissue, and blood, should be removed as part of this procedure. Intraoperative peritoneal lavage with saline solution will augment the debridement process. The addition of antibiotics to the lavage solution has not been shown of clear benefit. Drains are not generally necessary unless a well-defined abscess cavity is discovered at the time of abdominal exploration. Abdominal closure is performed in a single fascial layer, using either running or interrupted monofilament sutures. In heavily contaminated cases wound infection is avoided by leaving the skin and subcutaneous tissues open and closing them in a delayed fashion.

Intra-abdominal Abscess
Diagnosis

Abscesses are well-defined collections of purulent material that are walled off from the rest of the peritoneal cavity by inflammatory adhesions, loops of intestines, mesentery, the greater omentum, or other abdominal viscera. Intra-abdominal abscesses occurring outside of the solid viscera arise in two situations: (1) after resolution of diffuse peritonitis in which a loculated area of infection persists and evolves into an abscess and (2) after perforation of a viscus or an anastomotic breakdown that is successfully walled off by peritoneal defense mechanisms. In the latter situation the abscess most frequently is located in apposition to the defect in the GI tract.[19] Intermesenteric perforation of the colon or perforation of the retroperitoneal aspects of the GI tract may result in retroperitoneal abscesses.

The diagnosis of an intra-abdominal abscess is based on clinical suspicion with radiologic confirmation. Abdominal pain, localized tenderness, and a diffuse mass are characteristic of intra-abdominal abscess formation. However, the clinical findings may be somewhat more insidious and manifested only by anorexia and mild abdominal tenderness. As previously noted, a patient recovering from peritonitis who has a persistent fever or leukocytosis should be investigated for the presence of residual infection. Ultrasonography and CT scanning are clearly the examinations of choice for the diagnosis of intra-abdominal abscess formation.[20] Techniques such as gallium scans, white blood cell scans, and plain x-ray studies are of minimal value in this situation.

Management

The basic approach to management of intra-abdominal abscesses is very much the same as that for secondary peritonitis, with the exception that the abscess cavity frequently is drained by radiologically guided percutaneous catheters. The microbiology is similar, and antibiotic recommendations are the same (see box, p. 422, and Table 40-2).

Drainage, either percutaneous or surgical, represents the mainstay of the management of intra-abdominal abscesses. The ability to localize abscesses accurately not only allows the use of percutaneous techniques but also significantly facilitates the approach to abscess drainage when surgery is necessary. Percutaneous drainage is highly effective when the abscess is a single well-defined cavity without enteric communication.[21] In contrast, multiple abscesses, the presence of extremely viscous abscess contents such as those found in patients with fungal infections or pancreatic necrosis, and infected hematomas have a lesser chance of success by the percutaneous route. When approaching abscesses surgically, the accurate localization of the abscess by CT prevents the need for a general abdominal exploration and permits a direct (often extraserous) approach to the abscess. Drains, whether placed surgically or percutaneously, should be left in place until the patient is clinically improved and demonstrates minimal drainage from the catheter and there is radiologic evidence of resolution of the abscess by CT scan or sinogram. A sinogram also identifies a connection to the GI tract.

The results of percutaneous abscess drainage have not been compared to the surgical approach in a well-designed clinical trial. However, it appears that equivalent results can be achieved with each technique.[22] The outcome is optimized if the approach to the abscess is individualized for each patient and appropriate abscess drainage occurs early.

Tertiary Peritonitis

The combination of appropriate antibiotic therapy and timely surgical intervention is sufficient to effect complete resolution of an infection in the majority of patients presenting with secondary peritonitis. Even when infection persists or recurs, the ability of the host to localize the infection results in a discrete abscess that can be treated by percutaneous or surgical drain-

TABLE 40-3 Microbiology of Tertiary Peritonitis*

Organisms†	No. of Positive Cultures	No. of Patients
Aerobes		
Staphylococcus epidermidis	24	16
Enterococcus	14	8
Alpha-hemolytic streptococcus	4	3
Pseudomonas aeruginosa	16	12
Facultative Gram-negative bacilli		
Escherichia coli	11	6
Klebsiella pneumoniae and *K. oxytoca*	8	6
Enterobacter *cloacae* and *E. aerogenes*	16	8
Anaerobes		
Bacteroides fragilis	4	3
Clostridium perfringens, C. clostridiiforme, and unidentified clostridial species	5	3
Fungus		
Candida albicans	19	10
C. glabrata	10	5
C. tropicalis	2	2

*Modified from Rotstein OD, Pruett TL, Simmons RL. Microbiologic features and treatment of persistent peritonitis in the intensive care unit. Can J Surg 29:247, 1986.
†Isolates from the peritoneal cavity of 25 patients with persistent peritonitis.

age. Some patients, however, demonstrate an inability to wall off and resolve intraperitoneal infection and go on to the development of persistent diffuse peritonitis, or tertiary peritonitis. The clinical picture is characterized by occult sepsis with hyperdynamic cardiovascular response, low-grade fever, leukocytosis, and the development of organ dysfunction.[23] The microbiology of tertiary peritonitis differs significantly from that reported for secondary peritonitis (Table 40-3). Specifically, *Staphylococcus epidermidis, Pseudomonas* species, and *Can-*

dida species are the predominant microorganisms recovered from these patients.[24] Accordingly antimicrobial therapy should be focused, rather than empiric and broad spectrum as described for secondary peritonitis.

Optimal therapy for patients with tertiary peritonitis is limited by the poorly defined pathogenesis of this disease. Although microorganisms are regularly recovered from the peritoneal cavity, their precise contribution to the ongoing disease process is not well understood. Confounding observations include the fact that focused antimicrobial therapy is frequently unable to eradicate the microorganism, and the practice of performing repeat laparotomies to control residual infection has little impact on outcome in these patients and frequently does not reveal evidence of infection.[25] These discrepancies have led to the development of alternate hypotheses to explain the development of organ dysfunction associated with tertiary peritonitis. Specifically, the role of the GI tract as a source for bacteria and/or endotoxin has been the subject of recent interest.[26] Egress of bacteria and endotoxin from the GI tract in response to an inflammatory stimulus such as diffuse peritonitis has been postulated to lead to distant organ dysfunction. Altering this process by using techniques such as selective digestive decontamination[27] or enhancing the integrity of the mucosal barrier with specific nutrients[28] may become important components of the therapy for these patients. Other novel approaches, including the use of antibodies to endotoxin or to cytokines, as well as cytokine receptor antagonists, are presently being evaluated in this and other similar disease processes. At present, the best outcome in this patient population is achieved by providing aggressive hemodynamic monitoring and support, adequate nutrition, directed antibiotic therapy, and timely surgical intervention.

SUMMARY

- Patient with peritonitis:
  Resuscitate.
  Start therapy with broad-spectrum antibiotics active against Gram-negative enteric bacteria and anaerobic bacteria; continue antibiotic therapy until patient is afebrile and leukocyte count is normal for 48 hours (band count <3%).
  During surgical intervention, resect, close, or patch site of intestinal pathology.

- Patient with intra-abdominal abscesses:
  Resuscitate with crystalloids/colloids.
  Provide broad-spectrum antibiotic therapy as per peritonitis until culture results are available.
  Drain the abscess either percutaneously or surgically, depending on the clinical situation.

REFERENCES

1. Allen L, Weatherford T. Role of fenestrated basement membrane in lymphatic absorption from the peritoneal cavity. Am J Physiol 197:551, 1956.
2. Steinberg B. Infections of the Peritoneum. New York: Hoeber, 1944.
3. Hau T, Ahrenholz DH, Simmons RL. Secondary bacterial peritonitis: The biologic basis of treatment. Curr Probl Surg 16:1, 1979.
4. Dunn DL, Barke RA, Ewald DC, Simmons RL. Macrophages and translymphatic absorption represent the first line of host defense of the peritoneal cavity. Arch Surg 122:105, 1987.
5. Hau T, Hoffman R, Simmons RL. Mechanisms of the adjuvant effect of hemoglobin in experimental peritonitis. I. *In vivo* inhibition of peritoneal leukocytosis. Surgery 83:223, 1978.
6. Ford HR, Hoffman RA, Wing EJ, et al. Characterization of wound cytokines in the sponge matrix model. Arch Surg 124:1422, 1989.
7. Dunn DL, Simmons RL. Fibrin in peritonitis. III. The mechanism of bacterial trapping by polymerizing fibrin. Surgery 92:513, 1982.

8. Sinclair SB, Rotstein OD, Levy GA. Disparate mechanisms of induction of procoagulant activity by live and inactivated bacteria and viruses. Infect Immun 58:182, 1990.

9. Hau T, Payne WD, Simmons RL. Fibrinolytic activity of the peritoneum during experimental peritonitis. Surg Gynecol Obstet 148:415, 1979.

10. Lorber B, Swenson RM. The bacteriology of intraabdominal infections. Surg Clin North Am 55:1349, 1975.

11. Berne TV, Yellin AW, Appleman MD, Heseltine PNR. Antibiotic management of surgically treated gangrenous or perforated appendicitis. Comparison of gentamicin and clindamycin versus cefamandole versus cefoperazone. Am J Surg 144:8, 1982.

12. Bartlett JG, Louie TJ, Gorbach SL, Onderdonk AB. Therapeutic efficacy of 29 antimicrobial regimens in experimental intraabdominal sepsis. Rev Infect Dis 3:535, 1981.

13. Bohnen JMA, Solomkin JS, Dellinger EP, et al. Guidelines for clinical care: Anti-infective agents for intra-abdominal infection: A Surgical Infection Society policy statement. Arch Surg 127:83, 1992.

14. Fry DE, Berberich S, Garrison RN. Bacterial synergism between the enterococcus and *Escherichia coli.* J Surg Res 38:475, 1985.

15. Barie PS, Christou NV, Dellinger EP, et al. Pathogenicity of the enterococcus in surgical infections. Ann Surg 212:155, 1990.

16. Lennard ES, Dellinger EP, Wertz MJ, et al. Implications of leukocytosis and fever at conclusion of antibiotic therapy for intraabdominal sepsis. Ann Surg 195:19, 1982.

17. Stone HH, Bourneuf AA, Stinson LD. Reliability of criteria for predicting persistent or recurrent sepsis. Arch Surg 120:17, 1985.

18. Shrock TR, Deveney CW, Dunphy JE. Factors contributing to leakage of colonic anastomoses. Ann Surg 197:513, 1973.

19. Altemeier WA, Culbertson WR, Shook CD. Intraabdominal abscesses. Am J Surg 125:70, 1973.

20. Baker ME, Blinder RA, Rice RP. Diagnostic imaging of abdominal fluid collections and abscesses. Crit Rev Diagn Imaging 25:233, 1986.

21. Pruett TL, Rotstein OD, Fiegel VD, et al. Mechanism of the adjuvant effect of hemoglobin in experimental peritonitis. VIII. A leukotoxin is produced by *Escherichia coli* metabolism in hemoglobin. Surgery 96:375, 1984.

22. Olak J, Christou NV, Stein LA, et al. Operative vs. percutaneous drainage of intraabdominal abscesses. Arch Surg 121:141, 1986.

23. Rotstein OD, Meakins JL. Diagnostic and therapeutic challenges of intraabdominal infections. World J Surg 14:159, 1990.

24. Rotstein OD, Pruett TL, Simmons RL. Microbiologic features and treatment of persistent peritonitis in the intensive care unit. Can J Surg 29:247, 1986.

25. Norwood SN, Civetta JM. Abdominal CT scanning in critically ill surgical patients. Ann Surg 202:166, 1985.

26. Carrico CJ, Meakins JL, Marshall JC. Multiple-organ-failure syndrome: The gastrointestinal tract—The motor of "MOF." Arch Surg 121:197, 1986.

27. Poole GV, Muakkassa FF, Griswold JA. Pneumonia selective decontamination, and multiple organ failure. Surgery 111:1, 1992.

28. Wilmore DW, Smith RJ, O'Dwyer ST. The gut: A central organ of after-surgical stress. Surgery 104:917, 1988.

SUGGESTED READINGS

Ahrenholz DH, Simmons RL. Peritonitis and other intra-abdominal infections. In Simmons RL, Howard RJ, eds. Surgical Infectious Diseases. Norwalk, Conn.: Appleton & Lange, 1988.

Excellent comprehensive discussion of intra-abdominal infection.

Rotstein OD. Peritonitis and intraabdominal abscesses. In Wilmore DW, Brennan MF, Harken AH, Holcroft JW, Meakins JL, eds. Care of the Surgical Patient. New York: Scientific American Publications, 1992.

A comprehensive overview of the pathophysiology, diagnosis, and management of intra-abdominal infection, with many references.

CHAPTER 41

HIV/AIDS: Core Knowledge

Keith Henry

Human immunodeficiency virus (HIV), the etiologic agent linked to AIDS,[1] is a fairly heterogeneous virus, and its heterogeneity is manifest in a number of ways. Different viral strains have different cell tropisms, cytopathologies, latency periods, and genome sequence variations. HIV-1 contains 10 to 14 genes, and the protein products of these genes have been well characterized. HIV-2, another retrovirus linked with AIDS in Africa, is rare in North America at this time. Fewer than a dozen cases of HIV-2 have been reported in North America and all originated in Africa. Current screening for HIV-1 is likely to detect 50% to 60% of the cases of HIV-2.

TESTING FOR HIV

The ELISA (enzyme-linked immunosorbent assay) test is the initial serologic procedure used to detect antibodies to HIV-1. A major misconception is that a positive ELISA test alone indicates infection with HIV; the test is overly sensitive and has many false positive results. The confirmatory test of choice is the Western blot, which identifies antibodies generated to key proteins of the virus, such as gp120, gp41, p24 (the internal core protein), and the reverse transcriptase (RT) protein. Confusion persists about terminology relating to testing and clinical manifestations. "Exposure" means that a situation existed in which the HIV could have entered the other person's body. "Infection" with HIV is usually determined by serologic tests that detect antibody response to the virus.

Antibodies to HIV-1 are almost always detectable after sexual transmission. Exceptions include anal intercourse or needlestick transmission within 3 to 6 months after the infection has occurred. Once the test confirms the presence of antibodies to HIV, a person is said to be "actively infected" with HIV, presumably for life. HIV-1 can be recovered by culture techniques in essentially 100% of the cases of persons who have a positive HIV-1 serology.[2] Another technique that is becoming widely used to detect HIV-1 is the polymerase chain reaction, which is available through a number of research centers and appears to exhibit similar sensitivity and specificity to other available culture techniques.[3]

EPIDEMIOLOGY

HIV-1 is found in many body fluids, the most important being blood, semen, and vaginal secretions. The cumulative AIDS caseload is presently approaching 250,000 and will soon increase as a result of a change in the case definition. Previously, a person with HIV-1 infection was classified as representing an AIDS case if he/she developed one of the opportunistic infections, malignancies, dementia, or wasting syndromes associated with severe immunosuppression (see box, p. 428). The Centers for Disease Control (CDC) is considering a revision of the AIDS case definition to include persons with HIV who have a T-helper cell count (CD-4) $<200/mm^3$. At present, it is estimated that approximately 1 million Americans are infected

Diseases Indicative of AIDS*

Protozoan infections

PCP (may be fungus?)

Toxoplasma gondii encephalitis or disseminated infection

Chronic *Cryptosporidium* or *Isospora* enteritis

Viral infections

Chronic mucocutaneous herpes simplex

CMV other than liver or lymph node

Progressive multifocal leukoencephalopathy

Bacterial infections

Disseminated *Mycobacterium avium intracellulare*

Disseminated *Mycobacterium tuberculosis*

Salmonella (recurrent septicemia) infection

Fungal infections

Candidiasis, esophageal or pulmonary

Cryptococcal meningitis or disseminated infection

Disseminated histoplasmosis

Disseminated coccidioidomycosis

Malignancies

Kaposi's sarcoma

Primary brain lymphoma

Non-Hodgkin's lymphoma

Other

HIV encephalopathy (AIDS dementia)

HIV wasting syndrome

Chronic lymphoid interstitial pneumonia in children (under age 13)

T-helper cell (CD4) count $<200/mm^3$

*Data from Centers for Disease Control, Atlanta, 1987.
Note: Diseases listed are indicative of AIDS in conjunction with a positive test for HIV.

with HIV and that approximately 40,000 new HIV infections are occurring annually in the United States. The AIDS caseload among gay men is plateauing in many metropolitan areas, but it continues to rise significantly among intravenous drug users, heterosexuals, blacks and Hispanics.

The prevalence of HIV varies widely in the United States. A CDC study of hospital patients throughout the United States found that the rate of HIV infection in persons not suspected of being infected ranged from 0.1% to 8%.[4] In some areas, such as the Bronx, 18% to 22% of all men 25 to 44 years old were seropositive for HIV. These data strongly suggest that more routine use of HIV antibody testing is indicated in some populations. HIV-1 is expected to continue to move into inner-city populations, especially African-Americans and Hispanics.

HIV/AIDS IMMUNOPATHOGENESIS

New HIV-1 infection often results in a primary infection syndrome mimicking infectious mononucleosis. This period has been associated with an extremely high level of HIV-1 viremia that persists until antibodies targeting HIV-1 proteins are generated.[5] Then the HIV infection appears to settle into lymph nodes and be cleared from the plasma. Although HIV-1 can be detected in such places as lymph nodes or mononuclear cells, the next phase is often termed the "clinically latent phase." The person is asymptomatic during this interval. Although the person is asymptomatic, he/she can still transmit HIV-1 through high-risk behavior or through body fluid exposure to health care workers. The CD4 count is a major target for HIV-1. The normal CD4 count for adults is usually 800 to 1000 cells/mm^3. Although various patterns occur in the rate of decline of the CD4 count in HIV-1–infected individuals, the usual trend is a steady drop in CD4 counts of 5 to 10 per month, or 50 to 100 cells/mm^3 lost annually.

The average period from initial HIV infection to the development of AIDS ranges from 8 to 12 years. During that period, the person is often asymptomatic, although he/she may suffer from such early signs of HIV as fatigue, oral candidiasis, oral hairy leukoplakia, herpes zoster, seborrhea, and folliculitis. The risk for an AIDS-related infection goes up dramatically once the CD4 count falls below 200 cells/mm^3, or the percentage of CD4 cells drops to less than 20%.[6] The CDC recommends primary prophylaxis for *Pneumocystis carinii* pneumonia (PCP) for all HIV-1 infected persons with a CD4 count <200 or a CD4 percentage less than 20%. At present, it is expected that physicians caring for HIV-infected persons would know what the CD4 level is and offer prophylaxis when appropriate. A patient's immune status is relevant to surgical practices. One of the first questions a surgeon should ask of a patient infected with HIV-1 is the most recent CD4 count. This count helps quantify the risk for an HIV-related complication and to correctly evaluate such symptoms as fever or cough.

Full-blown AIDS can be the first sign that a person is infected with HIV since the clinically silent period can extend to the point when the person becomes acutely ill. The average survival of a person with AIDS after the diagnosis has been confirmed is 1 to 2 years if the individual is getting good care. Survival to 4 and 5 years with AIDS is now being seen. HIV infection should be viewed as a chronic infection that leads to attrition of the immune system and AIDS over a 10-year period of time. Early intervention with anti-HIV therapy can further significantly delay the development of AIDS and perhaps protect the immune system. One study from the San Francisco Clinic Cohort found that among men infected with HIV-1 for 12 years, 55% had progressed to AIDS and 45% were AIDS-free.[7] Approximately half of the people not yet developing AIDS at 12 years still were asymptomatic, and about half of those persons still had CD4 counts >500/mm^3.

ANTI-HIV THERAPY

Most authorities believe that AIDS is ultimately caused by HIV-1 and that viral replication is essential for the progression of disease. The life cycle of the virus provides numerous opportunities for intervention, although the major focus for drugs currently under development or available is the HIV-1 reverse transcriptase (RT). The one RT inhibitory drug that has proven beneficial and is widely available is zidovudine (AZT, otherwise known as Retrovir). AZT has been shown to delay the onset of AIDS-associated symptoms or the development of AIDS and to prolong the life of persons with AIDS. The benefits of AZT are probably transient in persons with advanced HIV disease as identified by a CD4 count <200/mm^3. Two large studies addressed the use of AZT to delay progression in mimimally symptomatic or asymptomatic patients.[8,9] In both studies, patients receiving AZT developed fewer than half the clinical endpoints when compared to placebo groups. These studies led to the expansion of treatment beyond severe AIDS-related complex and AIDS to persons with CD4 counts <500/mm^3. This is a significant point that should be recognized by surgical staff in the United States. AZT is recommended for persons with CD4 counts <500. The current recommended dosage for AZT is 500 mg a day divided into three doses (2-1-2). At that dosage, the toxicities are minimized but are nonetheless significant. During the first month of therapy, many persons have transient symptoms such as nausea, abdominal cramps, skin rash, and headache. The major late toxicities are anemia, granulocytopenia, and myopathy.

The current standard of care in persons infected with HIV-1 is to determine the CD4 count, and, if it is >600/mm^3, to repeat the count every 6 months.[10] If it is <500/mm^3 consistently, then AZT therapy is offered and the patient is checked every 1 to 2 months. If the CD4 count is <200/mm^3, PCP prophylaxis should be given. As the CD4 count falls progressively below 200, patients should be monitored monthly and carefully for the development of other opportunistic infections. AZT does not cure the patients, and breakthroughs (defined as progression of disease and/or development of new opportunistic complications) are typically encountered in patients with advanced disease. Breakthrough is probably related to the development of resistance to AZT, which is seen regularly in persons with low CD4 counts after they have received the drug for 6 months or more. AZT resistance is one of the major reasons that a need exists to expand the availability of other anti-HIV compounds such as dideoxyinosine (ddI) and dideoxycytosine (ddC). Isolates resistant to AZT are still sensitive to those two drugs.

DIDEOXYINOSINE AND DIDEOXYCYTOSINE

These nucleoside derivatives are close relatives to AZT and act by inhibiting RT. They generally do not have much toxicity in the bone marrow but at higher doses show significant peripheral neuropathy. Additionally, ddI appears to cause pancreatitis in persons with advanced HIV disease who often have *Mycobacterium avium intracellulare* (MAI) disease or cytomegalovirus (CMV) disease or who take medication with the propensity to induce pancreatitis. ddI is available for prescription use in patients who are intolerant to AZT or failing in AZT therapy. ddC is available for use in combination with AZT in patients with progressive disease who are taking AZT alone. One of the treatment options being actively explored is the use of nucleoside derivatives such as ddI or ddC combined with AZT. Preliminary data suggest that such combinations provide better immune stabilization and clinical outcome than either drug alone. This approach, which will be a major focus of studies in the near future, mirrors the experience of cancer, tuberculosis, and other antibacterial therapies.

AIDS-RELATED INFECTIONS

For HIV-infected persons, it is unusual to see any of the major HIV-associated infections other than oral candidiasis, vaginal candidiasis, or herpes zoster until the CD4 count is $<200/mm^3$. Once the CD4 count falls below 200, the person is at risk for PCP. In the CD4 count range of 75 to $125/mm^3$, one most frequently sees PCP, MAI disease, herpes simplex virus, toxoplasmosis, and esophageal candidiasis. Once the CD4 count drops below 50, CMV and MAI infections become much more common.[11] Thus two general stages of HIV-associated, AIDS-defining opportunistic infections are seen (see box). The early infections are relatively easy to diagnose and treat, which helps lengthen the life of the average person with AIDS. Unfortunately, since the immune system is not being reconstituted, the person next encounters late opportunistic infections, which are more difficult to diagnose and treat. Many patients succumb to a combination of infectious problems, wasting, and dementia.

Stages of AIDS by Indicator Disease or Infection

Early stage

T-helper cell (CD4) count $<200/mm^3$
Cutaneous Kaposi's sarcoma
PCP
Candida esophagitis
Extrapulmonary tuberculosis
Recurrent bacterial septicemia
Cryptococcal meningitis

Late stage

Recurrent PCP
CMV retinitis
Disseminated mycosis (cryptococcus, histoplasmosis, or coccidioidomycosis)
Mycobacterium avium intracellulare complex
Toxoplasma gondii brain abscess
Cryptosporidium/Isospora belli enteritis
Progressive multifocal leukoencephalopathy
AIDS dementia and wasting
CD4 count $<50/mm^3$
Advanced non-Hodgkin's lymphoma

Pneumocystis carinii Pneumonia

The most commonly occurring and defining HIV complication is PCP. Recommended treatment and prophylaxis options are summarized in Tables 41-1 and 41-2, respectively. Prophylaxis can be viewed as primary if the person has never had PCP and secondary if the patient already has had it. PCP should be suspected in HIV-infected persons with CD4 counts $<200/mm^3$ who seek treatment for fever, fatigue, cough, and headache and in those who have any type of infiltrate on CXR examination. The standard appearance on CXR examination is an alveolar pattern, although persons receiving aerosolized pentamidine prophylaxis often have an upper lobe distribution. A diagnosis can sometimes be made by vigorous induction of sputum with specific stain for *Pneumocystis* organisms, but often the patient needs bronchoscopy, brochoalveolar lavage, and analysis of lavage fluid with specific stains for *Pneumocystis* organisms. Standard stains for bacteria are unlikely to identify *Pneumocystis carinii*. The clinician must specifically request the stains

| TABLE 41-1 Therapy for *Pneumocystis Carinii* Pneumonia* |||

Agent	Regimen	Side Effects
Standard therapy		
Trimethoprim-sulfamethoxazole	15-20 mg/kg/day (based on tri-methoprim component) IV or po in three or four divided doses for up to 21 days	Anorexia, headache, nausea, vomiting, rash, neutro-penia, fever, hepatitis, thrombocytosis, nephri-tis, Stevens-Johnson syn-drome
Pentamidine isethionate (Pen-tam 300)	4 mg/kg/day infused over 1-2 hr IV (preferred) or IM for 14-21 days	Sterile abscesses (when given IM), hypotension, hypoglycemia, hypergly-cemia
Investigational therapy		
Dapsone and trimethoprim (Proloprim, Trimpex)	100 mg dapsone and 20 mg/kg trimethoprim po for 21 days	Anemia, methemoglobin-emia
Aerosolized pentamidine ise-thionate (NebuPent)	300-600 mg/day via jet nebulizer for 21 days	Cough, asthma
Clindamycin (Cleocin phos-phate) and primaquine phos-phate	900 mg clindamycin IV q 8 hr and 52.6 mg/day; primaquine (equivalent to 30 mg base) po for 21 days	Rash, leukopenia, nausea, diarrhea
566C80†	750 mg po tid	Fever, rash, nausea, anemia, liver function abnormali-ties

*Modified from Henry K. The evolving challenge of *Pneumocystis carinii:* A deadly opportunist in AIDS. Postgrad Med 87(3):45-56, 1990.
†Call 1-800-722-9292 for information.

| TABLE 41-2 Regimens for Continuous Prophylaxis of *Pneumocystis Carinii* Pneumonia* ||

Agent	Regimen
Standard therapies	
Trimethoprim-sulfamethoxazole	160 mg and 800 mg, respectively
Aerosolized pentamidine isethionate (NebuPent)	300 mg q 4 wk via Respirgard II jet nebulizer†
Investigational therapies	
Dapsone	25-50 mg po bid
Dapsone and trimethoprim (Proloprim, Trimpex)	25-50 mg dapsone and 200 mg trimethoprim po bid
Pentamidine isethionate (Pentam 300)	2-4 mg/kg IV or IM q 4 wk

*From Henry K, Thurn J. The evolving challenge of *Pneumocystis carinii:* A deadly opportunist in AIDS. Postgrad Med 87(3):45-54, 1990.
†Other doses, intervals, and nebulizers are being studied and may also be effective.

needed. The diagnosis is more difficult to make in persons receiving prophylaxis. Survival with PCP is about 85%. A recent major treatment advance is use of corticosteroids in persons who have a Po_2 at presentation of less than 65 mm Hg.[12] My major concerns about the use of aerosolized pentamidine for prophylaxis are its expense, its possible contribution to pneumothorax and extrapulmonary dissemination of *Pneumocystis* organisms, and its lack of effect against other AIDS-associated infections. Preliminary data suggest that trimethoprim-sulfamethoxazole (1 DS/day) is the preferred agent for PCP prophylaxis in the 75% of patients who can tolerate it.

Herpes Family Viruses

Herpes simplex infections can be severe and recurring in HIV disease and generally respond to acyclovir therapy. Mucosal infections can be treated with oral acyclovir, whereas more severe infections may necessitate the intravenous form. Some concern exists about resistance developing to acyclovir, and the recent approval of foscarnet provides an alternative therapy. Herpes zoster can be seen early in HIV infection. It sometimes recurs and generally responds well to acyclovir.

The most significant of the herpes family of viruses causing morbidity and mortality in AIDS is CMV. In some centers, CMV is now the leading infectious cause of death in AIDS patients. One of the major organs affected is the eye, where necrotizing retinitis is seen in up to 25% of patients. CMV infection will respond to ganciclovir 75% to 85% of the time, but therapy must be maintained. The major toxicity of ganciclovir is hematologic and resistance has also been reported. In cases of resistance, the patient may be switched to foscarnet[13] or intravitreal[14] ganciclovir. Ganciclovir plus GM-colony stimulating factor (GM-CSF)[15] and erythropoietin also have been used in an effort to minimize side effects. Blood cultures for CMV should be obtained in persons who are having fevers, wasting, and advanced HIV disease (CD4 counts <100/mm³).

Fungal Infections

The major fungal infections that clinicians should be aware of are *Candida* and crypto-coccal disease. *Candida* infection can be first seen as oral thrush and in later stages as a cause of esophagitis. The thrush can be treated with nystatin swish (5 ml three to five times a day), clotrimazole troches (10 mg three to five times a day), ketoconazole (200 mg a day), or fluconazole (100 mg a day). *Candida* esophagitis requires fluconazole orally or, occasionally, IV amphotericin B. Cryptococcal infection is often devastating to AIDS patients and still responds best initially to IV amphotericin B. After induction therapy with amphotericin B, maintenance therapy with fluconazole orally appears to result in improved long-term outcome. Fluconazole is now the maintenance regimen of choice,[16] a major treatment advance. In certain regions of the country, other disseminated fungal diseases are also a cause of significant morbidity and mortality (e.g., coccidioidomycosis in the Southwest and histoplasmosis in the Midwest).

Toxoplasmosis

Toxoplasma gondii causes cerebral abscess, usually in persons with low CD4 counts. *Toxoplasma* infections often respond to pyrimethamine and sulfadiazine. Alternative regimens include pyrimethamine and clindamycin. A new compound, 566C80, is a potentially promising oral agent. *Cryptosporidium* is another parasitic infection that can cause severe colitis and has evaded currently available therapies. Occasionally, symptoms can be addressed with hyperalimentation and drugs such as somatostatin.

Bacterial Infections

HIV-associated syphilis has a more virulent clinical course and is more difficult to diagnose and treat when compared to syphilis in non–HIV-infected patients. The incidence of *Mycobacterium tuberculosis* is increasing in the United States as a consequence of HIV infection and immunosuppression.[17] Inner-city minority populations have also seen a rise in this disease. Standard antituberculosis therapy is still successful in these cases. MAI is one of the most troublesome late-stage AIDS-associated infections and is one of the leading causes of death in major AIDS treatment centers at the present time. Combination treatment with IV amikacin and oral ciprofloxacin, ethambutol, clofazimine, and rifampin provides some benefit in many cases but constitutes for the patient a complex and difficult regimen.[18] Monotherapy with a macrolide antibiotic (azithromycin or clarithromycin) appears promising and would be another major treatment advance. Efforts are also under way to prevent MAI infections with drugs such as clarithromycin or rifabutin. The effectiveness of prophylaxis is currently unclear.

Pneumonia from encapsulated bacteria, such as *Haemophilus influenzae* and particularly *Streptococcus pneumoniae,* is seen more often in HIV-infected patients. Empiric therapy for a possible bacterial pneumonia should provide coverage for those organisms. Recently, an increase in often devastating infections from *Pseudomonas aeruginosa* in persons with advanced AIDS has occurred.[19] Empiric therapy for pneumonia in a late-stage AIDS patient should include coverage for *Pseudomonas* organisms. In persons who have indwelling catheters (e.g., Hickman catheters), catheter-related sepsis from *Staphylococcus aureus* or Gram-negative infections is always a threat and often necessitates aggressive therapy and removal of the catheter.[20]

AIDS-Dementia Complex

More persons are developing AIDS dementia as they survive their initial infections. Some data suggest that dementia may be delayed by anti-HIV therapy. At a late stage dementia is a common problem and difficult to treat.[21]

AIDS Wasting Syndrome

AIDS wasting syndrome is a diagnosis of exclusion and is frustrating to treat. Efforts to provide enteric hyperalimentation are often frustrated by gastrointestinal tract symptoms, and in some cases clinicians have resorted to total parenteral nutrition.[22] Treatment of some of the nutritional problems with somatostatin for diarrhea or megestrol acetate (Megace) for weight gain are still under study but appear to provide some promise.

ISSUES SPECIFIC TO THE SICU

A serious case of pneumonia resulting in respiratory compromise is the most likely reason for admitting a person infected with HIV to the SICU. Although a trend has been to avoid intubation of AIDS patients in the SICU during the late 1980s, more recent data suggest that these individuals can survive severe pneumonias and that intubation may be appropriate. Presently, clinicians are more aggressive about providing respiratory support for persons with respiratory compromise.[23] Good HIV/AIDS care should address a person's wishes about resuscitation status at an early stage of disease. For persons with late-stage AIDS, admission to the SICU and ventilatory support are often inappropriate. Since persons with HIV/AIDS can develop the regular medical problems of the general population, they may need the SICU for problems such as severe trauma, burns, or postoperative care.

Numerous articles discuss the experience in various centers with surgery for persons with HIV/AIDS.[24,25] In general, persons with early or midspectrum HIV infection do well with surgery, and their healing appears to be relatively unimpaired. Complication rates are higher in AIDS patients, but their ability to heal is still surprisingly intact, despite the severe insult to their cellular-mediated immunity. Again, the average survival from initial infection with HIV until death by AIDS currently is 10 to 12 years. Better therapy is likely to extend survival further. Therefore HIV/AIDS needs to be viewed as a chronic disease. The patient is not terminally ill until the late-stage condition has evolved.

INFECTION-CONTROL ISSUES

Infection control involves two issues: protection of the health care worker and protection of the patient. Available data suggest that the sterile technique practiced in operating rooms provides an excellent level of bidirectional protection for both the health care worker and the patient. In other clinical settings, compliance with universal precautions is not as strict, and the risk for HIV nosocomial transmission and other nosocomial infections subsequently increases. The risk of transmission from a sharps injury from an HIV-infected patient relates to the magnitude of the exposure and the clinical stage of the source patient. The level of viremia for HIV appears to range from 1 to 1000 infectious particles per milliliter, with higher levels

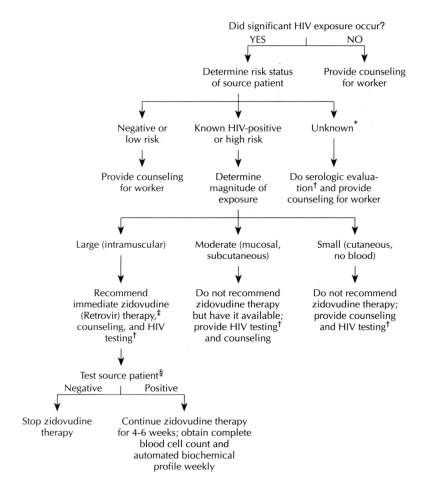

Did significant HIV exposure occur?

YES | NO

Determine risk status of source patient

Provide counseling for worker

Negative or low risk

Known HIV-positive or high risk

Unknown*

Provide counseling for worker

Determine magnitude of exposure

Do serologic evaluation† and provide counseling for worker

Large (intramuscular)

Moderate (mucosal, subcutaneous)

Small (cutaneous, no blood)

Recommend immediate zidovudine (Retrovir) therapy,‡ counseling, and HIV testing†

Do not recommend zidovudine therapy but have it available; provide HIV testing† and counseling

Do not recommend zidovudine therapy; provide counseling and HIV testing†

Test source patient§

Negative | Positive

Stop zidovudine therapy

Continue zidovudine therapy for 4-6 weeks; obtain complete blood cell count and automated biochemical profile weekly

*In high-incidence areas, such as New York City, consider voluntary testing of all source patients.
†Test at time of incident and then at 6 weeks, 3 months, and 6 months.
‡Administer 200 mg five times daily. Obtain baseline complete blood cell count and automated biochemical profile.
§If patient refuses testing, refer to local policy.

FIG. 41-1   Protocol for evaluation of health care workers exposed to HIV. (From Henry K, Thurn J. HIV infection in healthcare workers. How great is the risk? What can be done before and after exposure? Postgrad Med 89(3):30-38, 1991.)

in more advanced disease. The risk for HIV transmission from a hollow-bore needle injury is also higher than from a scalpel injury. The average volume of blood injected from a needlestick injury has been estimated to be 1.4 μL, and the average seroconversion rate from various studies has been approximately .03%, with an upper 95% conference interval around 1%.[26] In contrast, the seroconversion rate after needlestick exposure to a patient who is hepatitis B antigen positive ranges as high as 25% to 30%. Many studies have shown that the major risk for sharps injury involves inappropriate recapping or disposal of needles and not following recommended guidelines.

Current data suggest that double gloving provides additional protection from sharps injury. One study from San Francisco General Hospital clearly demonstrated a benefit from double gloving and also showed that prior knowledge of the patient's HIV status did not change significantly HIV exposure rates from injuries sustained in the operating room.[27] In areas of high HIV seroprevalence, double gloving should be routine when performing procedures on persons with known HIV or hepatitis B infection. Specific guidelines for infection control in the near future are likely to include requirements for double gloving and other modalities such as use of face shields and water-impermeable gowns (Fig. 41-1).

Current practice clearly suggests that the patient's best interest is served if the patient is aware of his/her HIV status and that clinical management of medical problems arising in an SICU can be best handled if a patient's HIV status is known by the medical/surgical team. In general, HIV testing of patients who are at risk for HIV should be encouraged. In general, such testing should be done with their consent and supported with counseling. Many states have specific laws regarding HIV testing of patients and the level of consent required.

The CDC has recently issued guidelines for prevention of HIV and hepatitis B virus trans-

---

Definition of Invasive Procedure*

Surgical entry into tissues, body cavities, or organs or repair of major traumatic injuries associated with any of the following:

1. An operating or delivery room, emergency department, or outpatient setting, including both physicians' and dentists' offices
2. Cardiac catheterization and angiographic procedures
3. A vaginal or cesarean delivery or other invasive obstetric procedure during which bleeding may occur
4. The manipulation, cutting, or removal of any oral or perioral tissues, including tooth structure, during which bleeding occurs or the potential for bleeding occurs

*From Centers for Disease Control. Recommendations for preventing transmission of human immunodeficiency virus and hepatitis B virus to patients during exposure-prone invasive procedures. MMWR 40:1-8, 1991.

---

mission to patients during exposure-prone invasive procedures[28] (see box). Recently, the CDC has decided to let each state develop its own guidelines pertaining to the HIV-infected health care worker rather than to further define any national standards. To date no cases of HIV transmission from a physician to a patient in any setting have been recorded. Approximately 30 well-documented cases of HIV infection have been reported among health care workers after exposure to patients. Almost all involved sharps injuries. Three cases of possible mucosal transmission have been recorded. A schema for the evaluation and possible treatment of the HIV-exposed health care worker is summarized in Fig. 41-1.

We all look forward to the time when an HIV vaccine will be available,[29] but that will not happen for many years. In the meantime, education and rigorous infection control practices remain the best defense against HIV transmission.

SUMMARY

- A positive ELISA screening test must be confirmed with Western blot test.
- Persons with HIV infection and a CD4 count <200 cells/mm³ are said to have advanced HIV/AIDS.
- New HIV-1 infection often mimics mononucleosis.
- Persons with latent HIV-1 infection can transmit HIV-1 virus.
- PCP prophylaxis should be provided for all HIV-1–infected persons with low CD4 counts.
- HIV infection is chronic and causes progressive immunodeficiency over approximately 10 years.
- AZT delays onset of AIDS and prolongs life in patients with AIDS. Use AZT in patients with CD4 <500 cells/mm³.
- Opportunistic infections are uncommon at CD4 counts >200 cells/mm³.
- PCP is the major HIV complication.
- Herpes simplex infections can be severe and recurrent.
- *Candida* and *Cryptococcus* are the major fungal infections.
- *MAI* infection is a late-stage occurrence and a leading cause of death.
- Persons with early or midspectrum HIV infections demonstrate satisfactory postsurgical healing.
- Careful surgical technique can provide protection for health care provider and patient.

REFERENCES

1. Barre-Sinoussi F, Chermann JC, Rey F, et al. Isolation of a T-lymphotropic retrovirus from a patient at risk for acquired immune deficiency syndrome. Science 220:868-871, 1983.
2. Jackson JB, Kwok SY, Sninsky JJ, et al. Human immunodeficiency virus type 1 detected in all seropositive symptomatic and asymptomatic individuals. J Clin Microbiol 28:16-19, 1990.
3. Ou C-H, Kwok S, Mitchell SW, et al. DNA amplification for direct detection of HIV-1 in DNA of peripheral blood mononuclear cells. Science 239:295-297, 1988.
4. St. Louis ME, Rauch KJ, Petersen LR, et al. Seroprevalence rates of human immunodeficiency virus infection at sentinel hospitals in the United States. N Engl J Med 323:213-218, 1990.
5. Daar ES, Moudgil T, Meyer RD, et al. Transient high levels of viremia in patients with primary human immunodeficiency virus type 1 infection. N Engl J Med 324:961-964, 1991.
6. Centers for Disease Control. Guidelines for prophylaxis against *Pneumocystis carinii* pneumonia for persons infected with human immunodeficiency virus. MMWR 38:1-9, 1989.
7. Rutherford GW, Lifson AR, Hessol NA, et al. Course of HIV-1 infection in a cohort of homosexual and bisexual men: An 11 year follow-up study. Br Med J 301:1183-1187, 1990.
8. Volberding PA, Lagakos SW, Koch MA, et al. Zidovudine in asymptomatic human immunodeficiency virus infection. A controlled trial in persons with fewer than 500 CD4-positive cells per cubic millimeter. N Engl J Med 322:941-949, 1990.
9. Fischl MA, Richman DD, Hansen N, et al. The safety and efficacy of zidovudine (AZT) in the treatment of subjects with mildly symptomatic human immunodeficiency virus type 1 (HIV) infection. A double-blind, placebo-controlled trial. Ann Intern Med 112:727-737, 1990.
10. Hoth DF Jr, Myers MW. Current status of HIV therapy. I. Antiretroviral agents. Hosp Pract 26:174-179, 183-184, 189, 197, 1991.
11. Crowe SM, Carlin JB, Stewart KI, et al. Predictive value of CD4 lymphocyte numbers for the development of opportunistic infections and malignancies in HIV-infected persons. J Acquir Immune Defic Syndr 4:770-776, 1991.
12. Bozette SA, Sattler FR, Chiu J, et al. A controlled trial of early adjunctive treatment with corticosteroids for *Pneumocystis carinii* pneumonia in the acquired immunodeficiency syndrome. N Engl J Med 323:1451-1457, 1990.
13. Jacobson MA, Drew WL, Feinberg J, et al. Foscarnet therapy for ganciclovir-resistant cytomegalovirus retinitis in patients with AIDS. J Infect Dis 163:1348-1351, 1991.

14. Cantrill HL, Henry K, Melroe NH, et al. Treatment of cytomegalovirus retinitis with intravitreal ganciclovir. Long-term results. Ophthalmology 96:367-374, 1989.

15. Hardy WD. Combined ganciclovir and recombinant human granulocyte-macrophage colony-stimulating factor in the treatment of cytomegalovirus retinitis in AIDS patients. J Acquir Immune Defic Syndr 4(Suppl 1):S22-S28, 1991.

16. Bozzette SA, Larsen RA, Chiu J, et al. A placebo-controlled trial of maintenance therapy with fluconazole after treatment of cryptococcal meningitis in the acquired immunodeficiency syndrome. N Engl J Med 324:580-584, 1991.

17. Barnes PF, Bloch AB, Davidson PT, et al. Tuberculosis in patients with human immunodeficiency virus infection. N Engl J Med 324:1644-1650, 1991.

18. Horsburgh CR Jr. *Mycobacterium avium* complex infection in the acquired immunodeficiency syndrome. N Engl J Med 324:1332-1338, 1991.

19. Nelson MR, Shanson DC, Barter GJ, et al. *Pseudomonas* septicaemia associated with HIV. AIDS 5:761-763, 1991.

20. Jacobson MA, Gellermann H, Chambers H. *Staphylococcus aureus* bacteremia and recurrent staphylococcal infection in patients with acquired immunodeficiency syndrome and AIDS-related complex. Am J Med 85:172-176, 1988.

21. Wiley CA, Nelson JA. Human immunodeficiency virus: Infection of the nervous system. Curr Top Microbiol Immunol 160:157-172, 1990.

22. Singer P, Rothkopf MM, Kvetan V, et al. Risks and benefits of home parenteral nutrition in the acquired immunodeficiency syndrome. J Paren Enter Nutr 15:75-79, 1991.

23. Wachter RM, Russi MB, Bloch DA, et al. *Pneumocystis carinii* pneumonia and respiratory failure in AIDS. Improved outcomes and increased use of intensive care units. Am Rev Respir Dis 143:251-256, 1991.

24. Ferguson CM. Surgical complications of human immunodeficiency virus infection. Am Surg 54:4-9, 1988.

25. Buehrer JL, Weber DJ, Meyer AA, et al. Wound infection rates after invasive procedures in HIV-1 seropositive versus HIV-1 seronegative hemophiliacs. Ann Surg 211:492-498, 1990.

26. Brown B, Steed DL, Webster MW, et al. General surgery in adult hemophiliacs. Surgery 99:154-159, 1986.

27. Gerberding JL. Reducing occupational risk of HIV infection. Hosp Pract 26:61-68, 73-76, 1991.

28. Centers for Disease Control. Recommendations for preventing transmission of human immunodeficiency virus and hepatitis B virus to patients during exposure-prone invasive procedures. MMWR 40:1-8, 1991.

29. Fauci AS. Optimal immunity to HIV—Natural infection, vaccination, or both? N Engl J Med 324:1733-1735, 1991.

CHAPTER 42

Burns, Electrical Injury, and Hypothermia and Frostbite

David H. Ahrenholz · Lynn D. Solem

BURNS

Burns are a major cause of morbidity and mortality in the United States. In 1985, fires were the cause of injury to 1.4 million persons; more than 54,000 patients required hospitalization for treatment of burns, and 5700 burn-related deaths occurred. Among burn patients, death is most commonly caused by carbon monoxide poisoning during a house fire.[1]

Four types of energy cause burn wounds: thermal, electrical, chemical, and radiation. Thermal injury accounts for 85% to 90% of burns in the United States. Chemical and electrical injuries comprise the vast majority of the remainder.

The severity of any burn is determined by the age of the patient, the depth of the burn, and the size of the wound measured as a percentage of total body surface area (TBSA). Burns are described as first-, second-, or third-degree (Fig. 42-1). A first-degree burn involves only the epidermis. This type of burn is erythematous but does not blister, and it heals in 3 to 6 days without sequelae. Sunburn is a typical first-degree burn. A superficial second-degree burn involves the entire epidermis and superficial portions of the dermis. The skin is blistered with a moist and weeping base. In children under 10 years, a superficial second-degree burn will heal in less than 2 weeks; in adults, healing takes less than 3 weeks. Second-degree burns produce minor color changes but not hypertrophic scarring. Patients with first-degree and superficial second-degree burns are usually treated as outpatients.

A deep second-degree burn extends through the epidermis and into deeper dermis. After blister removal, it is usually dry and demonstrates an ivory or mottled red base. This type of burn requires longer than 3 weeks to heal spontaneously and results in very significant scar formation. A third-degree burn destroys the entire thickness of the epidermis and dermis. A third-degree burn >3 cm in diameter will not heal spontaneously over its entire surface. Since both deep second-degree and third-degree burns produce marked scars, early excision and grafting is indicated after initial fluid resuscitation.[2]

The initial description of the burn includes an estimation of the percent of TBSA for second- and third-degree burns (first-degree burns are always excluded). Three methods can be used to calculate burn size: the "rule of the

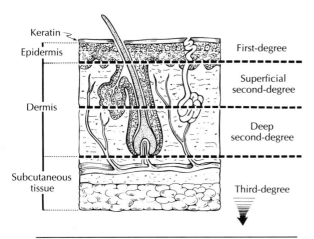

Keratin
Epidermis
Dermis
Subcutaneous tissue

First-degree

Superficial second-degree

Deep second-degree

Third-degree

FIG. 42-1 Simplified diagram of skin burn depth.

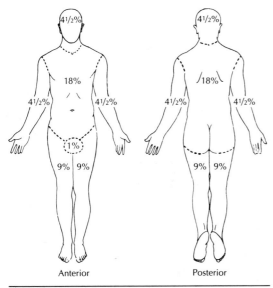

4½%

18%

4½% 4½%

1%

9% 9%

4½%

18%

4½% 4½%

9% 9%

Anterior

Posterior

FIG. 42-2 The "rule of nines" is easy to remember but inaccurate for use in children.

palm," the "rule of nines," and the Lund and Browder chart. For evaluation of small or scattered burns, the rule of the palm states that the patient's palm, excluding the fingers and the thumb, equals approximately 1% of the patient's TBSA. According to the rule of nines the major body surfaces can be expressed as multiples of 9% of TBSA in adults (Fig. 42-2). The head and the neck comprise approximately 9%, each arm and hand together represent 9%, the

anterior and the posterior trunk are 18% each (two nines), each leg is 18% (two nines), and the perineum comprises 1%. Since the rule of nines is very inaccurate for children under the age of 10, the Lund and Browder chart is a better tool for estimating burn size in that age group (Fig. 42-3).[3]

Initially, the burn patient's ABCs (airway, breathing, and circulation) are evaluated as for any trauma patient.[4] After the evaluation of ABCs and the primary survey, a short history is obtained and a rapid physical examination is performed. The medical history should include current medications, allergies, past and present medical illnesses, smoking history, use of drugs and/or alcohol, and the status of tetanus prophylaxis.

Next, a secondary head-to-toe survey is performed. Accidents can produce associated injuries that range from minor abrasions and lacerations, tympanic membrane rupture, or corneal abrasions to severe intra-abdominal, thoracic, and skeletal injuries. A burn injury alone does not acutely alter the patient's level of consciousness. Patients in a state of confusion or coma immediately after injury must be evaluated for significant smoke inhalation, closed head injury, or intoxication with alcohol or other drugs.

Initial laboratory evaluation for a major burn includes complete blood count (with platelet count), electrolytes, BUN, creatinine, liver function tests, and urinalysis. Measurements of ABG and carbon monoxide concentration are obtained for patients with suspected inhalation injury or a history of pulmonary dysfunction. Patients with a major burn injury (>40% TBSA in patients <60 years old and all patients >60 years old) require continuous cardiac monitoring.

Fluid Resuscitation

During the initial assessment of the patient, two large-bore intravenous catheters are inserted, preferably in an unburned upper extremity (Fig. 42-4). Lower extremity intravenous catheters or cutdowns should be avoided because they are associated with a high incidence of septic phlebitis.[5] We prefer that central venous catheter sites be reserved for later use.

AGE VS AREA

Area	Birth-1 yr	1-4 yr	5-9 yr	10-14 yr	15 yr	Adult	Second-degree	Third-degree	Total	Donor areas
Head	19	17	13	11	9	7				
Neck	2	2	2	2	2	2				
Ant. trunk	13	13	13	13	13	13				
Post. trunk	13	13	13	13	13	13				
R. buttock	2½	2½	2½	2½	2½	2½				
L. buttock	2½	2½	2½	2½	2½	2½				
Genitalia	1	1	1	1	1	1				
R. U. arm	4	4	4	4	4	4				
L. U. arm	4	4	4	4	4	4				
R. L. arm	3	3	3	3	3	3				
L. L. arm	3	3	3	3	3	3				
R. hand	2½	2½	2½	2½	2½	2½				
L. hand	2½	2½	2½	2½	2½	2½				
R. thigh	5½	6½	8	8½	9	9½				
L. thigh	5½	6½	8	8½	9	9½				
R. leg	5	5	5½	6	6½	7				
L. leg	5	5	5½	6	6½	7				
R. foot	3½	3½	3½	3½	3½	3½				
L. foot	3½	3½	3½	3½	3½	3½				
						TOTAL				

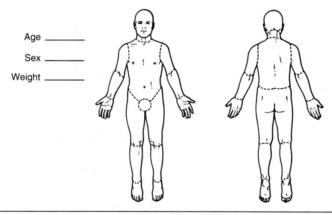

Age _____

Sex _____

Weight _____

FIG. 42-3 The Lund and Browder diagram accurately estimates burn size, especially in children less than 10 years old. (From Lund CC, Browder NC. The estimation of areas of burns. Surg Gynecol Obstet 79:352, 1944.)

Patients with a significant burn (>20% TBSA) require placement of a Foley catheter for monitoring of fluid resuscitation and urinary output. A nasogastric tube should be placed in patients with burns >25% to 30% of TBSA because such patients frequently develop an ileus and are at risk for vomiting and aspiration.

Patients with second- and third-degree burns that are >10% of TBSA usually require fluid resuscitation. The Parkland formula is the most widely used type, although several others are also very satisfactory. With the Parkland formula, 2 to 4 ml Ringer's lactate/kg/%TBSA burn is infused during the first 24 hours, with half given in the first 8 hours. The fluid infusion is titrated to maintain a urine flow of 0.5 to 1 ml/kg/hr.

Patients with >50% TBSA burns, significant inhalation injury (carboxyhemoglobin >10%), facial burns, or circumferential neck burns are at risk for developing airway com-

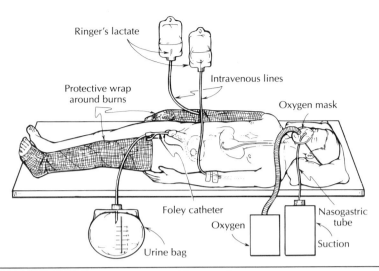

FIG. 42-4 Patient prepared for burn treatment and/or transfer.

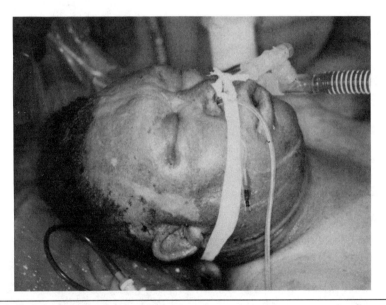

FIG. 42-5 Facial edema 24 hours after burn injury.

promise. Early endotracheal intubation will protect the patient's airway and reduce the risk of sudden airway occlusion by edema (Fig. 42-5).

The initial fluid resuscitation with Ringer's lactate solution is complete at 24 hours. The IV fluids are then changed to D$_5$W at a maintenance rate. Plasma replacement has been advocated in the first 8 hours of the second 24-

hour period, with 0.3 to 0.5 ml colloid/kg/% burn to replace the plasma losses of the first 24 hours. Because of the costs and the risk of infection associated with blood products, colloid replacement is not widely used.

Urine output, blood pressure, and pulse are monitored hourly during fluid resuscitation. Since all invasive monitoring is associated with infectious complications, it should be used sparingly.[6] The white blood cell count initially should be repeated every 6 hours since leukopenia often occurs in the first 48 hours.[7]

Treatment

The wound should be washed gently, and all blisters should be debrided. Silver sulfadiazine is the most commonly used topical antibiotic. However, for burns of the face and neck, or for small burns elsewhere, bacitracin is equally effective and less expensive. Selected superficial burns may be treated with pigskin or a nylon sheet (Biobrane).

In patients with large burns, silver sulfadiazine may induce transient neutropenia. Mafenide (Sulfamylon) is an excellent agent, but it causes metabolic acidosis and severe wound pain. Therefore sulfamylon is used less commonly than silver sulfadiazine.

Debridement and dressing of the burn wound cause severe pain, especially if the burn injury is superficial. Intravenous narcotics are used initially because absorption of subcutaneous and intramuscular injections is unpredictable. Oral narcotics and anxiolytic agents can be used later in selected patients. Nonnarcotic analgesics are ineffective when used alone in the treatment of burn pain.

Deeply burned skin is inelastic and does not accommodate the swelling from edema fluid during resuscitation. Circumferential burns of the extremities, trunk, or neck require early escharotomy with a scalpel, electrocautery, or a topical enzyme preparation such as sutilains ointment (Travase) to prevent impaired ventilation or blood flow. The patient is placed in the anatomic position (palms forward) when a medial or lateral escharotomy is performed on the extremities; the escharotomy must not cross the antecubital fossa or the olecranon (Fig. 42-6). On the dorsum of the hand, an escharotomy paralleling the extensor tendons should overlap a forearm escharotomy at the wrist to avoid constriction. Escharotomies of the index, long, and ring fingers are placed on the ulnar side of the fingers and the radial side of the small finger. An escharotomy on the thumb may be placed on either the radial or the ulnar side.

Incisions must divide all deep dermal bands to allow the involved part to swell freely. When deep second-degree burns require escharotomy, sutilains ointment is a highly satisfactory agent.

Metabolic Support

Nutritional support is critical to the survival of the patient with major burns.[8] Radiographic placement of a nasojejunal tube allows early enteral feeding without the complications of parenteral alimentation. Aggressive nutritional support improves survival, reduces infection, and prevents Curling's ulcer.[9] We estimate energy needs with the Harris-Benedict and Curreri formulas, measure nitrogen losses, add estimated wound losses, administer a calorie:nitrogen ratio feeding of 120 to 150:1, and chart nitrogen balance and body weight.[10,11] Enteral feedings are preferred, but parenteral supplementation is used for patients with marked ileus or diarrhea.

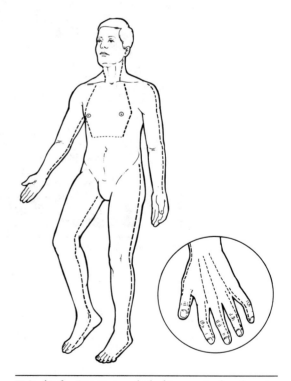

FIG. 42-6   Recommended placement of escharotomies.

Early Excision and Grafting

Wounds that are so deep that they will not heal within 3 weeks in the adult or 2 weeks in the child are best treated by early excision and grafting.[2] Excision (with a tourniquet placed) and immediate autografting or homografting have significantly reduced blood losses in grafting burns of the extremities. The deepest burns require excision to fascia, but the cosmetic results are poor.

Late Management

Once the wound has fully epithelialized, lengthy follow-up by the burn team is required to control hypertrophic burn scars. The use of continuous pressure garments and orthoses combined with an aggressive therapy program provide optimal functional and cosmetic outcome.[12] Grafting should not be performed by a team unable to provide such long-term care.

Itching and skin dryness are major problems associated with burns since burned skin or donor sites do not produce adequate natural oils and moisturizers. Commercially available lotions (e.g., Vaseline Intensive Care Lotion) significantly reduce pruritus. Antihistamines (e.g., diphenhydramine hydrochloride [Benadryl]) also reduce itching. Low-dose doxepin hydrochloride also can be helpful. More severe itching may respond to the use of a mechanical vibrator.

Skin hyperpigmentation is commonly associated with repeated injury (sunburn, windburn, or frostbite) in the first year after burn injury. Patients are advised to avoid any sun exposure while the burn areas remain erythematous since sunscreen agents do not prevent skin hyperpigmentation.

Burns may cause severe psychologic effects, and therefore early intervention is always indicated. Prompt return of the patient to his/her normal activities, including self-care, school, and vocational and avocational activities, is crucial.

Aggressive treatment of hypertrophic burn scars minimizes the need for further surgical treatment. Reconstruction of the burn, when indicated, is best undertaken after the hypertrophic scar has matured, usually at 18 to 24 months after healing. It is important to allow the patient, if of an appropriate age, to direct the timing and scope of these interventions.

ELECTRICAL INJURY

Electrical burns can result from conduction of electrical energy through tissue or from heat released as the current arcs through the air. Current arcs generate temperatures as high as 3000° C, secondarily ignite clothing, and add surface thermal injury to the conduction injury.

Low-voltage current can cause fatal cardiac dysrhythmias. Characteristically, survivors of injury caused by low-voltage current have minimal internal injuries. The current is concentrated at the entrance and exit sites; at these points, tissue may be charred. High-voltage current may damage tissue anywhere along its route, but the most severe damage typically occurs in the digits and distal extremities.

Serum creatine kinase (CK) is a sensitive indicator of total muscle damage after electrical burns.[13] In our series of 116 patients, patients with a total CK <400 IU had no significant tissue loss, whereas patients with a total CK >2500 IU were at risk for major amputation. The intermediate risk group of 400 to 2500 IU of CK had a less predictable course. Eighty-four percent of the 32 patients with a total CK >10,000 IU suffered major amputation or permanent neurologic deficits.

Because CK-MB is released by skeletal muscle after high-voltage electrical injury, myocardial injury must be diagnosed with ECG and clinical criteria.[14] Fortunately, significant cardiac injury is rare after electrical accidents.

The patient with an electrical injury requires the usual evaluation of ABCs,[3] insertion of large-bore intravenous lines, and placement of a Foley catheter. Adequate fluid resuscitation is begun immediately to maintain urine output at 75 to 100 cc/hr. Myoglobinuria, detectable through brownish-black urine, is easily treated with adequate fluid resuscitation, alkalinization of the urine, and, if necessary, intravenous administration of mannitol. Fasciotomy and operative wound debridement are performed immediately, and devitalized muscle is debrided. Carpal tunnel releases are performed on involved forearms. Early guillotine amputation, with care taken to salvage as much skin and subcutaneous tissue as possible, is required for extremities that remain nonperfused after fasciotomy. Wounds are packed open and debrided every 48 to 72 hours until only viable tissue remains. Skin grafts can be used to achieve closure of most wounds, but free tissue flaps may be necessary to cover exposed bone, tendons, joints, or neurovascular structures. This protocol minimizes tissue loss, avoids renal failure, results in early wound closure, and speeds rehabilitation. Despite these measures, many patients have prolonged psychologic and neurologic effects.[15]

HYPOTHERMIA AND FROSTBITE

Hypothermia is a clinical condition in which body temperature falls below 95° F (35° C). Hypothermia causes no long-term morbidity, whereas frostbite, in which tissue has been frozen, results in significant morbidity.[16] Moderate (<90° F or 32° C) to severe hypothermia (<82° F or <28° C) causes severe physiologic changes, including deterioration of mental function, decreased circulating blood volume, increased blood viscosity, and cold diuresis.

Treatment of hypothermia is outlined in the upper box. Mild hypothermia responds to external rewarming, but moderate and severe hypothermia respond best to internal warming measures, including peritoneal, gastric, or thoracic lavage. Unstable patients have been salvaged with cardiopulmonary bypass rewarming. Electrolytes, glucose, and blood gases (corrected for temperature) should be monitored during rewarming.

Frostbite occurs commonly in winter months, especially among homeless persons. The risk is increased with substance abuse or psychiatric illness. Acute frostbite injuries are treated with rapid local rewarming after correction of systemic hypothermia. Gentle local wound care and the use of antiprostaglandin agents (e.g., oral ibuprofen) are indicated (see lower box). Bone scans will aid in identification of poorly perfused digits at risk for amputation,

although tissue mummification usually takes several months. Amputation is always delayed until the tissue demarcates, unless infection supervenes. Following recovery, most patients have recurrent vasomotor symptoms in cold weather.

Emergency Treatment of Hypothermia*

Mild hypothermia: >90° F (32° C)
   Remove wet clothing
   Cover trunk with warm blankets
   Administer warm liquids by mouth
Moderate or severe hypothermia: ≤90° F (32° C)
   Infuse warmed IV fluids
   Begin peritoneal lavage with warmed fluid
     (104°-108° F) (40°-42° C)
   Intubate and ventilate with warm humidified air
   Consider extracorporeal bypass warming

---

*Modified from Ahrenholz DH. Frostbite. In Copeland EM III, Howard RJ, Warshaw AL, Levine BS, Sugarman H, eds. Current Practice of Surgery. New York: Churchill Livingstone [in press].

Frostbite Treatment Protocol*

1. Admit to hospital
2. Rewarm affected areas by immersing in 104°-108° F water (40°-42° C)
3. Debride ruptured blisters and apply aloe vera q 6 hr†
4. Elevate and splint affected parts; place lamb's wool between digits
5. Tetanus prophylaxis
6. Narcotic analgesics
7. Ibuprofen 12 mg/kg po every day for 1 week
8. Penicillin for evidence of infection
9. Daily wound cleansing
10. No smoking
11. Physical therapy once edema has resolved
12. Treatment of alcohol and drug addiction if present

---

*Modified from McCauley RL, Hing DN, Robson MC, et al. Frostbite injuries: A rational approach based on the pathophysiology. J Trauma 23:143, 1983.
†Many physicians substitute daily bacitracin or silver sulfadiazine dressing changes.

SUMMARY

- Four categories of energy cause burn injuries: thermal, electrical, chemical, and radiation.
- Burns are first-degree, superficial second-degree, deep second-degree, or third-degree (see Fig. 42-1).
- The rule of the palm, the rule of nines, or the Lund and Browder chart may be used to estimate the percent of total body surface area occupied by second- or third-degree burns.
- Patients with confusion or coma must be evaluated for significant smoke inhalation, closed head injury, intoxication, or poisoning.
- Patients with >10% TBSA burns require fluid resuscitation. A urinary bladder catheter should be placed in patients with >20% TBSA burn. A nasogastric tube should be used in patients with >25% TBSA burns.

- The Parkland formula provides adequate fluid replacement. Infuse 2 to 4 ml Ringer's lactate/kg/%TBSA burn during the first 24 hours. Half of the estimated volume is infused in the first 8 hours. Infusion is titrated to maintain a urine flow of 0.5 to 1 ml/kg/hr.
- Silver sulfadiazine is the most commonly used topical antibiotic for burns.
- Circumferential burns of the extremities, trunk, or neck require early escharotomy.
- Nutritional support is critical to patient survival, and enteral feedings are effective in providing such support.
- In electrical injuries, serum CK concentrations are sensitive indicators of total muscle damage.
- Hypothermia causes no long-term morbidity. Frostbite causes significant morbidity. The boxes on p. 444 describe treatment of hypothermia and frostbite.

REFERENCES

1. Rice DP, MacKenzie EJ, Jones AS. Cost of injury in the United States: A Report to Congress. San Francisco: Institute for Health and Aging. University of California, and Injury Prevention Center, Johns Hopkins University, 1989.
2. Herndon D, Barrow R, Rutan R, et al. A comparison of conservative versus early excision. Ann Surg 209:547, 1989.
3. Lund CC, Browder NC. The estimation of areas of burns. Surg Gynecol Obstet 79:352, 1944.
4. Advanced Burn Life Support Course [endorsed by the American Burn Association]. Lincoln, Neb.: Nebraska Burn Institute, 1987.
5. Pruitt BA, Stein JM, Foley FD, et al. Intravenous therapy in burn patients: Suppurative thrombophlebitis and other life-threatening complications. Arch Surg 100:399, 1970.
6. Ehrie M, Morgan A, Moore F, et al. Endocarditis with the indwelling balloon-tipped pulmonary artery catheter in burn patients. J Trauma 18:664, 1978.
7. Jarrett F, Ellerbe S, Demling RH. Acute leukopenia during topical burn therapy with silver sulfadiazine. Am J Surg 135:818, 1978.
8. Mochizuki H, Trocki O, Dominioni L, et al. Mechanism of prevention of postburn hypermetabolism and catabolism by early feeding. Ann Surg 200:297, 1984.
9. Watson L, Abston S. Prevention of upper gastrointestinal haemorrhage in burn patients. Burns 13:194, 1987.
10. Curreri PW. Assessing nutritional needs for the burned patient. J Trauma (Suppl 12) 30:S20, 1990.
11. Hildreth MA, Herndon DN, Desai MH, et al. Caloric needs of adolescent patients with burns. J Burn Care Rehabil 10:523, 1989.
12. Rivers E, Fischer SV. Rehabilitation for burn patients. In Kottke FJ, Lehmann JF, eds. Krusen's Hand Book of Physical Medicine and Rehabilitation. Philadelphia: WB Saunders, 1990, p 1070.
13. Ahrenholz DH, Schubert W, Solem LD. Creatine kinase as a prognostic indicator in electrical injury. Surgery 104:741, 1988.

14. McBride JW, Labrosse KR, McCoy HG, et al. Is serum creatine kinase-MB in electrically injured patients predictive of myocardial injury? JAMA 255:764, 1986.

15. Rosenberg D, Nelson M. Rehabilitation concerns in electrical burn patients: A review of the literature. J Trauma 28:808, 1988.

16. Ahrenholz DH. Frostbite. In Copeland EM III, Howard RJ, Warshaw AL, Levine BS, Sugarman H, eds. Current Practice of Surgery. New York: Churchill Livingstone [in press].

CHAPTER 43

Anaphylaxis

Paul Druck

DEFINITIONS

Anaphylaxis literally means a "reversal of protection," but the term is used to describe an unpredictable, rapid, generalized life-threatening reaction caused by exposure to an antigen to which the individual had been previously sensitized (see box, p. 448). Anaphylactoid reactions are clinically similar but are not antigen-IgE mediated. Idiopathic anaphylactic reactions occur without an identifiable pharmacologic or physical stimulus. The more general term "allergic reaction" includes anaphylactic and anaphylactoid reactions, as well as less dramatic, localized responses such as urticaria and isolated bronchospasm. The term "anaphylaxis" will be used generically in this chapter to encompass all anaphylactic and anaphylactoid reactions, unless otherwise specified.

EPIDEMIOLOGY

Anaphylaxis is estimated to occur in 1 of 2700 hospital admissions,[1] but the true incidence may be obscured by misdiagnosis. The two most common inciting agents, beta-lactam antibiotics and iodinated radiocontrast dyes, are each estimated to cause 500 deaths per year; iatrogenic anaphylaxis may thus account for more than 1000 fatalities annually.[1-3] In contrast,

only 60 to 80 deaths are attributed to insect or snake venom–induced anaphylaxis each year.[4]

No well-established risk factors for anaphylaxis exist other than a prior episode in response to the agent in question. A history of atopy (a genetic predisposition to immediate hypersensitivity reactions, present in 10% of the population, and typically manifest as allergic rhinitis, allergic asthma, or allergic dermatitis) does not clearly confer greater risk.[5] However, some retrospective reviews have noted an increased incidence of idiopathic[6,7] and radiocontrast dye–induced anaphylaxis[8] in patients with allergic asthma. Reexposure to the inciting agent does not invariably cause repeat anaphylaxis. The risk of recurrence is only about 10% to 20% with penicillin[6] and 17% to 35% for radiocontrast dye.[9] These findings may reflect historical and diagnostic inaccuracy.

INCITING AGENTS

By far the most common in-hospital causes are the beta-lactam antibiotics (75% of reported cases) and iodinated radiocontrast dyes[1,3] (see box, p. 448). The reported incidence of penicillin-related anaphylaxis ranges from 1 in 2500 to 1 in 25,000 courses, with a fatality rate of 1 per 100,000 courses.[6,10] Iodine-containing con-

Agents Capable of Causing Anaphylactic Reactions

Antibiotics (penicillins, cephalosporins, sulfonamides, erythromycin, vancomycin, streptomycin, polymyxins, tetracyclines)

Iodinated radiocontrast media

Blood and plasma products (transfusion components, antisera, and immunoglobulins)

Therapeutic peptides (insulin, pancreatic enzymes, growth hormone, adrenocorticotropic hormone, vasopressin, streptokinase, chymopapain [for discolysis])

Local anesthetics

Depolarizing and nondepolarizing neuromuscular relaxing agents

Opiates, salicylates, and NSAIDs

Anticancer chemotherapeutic agents

Complex polysaccharides (plasma expanders, iron-dextran complex)

Acetylcysteine

Chlorpropamide

Ethylene oxide

Fluorescein

Hydralazine

Hydrocortisone

Mannitol

Progesterone

Protamine

Quinidine

Thiopental

Thiazides

Seminal proteins

Parasitic infestations (e.g., rupture of echinococcal cyst)

Contact of blood with dialysis or oxygenation membranes

Foods (seafood, milk and egg proteins, wheat, sunflower seeds, mangoes, legumes [peanuts, soybeans])

Food additives (metabisulfites, benzoates)

Insect and snake venoms

Pollen, mold, animal dander

Vigorous exercise

Exposure to cold

Idiopathic (spontaneous?)

---

trast material causes major reactions in 1% to 2% of exposures.[8,9] Other significant causative agents include non–beta-lactam antibiotics, peptide hormones (e.g., insulin, growth hormone), streptokinase, chymopapain, blood products and antisera, opiates, salicylates, NSAIDs, neuromuscular blockers, barbiturates, and some complex polysaccharides (e.g., plasma expanders, iron-dextran). Foods, food additives, and Hymenoptera stings (bees, wasps) may affect hospitalized patients as well. Nonpharmacologic stimuli such as cold exposure and exercise may induce anaphylactoid reactions.[2,5,7,11]

Exposure may be effective by a variety of routes—intravenous, intramuscular, transcutaneous, or transmucosal (gastrointestinal, respiratory, genitourinary, or conjunctival mucosae). Prior exposure (sensitization) is necessary for true anaphylaxis, but may have not been apparent. Anaphylactoid reactions may occur on the first exposure (e.g., contrast dyes, salicylates, opiates, NSAIDs).[7,11]

MEDIATORS
Mechanisms of Response Propagation

True anaphylaxis is initiated when antigen binds to membrane-bound IgE on circulating basophils and connective tissue mast cells. Stimulated cells release preformed, granule-stored histamine and eosinophil chemotactic factor (ECF-a). These cells then rapidly synthesize and release arachidonic acid metabolites such as leukotrienes B4, C4, D4, and E4 (slow-reacting substance of anaphylaxis, or SRS-A) and prostaglandins (notably PGD_2, PGE_2, and $PGF_{2\alpha}$), as well as platelet-activating factor (PAF), heparin, chondroitin sulfate, and neutral proteases (chymase, tryptase). These primary mediators act on target tissues to produce the characteristic symptom complex of anaphylaxis and to stimulate release of secondary mediators such as lymphokines, interleukin-1, lysosomal enzymes, activated complement (C3a, C5a; anaphylatoxins), activated coagulation and fibrinolytic factors, and kinins. Endogenous catecholamines (tertiary mediators?) may be released in response to developing physiologic derangements. Additional substances that may limit the response are released by migrating eosinophils and neutrophils and include histaminase, phospholipase D (inactivates PAF), aryl–sulfatase B (inactivates leukotrienes), and membrane-stabilizing prostaglandins, which may prevent further mast cell degranulation.[2,5,11]

Anaphylactoid reactions are not initiated by IgE-antigen binding; the agent in question acts on basophils and mast cells either directly or through activated intermediates such as complement, kallikrein, or plasmin. A syndrome clinically indistinguishable from true anaphylaxis is then produced by the similar spectrum of released mediators.[2,11]

Idiopathic anaphylaxis may be initiated by the apparently spontaneous release of the newly discovered histamine-releasing factor that is produced by neutrophils, lymphocytes, monocytes, and platelets. Elevated plasma and urine histamine levels have been documented during episodes, suggesting typical mediators are involved.[7]

Specific Effects of Principal Mediators

The H_1 receptor effects of histamine include microvascular vasodilation, increased capillary permeability, bronchial smooth muscle contraction, increased pulmonary secretion, and coronary vasoconstriction. H_2 receptor effects include increased gastric secretion and positive cardiac inotropy and chronotropy.[2,9,11-14] The leukotrienes are by far the most potent bronchoconstrictors elaborated during anaphylaxis. Additional actions include increased pulmonary secretion, increased microvascular permeability, neutrophil chemotaxis, enhanced lysosomal enzyme release, coronary vasoconstriction, and depression of myocardial contractility.[2] The prostaglandins have complex and often opposing effects. PGD_2 and $PGF_{2\alpha}$ cause bronchoconstriction, whereas PGE_2 causes bronchorelaxation. The net effect is believed to be bronchospasm. Pulmonary hypertension, increased microvascular permeability, and vasodilation are also attributed to the prostaglandins.[2] Activated kinins have been implicated in vasodilation (especially bradykinin), increased microvascular permeability, and smooth muscle contraction. Activated complement can also cause increased capillary permeability and smooth muscle contraction, as well as stimulate chemotaxis and additional mediator release from mast cells and basophils.[2,11] A significant negative inotrope, platelet-activating factor decreases coronary blood flow and may depress atrioventricular conduction.[15]

PHYSIOLOGIC CONSEQUENCES

Manifestations of anaphylaxis may occur within seconds of exposure but generally occur within 15 minutes. In rare instances, the reaction is delayed for an hour or more, particularly after oral or cutaneous exposure. In a significant proportion of cases the reaction is biphasic or protracted, perhaps reflecting positive feedback loops between effector cells and secondary mediators or prolonged or episodic absorption or metabolism of the responsible agent.[1] The cardinal manifestations of anaphylaxis are respiratory failure secondary to upper or lower airway obstruction, profound cardiovascular collapse (shock), and generalized cutaneous reactions (see box, p. 450). Of patients dying from anaphylaxis, 70% succumb to respiratory complications and 24% to cardiovascular compromise.[4]

Respiratory Effects

Lower airway obstruction is primarily due to bronchospasm, perhaps aggravated by increased pulmonary secretions and small airway edema. Frank pulmonary edema is uncommon in the absence of *excessive* fluid resuscitation. Wheezing, coughing, dyspnea, and a sensation of tightness in the chest are early symptoms that can worsen rapidly.

Nasal congestion, dysphonia, tongue or buccal swelling, a sensation of a "lump" in the throat, and dyspnea herald the onset of upper airway obstruction, which can also progress rapidly. Intense edema of oropharyngeal structures causes the obstruction that may well be the most common cause of death.[4,16]

Signs and Symptoms of Anaphylaxis

Respiratory

Stridor
Dysphonia
Lump in throat sensation
Swelling of tongue, buccal muccosa
Dyspnea, tightness in chest
Wheezing
Cyanosis
If already receiving mechanical ventilation: increased airway pressure, increased peak/plateau pressure gradient, "auto-PEEP" (automatic positive end-expiratory pressure)

Cardiovascular

Hypotension
Tachycardia
Tachyarrhythmias and conduction disturbances
Myocardial ischemia
If pulmonary artery catheter in place: decreased cardiac filling pressures, decreased systemic vascular resistance, variable changes in cardiac output (usually increased) and pulmonary artery pressures

Cutaneous

Urticaria
Angioedema
Pruritus
Flushing
Pilomotor erection
Diaphoresis

Miscellaneous

Anxiety
Headache
Mental status changes (confusion to syncope)
Seizures
Gastrointestinal and urinary tract hypermotility
Uterine cramps

Cardiovascular Effects

Hypotension is initially due to peripheral vasodilation but is soon complicated by a reduction in circulating plasma volume as increased capillary permeability leads to leakage of plasma proteins and fluid. Decreased myocardial contractility and pulmonary hypertension may interfere with cardiac compensation. Myocardial ischemia, a result of coronary vasoconstriction, arterial hypotension, tachycardia, and hypoxia, can complicate both the diagnosis and the course of the episode. If a pulmonary artery catheter is in place, low cardiac filling pressures and low systemic vascular resistance are observed. Cardiac output may be elevated initially, then decreased as shock and ischemia supervene. Atrial and ventricular dysrhythmias and conduction disturbances may be observed. The most common ECG abnormalities are sinus tachycardia, atrial fibrillation, ST-T wave changes consistent with ischemia, and ectopy. In some cases, large doses of epinephrine may have produced these responses.[2,5,11,17]

Mucocutaneous Manifestations

Mucocutaneous effects are common but not invariable. They may include pruritus, urticaria (superficial, well-circumscribed, blanched, pruritic wheals with raised erythematous borders; hives), angioedema (localized, deep cutaneous, and subcutaneous nonpitting edema), flushing, conjunctival edema, pilomotor erection, diaphoresis, and cyanosis.[2,5]

Miscellaneous Findings

Other findings may include severe anxiety, headache, mental status changes ranging from confusion to syncope, seizures, nausea, vomiting, diarrhea, colicky abdominal pain, urinary urgency, and uterine cramps.[2,5]

TREATMENT

The concurrence of characteristic skin lesions with sudden hypotension and respiratory distress in a previously healthy individual should suggest anaphylaxis. The diagnosis may not be so obvious in a critically ill patient with cardiorespiratory instability, particularly if the syndrome is incomplete or if no temporal relation to administration of a suspicious agent is clear. The differential diagnosis is extensive (see box), but the most common alternatives are airway obstruction (secondary to asthma, chronic obstructive pulmonary disease, or mechanical obstruction), congestive heart failure, or hypovolemic or septic shock.

Initial Steps and Basic Support

With onset of symptoms, the patient should be returned to bed, given humidified oxygen by mask for respiratory distress, and placed in a supine or Trendelenburg position if significant hypotension exists. Continuous ECG and vital sign monitoring are essential; pulse oximetry is desirable. A medical, drug, and allergy history should be obtained, and adequate IV access should be assured. Whether the patient is receiving beta-blockers is particularly relevant with respect to use of non–beta-agonists or high-dose isoproterenol. The ongoing administration of blood products or new drugs should be stopped. Arterial blood gases should be checked as needed, and materials for endotracheal intubation or cricothyroidotomy must be on hand. Because anaphylaxis can progress rapidly, treatment should be aggressive rather than expectant.

Respiratory Compromise
Upper Airway Obstruction

Signs of impending upper airway obstruction require early endotracheal intubation once an upper airway foreign body has been ruled out. If advanced edema has made intubation impossible, prolonged attempts or trials of aerosolized epinephrine should be abandoned and cricothyroidotomy performed.

Bronchospasm

Bronchospasm may be caused by pulmonary vascular congestion, underlying bronchospastic disease, an inhaled foreign body, or occasionally, nebulized inhalers (e.g., acetylcysteine). If the patient is already intubated or tracheotomized, begin ventilation with a hand bag while

---

Differential Diagnosis of Anaphylaxis
Exacerbation of bronchospastic disease (asthma, chronic obstructive pulmonary disease)
Aspiration of foreign body
Hyperventilation syndrome
Globus hystericus
Vasovagal syncope
Septic or hypovolemic shock
Myocardial infarction, particularly if complicated by pulmonary edema or cardiogenic shock
Pulmonary embolus
Drug overdose
Hypoglycemia
Addisonian crisis
Seizure
Carcinoid syndrome
Pheochromocytoma
Systemic mastocytosis
Hereditary angioedema

---

checking for ventilator malfunction, endotracheal tube kinking, plugging, dislodgment or biting, and massive secretions.

If anaphylaxis is suspected, epinephrine is the first-line therapy and may be given subcutaneously for mild reactions or intravenously for severe reactions, particularly if associated hypotension is compromising absorption (see box, p. 452). If IV access is unavailable, intratracheal administration is effective.[2,18] Doses may be repeated at 5- to 10-minute intervals, but if frequent redosing is necessary to maintain a response, continuous infusion with intra-arterial pressure monitoring is indicated.[2,19] If the response to epinephrine is inadequate, IV aminophylline and inhaled bronchodilators should be added. Patients receiving beta-blockers may not respond to epinephrine,[19] and may require prompt doses of non–beta-agonist bronchodilators. If these are ineffective, a pure beta-agonist such as isoproterenol in sufficiently high doses may overcome the beta-blockade without incidental alpha side effects. The only contraindication to epinephrine or other beta-agonists is idiopathic hypertrophic subaortic stenosis. If the response, as assessed

Pharmacologic Therapy of Anaphylaxis

General supportive measures

See text discussion, p. 451.

Bronchospasm

Epinephrine: 1:1000, 0.1-0.3 ml sc q 10 min, if patient is stable

1:100,000, 10 ml slow IV injection if patient is unstable or hypotensive; intratracheal if no IV access available

If frequent redosing necessary:

Epinephrine: 4 μg/ml continuous infusion, beginning with 1 μg/ml*

If ineffective:

Aminophylline: 5-6 mg/kg IV over 20 min, then 0.2-0.9 mg/kg/hr

Metaproterenol: 0.5%, 0.3 ml in 2.5 ml saline via nebulizer

Ipratropium bromide: inhaler, two puffs (36 μg); onset of action occurs about 30 min after dose

Hypotension

See Chapter 2. Fluid rescuscitation (colloid preferred), guided by cardiac filling pressures, target pulmonary capillary wedge pressure = 16-18 mm Hg.

If ineffective:

Epinephrine: 4 μg/ml continuous infusion, beginning with 1 μg/min, titrate to mean arterial pressure ≥ 60 mm Hg* (alternative: isoproterenol, 4 μg/ml, beginning with 1 μg/min*)

If ineffective or patient has tachyarrhythmias, myocardial ischemia:

Norepinephrine: 4 μg/ml continuous infusion, beginning with 1 μg/min,* titrate to mean arterial pressure ≥ 60 mm Hg

Dopamine: 400-800 μg/ml continuous infusion, beginning with 5 μg/min*

For refractory hypotension:

Cimetidine: 300 mg IV injection (consider other causes: myocardial dysfunction, pneumothorax, profound acidosis)

For patient with beta-blockade:

Atropine: 0.5 mg IV q 5 min to relieve bradycardia (target heart rate = 60-80 beats/min

Glucagon: 1 mg IV, then 0.07 mg/kg/hr; monitor hyperglycemia (alternative: isoproterenol, 4 μg/ml, beginning with 1 μg/min to overcome beta-block; weigh risks of dysrhythmias, ischemia*)

Ancillary therapy

H_1-receptor antagonists: diphenhydramine, 1-2 mg/kg IV to maximum 50 mg (alternatives: chlorpheniramine, hydroxyzine)

Steroids: hydrocortisone, 100-200 mg IV q 4 hr, or prednisone, 25-50 mg po q 6 hr for 24 hours

*Requires continuous ECG and intra-arterial pressure monitoring.

by clinical judgment, vital signs, and arterial blood gases remains poor, intubation and mechanical ventilation are indicated. Respiratory rate, tidal volume, and inspiratory flow rate should be adjusted to provide adequate ventilation without excessive airway pressures (e.g., peak airway pressure >60 cm H_2O).[11] Steroids have no role in initial management,[5] but a patient receiving long-term steroid therapy may require stress supplementation.

Hemodynamic Compromise

Hypotension should be treated with recumbency, fluid resuscitation, and, if necessary, pressors (see box). Resuscitation with colloid rather than crystalloid may have the advantage of longer duration of action and lower effective volume.[2] Failure to respond to reasonable fluid loading, particularly in a patient with underlying cardiac disease, necessitates monitoring cardiac filling pressures, preferably with a pulmonary artery catheter. Persistent hypotension (mean arterial pressure <60 mm Hg) with evidence of adequate fluid loading (pulmonary capillary wedge pressure 16 to 18 mm Hg) requires the addition of pressors. If epinephrine administered for bronchospasm produced a favorable pressure response, continuous epinephrine infusion with arterial pressure monitoring should be intitiated. If epinephrine is ineffective or produces excessive tachycardia, or if the patient is receiving beta-blocking agents, norepinephrine is an alternative.[2,11] Dopamine has been somewhat less effective in this setting, but may be useful.[11] If pressors are ineffective, cardiac outputs should be measured to rule out primary myocardial dysfunction, which may be a result of ischemia or the negative inotropic effects of anaphylactic mediators. In this circumstance, ischemia should be relieved or inotropic support instituted as appropriate. Dobutamine is the inotrope of choice (beware of vasodilation at low doses); amrinone also may be effective and may cause less of an increase in myocardial oxygen consumption. If necessary, isoproterenol can be used to raise the heart rate to 60 to 80 beats/ min in a patient with bradycardia and beta-blockade. Glucagon, a nonadrenergic inotrope, may also be useful in the face of adrenergic blockade.[2,5] Finally, if hypotension is unremitting (usually because of profound peripheral vascular collapse) cimetidine may help oppose peripheral H_2-receptor–mediated vasodilation.[2,20]

Adjunctive Measures and Recovery Phase

Additional measures that may help limit the extent or duration of reaction, but are not considered urgent or first-line therapy are parenteral antihistamines such as diphenhydramine and local subcutaneous injection of epinephrine or the intermittent application of a tourniquet at *venous occlusion pressure* to limit antigen absorption from an injection site.[5,11]

Once the patient is stabilized, the principal considerations are preventing relapse (late-phase reaction), identifying the causative agent, and excluding complications such as myocardial infarction, pneumothorax, and aspiration. Late-phase reactions can be prevented by giving high-dose glucocorticoids for 24 hours, followed by rapid taper. Patients should remain under observation for at least 24 hours.[1,5]

PREVENTION

The histories of patients must clearly document all adverse reactions to drugs and foods since

---

Pretreatment Protocol: Emergency Administration of Radiocontrast Media in High-Risk Patients

1. Hydrocortisone: 100-200 mg IV q 4 hr until procedure completed (first dose administered no less than 1 hour before procedure)
2. Diphenhydramine: 50 mg IV 1 hour before procedure
3. Ephedrine (optional): 25 mg po 1 hour before procedure; omit this step for patients with history of ischemic heart disease, history of tachyarrhythmias, significant hypertension, suspected coexistence of aortic dissection
4. Preliminary evidence suggests increased incidence of reactions with H_2-receptor antagonists; there may be potential benefit to holding last dose of a regularly scheduled H_2-blocker before procedure if risk does not outweigh potential benefit.

---

anaphylaxis can be reliably prevented only when sensitivity is known beforehand and reexposure avoided. The two most common situations of intentional reexposure and their management follow.

Iodine-Containing Radiocontrast Material

New imaging modalities frequently offer alternatives to contrast studies in sensitive patients: those with a history of major anaphylactic reactions, unexplained hypotension, wheezing, oropharyngeal-laryngeal edema, angioedema, or urticaria. In those rare instances when the benefit may outweigh the risk, pretreatment regimens (see box) can reduce the risk of recurrent anaphylaxis from the reported range of 17% to 35% to as low as 3% (vs. 1% to 2% for the general population).[21] One study observed an *increased* incidence of major reactions when an H_2-receptor antagonist was added to the pretreatment protocol. In view of this preliminary information, these agents should not be used prophylactically. It may be prudent to withhold doses from patients who are chronically receiving such drugs until the study is completed uneventfully.[9]

Beta-Lactam Antibiotic Desensitization

1. Contraindicated in patients with history of Stevens-Johnson syndrome or exfoliative dermatitis.
2. Perform in consultation with allergy/immunology specialists.
3. Obtain informed consent.
4. Perform in monitored setting with IV access established and all materials necessary to treat full-scale anaphylaxis available.
5. Antiallergic premedication is controversial.
6. Hold beta-blockers if clinically advisable.

Specific procedures:

1. Able to take po: 100 U penicillin (or equivalent dose of other antibiotic)
   a. Administer successive double doses q 15 min until 400,000 U achieved
      (1) For mild cutaneous reaction, repeat dose
      (2) For marked reaction, repeat lower dose after patient stabilizes
   b. Administer 200,000, 400,000, 800,000, then 1,000,000 U IV at 15-minute intervals, as tolerated
2. Unable to take po:
   a. Prepare series of tenfold dilutions of antibiotic and determine lowest reactive concentration on scratch test (<4 mm wheal)
   b. Administer 0.02 ml intradermally of next lower concentration; if no reaction occurs, proceed
   c. Administer successive doubled doses sc q 20 min until therapeutic concentration achieved; repeat dose if reaction occurs
   d. Repeat challenge with therapeutic concentration IM, then IV

NOTE: Once full therapy has begun, avoid lapses in treatment schedule; resensitization may occur rapidly.

Beta-Lactam Antibiotics

In those unusual circumstances when microbiologic sensitivity testing offers no alternative to a penicillin-family antibiotic for a life-threatening infection, desensitization protocols based on the lower antigenicity of enterally absorbed penicillins[22-24] may be followed (see accompanying box).

Estimates of the cross-reactivity between penicillins and cephalosporins varies widely, with 15% being an often quoted but poorly documented figure. If minor reactions are excluded, most studies have demonstrated an extremely low incidence. Generally, cephalosporins exhibit less cross-reactivity among themselves than do the penicillins. Of the newer penicillins, the monobactams (prototype: aztreonam) have demonstrated negligible cross-reactivity with penicillin, whereas the carbipenems (prototype: imipenem) have shown significant cross-reactivity and should be avoided in penicillin-sensitive patients.[6,25,26]

Because antibiotic metabolites are often responsible for allergic reactions, intradermal skin testing with the antibiotic in question is frequently falsely negative and of limited value. If the clinical situation demands a potentially reactive antibiotic and time permits, consultation with allergy/immunology personnel for skin testing with a full panel of antibiotic determinants may offer a higher degree of test sensitivity.[27]

SUMMARY

- Anaphylaxis is an unpredictable, rapidly progressive, life-threatening reaction that may occur without a clear allergic history.
- Death may result from upper airway edema and obstruction, intractable bronchospasm, or cardiovascular collapse.
- Associated clinical features are pruritus, urticaria, angioedema, tachyarrhythmias, cardiac conduction disturbances, and mental status changes.
- Initial therapy includes ensuring a patent airway, administering epinephrine (sc or IV), stopping administration of suspicious agents, and continuous monitoring in the intensive care unit.
- Bronchospasm is treated with epinephrine, aminophylline, inhaled bronchodilators, and mechanical ventilation.
- Hypotension is treated with fluid resuscitation, monitoring cardiac filling pressures, pressors (norepinephrine, dopamine), and inotropes.
- Patients with beta-blockade may not respond to conventional (or any) doses of beta-agonists.
- Adjunctive therapy includes antihistamines; steroids to prevent prolonged or biphasic reactions; exclusion of complications such as myocardial infarction, pneumothorax, and aspiration; postreaction observation, and identification of responsible agent.
- Pretreatment protocols reduce risk of anaphylaxis during life-saving administration of high-risk agents.

REFERENCES

1. Stark BJ, Sullivan TJ. Biphasic and protracted anaphylaxis. J Allergy Clin Immunol 78:76, 1986.
2. Haupt MT, Carlson RW. Anaphylactic and anaphylactoid reactions. In Shoemaker WC, Ayres S, et al. Textbook of Critical Care Medicine. Philadelphia: WB Saunders, 1989, p 993.
3. Lasser EC, Lang J, Sovak M. Steroids: Theoretical and experimental basis for utilization in prevention of contrast media reactions. Radiology 125(1):1, 1977.
4. Barnard JH. Studies of 400 Hymenoptera sting deaths in the United States. J Allergy Clin Immunol 52:259, 1973.
5. Bochner BS, Lichtenstein LM. Anaphylaxis. N Engl J Med 324:1785, 1991.
6. Weiss ME, Adkinson NF. Immediate hypersensitivity reactions to penicillin and related antibiotics. Clin Allergy 18:515, 1988.
7. Wiggins CA, Dykewicz MS, Patterson R. Idiopathic anaphylaxis: A review. Ann Allergy 62:1, 1989.
8. Ansell G, Tweedie MCK, West CR, et al. The current status of reactions to intravenous contrast media. Invest Radiol 15(6):S32, 1980.
9. Greenberger PA, Patterson R, Tapio CM. Prophylaxis against repeated radiocontrast media reactions in 857 cases. Adverse experience with cimetidine and safety of β-adrenergic antagonists. Arch Intern Med 145:2197, 1985.
10. Idsoe O, Guthe T. Willcox RR, et al. Nature and extent of penicillin side reactions with particular reference to fatalities from anaphylactic shock. Bull World Health Organ 38:159, 1968.
11. Carlson RW, Bowles AL, Haupt MT. Anaphylactic, anaphylactoid, and related forms of shock. Crit Care Clin (2)2:347, 1986.
12. Capurro N, Roberto L. The heart as a target organ in systemic allergic reactions. Circ Res 36:520, 1982.
13. Feigen GA, Prager DJ. Experimental cardiac anaphylaxis. Am J Cardiol 24:474, 1969.
14. Levi R, Allan G. Histamine-mediated cardiac effects. In Bristow MR. Drug Induced Heart Disease. Amsterdam: Elsevier-North Holland Biomedical Press, 1980, p 377.
15. Levi R, Burke JA. Acetylglyceryl ether phosphorylcholine (AGEPC): A putative mediator of cardiac anaphylaxis in the guinea pig. Circ Res 54:117, 1984.
16. Delage C, Irey NS. Anaphylactic deaths: A clinicopathologic study of 43 cases. J Forensic Sci 17(4):525, 1972.
17. Moss J, Fahmy NR, Sunder N. Hormonal and hemodynamic profile of an anaphylactic reaction in man. Circulation 63:210, 1981.

18. Heilburn H, Hjemdahl P, Daleskog M. Comparison of subcutaneous injection and high dose inhalation of epinephrine—Implications for self-treatment to prevent anaphylaxis. J Allergy Clin Immunol 78:1174, 1986.

19. Barach EM, Nowak RM, Lee TG, et al. Epinephrine for treatment of anaphylactic shock. JAMA 251:2118, 1984.

20. Mayumi H, Kimura S, Asano M, et al. Intravenous cimetidine as an effective treatment for systemic anaphylaxis and acute allergic skin reactions. Ann Allergy 58:447, 1987.

21. Greenberger PA, Halwig JM, Patterson R. Emergency administration of radiocontrast media in high risk patients. J Allergy Clin Immunol 77:630, 1986.

22. Sogn DD. Prevention of allergic reactions to penicillin. J Allergy Clin Immunol 78:1051, 1986.

23. Sullivan TJ, Yecies LD, Shatz GS, et al. Desensitization of patients allergic to penicillin using orally administered β-lactam antibiotics. J Allergy Clin Immunol 69:275, 1982.

24. Wendel GD, Stark BJ, Jamison RB, et al. Penicillin allergy and desensitization in serious infections during pregnancy. N Engl J Med 312:1229, 1985.

25. Saxon A. Immediate hypersensitivity reactions to β-lactam antibiotics. Ann Intern Med 107:204, 1987.

26. Saxon A. Immediate hypersensitivity reactions to β-lactam antibiotics. Rev Infect Dis 5:S368, 1983.

27. Solley GO, Gleich GL, Van Dellen RG. Penicillin allergy: Clinical experience with a battery of skin test reagents. J Allergy Clin Immunol 69:238, 1982.

CHAPTER 44

Disorders of Coagulation

Kathleen V. Watson • Gregory M. Vercellotti

Timely recognition and management of hemorrhage and thrombosis are fundamental to surgical critical care. Bleeding is an obligate complication of almost every surgical procedure, and when appropriately anticipated, it can be managed easily. This chapter reviews aspects of the physiology and pathophysiology of bleeding and thrombosis that are important to the critical care surgeon.

PHYSIOLOGY OF CLOT FORMATION

Cessation of bleeding requires three functional components: platelets, blood vessel wall, and clotting proteins. Each component serves a unique and cooperative role in hemostasis. A severe abnormality of one component or a modest abnormality of two or more of these components is likely to result in a bleeding disorder postoperatively.

Incisional (surgical) trauma to blood vessels uncovers vascular subintimal tissue and activates a sequence of catalytic events that culminate in clot formation. *Primary hemostasis* is initiated when circulating platelets are exposed and adhere specifically to vascular subendothelium and its rich content of procoagulant sub-

stances, such as von Willebrand factor, collagen, and fibronectin. Once adherent, the platelets undergo an energy-dependent shape change and release preformed substances that serve several functions: (1) vasoconstriction to control local hemorrhage (mediated by substances such as thromboxane A_2, epinephrine, and serotonin), (2) local activation of clotting proteins to form the fibrin clot, and (3) initiation of blood vessel wall repair (by platelet-derived growth factor and angiogenesis factors).

Secondary hemostasis, or fibrin clot formation, ensues via a highly regulated and interdependent series of catalytic reactions that comprise the extrinsic and intrinsic pathways (Fig. 44-1). The chief and immediate function of the plasma clotting proteins is to form fibrin clot from circulating fibrinogen via the action of thrombin. Thrombin is generated from factor II, prothrombin, by the enzymatic action of the prothrombinase complex (activated factors V, X, VIII, IX), which is linked via a calcium bridge to activated platelet membranes. Under physiologic conditions, either the extrinsic or the intrinsic pathway can independently activate the prothrombinase complex. Laboratory measurement of these clotting proteins is outlined in Table 44-1.

Once liberated, thrombin serves three key roles in hemostasis: (1) cleavage of fibrinogen to fibrin clot (fibrin monomers assemble into a loose reticulum overlying the bleeding site, which is strengthened by covalent cross-linkage under the specific influence of factor XIII; the fibrin clot serves not only as a mechanical barrier to bleeding but also as a template for vessel repair); (2) activation and recruitment of circulating platelets onto the growing thrombus; and (3) modeling and degradation of the clot, or fibrinolysis.

PHYSIOLOGY OF FIBRINOLYSIS

In order for the hemostatic system to work effectively, clot formation must be restricted to the site of hemorrhage. An inordinately large thrombus may obstruct venous blood flow, causing local pain and edema and resulting in the syndrome of phlegmasia cerulea dolens. Complete venous obstruction may increase tissue/compartment pressure to the degree that arterial circulation is compromised. Vascular thrombi also can embolize, with disastrous consequences to the distal vascular beds (e.g., pulmonary embolism). Unopposed activation of clotting systemically in the postoperative setting may lead to the potentially catastrophic complications of disseminated intravascular coagulation.

Limitation of the size and extent of the thrombus is affected by the process of fibrinolysis, a process ultimately regulated by the potent serine protease, plasmin. Plasmin binds and digests fibrin and fibrinogen, and it inactivates factors Va and VIIIa (Fig. 44-2). It circulates as the inactive zymogen, plasminogen, which is, in turn, cleaved into the catalytically active form under the influence of plasminogen activators. Tissue plasminogen activator (t-PA), the most important regulator of plasmin, is secreted constitutively by vascular endothelium and is released in abundance by both thrombin and vasoconstrictors. Plasmin activation by t-PA is enhanced in the presence of both fibrin and fibrin degradation products, thus providing a positive feedback loop for limitation of clot size locally on the luminal surface of the blood vessel.

TABLE 44-1 Commonly Used Laboratory Tests for Hemostasis

Test	Hemostatic Component
PT (prothrombin time)	Factors II, V, VII, X, and fibrinogen
PTT (partial thromboplastin time)	Factors II, V, VIII, IX, X, XII, and fibrinogen
TT (thrombin time)	Fibrinogen
BT (template bleeding time)	Platelet count, platelet function, capillary wall integrity

Naturally Occurring Anticoagulants

Plasminogen activators
Tissue plasminogen activator (t-PA)
Urokinase (UK, SCUPA)
Activated protein C (APC)
Protein S
Antithrombin III (AT III)
Heparin cofactor II
Plasminogen/plasmin
Heparans
Thrombomodulin
Extrinsic pathway inhibitors (LACI, EPI)

Other naturally occurring plasminogen activators include (1) urokinase, which circulates as an inactive single chain (SCUPA, or single-chain urokinase plasminogen activator) complexed to a competitive inhibitor, and (2) the intrinsic pathway, which can work directly (via a complex of factor XIIa, kallikrein, and factor XIa), or indirectly (by high-molecular-weight kininogen-induced release of bradykinin) (Fig. 44-3).

Both free and fibrin-bound plasmin are specifically and rapidly inactivated by alpha-2 antiplasmin. In addition, plasminogen activator inhibitors (PAIs) are abundant in the endothelial matrix and inactivate both t-PA and urokinase.

The body has many other naturally occurring

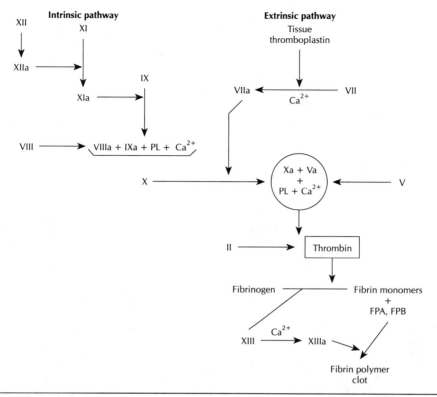

FIG. 44-1 Plasmatic coagulation cascade. PL, phospholipid; FPA, fibrinopeptide A; FPB, fibrinopeptide B.

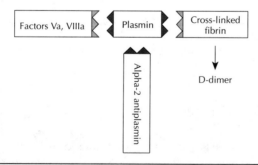

FIG. 44-2 Fibrinolysis. Plasmin inactivates factors Va and VIIIa and degrades cross-linked fibrin, releasing the D-dimer. Plasmin is inhibited by alpha-2 antiplasmin.

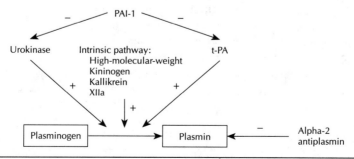

FIG. 44-3 Plasminogen activators (+) and inhibitors (−). PAI-1, plasminogen activator inhibitor; t-PA, tissue plasminogen activator.

anticoagulant devices (see box, p. 458). Whereas free, unbound thrombin is a procoagulant enzyme, thrombin bound to vascular endothelial cells triggers events that limit thrombosis. Thrombin binds specifically and reversibly to thrombomodulin, a glycoprotein present on the vascular endothelial cell luminal surface, and causes (1) activation of protein C (APC) from its inactive circulating zymogen, and (2) release of t-PA. Protein S complexes with activated protein C on the surface of platelets and endothelial cells to proteolytically inactivate factors Va and VIIIa, thus preventing further clot formation.

Free thrombin in the circulation is rapidly and potently inhibited by antithrombin III (AT III). AT III also inactivates factors IX, X, XI, and XII. Its inhibitory activity is greatly accelerated in the presence of exogenous heparin or endogenous heparinoids (present on the vascular luminal surface).

Role of vascular endothelium. Recent biomedical research has elucidated the role of several substances synthesized by vascular endothelial cells in the physiology of hemostasis[1] (Table 44-2).

Although the therapeutic applications of these substances are currently limited, they may play a key role in future postoperative management of bleeding and thrombosis in the SICU.

PATHOPHYSIOLOGY OF HEMORRHAGE AND THROMBOSIS

The elements of normal hemostasis are platelets, clotting proteins, blood vessel wall, and circulating inhibitors. Considering the complexity of the system, the potential for disregulation is great. In general, two serious complications may arise in the postoperative setting: excessive bleeding or thrombosis. Either may be the result of deficiency or malfunction in individual or collective components of hemostasis.

Bleeding Disorders
Preoperative detection

A careful medical history and physical examination are crucial elements for detection of

TABLE 44-2 Endothelial Cell Regulation of Clotting

Factor	Function
von Willebrand factor	Promotes platelet adhesion
Thrombomodulin	Activates protein C
PAI-1	Inhibits fibrinolysis
t-PA	Promotes fibrinolysis
Tissue factor	Activates extrinsic pathway
Prostacyclin (PGI$_2$)	Impairs platelet aggregation (vasodilator)
Endothelial-derived factor	Impairs platelet aggregation (vasodilator)
Relaxation factor (EDRF, NO)	Vasodilator
Endothelins (ET 1, 2, 3)	Vasoconstrictors
Heparan sulfate	Increases antithrombin III activity
	Permeability barrier

bleeding defects. It is necessary to have at least a working knowledge of the fundamental components of hemostasis: (1) formation of the platelet plug on the vascular wall (primary hemostasis), (2) formation of the fibrin clot by a carefully controlled activation of thrombin in the plasma (secondary hemostasis), and (3) degradation and modeling of the fibrin clot (fibrinolysis) (see Figs. 44-1 through 44-3). Disruption of any of these aspects of hemostasis may result in a bleeding tendency.

The medical history must be tailored to the individual patient's illness and anticipated surgical procedure, but in each case particular inquiry should be made about previous complications of surgery, bleeding as a result of trauma, family history, and drug ingestion (see box, p. 462). It is easy to discount excessive bleeding that follows dental extraction or excisional biopsy as a local complication of the procedure when, in fact, it may be a clue to impaired primary hemostasis (e.g., thrombocytopenia, drug-induced platelet dysfunction, capillary fragility). Excessive swelling of the

TABLE 44-3   Hereditary Bleeding Disorders

Disorder	Screening Laboratory Abnormality
Hemophilia A (factor VIII deficiency)	PTT
Hemophilia B (factor IX deficiency)	PTT
von Willebrand's disease	PTT, BT
Rendu-Osler-Weber syndrome	None
Glanzmann's thrombasthenia	BT
Bernard-Soulier syndrome	BT, platelets
Wiskott-Aldrich syndrome	BT

Drugs That Impair Platelet Function

Aspirin	Cephalosporins
NSAIDs	Hydroxychloroquines
Dipyridamole	Miscellaneous (ethanol, antihistamines, garlic, ginger)
Sulfinpyrazone	
Ticlopidine	
Eicosapentaenoic acid	Beta-blockers
Penicillins, semisynthetic penicillins	Methylxanthines (caffeine, theophylline)

muscles or joints following athletic trauma might be attributed to the fervor of the activity when it actually indicates muscle bleeding or hemarthrosis due to a plasmatic clotting protein deficiency such as hemophilia. Details of the family history may disclose a hereditary predisposition to von Willebrand's disease, hemophilia, or other hereditary bleeding disorders (Table 44-3).

The history should focus specifically on ingestion of drugs that may cause a bleeding tendency. A partial listing of such drugs is shown in the box. More extensive lists of offending drugs are available in several review articles.[2,3] Defective platelet function accounts for as much as 50% of nontechnical postoperative hemorrhage. In most cases acquired or drug-induced dysfunction accounts for this abnormality. Drugs may inhibit platelet function by a variety of mechanisms. Aspirin irreversibly inactivates platelet cyclooxygenase by acetylation, preventing generation of thromboxane A_2 and the platelet-release reaction. Other nonsteroidal drugs inhibit cyclooxygenase only transiently and can be discontinued shortly before surgery.

Aspirin and other NSAIDs are used by more than half of patients who undergo unexpected surgery.[4] Although the likelihood of inducing a serious bleeding disorder by the use of NSAIDs alone is very low, their use will magnify the hemostatic defect of almost any other bleeding disorder, for example, von Willebrand's disease or mild hemophilia. Furthermore, in any pathologic state in which hemostasis is compromised, such as uremia or liver disease, NSAIDs will enhance the effect and thereby increase the risk of perioperative bleeding (see upper left box, p. 462). Most of the hereditary platelet functional defects, such as Glanzmann's thrombasthenia and Bernard-Soulier syndrome, are very rare and are best screened for by preoperative medical history.

Screening laboratory tests have an important role in preoperative evaluation in combination with a general evaluation of the patient's clinical status. However, they offer limited predictive value. A normal test will not ensure normal hemostasis. An abnormal test will not accurately predict the severity of bleeding.

Previously unrecognized hemostatic disorders, such as deficiency of factor XIII, which promotes stabilization of the fibrin clot, may not be manifested preoperatively. Conditions such as amyloidosis and scurvy may be associated with profound bleeding despite normal screening laboratory test results (see lower left box, p. 462).

There are very few well-designed clinical studies that document the incidence of perioperative bleeding in comparison to preoperative laboratory screening tests. Rapaport[5] recommends a directed medical history to determine the extent of laboratory testing necessary

Acquired Bleeding Disorders	
Liver disease	Lymphoproliferative disease
Renal disease	Acute leukemia
Malabsorption	Systemic lupus erythematosus
Amyloidosis	
Paraproteinemia	
Myeloproliferative disease	Cushing's syndrome
	Scurvy

Bleeding Disorders Possible With Normal Screening Tests	
Simple purpura	Amyloidosis
Vasculitic purpura	Rendu-Osler-Weber syndrome
Hypercortisolemia	Scurvy
Multiple myeloma	Ehlers-Danlos syndrome
Factor XIII deficiency	
Alpha-2 antiplasmin deficiency	Henoch-Schönlein purpura
Mild deficiency of factors VIII, IX	

Medical Questionnaire for Preoperative Assessment of Hemostatic Function*
1. Have you ever bled excessively or developed swelling after biting your tongue, cheek, or lip?
2. Do you develop large bruises spontaneously?
3. How long have you bled after a dental extraction? Has bleeding ever resumed the day after an extraction?
4. What operations have you had, including minor surgery such as skin biopsies? Was bleeding after surgery ever hard to stop? Did it require a transfusion? Have you ever had unusual bruising in the skin around an area of surgery or injury?
5. Have you had a medical problem within the past 5 years requiring a doctor's care? If so, what was its nature?
6. What medications, including aspirin or any other remedies for headaches, colds, menstrual cramps, or other pains, have you taken within the past 10 days?
7. Has any blood relative had a problem with unusual bruising after surgery? Were blood transfusions required to control this bleeding?

*Modified from Rapaport SI. Preoperative hemostatic evaluation: Which tests, if any? Blood 61:229-231, 1983.

preoperatively (see box at right). On the basis of medical history and physical examination, a hierarchy of recommendations for preoperative laboratory screening for hemostatic disorders is summarized in Table 44-4.

Preoperative management of generalized bleeding condition

Identification of generalized bleeding diathesis portends major risk for intraoperative bleeding and its attendant complications (wound infection, disability from hematomas of joints and muscles, and pressure necrosis as a result of hematoma formation).

Quantitative and qualitative abnormalities of the hemostatic system usually can be identified and treated before surgery with specific component therapy. For example, if the defect is determined to be one of plasmatic phase coagulation, then factors can be replaced with either specific factor concentrates, fresh frozen plasma, or cryoprecipitates to restore a level sufficient for almost normal hemostasis[6] (Table 44-5).

Adjunctive administration of the anabolic steroid danazol may sufficiently raise levels of factor VIII in mild hemophiliacs without the potential infectious hazards of plasma component therapy.

Cryoprecipitate is useful for the management of hypofibrinogenemia, dysfibrinogenemia, and von Willebrand's disease. Patients with mild hemophilia A and those with von Willebrand's disease may benefit from preoperative use of deamino-D-arginine vasopressin (dDAVP), which promotes release of preformed von Willebrand factor from the vascular endothelial cells. This approach also may be taken in patients with uremia and other conditions in which it has been shown to improve hemostasis both in vitro (as measured by increased levels of factor VIII:C, factor VIII:Ag,

TABLE 44-4 Preoperative Laboratory Screening for Bleeding Disorders*

Bleeding Risk	Bleeding History	Surgical Procedure	Laboratory Tests
Minimal (I)	Negative	Minor (e.g., dental extraction)	None
Moderate (II)	Negative	Major, but not high risk (e.g., cholecystectomy, bowel resection)	PT,† PTT, platelet count
High (III)	Questionable or negative	High-risk (e.g., CNS surgery, procedures using cardiopulmonary bypass, prostatectomy)	PT, PTT, TT, BT
Very high (IV)	Positive	Minor or major	Same as for level III If results are normal, BT after ingestion of aspirin‡ Platelet aggregation studies Factor VIII and IX assays TT If these tests are normal, measure plasma alpha-2 antiplasmin, dilute whole blood clot lysis time

*Modified from Rapaport SI. Preoperative hemostatic evaluation: Which tests, if any? Blood 61:229-231, 1983.
†PT necessary only in presence of liver disease, vitamin K deficiency due to poor diet, malabsorption, or use of broad-spectrum antibiotics.
‡Should not be performed on patient who must go to surgery without delay regardless of outcome of test.

and factor VIII:RCo [ristocetin cofactor activity, which is deficient or abnormal in von Willebrand's disease]) and in vivo (in which bleeding time and incidence of bleeding are reduced).[7,8]

Platelet functional defects are managed readily with transfusion of platelet concentrates. For preoperative template bleeding times >15 minutes, transfusion of 6 to 8 units of platelets preoperatively with availability of 6 to 8 units for infusion during the operative procedure is usually adequate.[9]

Transfusion of platelets clearly corrects the disorders of thrombocytopenia when caused by a reduced megakaryopoiesis (e.g., aplastic anemia) but is of limited value alone for the management of destructive idiopathic thrombocytopenic purpura or sequestrative thrombocy-

TABLE 44-5 Plasma Clotting Factors

Factor	In Vivo Half-Life	Level Required for Hemostasis*
Fibrinogen	3-4 days	100 mg/dl
II	2-5 days	20%-40%
V	15-36 hr	<25%
VII	4-7 hr	10%-20%
VIII	9-18 hr	25%-30%
IX	20-24 hr	25%-30%
X	32-48 hr	10%-20%
XI	40-80 hr	15%-25%
XII	48-52 hr	0%
XIII	12 days	<5%
von Willebrand	<6 hr	25%-50%

*Percentage values expressed as percent of normal.

topenia (hypersplenism). In such cases treatment of the underlying condition is imperative. Platelet transfusions can be useful for the rare patient with a hereditary thrombasthenia (e.g., Glanzmann's thrombasthenia, gray platelet syndrome, Wiskott-Aldrich syndrome, Bernard-Soulier syndrome) and even for management of acquired platelet functional defects (e.g., aspirin-induced defects) when bleeding is uncontrolled.

Postoperative management

Prevention of postoperative thrombotic complications has been the topic of medical and surgical literature for decades. The ideal management of them remains controversial.

Full anticoagulation with heparin is associated with a high incidence of postoperative bleeding complications and is inappropriate for prophylactic use. One review has summarized the results of more than 70 randomized trials of perioperative prophylaxis using subcutaneous ("minidose") heparin for patients undergoing general, urologic, orthopedic, or traumatic orthopedic surgery.[10]

Administration of heparin perioperatively reduced the incidence of deep venous thrombosis by 67% for general surgery, 68% for orthopedic surgery, and 75% for urologic surgery. Overall, the estimated risk of pulmonary embolism was reduced 47% when heparin was administered perioperatively. In the untreated control groups, there were 55 deaths attributed to pulmonary embolism, compared to 19 deaths in the treated groups. Results were comparable among general surgical and orthopedic trials. Risk of fatal bleeding was very low and virtually identical for the two groups. There was no evidence that administration of heparin every 8 hours was more favorable than administration every 12 hours (see Chapter 12).

Oral anticoagulation with warfarin is the only therapy that provides adequate protection from progression of thrombosis in patients with preexisting venous thrombosis. The usefulness of oral anticoagulation is limited by the frequency of bleeding complications, the relative difficulty of achieving stable therapeutic values, and the necessary delay in obtaining sufficient

anticoagulation. A target prothrombin time of 1.5 times the control value is now considered to provide adequate anticoagulation while minimizing the risk of hemorrhage in surgical patients. Recently, many hospital laboratories have begun to report the International Normalized Ratio (INR) along with the prothrombin time for patients receiving warfarin.[11] The INR is determined by comparing the patient's prothrombin time (PT) to a mean normal prothrombin time (MPT) based on the International Sensitivity Index (ISI) for the particular thromboplastin and instrument being used, where $INR = (PT/MPT)^{ISI}$. INRs should improve the standardization of oral anticoagulant therapy. Yet the INR is applicable only to patients taking warfarin.

Dextrans have been widely used to prevent postoperative thrombosis. They are branched polysaccharides that, when administered intravenously, are thought to inhibit platelet function by direct absorption and to interfere with the polymerization of fibrin. Although dextrans may be effective for prevention of thrombosis in high-risk patients, their complication rate and cost are considerable. Complications include bleeding, allergic reaction, renal failure, and pulmonary edema from volume overload. Dextrans probably offer no advantages over warfarin for use in the high-risk patient.

Many imaginative physical methods of preventing venous thromboembolism have been developed. These include simple elastic stockings, electrical stimulation of calf muscles, and intermittent external pneumatic compression of the calves. Of these, only external pneumatic compression has been demonstrated to effectively prevent deep venous thrombosis. This relatively new method may prove to be very useful when used in combination with other means of thrombosis prophylaxis, particularly since it carries no risk of bleeding.

The American College of Chest Physicians recommends the following prophylactic measures for venous thromboembolism[12]:

1. Moderate- to high-risk patients should be treated with heparin, 5000 units subcutaneously every 12 hours, or with intermittent pneumatic compression.

2. Patients undergoing neurosurgical procedures, urologic surgery, and major knee surgery should be treated with intermittent pneumatic compression.
3. Patients undergoing elective hip surgery should be treated prophylactically with adjusted-dose heparin (to prolong the activated PTT in the upper half of the normal range) or moderate-dose warfarin sodium (to prolong the PT to 1.3 to 1.5 times control).
4. Patients undergoing surgery for fractured hips should be treated prophylactically with moderate-dose warfarin sodium.

Thrombotic Disorders

Surgery is a major risk for thrombosis with subclinical deep venous thrombosis, occurring in 20% to 30% of patients. Surgery is thrombogenic for a number of reasons: obligate release of tissue factor during even the cleanest incision of tissue, venous stasis immobilization, and decreased fibrinolytic activity occurring within 24 hours of surgery. Most thrombotic complications can be anticipated preoperatively through a careful medical history and physical examination. Causes of hereditary and acquired thrombotic disorders are listed in the upper and middle boxes.

Acute disseminated intravascular coagulation

Acute disseminated intravascular coagulation (DIC) is a common postoperative complication. This condition can be described clinically and pathologically as a complex and paradoxical picture of concurrent hemorrhage and microvascular thrombosis, resulting from acquired abnormalities of all three functional components of hemostasis: platelets, clotting proteins, and blood vessel.[13] Rapid identification of the underlying cause of DIC is imperative for its successful management (see lower box).

Chief among the causes of DIC in the SICU is Gram-negative bacterial sepsis, which has a mortality of 40% to 90%. Endotoxin, a component of the outer cell wall of Gram-negative bacteria, is responsible for the animal model analog of DIC, the Shwartzman reaction. Injection of endotoxin into animals causes hypotension, leukopenia, thrombocytopenia, microvascular thrombosis, and organ failure. Activation of DIC during endotoxinemia has been attributed to several causes, including (1) induction

---

Causes of Hereditary Thrombotic Disorders

Protein C deficiency
Protein S deficiency
Antithrombin III deficiency/abnormality
Heparin cofactor II deficiency
Dysfibrinogenemia
Plasminogen deficiency
Diminished plasminogen activator activity

Acquired Predisposition to Thrombosis

Malignancy	Myeloproliferative disease
Congestive heart failure	Sickle cell disease
Trauma	Paroxysmal nocturnal hemoglobinuria
Pregnancy	
Oral contraceptives	Lupus inhibitor
Cigarette use	Nephrotic syndrome

Causes of Acute DIC

Obstetric complications	*Infection*
Eclampsia/pre-eclampsia	Sepsis
Amniotic fluid embolism	Toxic shock syndrome
	Viremia
Cardiovascular disease	Fungemia
Aneurysm	
Acute myocardial infarction	*Malignancy*
	Hematologic malignancies
Trauma	Solid organ tumors
Massive blunt trauma	
Burns	
Heat stroke	

of tissue factor expression by vascular endothelial cells and monocytes; (2) depletion of AT III; (3) activation of the intrinsic pathway via factor XII; (4) stimulation of platelet activating factor; (5) inhibition of the release of prostacyclin; (6) down-regulation of thrombomodulin and decrease in activated protein C; (7) release of the monokines, tumor necrosis factor (TNF) and interleukin 1 (IL-1); (8) and interference with plasminogen activator (PAI-1).[14]

Laboratory diagnosis of acute DIC should include evaluation of clotting proteins plus complete blood counts and peripheral blood morphology (see box). Thrombocytopenia is a seminal complication of DIC. It occurs in the early stage of this condition and, if severe, presages major problems. Thrombocytopenia occurs as a result of decreased platelet survival from immune destruction and rapid consumption when thrombin is generated in excess.

Clotting factors II, V, X, and XIII, fibrinogen, and AT III are rapidly depleted by thrombin proteolysis. Depletion of these factors is determined by both the plasma half-life (see Table 44-5) and the rate of factor synthesis by the liver. When hepatic function is impaired by hypoperfusion, trauma, medication, or infection, clotting protein production is suboptimal, resulting in a hemostatic imbalance that leads to bleeding and thrombosis.

Measurement of factor V, which is rapidly degraded by plasmin and is often the first factor to fall in acute DIC, can be very useful. D-dimer is a specific cleavage product of plasmin-mediated proteolysis of cross-linked fibrin, unlike fibrin degradation products, which are derived from both fibrin or fibrinogen. Levels of D-dimer may be elevated in any state of thrombosis but are uniformly very high in DIC.

Rapid recognition and treatment of the primary underlying disease is crucial for successful management of DIC. Regardless of the etiology—sepsis, malignancy, vasculitis, trauma, vascular injury, or catastrophic complications of pregnancy—the coagulopathic condition can be contained only when the initiating process is controlled. Vitamin K should be administered in all cases. If the plasma fibrinogen falls

---

Laboratory Diagnosis of Acute DIC

Abnormal screening tests: PT, PTT, TT
Decreased platelets
Decreased fibrinogen
Fragmented red blood cells (schistocytes)
Increased D-dimer
Elevated fibrin degradation products

---

rapidly or falls below 100 mg/dl, cryoprecipitate should be infused. Platelet transfusion requirements may vary greatly among patients; in general platelet transfusions are indicated to prevent bleeding complications. Heparin may be useful, but because of the concomitant hazards of bleeding and heparin-associated thrombocytopenia, its use must be individualized. Newer approaches to management of DIC include infusions of alpha-2 antiplasmin or epsilon-aminocaproic acid plus heparin, and the use of hirudin.

Heparin-associated thrombocytopenia

Heparin is ubiquitous in the SICU—as an anticoagulant for intra-arterial catheters, for hemodialysis, and for routine perioperative anticoagulation. Thrombocytopenia develops in as many as 10% of patients who are treated with heparin, and platelet dysfunction, manifested as a prolonged bleeding time, may develop even more often.[15-17] Platelet counts may fall as low as $20,000/mm^3$, but spontaneous bleeding rarely results. Instead, disseminated or localized venous and arterial thrombosis may occur in as many as 20% of patients with heparin-associated thrombocytopenia (HAT). The morbidity and mortality of arterial thrombosis in HAT is very high.

Thrombocytopenia typically appears 5 to 10 days after the initiation of heparin therapy. Several factors increase the likelihood of HAT: (1) an animal source of heparin (bovine heparin is more likely than porcine heparin to cause thrombocytopenia), (2) previous treatment with heparin, and (3) administration of high-molecular-weight heparins, which are more immunogenic and therefore more likely to induce HAT. Establishing the pathogenesis of HAT has been difficult. A wealth of evidence supports the view that the disorder is immunologically mediated. Platelet-associated immunoglobulin can be detected in many patients, but it is a nonspecific finding that may occur during sepsis.

There is no specific diagnostic test for HAT. A decrease in the platelet count below 100,000/mm^3 (or 50% of baseline) as well as the occurrence of unexplained arterial or venous thrombosis during heparin therapy should be viewed as highly suspicious for the disorder. Studies of in vitro platelet aggregation and serotonin release that were done in the presence and absence of heparin may be useful but are not sensitive.

Despite the lack of conclusive evidence that cessation of the use of heparin will be beneficial, most clinicians who treat HAT immediately stop administration of heparin. Whenever possible, alternative therapeutic anticoagulation with warfarin, thrombolytic agents, dextran, or experimental treatments such as prostaglandin analogs and plasmapheresis have been used. Low-molecular-weight heparin may prove to be useful in the management of HAT.[18] Platelet transfusion should be avoided because it can precipitate arterial thrombosis. Mechanical interruption of the vena cava with intravenous filters also may be helpful.

Bleeding after cardiopulmonary bypass

Cardiopulmonary bypass (CPB) circuits are used routinely for open heart surgery throughout the world. More than 250,000 open heart procedures are performed annually in the United States alone. Although postoperative bleeding occurs infrequently (0.8% to 5%) following CPB, it may be profound and often requires reoperation. Many hemostatic abnormalities have been identified, and they account for deranged hemostasis, including impaired platelet function, thrombocytopenia, decreased levels of clotting factors, and accelerated fibrinolysis (see box). Further discussion of this

---

Causes of Bleeding After Cardiopulmonary Bypass

Common (95%-98%)

Defective surgical hemostasis
Acquired transient platelet dysfunction

Uncommon (1%-5%)

Drug-induced platelet dysfunction (aspirin)
Thrombocytopenia (HAT, sepsis, posttransfusion purpura, fat emboli)
Vitamin K–dependent factor deficiencies (warfarin, liver dysfunction)
Consumptive coagulopathy (sepsis, cardiogenic shock)
Inherited clotting factor deficiencies or platelet dysfunction

Doubtful significance

Primary fibrinolysis
Heparin (inadequate neutralization, rebound)
Protamine excess

---

topic is beyond the scope of this chapter, but several excellent reviews are available.[9,19]

Management of bleeding complications after CPB includes supportive care with the use of cryoprecipitate, fresh frozen plasma, and vitamin K for patients with acquired deficiencies of vitamin K–dependent factors caused by warfarin or liver dysfunction. Patients with hereditary deficiencies of factors V, VII, X, or XI may be treated with fresh frozen plasma, and cryoprecipitate may be needed for patients with von Willebrand's disease who are undergoing CPB. To date, studies have not demonstrated a beneficial effect of platelet transfusions, and the 1987 National Institutes of Health consensus conference recommended that prophylactic platelet transfusions not be routinely administered after CPB.[20] Other therapies that may have some efficacy following CPB include fibrin glues, aprotinin, desmopressin, epsilon-aminocaproic acid, and the prostacyclin analog Iloprost (Berlex Laboratories Inc., Cedar Knolls, N.J.).

SUMMARY

- Hemostasis requires functional platelets, vascular endothelium, clotting proteins, and circulatory inhibitors.
- Primary hemostasis begins when circulating platelets adhere to endothelium.
- Secondary hemostasis requires a highly coordinated series of catalytic reactions, the extrinsic and intrinsic pathways.
- Fibrinolysis limits the size and extent of thrombosis.
- Plasmin is an important regulator of fibrinolysis. Secreted by endothelium, t-PA regulates plasmin.
- Protein C and protein S are other naturally occurring anticoagulants.
- Vascular endothelial cells regulate clotting (see Table 44-2).
- A careful medical history remains crucial in preoperative detection of bleeding disorders (see box, p. 462).
- Aspirin, NSAIDs, beta-blockers, and dipyridamole are commonly used drugs that inhibit platelet formation.
- The history, physical examination, and proposed surgical procedure should be used to guide preoperative laboratory screening.

- Appropriate clotting factors should be administered preoperatively to patients with deficiencies (see Table 44-5).
- Platelets should be checked preoperatively for platelet deficiency or functional platelet defects.
- Prophylaxis for thrombosis can reduce postoperative thrombotic complications (see also Chapter 12).
- Since surgery is thrombogenic, it poses a major risk for patients with subclinical deep venous thrombosis.
- Acute DIC results from simultaneous abnormalities of platelets, clotting proteins, and vascular endothelium.
- Gram-negative sepsis is the chief cause of DIC in the SICU.
- Control of the initiating process is the most effective treatment for DIC.
- HAT develops in 10% of patients receiving heparin. When HAT is detected, most clinicians discontinue heparin.
- Many hemostatic abnormalities occur after CPB and may cause bleeding complications.

REFERENCES

1. Vane JR, Anggard EE, Botting RM. Regulatory functions of the vascular endothelium. N Engl J Med 323:27-36, 1990.
2. Fuster V, Badimon L, Basfimon J, et al. Drugs interfering with platelet functions: Mechanisms and clinical relevance. In Verstraete M, Vermylen J, Lijnen HR, et al., eds. Thrombosis and haemostasis (Eleventh Congress), 1987, p 349.
3. Triplett DA. Quantitative or functional disorders of platelets. In Triplett DA, ed. Platelet Function. Chicago: American Society of Clinical Pathology, 1978.
4. Ferraris VA, Swanson E. Aspirin usage and perioperative blood loss in patients undergoing unexpected operations. Surg Gynecol Obstet 156:439-442, 1983.
5. Rapaport SI. Preoperative hemostatic evaluation: Which tests, if any? Blood 61:229-231, 1983.
6. Rizza CR. The treatment of hereditary and acquired bleeding disorders. In Bowie EJW, Sharp AA, eds. Hemostasis and Thrombosis. London: Butterworth, 1985, p 259.
7. Kobrinsky NL, Israels ED, Gerrard JM, et al. Shortening of bleeding time by 1-deamino-8-D-arginine vasopressin in various bleeding disorders. Lancet 1:1145-1148, 1984.
8. Mannucci PM, Remuzzi G, Pusineri F, et al. Deamino-8-D-arginine vasopressin shortens the bleeding time in uremia. N Engl J Med 308:8-12, 1983.
9. Bick RL. Hemostasis defects associated with cardiac surgery, prosthetic devices and other extracorporeal circuits. Semin Thromb Hemost 11:249-280, 1985.
10. Collins R, Scrimgeour A, Yusut S, Peto R. Reduction in fatal pulmonary embolism and venous thrombosis by perioperative administration of subcutaneous heparin: Overview of results of randomized trials in general orthopedic and urologic surgery. N Engl J Med 318:1162-1173, 1988.
11. Hirsh J. Oral anticoagulant drugs. N Engl J Med 324:1865-1875, 1991.

12. Sackett DL. Rules of evidence and clinical recommendations on the use of antithrombotic agents. Chest 95 (Suppl 2):2S-4S, 1989.

13. Bick RL. Disseminated intravascular coagulation and related syndromes: A clinical review. Semin Thromb Hemost 14:299-338, 1988.

14. Muller-Berghaus G. Septicemia and the vessel wall. In Verstraete M, Vermylen J, Lijnen HR, et al., eds. Thrombosis and Haemostasis. Leuven, Belgium: Leuven University Press, 1987, p 619.

15. Kelton JG, Levine MN. Heparin-induced thrombocytopenia. Semin Thromb Hemost 12:59-66, 1986.

16. Warkentin TE, Kelton JG. Heparin and platelets. Hematol/Oncol Clin North Am 4:243-264, 1990.

17. Clines DB, Tomaski A, Tannenbaum S. Immune endothelial-cell injury in heparin-associated thrombocytopenia. N Engl J Med 316:581-589, 1987.

18. Hirsh J, Levine MH. Low molecular weight heparin. Blood 79:1, 1992.

19. Woodman RC, Harker LA. Bleeding complications associated with cardiopulmonary bypass. Blood 76:1680-1697, 1990.

20. National Resource Education Program. Indications for the use of red blood cells, platelets and fresh frozen plasma. In Transfusion Alert. Pub. no. 9-297a [abstract]. Bethesda, Md.: National Institutes of Health, 1989.

CHAPTER 45

Transfusions

Elizabeth H. Perry

In the critically ill patient, blood components are transfused for two main reasons: to increase oxygen-carrying capacity and to improve hemostasis. Products derived from plasma such as albumin and plasma protein fraction (PPF) are transfused to increase intravascular volume and are discussed briefly. Blood components are made from donations of whole blood that have been collected in an anticoagulant-preservative solution and made into blood components at a blood center or hospital blood bank (Fig. 45-1). Indications for transfusion and the amount of blood component to transfuse for a desired end result are well established for routine transfusion episodes. The critically ill unstable patient may, however, have unique indications for transfusion that are not covered by standard transfusion criteria. It is the responsibility of the hospital transfusion committee to examine transfusion practices in the SICU to ensure that the practices for transfusion in these patients are acceptable and that the risks of transfusion do not outweigh the benefits (Table 45-1).

BLOOD COMPONENTS AND INDICATIONS FOR TRANSFUSION
Components for Increasing Oxygen-Carrying Capacity

Advances in blood component therapy have made whole blood transfusion less common. The use of whole blood is indicated when a patient needs simultaneous replacement of oxygen-carrying capacity and volume. Hospitals specializing in trauma often carry an inventory of whole blood to use after crystalloid solution resuscitation. Whole blood is stored at 1° to 6° C and contains both RBCs and stable coagulation factors. After refrigerated storage, it does not contain functional granulocytes or platelets, and the labile coagulation factors V and VIII are markedly reduced. Whole blood does contain viable lymphocytes, which may cause graft-vs.-host disease in the severely immunocompromised patient. The main indication for transfusion of whole blood is for active bleeding in patients who have lost more than 25% of their blood volume. Whole blood has a volume of 500 ml/U and contains plasma so that if the patient needs oxygen-carrying capacity alone, RBCs would be a more suitable choice. Because of the anticoagulant-preservative solution that is needed for storage, the hematocrit value of whole blood is 36% to 44%, slightly lower than that of the donor. The transfusion of 1 U of whole blood will increase the hematocrit value in a stable adult by approximately 3%.

RBCs are indicated for increasing oxygen-carrying capacity in anemic patients. One unit of RBCs has the same RBC mass as a unit of whole blood. The hematocrit level of packed RBCs collected in standard anticoagulant-preservative solutions ranges from 70% to 80%, whereas the hematocrit level of RBCs stored in additive solutions to extend the shelf life ranges from 52% to 60%. As with any transfusion, the

TABLE 45-1 Risks and Benefits of Blood Transfusions				
Component	**Description**	**Benefits**	**Risks**	**Expected Result**
Whole blood	500 ml/U Stored at 1°-6° C	Increases oxygen-carrying capacity and replaces blood volume simultaneously	Volume overload; transfusion reactions; disease transmission iron overload; graft vs. host disease	Increases hematocrit (HCT) 3%/U in stable 70-kg adult
Red blood cells	250-300 ml/U Stored at 1°-6° C	Increase oxygen-carrying capacity	Transfusion reactions; disease transmission; iron overload; graft-vs.-host disease; alloimmunization	Increase HCT 3%/U in stable 70-kg adult
Platelets	50 ml/U Stored at room temperature	Control or prevent bleeding from decreased or dysfunctional platelets	Transfusion reactions; disease transmission	Increase platelets 5000-7500 µL/U in stable adult
Fresh frozen plasma	200-250 ml/U Noncellular	Increases level of deficient coagulation factors	Same as platelets	Increases factor 2%-3%/U in adult
Cryoprecipitate	10 ml/U; contains factor VIII, von Willebrand's factor (vWF), fibrinogen, factor XIII, fibronectin	Controls or prevents bleeding in patients with hemophilia A, deficiency of vWF, factor XIII deficiency, or afibrinogenemia, hypofibrinogenemia, or dysfibrinogenemia	Same as platelets	Factor VIII: 80-120 U/bag Fibrinogen: 250 mg/bag

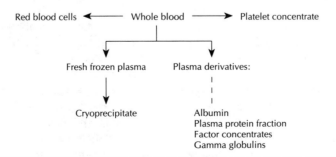

FIG. 45-1   Production of blood components from whole blood.

decision to transfuse RBCs must be made on clinical grounds rather than on any preset transfusion trigger.

Components for Hemostasis

Blood components used to improve hemostasis include platelets, fresh frozen plasma (FFP), cryoprecipitate, and factor concentrates. Platelet transfusions are administered to control or prevent bleeding associated with thrombocytopenia or platelet dysfunction. Platelet concentrates are made from whole blood and are stored at room temperature on a rotator for up to 5 days. The standard dose for platelet concentrates is 1 U (5.5×10^{10} platelets) per 10 kg of body weight. Some blood banks supply platelets in standard pools for adult patients (e.g., "six pack" or "eight pack" of platelet concentrates), whereas other blood banks pool the appropriate dose for each patient at the time transfusion is requested. The former procedure has the benefit that a standard dose is immediately ready for transfusion, whereas the latter has the benefit that the patient gets neither too many or too few donor exposures.

Platelets may also be collected by apheresis, a procedure that provides a number of platelets equivalent to six platelet concentrates (3×10^{11} platelets) collected from a single volunteer donor. This method is used to minimize donor exposures in a patient who is receiving platelet transfusions. Human leukocyte antigen (HLA)–matched platelets are also collected by apheresis. Their use may be indicated in patients who are alloimmunized and refractory to transfusion with platelet concentrates. HLA–matched platelets must be ordered from a blood collection center after consultation with the blood bank or transfusion service.

Guidelines for platelet transfusion have been developed because of the cost of platelet transfusion therapy, the risks associated with unnecessary transfusion, and the need for appropriate use of donated resources. Guidelines usually are developed by each transfusing facility based on data in the literature and are approved by appointed transfusion committees. In general, 1 U of platelet concentrate is expected to increase the platelet count by 5000 to 7500/μl in an adult patient. If the expected

Use of Corrected Count Increments to Determine Responsiveness to Platelet Transfusions

$$\text{Corrected count increment (CCI)}^* = \frac{(\text{Posttransfusion platelet count} - \text{Pretransfusion platelet count}) \times \text{Body surface area}}{\text{Number platelets transfused} \times 10^{10}}$$

Example

Posttransfusion count = 50,000/μL
Pretransfusion count = 20,000/μL
Body surface area = 1.73 m²

7 platelet concentrates transfused = $(7)(5.5 \times 10^{10}$ platelets/platelet concentrate) = $35.5 \times 10^{10} = 3.55 \times 10^{11}$ platelets

$$\text{CCI} = \frac{(50,000 - 20,000) \times 1.73}{3.55} = 14,620$$

This is an adequate response to the platelet transfusion given, and administration of HLA platelets is not indicated.

*An adequate CCI >7,500.

increment is not obtained with an appropriate number of platelet concentrates, HLA-matched platelets are administered after other causes of refractoriness such as splenomegaly, bleeding, sepsis, and disseminated intravascular coagulation (DIC) have been excluded. A corrected count increment, using pretransfusion and 1-hour posttransfusion platelet counts, is a useful tool for determining refractoriness to platelet transfusion (see box). Prophylactic platelet transfusions (i.e., platelet transfusions given to prevent bleeding) may be indicated if the platelet count is <15,000 to 20,000/μL.

FFP is plasma separated from whole blood and frozen within 8 hours of collection. FFP contains 100% of all normal plasma constituents, including coagulation factors, complement components, and other plasma proteins. FFP is indicated for replacement of coagulation factors in patients with documented or suspected deficiency. Each unit of FFP contains 200 to 250 ml of plasma and 1 U of coagulation factor per 1 ml of plasma. FFP is not indicated for volume expansion or replacement of colloidal losses in postoperative patients because the risk of possible transfusion reactions and transmission of viral infections outweighs potential benefits. Alternatives to FFP for these indications include the plasma derivatives albumin and PPF and the synthetic colloids such as hetastarch and dextran.

Cryoprecipitate is another component that is useful for hemostasis. Cryoprecipitate is made from FFP that is allowed to thaw in the cold, forming a white precipitate, which can be separated by centrifugation and stored. Cryoprecipitate contains factor VIII (80 to 120 U/bag), von Willebrand factor (vWF), factor XIII, fibrinogen (250 mg/bag), and fibronectin. Bleeding in patients with hemophilia A (factor VIII deficiency), von Willebrand's disease, inherited deficient or abnormal fibrinogen, and factor XIII deficiency can be treated with cryoprecipitate. It also can be used as a source of fibrinogen for hypofibrinogenemic patients with DIC and for fibrin glue. Cryoprecipitate has been reported to shorten the prolonged bleeding time in patients with uremia; reports of the beneficial effects of using conjugated estrogens and synthetic vasopressin (DDAVP) in patients with uremic platelet dysfunction show a similar reduction in the bleeding time and clinical bleeding without the risk associated with transfusion of blood components.

Factor concentrates are special blood components and include factor VIII and IX concentrates for treatment of hemophilia A and B, respectively, and antithrombin III concentrate, which is used for prevention and treatment of thrombosis in patients with inherited antithrombin III deficiency. Consultation with a hematologist or specialist in the use of these products is necessary before their use.

Volume Expanders

Blood derivatives can be used to restore intravascular volume. Five-percent albumin frequently is used for restoration of intravascular volume in the emergency department and operating room. It is also a useful volume expander in the critically ill hypovolemic patient in the SICU. Albumin is prepared by cold ethanol fractionation and heat inactivation and does not carry the same risks of viral disease transmission as blood components. However, albumin can cause allergic and febrile transfusion reactions. PPF is another plasma derivative made by fractionation and heat treatment, and it contains 83% albumin and 17% globulins. New manufacturing processes have resolved the problem of hypotensive episodes from activation of the kinin system, which had been reported to occur with rapid infusion of PPF. Synthetic colloids such as hetastarch and dextran also may be used to restore intravascular volume. Both of these agents can cause abnormalities in the coagulation screening tests, prolongation of the prothrombin time (PT) and partial thromboplastin time (PTT), and marked shortening of the thrombin time. Anaphylactic reactions and bleeding have been reported with the use of dextrans.

BLOOD TYPING AND SCREENING BEFORE TRANSFUSION

After blood has been collected from volunteer donors, samples undergo testing at the processing facility. These tests include typing of the blood for ABO and Rh blood groups and screening of the donor plasma for unexpected antibodies. These same tests are done on blood from patients for whom a transfusion has been ordered. Blood for transfusion is matched to both the ABO and Rh blood types.

ABO blood group. The ABO blood group is the most important blood group in a transfusion because the naturally occurring antibodies in the ABO group are IgM and they bind complement. Consequently, if ABO incompatible blood is transfused, intravascular hemolysis results. There are two major antigens in the ABO blood group system, A and B, and four major ABO blood groups: A, B, AB, and O. Antibodies to the ABO blood group are formed by exposure to antigens in the gut flora and environment rather than by direct stimulation from incompatible RBC antigens. Therefore they are called *naturally occurring antibodies*. If the A antigen is on an individual's RBCs, he/she cannot make natural antibodies to the A antigen but can make anti-B antibodies to the absent B antigen. A normal person with type A blood has the A antigen easily demonstrable on RBCs and

TABLE 45-2　ABO Blood Group System

Blood Group	Red Cell Antigens	Red Cell Antibodies	Compatible Red Cells
A	A	Anti-B	A, O
B	B	Anti-A	B, O
AB	A, B	None	A, B, AB, O
O	None	Anti-A and anti-B	O

anti-B antibody circulating in the plasma. Table 45-2 shows ABO blood antigens, antibodies, and compatible RBCs.

In emergency situations, if time does not permit determining the ABO blood type of an exsanguinating patient, group O RBCs can be transfused because they do not carry the A or B antigen. Potential serious side effects exist if group O whole blood is transfused to a non-O patient because whole blood also contains plasma, which in a type O blood donor contains naturally occurring anti-A and anti-B antibodies. The likelihood of complications is related to the concentration of antibody in the plasma. If these antibodies are present in low titer, there may be no complications. However, if the antibodies are present in high titer, and the patient is type A, B, or AB, a significant hemolytic transfusion reaction can occur. If emergency transfusion is necessary and there is not time to determine the ABO type, the best approach is to transfuse only group O RBCs until the patient's actual blood type has been determined.

Rh antigen. After ABO, the next most important RBC antigen is the Rh, or D, antigen. The terms *Rh positive (D+)* and *Rh negative (D−)* refer to the presence or absence of the D antigen. Unlike the ABO blood group, antibody to Rh (D) occurs in Rh-negative individuals only after exposure through transfusion or pregnancy to Rh-positive RBCs. The Rh blood group is important because of its immunogenicity. An Rh-negative person who is transfused with Rh-positive blood has a 50% to 100% chance of mounting an immune response and producing anti-D antibody. This antibody is responsible for delayed hemolytic transfusion re-

actions and is the major antibody implicated in hemolytic disease of the newborn. When uncrossmatched blood is released for transfusion, Rh-negative blood is given, if available, until Rh typing can be done on the patient. Once the patient has been confirmed as Rh positive, type-specific blood can be given.

Unexpected antibodies. A third laboratory test done on all donors and patients before a routine transfusion is a "screen" on the plasma for clinically significant "unexpected" antibodies. Antibodies to ABO are "expected" antibodies and are sought in this test. Therefore the screening cells must be group O so that anti-A and anti-B antibodies are not detected.

This test is performed by incubating plasma from the donor or patient with two different screening RBCs that have been selected because they carry the specific RBC antigens necessary to detect the most clinically significant unexpected antibodies. Agglutination or hemolysis in the test tube that contains the screening cells and plasma indicates a positive antibody screen. After incubation at room temperature and at 37° C, the cells are washed with normal saline solution to remove unbound globulins, and anti-human globulin serum (Coombs' serum) is added to the cells. This serum detects nonagglutinating antibody or complement coating the cells. The Coombs' test result is negative if no agglutination occurs. If the result of the entire antibody screening test is negative, a donated unit of blood may then be labeled and put in the blood bank for transfusion if all the required tests for infectious diseases are also negative. If an unexpected antibody is detected by the screening procedure, the donor's RBCs can be used if they have been labeled as having a specific antibody present in the small amount of plasma in a packed RBC unit. The FFP and cryoprecipitate cannot be used for transfusion but can be sent for processing into plasma derivatives such as albumin and gamma globulin. If the antibody screen is negative for a patient, crossmatching can begin to select a unit of blood for transfusion.

Pretransfusion compatibility testing is performed in the laboratory by crossmatching. A major crossmatch is done by mixing the donor's RBCs with the patient's serum. This procedure detects agglutination or hemolysis of donor RBCs by an antibody that might be present in the patient's plasma. If the antibody screen is negative, the main reason for a crossmatch is to ensure ABO compatibility since ABO incompatibility can result in intravascular hemolysis and possibly death. If unexpected antibodies are detected in the patient's antibody screen, the RBCs selected for crossmatching must be negative for the antigen to which the patient has made an antibody. In that case a complete crossmatch through the Coombs' phase must be done. A full crossmatch may take up to 1 hour to perform, and extra time must be allowed if a patient is known to have an antibody.

ORDERING TRANSFUSIONS

When a physician decides that transfusion is needed, an order is written for the specific blood component, number of units, and indication for transfusion. In some hospitals documentation of informed consent to allow transfusion is also required. The length of time for the transfusion should be specified. Routine RBC typing, the screening for clinically significant antibodies, and crossmatch requires 60 to 90 minutes if no unexpected antibodies are identified. In emergency situations type-specific (e.g., A positive) RBCs can be available 10 to 20 minutes after a blood specimen is received in the laboratory. If ABO and Rh types are already on file in the blood bank, release of type-specific units requires even less time. In patients with life-threatening hemorrhage who do not have a blood type on record, group O Rh-negative RBCs may be released uncrossmatched from the blood bank and transfused. A properly labeled tube of blood should be sent to the laboratory as soon as possible. After the provided sample has been crossmatched, type-specific RBCs can be provided and an antibody screen done to ensure that no clinically significant RBC antibodies are present.

FFP and cryoprecipitate do not require a crossmatch before release from the blood bank. These components are stored frozen, and 45 minutes should be allowed for thawing or pooling of units. Both FFP and cryoprecipitate should be type specific to prevent immune hemolysis.

Patients may also have requirements for specialized components. When necessary and specifically ordered by a physician, cytomegalovirus (CMV) antibody–negative cellular components or irradiated components can be provided. CMV antibody–negative cellular components (i.e., RBCs and platelets) decrease the incidence of transfusion-transmitted CMV disease in patients without evidence of previous CMV disease (i.e., patients with negative CMV-antibody tests). FFP and cryoprecipitate are not thought to transmit CMV. CMV disease can be a serious problem in patients who have received bone marrow and solid organ transplants. Recent studies suggest that CMV can also be prevented by using leukocyte-reduction filters, which remove 99% to 99.9% of WBCs. In areas where CMV antibody–negative donors are rare, the use of leukocyte-reduction filters has become one alternative in reducing the incidence of transfusion-transmitted CMV.

Gamma-irradiated blood components are indicated for prevention of transfusion-associated graft-vs.-host disease in severely immunocompromised patients. It is necessary for the physician to order irradiated blood components for patients who are at high risk for transfusion-associated graft-vs.-host disease. Absolute indications for provision of irradiated components include patients with congenital immunodeficiency syndromes, intrauterine transfusions, bone marrow transplants, and certain hematologic malignancies.

Other special requirements include leukocyte-reduced cellular components for patients with two or more documented febrile nonhemolytic transfusion reactions. Febrile reactions generally are due to antibodies to WBCs in the recipient or donor. Use of leukocyte reduction may prevent these reactions. Other methods of leukocyte reduction include buffy coat removal, washing, and deglycerolizing cryopreserved RBCs.

The use of washed RBCs and platelets is indicated for patients with anaphylaxis from IgA deficiency or severe allergic reactions from unspecified plasma proteins. In the case of IgA deficiency with anaphylaxis, if FFP and cryoprecipitate transfusions are needed, the blood must be collected from IgA-deficient donors.

Frozen-thawed-deglycerolized RBCs were transfused commonly in the recent past to provide leukocyte-reduced RBCs for prevention of CMV infection or to prevent alloimmunization to HLA antigens. With the use of the new generation of leukocyte-reduction filters, RBC cryopreservation now is limited to storage of rare and selected RBC units. Once these units are thawed and deglycerolized, they must be used within 24 hours since they are no longer in a closed system.

TRANFUSION REACTIONS

Transfusion reactions are classified in several ways, including acute and delayed, hemolytic and nonhemolytic, immunologic and nonimmunologic, and combinations of these categories. Immediate reactions generally occur within 2 to 4 hours of the tranfusion, whereas delayed reactions occur days to years later. Patients being transfused must be monitored closely to identify quickly a transfusion reaction and to indicate promptly appropriate management. Symptoms such as fever and chills may signal the onset of a hemolytic transfusion reaction or a less serious febrile nonhemolytic transfusion reaction.

When an alteration in the patient's vital signs occurs or if symptoms develop during a transfusion, the transfusion must be stopped immediately. The IV line should be kept in place until the situation has been fully assessed. Shock, anaphylaxis, pulmonary edema, and circulatory overload must be treated aggressively.

After the patient has been stabilized, the labels on the blood bag must be rechecked against the patient's identification bracelet to make certain that a clerical error has not occurred. The discontinued bag of blood, the entire transfusion set, and all forms and labels are sent to the blood bank with a report of suspected transfusion reaction.

Immediate hemolytic transfusion reactions occur by immune and nonimmune mechanisms. Fifty-one percent of transfusion-associated deaths reported to the Food and Drug Administration (FDA) from 1976 to 1985 were a consequence of acute hemolysis resulting from ABO incompatibility. Immediate hemolysis of RBCs after ABO-incompatible transfusion results from IgM antibodies binding to RBC antigens. With binding of the IgM antibodies, subsequent activation of the complement, coagulation, and kinin systems occurs and can lead to shock, acute renal failure, and DIC. The possibility of hemolysis must always be considered when fever is associated with transfusion since fever is present in approximately 75% of patients with hemolytic transfusion reactions. Other signs and symptoms of immediate hemolytic transfusion reactions include hemoglobinuria, chills, flank pain, nausea, vomiting, tachycardia, tachypnea, and hypotension. The risk of death from a hemolytic transfusion reaction is estimated as 1 in 100,000 transfusion episodes. The major cause is ABO incompatibility attributable to clerical error in patient identification or to error in labeling of crossmatch tubes or blood components. Nonimmune hemolysis of RBCs is rare and can result from simultaneous infusion of hypotonic or hypertonic solutions, mechanical damage from pumps or needles, overwarming of blood, or bacterial contamination.

The most common immediate transfusion reactions are febrile nonhemolytic and allergic transfusion reactions. Febrile nonhemolytic transfusion reactions occur with 1% to 2% of transfusions and are caused by antibodies in the patient's plasma to HLA or granulocyte antigens in the transfused component. These reactions occur most often in patients who have been transfused previously or who are pregnant. Febrile nonhemolytic transfusion reactions recur in 10% to 12% of patients, and the use of leukocyte-reduced RBCs is recommended when a patient has had two or more of these reactions. It cannot be assumed that a febrile reaction is a nonhemolytic reaction, and the transfusion must be stopped to evaluate the possibilities of a hemolytic reaction or bacterial contamination of the unit. The transfusion cannot be restarted.

Allergic reactions occur in 1% to 4% of transfusion episodes. If urticaria is the only manifestation of an allergic reaction, the transfusion can be restarted after an antihistamine has been given and the hives have disappeared. Even if the transfusion reaction is mild and the transfusion is completed without further incident, a report of suspected transfusion reaction should be sent to the blood bank both to evaluate the severity and to document the occurrence. Anaphylactic reactions must be evaluated thoroughly to minimize the possibility of further reactions. Most allergic reactions are due to antibodies to plasma proteins in the donor units.

Noncardiogenic pulmonary edema is a rare transfusion reaction that results from passive transfer of donor antibody directed against the patient's WBCs. Leukoagglutination and stasis in the pulmonary microvasculature then occur. Appropriate management includes intubation, positive pressure ventilation, and fluid resuscitation.

Delayed hemolytic transfusion reactions frequently are detected by the blood bank when an unexpected antibody is identified in a blood specimen sent to the laboratory for type, screen, and crossmatch 1 to 10 days after transfusion. In these cases an RBC antibody had been formed some time in the past as a response to transfusion or pregnancy and had fallen to undetectable levels at the time of the initial antibody screening test before transfusion. Because the antibody was undetectable and no documentation of the antibody was present in the blood bank, RBCs with the antigen were transfused, and an anamnestic response of antibody production followed. Delayed reactions may also occur after primary exposure to a foreign RBC antigen. The patient generally demonstrates fever, anemia, and indirect hyperbilirubinemia. In general, the transfused RBCs are destroyed extravascularly in the spleen.

INFECTIOUS COMPLICATIONS OF TRANSFUSION

Viral, bacterial, and protozoal infections can be transmitted by transfusion. The most common disease causing serious clinical problems is viral hepatitis. Up to 10% of cases of posttransfusion hepatitis are caused by hepatitis B despite sensitive screening tests for hepatitis B surface antigen. The other 90% are caused by non-A, non-B hepatitis, with 85% to 90% of them caused by the recently discovered hepatitis C virus (HCV). Infection with HCV may not be clinically apparent in the months following transfusion since as many as 75% of cases are anicteric. Up to half of patients with HCV develop chronic hepatitis, and of them, 10% to 15% develop cirrhosis that becomes a major health problem. Blood collection centers started screening for antibody to HCV in 1990. With the introduction of this test, the risk of transfusion-transmitted hepatitis is expected to decrease. The blood bank or transfusion service must be notified if a patient who has been transfused develops hepatitis. Alerting the blood bank allows investigation of donors to begin.

AIDS is transmitted by transfusion, and all blood donors are asked specific questions related to risk of HIV exposure to exclude donors in high-risk groups. The blood is also tested for antibody to HIV-1 and HIV-2. The risk of acquiring AIDS from a blood transfusion ranges from 1 in 40,000 to 1 in 100,000 per donor exposure. For transfusion recipients, this risk is present because a window between the time the donor is exposed to the virus and the time that seroconversion occurs exists. No test consistently detects infectious donors in this interval; therefore blood collection centers rely on volunteer donors who do not have known risk factors for infection. Transmission of malaria is rare in the United States but is a major issue in endemic areas.

Bacterial contamination of RBCs and platelets is a rare occurrence, but fatal complications have been reported. Deaths related to bacterial contamination have increased from 4% to 10% of deaths related to transfusion over the past 10 years. Contamination of platelets most often is caused by skin flora that grow while the platelets are stored at room temperature. Contamination of RBCs most often is caused by Gram-negative bacteria, which proliferate at refrigerator temperature. Bacterial contamination should be suspected in patients who have a transfusion reaction that consists of fever, chills, and hypotension. If bacterial contamination is suspected, the patient's blood and the donor blood remaining in the bag are sent for culture. Broad-spectrum antibiotic therapy is given until transfusion-associated sepsis is excluded.

TABLE 45-3   Current Estimated Transfusion Risks

Complication	Risk per Unit Transfused
Fever, chills, urticaria	1:100
Posttransfusion hepatitis (liver function tests)	1:140-1:500
Posttransfusion hepatitis (reported)	1:5,000-1:10,000
Acute hemolysis	1:6,000
Fatal hemolytic transfusion reaction	1:100,000
HIV infection	1:60,000

SUMMARY

- The main indications for transfusion of blood components are to increase oxygen-carrying capacity and improve hemostasis.
- When intravascular volume expansion is necessary, use of albumin and PPF derived from plasma may be indicated.
- FFP should not be used for intravascular volume expansion. It is used to replace deficient clotting factors.
- Use of whole blood is indicated for simultaneous replacement of oxygen-carrying capacity and intravascular volume only. Use of whole blood is considered for patients actively bleeding who have lost 25% of blood volume.
- Packed RBCs are used for increasing oxygen-carrying capacity of anemic patients. Threshold for transfusion depends on the clinical state of the patient.
- Platelet transfusion is used to control or prevent bleeding resulting from deficient numbers of platelets or from dysfunctional platelets.
- FFP contains 100% of all normal plasma constituents, including coagulation factors and complement. It is used to replace deficient clotting factors.
- Cryoprecipitate contains factor VIII, vWF, factor XIII, fibrinogen, and fibronectin. It is used for patients with hemophilia A, von Willebrand's disease, factor XIII deficiency, abnormal fibrinogen, or deficient fibrinogen.
- Albumin can cause allergic and febrile transfusion reactions.
- Major blood groups are A, B, AB, and O.
- In emergencies group O, Rh-negative blood is used for transfusion until type and crossmatch are complete.
- For specific indications, CMV antibody-negative, gamma-irradiated, leukocyte-reduced, and washed blood components are available.
- When an alteration in vital signs, fever, chills, flank pain, nausea, vomiting, tachycardia, tachypnea, or hypotension occurs, a transfusion reaction should be suspected and the ongoing transfusion stopped.
- Febrile nonhemolytic and allergic reactions are the most common transfusion reactions.
- Hepatitis B comprises 10% of posttransfusion hepatitis. Non-A, non-B hepatitis accounts for 90%. Eighty-five percent to 90% of posttransfusion hepatitis is associated with hepatitis C.
- Current estimated transfusion risks are shown in Table 45-3.

SUGGESTED READINGS

Alexander MR, Stumpf JL, Nostrant TT, Khanderia U, Eckhauser FE, Colvin CL. Albumin utilization in a university hospital. DICP 23:214-217, 1989.

Alving BM, Hojima Y, Pisano JJ, et al. Hypotension associated with prekallikrein activator (Hageman-factor fragments) in plasma protein fraction. N Engl J Med 299:66-70, 1978.

Anderson KC, Weinstein HJ. Transfusion-associated graft-versus-host disease. N Engl Med 323:315-321, 1990.

Barnes A. The blood bank in hemotherapy for trauma and surgery. In Barnes A, Umlas J, eds. Hemotherapy in trauma and surgery. Washington, D.C.: American Association of Blood Banks, 1979.

Blumberg N, Bove J. Un–cross-matched blood for emergency transfusion. JAMA 240:2057-2059, 1978.

Centers for Disease Control. Public Health Service Inter-Agency guidelines for screening donors of blood, plasma, organs, tissues, and semen for evidence of hepatitis B and hepatitis C. MMWR 40(No. RR-4), 1991.

Coffin CM. Current issues in transfusion therapy: Indications for use of blood components. Postgrad Med 81:343-350, 1987.

Counts RB, Haisch C, simon TL, Maxwell NG, Heimbach DM, Caprico CJ. Hemostasis in massively transfused trauma patients. Ann Surg 190:91-99, 1979.

Dzik WH, Kirkley SA. Citrate toxicity during massive blood transfusion. Transfusion Med Rev 2:76-94, 1988.

Hillyer CD, Snydman DR, Berkman EM. The risk of cytomegalovirus infection in solid organ and bone marrow transplant recipients: Transfusion of blood products. Transfusion 30:659-666, 1990.

Hogman CF, Bagge L, Thorer L. The use of blood components in surgical transfusion therapy. World J Surg 11:2-13, 1987.

Holland PV, ed. Standards for blood banks and transfusion services, 13th ed. Arlington, Va.: American Association of Blood Banks, 1989.

Honig CL, Bove JR. Transfusion-associated fatalities: Review of Bureau of Biologics reports 1976-1978. Transfusion 20:653-661, 1980.

Kickler TS. The challenge of platelet alloimmunization: Management and prevention. Transfusion Med Rev 4:8-18, 1990.

Leikola J, Myllyla G. The clinical use of red blood cell components. In Summers SH, Smith DM, Agranenko VA, eds. Transfusion therapy: Guidelines for practice. Arlington, Va.: American Association of Blood Banks, 1990, pp 1-25.

McCullough J, Steeper TA, Connelly DP, Jackson B, Huntington S, Scott EP. Platelet utilization in a university hospital. JAMA 259:2414-2418, 1988.

Mollison PL, Engelfriet CP, Contreras M, eds. Blood transfusion in clinical medicine, 8th ed. Oxford: Blackwell Scientific Publications, 1987.

Ness PM, Perkins HA. Cryoprecipitate as a reliable source of fibrinogen replacement. JAMA 241:1690-1691, 1979.

NIH Consensus Conference. Fresh frozen plasma: Indications and risks. JAMA 253:551-553, 1985.

NIH Consensus Conference. Perioperative red blood cell transfusion. JAMA 260:2700-2703, 1988.

NIH Consensus Conference. Platelet transfusion therapy. JAMA 257:1777-1780, 1987.

Pineda AA, Brzica SM, Taswell JG. Hemolytic transfusion reaction: Recent experience in a large blood bank. Mayo Clin Proc 53:378, 1978.

Pineda AA, Taswell HF. Transfusion reactions associated with anti-IgA antibodies: Report of four cases and review of the literature. Transfusion 15:10-15, 1975.

Pineda AA, Taswell HF, Brzica SM. Delayed hemolytic transfusion reaction: An immunologic hazard of blood transfusion. Transfusion 18:1-7, 1978.

Propp DA. Blood component therapy. J Emerg Med 6:151-159, 1988.

Reed LR, Heimbach DM, Counts RB, et al. Prophylactic platelet administration during massive transfusion. Ann Surg 203:40-47, 1986.

Sazama K. Reports of 355 transfusion-associated deaths: 1976 through 1985. Transfusion 30:583-590, 1990.

Snyder EL, ed. Blood transfusion therapy: A physician's handbook, 2nd ed. Arlington, Va.: American Association of Blood Banks, 1987.

Snyder EL. Clinical use of albumin, plasma protein fraction and isoimmune globulin products. In Kolins J, Britten AFH, Silvergleid AJ, eds. Plasma products: Use and management. Arlington, Va.: American Association of Blood Banks, 1982, pp 87-107.

Snyder EL. Clinical use of white cell–poor blood components. Transfusion, 29:568-571, 1989.

Tegtmeier GE. Posttransfusion cytomegalovirus infections. Arch Pathol Lab Med 113:236-245, 1989.

Walker RH, ed. Technical manual, 10th ed. Arlington, Va.: American Association of Blood Banks, 1990.

Wilson RF, Dulchavsky SA, Soullier G, Beckman B. Problems with 20 or more blood transfusions in 24 hours. Am Surg 53:410-417, 1987.

CHAPTER 46

Fluids and Electrolytes

Roderick A. Barke

BODY COMPARTMENTS AND DISTRIBUTION OF WATER AND ELECTROLYTES

Insight into the normal distribution of water and electrolytes in the unstressed state is necessary for an understanding of disordered fluid and electrolyte balance in the critically ill patient. The distribution of the extracellular fluid (ECF) and intracellular fluid (ICF) spaces in the normal state are described by the Yannet-Darrow diagram, as is the normal electrolyte distribution of the plasma and intracellular fluid (Fig. 46-1). Normal fluid homeostasis assumes both the ability to take fluid orally as desired and normal kidney function. Assuming normal activity, temperature, and humidity, fluid balance for a 70-kg adult in the normal state is outlined in Table 46-1. Critical illness alters the input-output equation, with resultant effects on volume, concentration, and composition of the body compartments. For example, insensible respiratory free water loss effectively is minimized during mechanical ventilation. Common measurable losses in terms of GI secretions are outlined in Table 46-2. The mechanisms by which injury alters salt and water balance during critical illness, surgery, and trauma are important in managing critically ill patients.

EFFECT OF STRESS OF SURGERY OR TRAUMA ON FLUID HOMEOSTASIS

Although anesthesia alone is associated with decreased renal plasma flow, glomerular filtration rate (GFR), and urinary volume, the anesthesia-related renal effects return to normal rapidly after the termination of anesthesia. The addition of a surgical procedure to the effect of anesthesia markedly alters the homeostatic response. The depression in renal function that results in salt and water retention lengthens and persists 3 to 10 days. Compromise of renal function depends on the magnitude of the stress. Sodium and water retention after surgery and trauma has been attributed to a change in the hormonal environment following stress. However, the relationship between the alterations in salt and water physiology and the associated change in the hormonal environment do not fully answer the question of whether surgical stress results in an obligate hormonal response with increased production of 17-hydroxycorticosteroids, aldosterone, and antidiuretic hormone (ADH). Rather, the major factor may relate to a redistribution of the ECF to the intracellular and interstitial space. The next section reviews the evolution of present thinking on this relationship.

TABLE 46-1 Fluid Balance in the Normal State

Input	Amount (ml)	Output	Amount (ml)
Oral fluid	1300-2300	Urine	800-1600
Water of oxidation	300	Feces	100
		Insensible loss	
		Skin	300-400
		Respiratory	300-400
		Sweat	100
TOTAL GAIN	1600-2600	TOTAL LOSS	1600-2600

TABLE 46-2 Composition of Common Gastrointestinal Secretions

Secretion	Sodium (mEq/L)	Potassium (mEq/L)	Chloride (mEq/L)	HCO_3^- (mEq/L)
Saliva	60	20	15	50
Stomach	30-90	4-12	50-150	70-90
Pancreatic	135-155	4-6	60-110	70-90
Bile	135-155	4-6	80-110	35-50
Jejunal	70-125	3.5-6.5	70-125	10-20
Ileostomy	90-140	4-10	60-125	15-50
Diarrhea	25-50	35-60	20-40	35-45

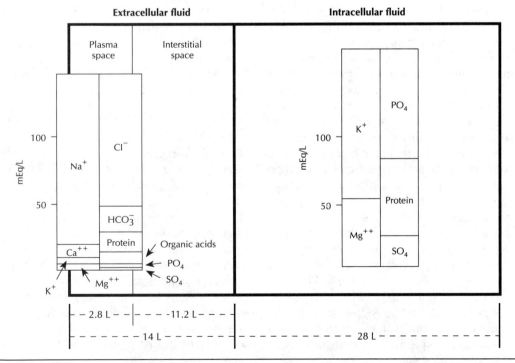

FIG. 46-1 Yannet-Darrow diagram of distribution of extracellular fluid and intracellular fluid volumes in the normal state. Values are for a 70-kg person with 60% water content.

Evolution of Understanding of Hormonal Response

At the time of Coller and Hardy,[1,3] surgeons thought that surgical stress or trauma evoked an adrenocortical response, the so-called classic stress response. This concept led to a recommendation that salt and water be restricted after surgical stress. Further study of the adrenal response to surgery and trauma led to remarkable contradictory data challenging this concept. Although some temporal correlation between the alteration in renal fluid and electrolyte handling and 17-hydroxycorticosteroid response exists, the correlation was out of phase with respect to the real-time retention of salt and water after injury. In fact, data from animals[4] or Addisonian patients[5] who had undergone an adrenalectomy suggested that an increased 17-hydroxycorticosteroid response was not necessary for poststress fluid and sodium retention. These and other data cast doubt on 17-hydroxycorticosteroid response as a principal mechanism of altered renal response after injury. The discovery of aldosterone and insight into the renin-angiotensin-aldosterone response provided another possible mechanism for altered renal function after stress. On careful analysis, although the adosterone level increases after surgery or trauma, the temporal relationship between plasma aldosterone concentration and renal salt and water retention correlated only initially during the postoperative course.[6-8] As in the 17-hydroxycorticosteroid case, patients who had undergone an adrenalectomy had a degree of fluid and electrolyte retention similar to that of normal patients. These findings suggest that a factor other than aldosterone may be active. ADH was an attractive possibility. Although ADH activity was noted to increase after stress, data collected from surgical patients with diabetes insipidus suggested the renal fluid–handling after stress was not wholly consistent with increased ADH activity alone.[9-11] These data suggested that the altered renal response to stress should not be interpreted solely as an adrenocortical response to injury, but that it may represent a homeostatic mechanism in response to a deficit in ECF volume.

The thesis that inadequate resuscitation in response to injury decreases plasma volume and renal plasma flow by internal redistribution of fluid to the interstitial space and intracellular space was tested using numerous dilution techniques. The measurement of the functional ECF volume (FECV), as determined by the sulfate dilution equilibrium volume after hemorrhagic shock and resuscitation,[12] demonstrated that simple isovolemic replacement based on shed blood led to a marked deficit in FECV. These and other studies suggested the adrenal response to surgical stress and trauma may be secondary to decreased circulating plasma volume and could not be assumed to be strictly an adrenal phenomenon. Currently, fluid therapy after injury should be directed at repletion of the fluid internally redistributed plus insensible and sensible losses.

This discussion may be expanded from surgery or trauma to critical illness in general. Critical illness such as sepsis, unrelated to operative or traumatic injury, can result in a loss of ECF to the intracellular and interstitial spaces by altering endothermal and cell membrane permeability. This mechanism results in a similar condition of low renal plasma flow from both decreased circulating plasma volume and depleted FECV. The approach to fluid and electrolyte therapy in critical illness, in general, should also correct possible losses, insensible losses, and internally redistributed fluid.

GOAL OF FLUID AND ELECTROLYTE THERAPY

From the foregoing discussion, a proper treatment plan after injury or critical illness should restore renal plasma flow by replacement of the FECV deficit. Intravenous replacement solutions, the tools available to accomplish this goal, may be divided into crystalloid or colloid groups. Table 46-3 lists commonly used crystalloid solutions. Colloid solutions are used for special purposes as indicated in the management of fluid and eletrolytes. Table 46-4 lists commonly used colloid solutions. Fluid and electrolyte therapy may be analyzed further according to disorders common to the critical care setting.

TABLE 46-3   Crystalloid Solutions

Solutions	Glucose (g/L)	Sodium (mEq/L)	Chloride (mEq/L)	Potassium (mEq/L)	Calcium (mEq/L)	Lactate (mEq/L)
D5%/W	50					
D10%/W	100					
D5%/0.2% NaCl	50	34	34			
D5%/0.33% NaCl	50	56	56			
D5%/0.45% NaCl	50	77	77			
D5%/0.9% NaCl	50	154	154			
0.9% NaCl		154	154			
Lactated Ringer's		130	109	4	3	28
3% NaCl		513	513			

TABLE 46-4   Colloid Solutions

Solutions	Glucose (g/L)	Sodium (mEq/L)	Chloride (mEq/L)
5% Albumin	5	130-160	130-160
25% Albumin	25	130-160	130-160
5% Hetastarch	5	154	154

HYPEROSMOLALITY, HYPERTONICITY, AND HYPERNATREMIA

Although osmolality and tonicity both describe plasma solute concentration, they represent fundamentally different concepts that are important to the understanding of altered fluid and electrolyte homeostasis. Hypertonicity or hypotonicity describes the relationship between total solutes and water in either serum or plasma. Tonicity can be measured directly by freezing point depression or vapor pressure measurement or indirectly by using the serum sodium concentration. The relationship of serum sodium concentration to water balance makes several important assumptions:

- The total amount of crystalloids is constant. Important exceptions include hyperglycemia and azotemia.
- No significant water-insoluble substances exist in the plasma. Clinical exceptions include hyperproteinemia (e.g., with multiple myeloma) or hyperlipidemia.

- The relationship of sodium ions to total cations is normal (normal ratio, 142 mEq of sodium ions to 155 mEq total cations).

With these assumptions, the plasma osmolarity can be estimated from measurement of plasma sodium, glucose, and BUN concentration by using the following equation:

$$\text{Serum osmolarity (mOsm/L)} = 2\,Na^+\,(mEq/L)_{plasma} + \text{Glucose (mg\%)}/18 + \text{BUN (mg\%)}/2.8$$

Assuming no other osmotically active solutes, the measured osmolarity will be less than 10 mOsm/L greater than the calculated osmolarity. Although plasma osmolarity can be calculated in hyperproteinemic and hyperlipidemic states, plasma osmometry should be performed if the diagnosis of a hypertonic or hypotonic (the most common case) state will be seriously considered.

Sodium and glucose are distributed in the ECF, whereas urea is distributed in total body water. Solute can be classified as "effective" or "ineffective." Effective solute is distributed only in the ECF, whereas ineffective solute is distributed in total body water. Effective solutes include sodium, glucose, mannitol, and glycerol. Ineffective solutes include urea, ethanol, methanol, and ethylene glycol. Tonicity is calculated by modifying the previous equation as follows:

$$\text{Serum tonicity (mOsm/L)} = \\ 2\,Na^+\,(mEq/L)_{plasma} + \\ Glucose\,(mg\%)/18$$

The distinction between osmolality and tonicity is important to differentiate a hyperosmolar hypertonic state from a hyperosmolar nonhypertonic state. In the hyperosmolar hypertonic state, ICF water is redistributed to the ECF. Consequently, the ICF compartment decreases in size. The signs and symptoms of decreased ICF compartment are a consequence of cellular dehydration and are expressed primarily as neurologic signs and symptoms (e.g., weakness progressing to lethargy, disorientation or delusional states, obtundation, coma).[13] Acute rapid changes in ICF can result in mechanical disruption of the cerebral blood vessels (i.e., subarachnoid and subcortical hemorrhage).

To compensate for changes in osmolality, the brain generates "idiogenic osmols," which are isolated to the brain. These idiogenic osmols represent a partial compensation for the changes in brain parenchymal volume and occur within hours (hyperglycemia) to days (hypernatremia) of the onset of the abnormal tonicity. In the hyperosmolar nonhypertonic state, the change in ICF volume is minimized. Since the solute is distributed in total body water, CNS alteration is produced by the solute toxicity itself (i.e., ethanol) and not by the change in the ICF volume.

Hyperosmolar, hypertonic states can result from pure water loss, hypotonic water loss, or an increase in effective solute. Pure water loss results in a decrease in both the ICF and the ECF, according to the distribution of solute. Pure water loss can result from exaggerated insensible losses through the skin and lungs as a result of environmental conditions or extensive burns, hyperpyrexia, or mechanical hyper-

ventilation. Since critically ill patients generally cannot correct losses through thirst mechanisms, careful monitoring is necessary in patients with these conditions to prevent and correct fluid loss.

Another cause of almost pure water loss is diabetes insipidus—either central or nephrogenic (Fig. 46-2). Central diabetes insipidus can occur as a result of blunt head trauma, anoxic encephalopathy, vascular disorders (e.g., intraventricular hemorrhage, cerebral aneurysms), hypophysectomy, brain tumors (especially metastatic breast cancer), infectious causes (e.g., encephalitis, meningitis) or drug use (e.g., ethanol, opiate antagonist, clonidine). The presentation of central diabetes insipidus may be partial or complete. With access to water as desired, patients who are affected with complete central diabetes insipidus generally have urinary osmolality <100 mOsm/L and massive polyuria.[14]

Nephrogenic diabetes insipidus results from insufficient water conservation by the kidney despite a normal ADH signal.[15] Nephrogenic diabetes insipidus can result from interruption of the normal corticomedullary gradient or from acquired insensitivity of the distal tubule and collecting duct to ADH. Interruption of the normal corticomedullary gradient occurs with protein or caloric malnutrition, diuretic use, and renal failure. Acquired insensitivity to ADH can result from nephrotoxic drugs (e.g., aminoglycosides), hypercalcemia, and hypokalemia. The diagnosis of either nephrogenic or central diabetes insipidus is made clinically under the conditions of controlled dehydration. Demonstration of inappropriate urinary volume and hypo-osmolality (<200 mOsm/kg) in the presence of increasing plasma hyperosmolality (>300 mOsm/kg) over the period of 12 to 18 hours confirms the presence of diabetes insipidus.

Differentiation of nephrogenic diabetes insipidus from central diabetes insipidus is made by administration of aqueous vasopressin (Pitressin) (5 U sc), In patients with central diabetes insipidus urinary osmolality will concentrate to 800 to 1200 mOsm/kg after vasopressin administration, whereas in patients with nephrogenic diabetes insipidus little or no increase

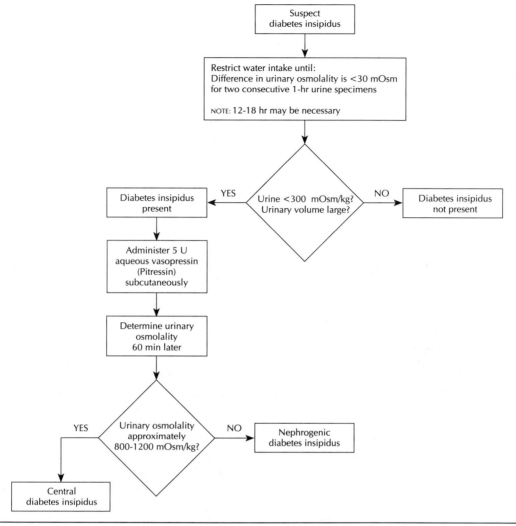

FIG. 46-2 Diagnosis of diabetes insipidus.

in urinary osmolality occurs. Compromised renal function may make the diagnosis of diabetes insipidus difficult since the usual endpoints cannot be reached.

The time needed for rehydration of the patient with pure water loss should approximate the time it took to develop the dehydrated state. Too rapid and potentially hazardous volume loading must be avoided. The volume loss is approximated as follows[16]:

Water deficit (L) =

0.6 body weight in kilograms × (Plasma Na⁺

$(mEq/L)/140 \ mEq/L - 1)$

The first half of the calculated deficit is administered over one third of the interval thought to produce the dehydration. Electrolyte values are measured at the end of this period, and the water deficit again is calculated at this time.

Hypotonic fluid losses result in marked decreases in the ECF and in plasma volume. As opposed to pure water loss, hypotonic fluid loss is associated with hypovolemia, hypotension, tachycardia, azotemia, and oliguria. Renal mechanisms are the most common causes of the clinical findings that occur with hypotonic losses. Hyperglycemia (e.g., hyperosmolar, hyperglycemic, nonketotic coma), polyuric acute tubular necrosis, postobstructive uropathy, loop diuretic administration, or mannitol administration is commonly implicated. Urinary losses are diagnosed by measuring the urinary sodium concentration. Generally, for hypotonic fluid loss of renal origin the sodium level is >40 mEq/L, and for that of nonrenal origin it is <20 mEq/L. Hypovolemia and hypotension are corrected by replacement of volume deficits; hypertonicity is corrected once the volume deficit is corrected.

The most common cause of hypertonicity (effective solute gain) is hypernatremia (Table 46-5) resulting from the administration of sodium bicarbonate during cardiac arrest. The osmolal gap (osmolality minus tonicity) is <10 mOsm/kg in this state. Another cause for hypertonic solute gain is the treatment of cerebral edema with administration of mannitol or glycerol. In this state the osmolal gap is >10 mOsm/kg since mannitol or glycerol is usually an unaccounted effective solute. The administration of osmotic diuretics results in further hypotonic fluid loss and increased hypertonicity.

Finally, hyperosmolality without hypertonicity is by default associated with the presence of an ineffective solute such as azotemia that complicates acute renal failure. In the proper clinical context in patients with increased plasma osmolality, normal tonicity, an osmolal gap >10 mOsm/kg, and the presence of a BUN concentration <40mg%, ingestion of ethanol, methanol, or ethylene glycol is suspected because these solutes distribute in total body water.

Hypo-osmolality and Hyponatremia

Water excess is produced when either excess water is administered or renal water clearance is insufficient (e.g., in a patient with syndrome of inappropriate antidiuretic hormone [SIADH]). The symptoms of water intoxication are related to the shifting of water from the extracellular space into the intracellular space. In a closed space such as the skull, the edema produced can be life-threatening. The symptoms of hypotonicity are, consequently, mainly neurologic and ophthalmologic:

Neurologic:
Headache
Nausea and vomiting
Muscle fasciculation
Hyperactive reflexes (early)
Loss of reflexes (late)
Obtundation
Convulsions
Hypertension or bradycardia

Ophthalmologic:
Blurred vision
Blindness
Papilledema

The severity of symptoms is related more to the rate at which the hypotonicity is produced than to the serum sodium concentration. The more gradual the process, the more mild are the signs and symptoms. In addition, the hypotonic state is almost never one of pure water excess at a constant solute concentration. Mixed states are the rule rather than the exception. The differential diagnosis of hypotonic states common to the SICU includes the following:

- The administration of excess hypotonic fluid during states with excess ADH (e.g., in the postoperative period with inadequate resuscitation)
- SIADH (e.g., with carcinoma of the lung, Hodgkin's disease, leukemia, CNS disorders)
- Hypertonic fluid loss with hypotonic fluid replacement
- The clinical use of oxytocin
- Patients admitted to the SICU with cardiovascular or hypertensive diagnoses who are receiving diuretic therapy

In some conditions such as pregnancy, mild to moderate hypotonicity is a normal response and requires no action by the physician. The diagnosis is established by evidence of hypotonicity (decreased osmolality) and hyponatremia (Table 46-6). Other laboratory findings are of little value unless one of the previously mentioned conditions is present. Treatment depends on the severity of the symptoms and the acid-base disorder present in association with the dilutional disorder. In many cases simple water restriction is all that is required. In moderate to severe situations hypertonic salt solution may be given. Generally the hypotonic state

| TABLE 46-5   Causes and Treatment of Hypernatremia |

Water Loss	Hypotonic Fluid Loss	Effective Solute Increase
Mechanism		

Renal losses
  Diabetes insipidus
    Central
    Nephrogenic
	Renal losses
	  Acute tubular necrosis
	    with polyuria
	  Postobstructive uropathy
	  Loop diuretics
	  Mannitol
		Hypertonic sodium and sodium
		  bicarbonate
		Primary hyperaldosteronism
		Cushing's syndrome

Increased insensible losses
  Burns
  Respiratory infection or injury
  Fever		

Treatment		

Judicious water replacement	Hypotonic saline solution
	  replacement
		Diuretics and judicious water
		  replacement

| TABLE 46-6   Causes and Treatment of Hyponatremia* |

Mechanism	ECF Changes	Causes	Urinary Sodium	Treatment

Excess total body water	ECF increase, no edema	SIADH
		Glucocorticoid in-
		  sufficiency
		Thyroid insuffi-
		  ciency
			>20 mg/L	Water re-
				  striction

Total body water deficit and larger total body sodium deficit	ECF volume de-
	pletion
		Renal
		  Diuretics
		  Mineralocorticoid
		    insufficiency
		  Salt-wasting ne-
		    phropathy
		  Renal tubular aci-
		    dosis
		  Osmotic diuresis
		Nonrenal
		  Vomiting
		  Diarrhea
		  Third-space
		    losses
			Renal >20 mg/L
			Nonrenal, <10
			  mg/L
				Isotonic
				  saline
				  solution

Total body so-
dium excess and larger to-
tal body water excess
	ECF increase, edema	CHF
		Cirrhosis
		Nephrotic syn-
		  drome
		Chronic renal failure
			<10 mg/L
			If chronic renal
			  failure, >20
			  mg/L
				Water re-
				  striction

*Modified from Berl T, Anderson RJ, McDonald KM, et al. Clinical disorders of water metabolism. Kidney Int 10:117-132, 1976.

should be corrected over a length of time similar to that which produced the hypotonic state. Rapid correction of a hypotonic state can be lethal and must be avoided. The serum concentration should not be increased more than 2 mEq/L/hr unless severe symptoms exist (convulsions). In the presence of normal acid-base balance, a 50-50 mixture of 3% normal saline solution and sodium lactate solution may be given. In the presence of alkalosis 3% normal saline solution should be administered. With acidosis, 0.5 or 1 M sodium lactate may be given in a 50-50 mixture with 3% normal saline solution. Critically ill patients may not tolerate the fluid shifts that result from hypertonic fluid loading, and another strategy should be used. One such strategy uses a loop diuretic (e.g., furosemide) and replaces the urinary loss with hypertonic saline solution while cardiovascular status is carefully monitored invasively (i.e., with a Swan-Ganz catheter).

Potassium

Hyperkalemia and hypokalemia are common electrolyte disturbances in the critically ill. Hypokalemia is common in the SICU and can result from many causes, including the following:

- Nasogastric suction, which removes gastric acid secretion containing approximately 20 mEq/L potassium
- Insulin-mediated glucose transport and glycogen synthesis, which involve an obligate intracellular potassium store (i.e., the treatment of diabetic hyperglycemia and ketoacidosis)
- Alkalosis, which results in a shift of potassium from the ECF to the ICF. GI losses (e.g., from diarrhea, ileostomy), pancreatic juice losses (pancreatic fistuli), and biliary losses (biliary fistula, T-tube drainage), which can contain 5 to 15 mEq/L of potassium

Renal losses of potassium are prominent (1) because obligate urinary potassium losses occur even in the presence of hypokalemia and (2) because of the frequent use of thiazide and loop diuretics. Hypokalemia can be secondary to other electrolyte disorders such as hypomagnesemia. Beta-adrenergic agonists de-

crease serum potassium through beta-2–mediated stimulation of cellular potassium uptake. Epinephrine therapy in patients with acute myocardial infarction or terbutaline-albuterol therapy in obstetric patients with premature labor has been associated with hypokalemia.

Hyperkalemia can occur from (1) a shift of potassium from the ICF to the ECF, as in acidosis; (2) massive cell lysis (chemotherapy with extensive rapid cell death); (3) rhabdomyolysis (crush injury and extreme exercise); (4) rapid hemolysis; and (5) iatrogenic mechanisms. Finally, the most common cause of hyperkalemia in the critically ill is renal failure.

The signs and symptoms of hypokalemia may be subtle and depend on whether the deficit is acute or chronic. The clinical signs and symptoms of hypokalemia are as follows:

Cardiovascular: depression of the ST segment; lengthening of the QT interval; inversion of the T wave; presence of a U wave; cardiac arrest with the heart in diastole
Gastrointestinal: paralytic ileus
Renal: impaired ability to concentrate urine; increased hepatic encephalopathy (increased renal ammoniagenesis)
Skeletal muscle: weakness; decreased reflexes
Metabolic: glucose intolerance
Central nervous system: confusion

In patients with chronic hypokalemia the ECG signs are often absent, and skeletal muscle weakness is the most prominent finding. Knowledge of the nature of the signs and symptoms and the magnitude of the potassium deficit is needed to treat hypokalemia. Treatment of serious cardiac or neurologic signs constitutes an emergency. However, the calculation of the actual potassium deficit is at best a crude estimation since total potassium stores and serum potassium concentrations can vary independently. As mentioned previously, severe hypokalemia often is accompanied by metabolic alkalosis from renal tubular conservation of potassium and obligate retention of bicarbonate. Thus the more profound the metabolic alkalosis, the greater is the potassium deficit. It is better to know that hypokalemia with metabolic alkalosis is often associated with a deficit as large as 450 to 600 mEq of potassium than to use one of the many mathematic approaches to the calculation of the potassium deficit based on serum potassium and serum pH levels. In patients with severe hypokalemia treatment should be parenteral through a centrally placed catheter with cardiac monitoring. In the critically ill adult patient 20 mEq of potassium chloride in 100 ml of 0.9% normal saline solution may be administered safely over 1 hour. Infusions >20 mEq potassium chloride over 1-hour periods must be adminsitered only with great care and monitoring in patients with severe symptomatic hypokalemia. Obtaining serial measurements of serum potassium concentration is imperative.

Certain special situations should be noted in the treatment of hypokalemia. Hypokalemia in the presence of metabolic acidosis should be treated before treatment of the acid-base disorder since bicarbonate therapy will exacerbate the potassium deficit. Digoxin inhibits the transport of potassium into the cell. Patients receiving cardiac glycoside therapy are more likely to have transient hyperkalemia during potassium administration. Potassium administration in the patient with impaired renal function must be done with extreme caution.

The clinical signs and symptoms of hyperkalemia are as follows:

Cardiovascular (in order of appearance): peaking of the T wave; widening of the QRS complex; loss of the P wave; "sine-wave" configuration; cardiac arrest with asystole
Renal: decreased renal ammoniagenesis and mild metabolic hyperchloremic acidosis
Skeletal muscle: weakness progressing to flaccid paralysis; decreased reflexes

As with hypokalemia, the treatment of hyperkalemia should be matched to the severity of the signs and symptoms. Emergency treatment is necessary if ECG signs of hyperkalemia are present (independent of the serum potassium concentration) or if the serum potassium concentration is greater than 6 mEq/L. Treatment of hyperkalemia is divided into several categories: membrane antagonism, temporary potassium redistribution, and potassium removal. The mainstay of membrane antagonism is cal-

cium treatment (gluconate or chloride, 10 to 20 ml IV of 10% solution). The effect is immediate, and calcium adminstration should be the initial treatment unless special circumstances such as cardiac glycoside therapy or associated hypercalcemia exist. Temporary redistribution of potassium from the ECF to the ICF is accomplished with either sodium bicarbonate (50 to 150 mEq IV over 5 minutes) or insulin-glucose therapy (10 U regular insulin in 50 ml $D_{50}W$ over 30 to 60 minutes). Temporary redistribution by these methods results in an onset of action of 5 to 30 minutes, with a duration of action of approximately 1 to 2 hours in the case of bicarbonate therapy or 4 to 6 hours with insulin-glucose therapy. Profound alkalosis, hyperglycemia, or hypoglycemia would limit such therapy. The foregoing treatments provide only a temporary reprieve from severe hyperkalemia. These treatments must be followed by potassium removal. Potassium elimination is accomplished by diuretic therapy (furosemide, 40 to 80 mg IV, or bumetanide [Bumex], 1 to 2 mg IV), use of cationic exchange resins (sodium polystyrene sulfonate [Kayexalate], 50 g in 500 to 1000 cc 70% sorbitol solution orally or as a retention enema), and dialysis (hemodialysis or peritoneal dialysis) (see box).

Treatment of Hyperkalemia

Membrane antagonism

Calcium gluconate or calcium chloride, 10-20 ml 10% solution IV

Temporary redistribution of potassium from ECF to ICF

Sodium bicarbonate, 50-150 mEq IV over 5 min
Insulin and glucose, 10 U regular insulin in 50 ml $D_{50}W$ IV over 30-60 min

Potassium removal

Dialysis
Cationic exchange resins (sodium sulfonate, 50 g in 500-1000 ml 70% sorbitol solution orally or as retention enema)
Diuretic therapy

SUMMARY

- Anesthesia and surgery result in salt and water retention. Corticosteroid, aldosterone, and ADH increases exist after surgery, but they do not fully explain salt and water retention.
- A major goal of fluid therapy is replacement of the FECV deficit to restore renal and other organ plasma flow.
- Hyperosmolar, hypertonic states result from pure water loss, hypotonic water loss, or effective solute increase (see Table 46-5).
- Pure water loss can result from diabetes insipidus (see Fig. 46-2).

- Excess water administration or deficient renal water clearance causes hyponatremic, hypotonic states. Hyponatremia should be corrected gradually (increase sodium no more than 2 mg/L/hr unless severe symptoms exist).
- Treat hypokalemia before metabolic acidosis when both conditions exist. Use caution when administering potassium to patients with renal failure.
- Treatment of hyperkalemia includes membrane antagonism, potassium redistribution, or potassium removal (see box, p. 489).

REFERENCES

1. Coller FA, Campbell KN, Vaughan HH, et al. Postoperative salt intolerance. Ann Surg 119:533, 1944.
2. Hardy J. The role of the adrenal cortex in the postoperative retention of salt and water. Ann Surg 132:189, 1950.
3. Hardy J, Ravdin I. Some physiological aspects of surgical trauma. Ann Surg 136:345, 1952.
4. Ingle DJ, Meeks RC, Thomas KE. The effect of fractures upon urinary electrolytes in non-adrenalectomized and in adrenalectomized rats treated with adrenal cortex extract. Endocrinology 49:703, 1951.
5. Rosenbaum JD, Paper S, Ashley MM. Variations in renal excretion of sodium independent of change in adrenocortical hormone dosage in patients with Addison's disease. J Clin Endocrinol Metabol 15:1459, 1955.
6. Moran WH Jr, Rosenberg JC, Schloff L, et al. The relationship of adrenal steroids to postoperative electrolyte metabolism. Surgery 46:109, 1959.
7. Jepson RP, Jordon A, Levell MJ, et al. Metabolic response to adrenalectomy. Ann Surg 145:1, 1957.
8. Mason AS. Metabolic response to total adrenalectomy and hypophysectomy. Lancet 2:632, 1955.
9. Ariel IM. Effects of a water load administered to patients during the immediate postoperative period. Arch Surg 62:303, 1951.
10. Kennedy JH, Sabga GA, Hopkins RW, et al. Urine volume and osmolality. Arch Surg 88:155, 1964.
11. Hayes MA, Coller RA. The neuroendocrine control of water and electrolyte excretion during surgical anesthesia. Surg Gynecol Obstet 95:142, 1952.
12. Shires GT, Carrico CT, Cohn D. The role of extracellular fluid in shock. Int Anesthesiol Clin 2:435, 1964.
13. Feig PU, McCurdy DK. The hypertonic state. N Engl J Med 297:1444-1454, 1977.
14. Miller M, Dalakos T, Moses AM, et al. Recognition of partial defects in antidiuretic hormone secretion. Ann Intern Med 73:731-729, 1970.
15. Cox M, Geheb M, Singer I. Disorders of thirst and renal water excretion. In Arieff AL, DeFronzo RA, eds. Fluid, Electrolyte, and Acid-Base Disorders. New York: Churchill Livingstone, 1985, pp 119-183.
16. Geheb MA. Clinical approach to the hyperosmolar patient. Crit Care Clin 3:805, 1987.

SUGGESTED READINGS

Bernards WC. Fluid therapy in surgery, shock, and trauma: An historical survey. Crit Care Updates 2:1-9, 1991.

Vanatta JC, Fogelman MJ. Moyer's Fluid Balance, A Clinical Manual, 4th ed. Chicago: Year Book Medical Publishers, 1988.

CHAPTER 47

Infection in the Immunocompromised Patient

David L. Dunn

Surgical patients develop compromise of various components of their host defense system for many different reasons. The underlying causes, however, can be grouped into three general categories: (1) the presence of one or more underlying disease states (e.g., diabetes mellitus, renal failure, congestive heart failure), (2) exogenous immunosuppression (e.g., administration of immunosuppressive drugs for the purpose of solid organ or bone marrow allograft maintenance or chemotherapy for the treatment of malignancy); and (3) an insult associated with a major burn, polytrauma, or a major operative event. Although patients who undergo major surgery most commonly develop infection at the operative site, the immunocompromised patient is particularly prone to the development of localized specific-site infection, infection at distant sites, and disseminated systemic infection. In this chapter the evaluation and treatment of different types of infection that occur in the immunocompromised surgical patient are discussed.

HOST DEFENSES AND THE IMMUNOCOMPROMISED PATIENT

Invading microorganisms encounter several different types of host defenses that act alone and together to prevent infection. The most obvious type of host defense is that of the epithelial membranes (skin, respiratory, gut, urogenital) that create barriers to prevent microbes from invading sterile areas of the body. At many barrier sites ancillary mechanisms act in concert with the physical barrier to augment host defenses. Three general categories of these mechanisms exist (Table 47-1). Unfortunately, barrier function is imperfect, and direct trauma and disease states that diminish barrier integrity may allow microorganisms entry into the sterile host tissues. Invading microorganisms then encounter several different types of host defenses: (1) humoral, (2) cellular, and (3) monokine.

Humoral host defenses consist of complement and antibody.[1] The cell surface of many bacteria and fungi may trigger both classic and alternative complement pathway activation, resulting in enhanced phagocytosis (via C3b deposition), augmentation of the inflammatory response (via C3a- and C5a-mediated increased vascular permeability plus C5a and C5b67 leukocyte chemoattraction), and microbial death (via C789 deposition, causing microbial cell lysis). Most mammalian species possess preformed or natural antibody directed against many microorganisms, and this antibody acts

TABLE 47-1 Host Defenses

Mechanism	Example
Secretion of chemical compounds that inhibit microbacterial growth	Sebaceous gland secretions of skin
Physical removal of microorganisms	Respiratory ciliary action
Presence of resident microflora that prevent adherence, proliferation, and penetration of pathogens at barrier-host interface, that is, colonization resistance	Skin and gut autochthonous microflora

to bind microbes and microbial toxins. Antibody binding (human IgM, IgG1, and IgG3) triggers classic complement pathway deposition on the microbial cell surface in an extremely efficient fashion.

Simultaneously, resident macrophages engulf invading microbes, and phagocytic polymorphonuclear phagocytes (PMNs) are recruited into the area of incipient infection in large numbers, with the influx beginning 2 to 4 hours after invasion.[2] Both macrophages and PMNs possess receptors for the Fc region of immunoglobulins of the IgG class and C3b, both of which serve to target and markedly enhance phagocytic activity. Simultaneously, macrophages secrete a variety of monokines (i.e., interleukin-1 [IL-1], tumor necrosis factor [TNF], interleukin-6 [IL-6], and interferon) that appear to enhance the activity of cellular host defenses within the local environment. Unfortunately, these monokines are capable of concurrently exerting deleterious effects on the host should the local response be so exuberant that dissemination into the systemic circulation occurs. The triggering of local and systemic host defenses by invading microorganisms also serves to stimulate cellular immunity and immunologic memory. Should invasion occur after resolution of the initial infection, large amounts of high-affinity antibody are synthesized, and a more rapid (so-called "second set") humoral and cellular immune response will occur.

Despite current knowledge about the various components of the immune system and host defenses, precise quantification of the overall status of host defense and of specific host defense compartments is a difficult problem and does not constitute part of the current diagnostic armamentarium. Although the activity of various components of host defense (e.g., complement, phagocytosis) can be measured in vitro, these requirements remain largely an investigational tool, and few studies have provided evidence of correlations of the results of these tests with either infectious complications or overall outcome. Determination of the presence or absence (anergy) of delayed hypersensitivity by placement of skin tests to a variety of antigens and measurement of in vitro PMN phagocytic function have provided some interesting data and an approximate correlation with infectious complications in some groups of patients.[3] Unfortunately, the complexity of the immune response in a given individual probably would require sequential monitoring of all the different components of host defense, an area that is currently being investigated intensively in the research laboratory.

DIAGNOSIS OF INFECTION

Intensivists evaluating the immunocompromised patient for infection should immediately consider the following two observations: (1) critically ill patients may not mount a normal response to an infection, and (2) virtually all pathogens (bacterial, fungal, viral, and parasitic) must be considered as potentially causative organisms. Immunocompromised patients may not exhibit a normal response to infection because the above-mentioned host defenses that cause fever and leukocytosis are depressed. Thus the normal inflammatory response does not invariably occur in this patient population. For example, the immunocompromised patient who develops severe infection such as that which results after perforation of an intra-abdominal viscus may develop little if any fever, elevation of the white blood cell count, or even abdominal pain.[4] Furthermore, low-virulence pathogens that would not cause infection in the normal host may produce a significant infection in the immunocompromised individual, and virulent pathogens may cause overwhelming infection in this group of patients.[5-7] Thus the clinician must always suspect the presence of infection in the immunocompromised patient and should pursue an aggressive diagnostic regimen in an attempt to ascertain the precise site of infection and the causative pathogen(s).

Any sign of infection (e.g., fever, leukocytosis, hypotension, organ dysfunction) mandates a diagnostic evaluation to determine whether or not the infection is disseminated while simultaneously attempting to locate a specific nidus of infection and identify the causative pathogen. These steps should be done:

- Discuss with the patient and any relatives or knowledgeable friends the series of events that led to the current illness. Symptoms and signs of infection such as fever, chills, night sweats, myalgias, and lethargy should be documented with regard to severity and temporal course. The possibility of communicable diseases, travel-related disease, and disease obtained from pets or animals should be considered.
- Obtain a complete blood count with differential, a urine specimen for analysis and culture, and a specimen of blood for cultures. The procedures for culture should allow identification of aerobic, anaerobic, and acid-fast bacterial, fungal, and viral pathogens. During episodes of severe bacteremia, a Gram's stain or Wright's stain of the blood may reveal the presence of intraphagocytic organisms.
- Attempt to determine if the symptoms and signs should direct attention to a particular site. Focus on any suspicious site, both in the history and the physical examination. Perform specific diagnostic tests to evaluate the suspicious area completely.
- Intensively evaluate the suspected site (Figs.

47-1 and 47-2). Specimens obtained through invasive means (e.g., bronchoscopy, tissue biopsy, percutaneous drainage) should be sent for several different types of stains: (1) Gram's stain for aerobic and anaerobic bacteria; (2) potassium hydroxide, methenamine silver, and India ink stains to identify fungi, (3) Giemsa stain to identify organisms such as *Pneumocystis carinii* and some fungi; (4) Ziehl-Neelsen stain to identify acid-fast bacilli such as *Mycobacterium* species; (5) Tzanck smear for herpes simplex virus (HSV) and varicella-zoster virus (VZV); and (6) immunofluorescence stain to detect cytomegalovirus (CMV). Procedures for culture should allow identification of aerobic, anaerobic, and acid-fast bacterial, fungal, and viral pathogens.

TREATMENT OF INFECTION

Once diagnostic studies are complete, the clinician must decide on treatment. A considered decision is based on the available information. Three different cases are common: (1) a general type of pathogen (bacterial, fungal, or viral) has been identified based on the initial results; (2) no pathogen has been identified, and the patient is ill, possibly in extremis; and (3) no pathogen has been identified, and the patient is not particularly ill. Cases 1 and 2 allow the intensivist to institute therapy in an empiric fashion. In case 2 the use of empiric antimicrobial therapy is indicated in many cases because morbidity and mortality associated with infection in this group of patients is high. Appropriate empiric therapy depends on (1) a knowledge of the most common offending pathogens (based on the suspected site, the type of patient, and the time course after operative or immunosuppressive event(s)); (2) a willingness to pursue an ongoing diagnostic protocol coupled with institution of routine supportive measures; and (3) daily reevaluation of the effects and side effects of empiric therapy in relation to the accumulating microbiologic information and clinical course of the patient.

Bacterial Infections

Immunocompromised patients commonly develop bacterial infections caused by bacterial microorganisms that also are cultured fre-

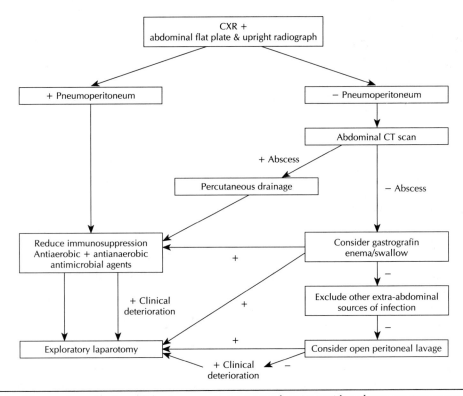

FIG. 47-1 Diagnostic evaluation of the immunocompromised patient with pulmonary symptoms or signs.

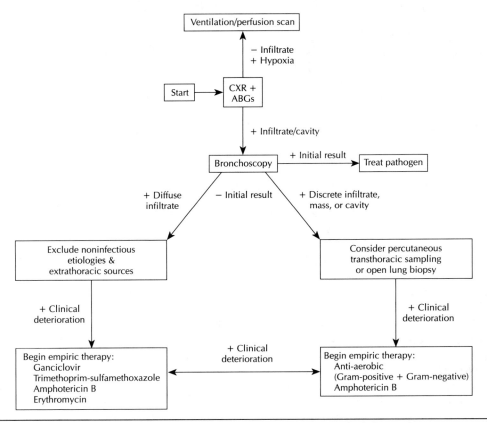

FIG. 47-2 Diagnostic evaluation of the immunocompromised patient with abdominal symptoms or signs.

quently from normal individuals. They are more likely to develop infection from organisms that normally are considered to possess a relatively low degree of virulence (e.g., *Staphylococcus epidermidis, Streptococcus faecalis* [enterococcus], and *Candida albicans*).[8] Several specific points, however, should be made regarding the former types of infections:

1. Urinary tract infections caused by Gram-negative bacilli remain the most common cause of nosocomial infections overall but are identified as associated with increased lethality in immunosuppressed patients, particularly in transplant patients when they occur in the first several weeks after transplantation.[9]

2. Bacterial (Gram-negative, Gram-positive, and polymicrobial) pulmonary infections are still common and are associated with high mortality rates, particularly in heart-lung and lung transplant patients.[10]

3. Most likely, patients who develop these particular types of infection are more prone to bacteremic episodes.

The mortality associated with nosocomial Gram-negative bacteremia is in excess of 30% in most studies of immunosuppressed individuals.[11,12]

Unusual bacterial infections can also occur in these patients. Low-virulence pathogens such as *Nocardia asteroides, Listeria monocytogenes, Legionella pneumophila* or *Legionella micdadei,* and *Actinomyces israelii* can all cause infections in this group of patients and deserve special mention. Nocardial infections can involve the lung, CNS, and subcutaneous tissue. A patient who develops nocardial infection may present with one or all sites involved and may complain of headache, cough, and the recent onset of one or more subcutaneous masses. Nocardial infection should be treated with IV sulfisoxazole. The addition of one or more agents in combination (e.g., trimethoprim, amikacin, ceftriaxone, ampicillin plus clavulinic acid, or a tetracycline) may facilitate recovery. Infection caused by *L. monocytogenes* typically presents with CNS involvement. Cerebritis, meningitis, or both may be present. Headache and photophobia are the most common presenting symptoms of this disease. Listerial infections should be treated with ampicillin plus

an aminoglycoside. The patient infected with *L. pneumophila* most commonly develops a persistent nonproductive cough and malaise that may proceed rapidly to the development of pulmonary failure and death. *Legionella* infections should be treated with erythromycin or a tetracycline. *Actinomyces* species can cause either soft tissue (frequently cervicofacial), pulmonary, or disseminated infection and are diagnosed by observing the gross appearance of "sulfur granules" at the site of infection and by characteristic anaerobic growth. Treatment consists of high-dose penicillin.

Interestingly, many of these unusual infections can be eliminated by the prophylactic adminstration of trimethoprim-sulfamethoxazole. All patients in the transplant program at the University of Minnesota start oral trimethoprim-sulfamethoxazole therapy immediately after transplantation and continue it for life. The only patients who develop several types of unusual infections *(Nocardia, Listeria, Legionella, Pneumocystis)* are those who do not receive this agent as a result of either allergy or noncompliance. The knowledge of whether or not the patient is taking trimethoprim-sulfamethoxazole facilitates the diagnostic evaluation because the above-mentioned unusual pathogens can be virtually excluded if the patient is receiving the drug.

The treatment of bacterial infection in the immunocompromised patient requires identification of the region of the body that is the source. Empiric therapy can be directed against those pathogens that frequently occur in that region of the body while culture results are being obtained. For example, intra-abdominal sepsis from secondary bacterial peritonitis almost invariably is caused by polymicrobial aerobic and anaerobic organisms derived from the gut microflora, whereas bacterial pneumonia can result from monomicrobial Gram-negative or Gram-positive pathogens. Empiric therapy and subsequent treatment regimens more commonly use broad-spectrum, single antimicrobial agents that lack organ toxicity.[13] A third-generation cephalosporin or a carbapenem such as imipenem-cilastatin sodium may be chosen over multi-drug regimens that use an aminoglycoside. Alternatively, the aminoglycoside component may be replaced with a monobactam (Fig. 47-3). Once specific culture and sensitivity results are available, a decision must be made whether or not to convert the empiric therapy regimen to agents that are precisely targeted against the offending pathogen. This decision should be based on both the culture and sensitivity results and, more importantly, on the clinical course of the patient. If the patient is doing extremely well, it makes little sense to alter an empiric therapy regimen as long as those agents chosen for empiric therapy demonstrate some reasonable degree of efficacy against the isolated organism. In transplant recipients the severity of these infections frequently mandates an absolute reduction in the number and dosage of immunosuppressive agents that are administered. In virtually all cases the patient should receive only low-dose steroid therapy for immunosuppression. Elimination of other immunosuppressive drugs such as cyclosporine, FK-506, and azathioprine is necessary to eradicate severe infection and to maximize survival. Although the potential for allograft rejection in transplant patients exists, rejection during severe infection rarely occurs.

Fungal Infections

Fungal infections represent an increasingly common cause of nosocomial infection in normal and immunocompromised patients. These infections are frequently life threatening, and for that reason administration of empiric antifungal therapy has become standard in many SICUs during the diagnostic evaluation of severe infection in the immunosuppressed individual. Fungal infections occur frequently in the presence of infection from other bacterial and viral pathogens. In many cases it is difficult to determine the precise impact of each co-pathogen on the host.

Candida species *(C. albicans, C. parapsilosis, C. tropicalis,* and *C. glabrata)* are increasingly common agents of nosocomial infections. An

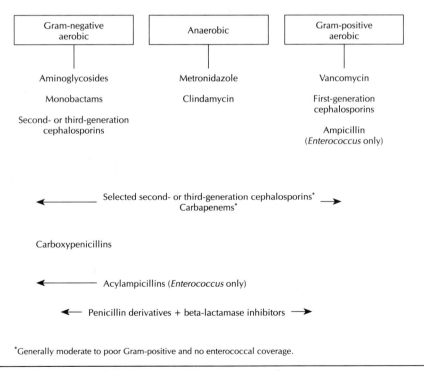

FIG. 47-3   Empiric antimicrobial therapy in immunocompromised patients.

exponential rise in the incidence of *Candida* fungemia, pneumonia, and urinary tract infections has been observed in many burn units and SICUs. Most candidal infections, particularly candidemia, are associated with three factors, frequently in combination: (1) the presence of immunosuppression (e.g., associated with diabetes, antirejection therapy), (2) prolonged (often empiric) broad-spectrum antibacterial therapy, and (3) the placement of and prolonged use of indwelling tubes or catheters. For these reasons, empiric and directed antibacterial therapy, the use of invasive monitoring catheters, IV access lines and sites, and other indwelling catheters must be reassessed daily. Candidemia causes a symptom complex very similar to that of Gram-negative bacteremia. Current evidence suggests that the toxic Gram-negative bacterial cell wall component lipopolysaccharide (LPS, endotoxin) may markedly potentiate the effects of *Candida* within the bloodstream.[14] Less commonly, *Candida* species can cause more aggressive infections at a specific site and produce abscesses within the native liver or kidney or a transplanted organ. Alternatively, *Candida* species can act as a single pathogen or as co-pathogens that are components of an extremely virulent necrotizing soft tissue infection.

A large number of other fungal pathogens can also cause infection in the immunocompromised patient. Infections caused by *Aspergillus* species (*A. fumigatus, A. flavus, A. terreus,* and *A. nidulans)* occur sporadically, although small clusters of cases correlated in time with building construction in the surrounding environs of a hospital that contains immunocompromised patients have been observed on several occasions. Most commonly, *Aspergillus* infection involves the bronchopulmonary tree. Either diffuse bilateral bronchopneumonia or a discrete unilateral infiltrate occurs. Patients often present with very nonspecific symptoms and signs such as a mild cough and fever. These infections are aggressive; thus rapid diagnosis is extremely important. Because these organisms are also frequently normal inhabitants of the oropharynx, sputum cultures are not par-

ticularly helpful. Bronchoscopy with bronchoalveolar lavage, percutaneous needle sampling of a discrete mass within the lung parenchyma, or occasionally open biopsy should be considered to establish the diagnosis. The presence of septate hyphae on methenamine silver stain of the specimen indicates that this organism may be present.

Aspergillus infection can also involve the CNS as either meningitis or a brain abscess. These organisms can also cause abscesses or diffuse infection within other organs of the body and necrotizing soft tissue infection, particularly in patients with severe neutropenia. Several other fungi also cause infection in the immunocompromised patient, although less frequently than *Candida* and *Aspergillus* species. *Pseudallescheria, Mucor,* and *Rhizopus* species cause aggressive soft tissue, craniofacial, pulmonary, and other types of infections, particularly in immunocompromised diabetic patients. These organisms are typically extremely aggressive, and the infection spreads so rapidly that aggressive surgical extirpation of the infected site in combination with antifungal agents is warranted in each and every case whenever the site and extent of involvement allow such measures. Skin and soil saprophytes such as *Trichophyton* species cause mild to moderate infection intermittently in the immunocompromised patient, and rarely unusual soil organisms such as *Paecilomyces* and *Fusarium* are observed.

The treatment of fungal infections is largely empiric, and in the majority of cases amphotericin B, which is the most effective agent, should be administered. Mild infections such as *Candida* line sepsis with minimal systemic symptoms should be treated by removal of any infected prosthetic device and administration of approximately 350 mg of amphotericin B. More aggressive infections such as *Candida* peritonitis or cryptococcal meningitis require more prolonged therapy (≥ 1 g). Frequently, the addition of a second agent such as 5-fluorocytosine (5-FC) is of benefit. Extremely aggressive infections require very long courses of amphotericin B therapy, the addition of 5-FC, and frequently a third agent such as rifampin to obtain maximum benefit. Because these infections occur sporadically and in extremely ill patients, few randomized trials have been performed to determine the precise dosing requirements for each type of infection. Only general guidelines can be provided, and the extent of therapy, interpretation of antifungal agent sensitivity patterns for specific organisms, and the usefulness of two or more agents in combination for more aggressive infection have not been established entirely.

Over the last several years, a number of antifungal agents have been developed that are based on an imidazole ring structure. Evidence suggests use of oral pharyngeal swish-and-swallow antifungal agents such as miconazole may be helpful in reducing the incidence of fungal infections in immunocompromised patients. Ketoconazole is an effective agent for *Candida,* blastomycosis, and several other types of infections, but it interferes with the hepatic metabolism of many drugs, including cyclosporine. For that reason, its use in the transplant patient population has been somewhat limited. Fluconazole is a triazole drug that can be used in IV and oral formulations. It exhibits good efficacy against *Candida* and some other fungi, but overall it is probably inferior to amphotericin B. It may represent an ideal drug for empiric treatment of the patient with a suspected mild candidal infection or for prophylaxis during prolonged antibacterial chemotherapy in the immunosuppressed patient population. Several clinical trials are currently underway to determine whether or not benefit is achieved from the prophylactic use of this agent in this setting. Itraconazole and several other antifungal agents are currently being tested for the treatment of fungal infections in immunocompromised patients, and efficacy has been reported in some cases, particularly when amphotericin B resistance was noted initially. Finally, less toxic liposomal formulations of amphotericin B are being evaluated.

Viral Infections

Viruses have been identified as pathogens that cause significant morbidity and mortality in the immunocompromised patients. The majority of this information is derived from studies of patients undergoing solid organ or bone marrow transplantation. Viruses belonging to the Herpesviridae group are HSV, VZV, Epstein-Barr virus (EBV), and CMV. All cause infections frequently during periods of maximal immunosuppression, with the highest incidence noted within the first 2 to 3 months after transplantation and subsequent to antirejection therapy. HSV most commonly causes epidermal vesicular lesions or oropharyngeal sores that are painful and can become secondarily infected with bacterial or fungal pathogens. Rarely fulminant pneumonitis, hepatitis, or meningoencephalitis occurs. VZV infection typically occurs as reactivation disease in a patient who has experienced chicken pox as a child. Reactivation consists of herpes zoster within a defined dermatomal distribution (shingles). Occasionally massive dissemination can occur throughout a large portion of the skin surface area. Dissemination is more common in patients who have not previously been exposed to VZV, and primary disease in the seronegative, immunosuppressed host can be life-threatening. In this situation manifestations typically include severe pneumonia, encephalitis, and massive epidermal dissemination. Both HSV and VZV infections are treated with acyclovir. Oral acyclovir should be administered to those patients with mild manifestations, whereas more severe disease mandates IV therapy with a concomitant reduction in immunosuppressive therapy. Should evidence of progression of disease occur while the patient is receiving high-dose IV acyclovir, all immunosuppression with the exception of a very low dose of prednisone should be halted. The patient should receive IV ganciclovir or foscarnet in place of acyclovir, and antiviral agent sensitivity testing should be performed. Zoster immunoglobulin also can be administered.

EBV can cause a mild, moderate, or severe mononucleosis type syndrome as the primary disease in the immunosuppressed patient. The treatment of choice for this process is also acyclovir. EBV has been closely associated and is most likely causal in the development of many posttransplant lymphomas. This virus causes alterations in B lymphocyte growth regulation, and, in some patients unchecked B-cell proliferation can lead to the development of polyclonal B-cell hyperplasia, after which malignant monoclonal B lymphocyte clones arise and cause organ invasion and systemic dissemination. EBV-induced posttransplant lymphomas are unusual in that they often involve visceral organs (including the transplanted organ) very early in their course, and approximately 25% to 30% of the patients have CNS involvement initially. No standardized treatment regimens exist for this disease process, although high-dose IV acyclovir, ganciclovir, and the use of interferon-α2b in conjunction with immunoglobulin, with or without a concomitant reduction in immunosuppression, have shown some promise.

Among all the herpesvirus infections, those caused by CMV have been most clearly associated with a significant impact on patient survival. CMV infection is difficult to diagnose because the patient may develop only very subtle mild systemic manifestations and because the disease can involve so many different organ systems and produce manifestations that vary markedly from patient to patient. Patients who develop CMV commonly exhibit systemic manifestations such as fever, malaise, and leukopenia. The most common organ system this virus targets is the lung, and pulmonary manifestations typically include shortness of breath, cough, and hypoxia. The CXR may show mild to moderate interstitial changes or, occasionally, a fluffy nondiscrete infiltrate. In more severe cases, diffuse, severe interstitial changes similar to those seen with the adult respiratory distress syndrome occur. Other manifestations of CMV infection include GI bleeding from mucosal ulceration, hepatitis, pancreatitis, and retinitis. Currently, most patients develop mild to moderate disease, although an occasional case of severe, lethal CMV consisting of severe hypotension, organ failure, and death occurs.

Only within the last several years has it been possible to diagnose and treat this disease process more effectively. Body fluid samples should be obtained from blood, urine, and sputum in all patients in whom a herpesvirus infection is suspected. Specific tissue sites should also be sampled. Bronchoscopy with bronchoalveolar lavage is an effective means of determining whether or not active infection is present within the lung, and abnormal areas of mucosa or obvious mucosal ulceration within the GI tract should be biopsied. Other sites of involvement, such as the liver, are amenable to percutaneous biopsy, and occasionally evidence of CMV infection is observed during examination of renal allograft biopsies. Tissue specimens should be pathologically examined for the presence of CMV inclusion bodies. Routine virologic cultures using a lytic fibroblast assay should also be performed on all specimens, but culture results are often not available for several weeks. Samples should be analyzed through the enhanced shell vial (so-called "rapid antigen") assay that uses growth of the specimen with fibroblasts for 14 to 18 hours, followed by staining with an immunofluorescence-tagged monoclonal antibody directed against CMV early capsid antigens and direct microscopic observation. This rapid test can markedly facilitate the diagnosis of CMV disease.

Both oral or IV acyclovir and anti-CMV immunoglobulin are efficacious in the prevention of CMV disease in solid organ and bone marrow transplant recipients.[15,16] Patients at highest risk for the development of CMV disease include recipients of both living related and cadaveric allografts who receive tissue or bone marrow from a CMV seropositive donor and are themselves CMV seronegative. Patients who receive cadaveric organs and those who suffer one or more episodes of rejection require antirejection therapy (particularly with antilymphocyte globulin preparations such as Minnesota antilymphocyte globulin and the murine monoclonal antibody OKT3). Older patients are at higher risk to develop CMV. Most patients present with vague symptoms, typically consisting of fever, malaise, leukopenia, shortness of breath, or a combination of these symptoms and signs. Determining the presence of CMV through serologic and culture techniques often requires days to weeks. Therefore aggressive diagnostic evaluation in which blood, urine, sputum, bronchoalveolar lavage, GI, and/or tissue biopsies are obtained and evaluated by the rapid antigen technique is mandatory to determine whether or not CMV or some other pathogen is responsible for the patient's systemic manifestations.

In all cases the presenting complex of symptoms and signs should be reviewed in conjunction with the information obtained from these assays. Should a tissue-invasive site be identified in conjunction with one or more of the above-mentioned symptoms, a 14-day course of IV ganciclovir therapy should be instituted.[17,18] This drug exhibits excellent in vitro activity against CMV compared to acyclovir and many other antiviral agents. Administration can be associated with toxic effects that most commonly consist of bone marrow suppression and hepatitis. Because the drug is excreted by the kidney, the dosage should be adjusted in the presence of renal dysfunction. Patients who exhibit severe manifestations compatible with CMV disease should receive ganciclovir on an empiric basis, often in conjunction with a reduction in immunosuppression. Those individuals with moderate signs and symptoms compatible with CMV, who have only blood or urine samples positive for this organism, should also receive therapy. Asymptomatic patients who exhibit CMV shedding should not receive ganciclovir therapy. Overall, ganciclovir is effective, safe, and appears to improve patient and allograft survival.[17] Recently we have successfully identified a group of patients in whom mild to moderate CMV disease and mild to moderate rejection can be treated simultaneously with success.

Protozoan and Parasitic Infections

P. carinii can produce significant pulmonary symptoms (e.g., dyspnea), and the CXR often demonstrates bilateral diffuse alveolar or interstitial abnormalities. Patients receiving trimethoprim-sulfamethoxazole prophylaxis rarely develop infection caused by this pathogen. High-dose trimethoprim-sulfamethoxazole, pentamidine isthionate, trimethoprim-dapsone, or trimetrexate is used for treatment. *Toxoplasma gondii* infection can cause necrotizing encephalitis, myocarditis, or pneumonitis, and transmission through transplantation of cardiac allograft tissue has been documented. Treatment should be instituted with pyrimethamine and sulfadiazine. Other parasitic diseases (e.g., strongyloidiasis, amebiasis, malaria, schistosomiasis) are seen rarely outside of tropical environments.

NEW THERAPEUTIC MODALITIES

Three emerging areas of therapeutic intervention deserve discussion: (1) selective gut decontamination, (2) use of antiendotoxin antibodies, and (3) use of monokine antagonists. Selective gut decontamination uses oral antibacterial and antifungal agents to prevent nosocomial infections, particularly in the immunocompromised individual. This concept arose from two observations: (1) when patients with hematologic malignancies became severely neutropenic, episodes of Gram-negative bacterial sepsis were more frequent and were caused by organisms that could be isolated concurrently from the stool[19]; and (2) patients in SICUs became rapidly colonized with Gram-negative aerobic isolates—first in the nasopharynx, then in the upper GI tract—and these same organisms frequently were isolated from the pulmonary tree and appeared to cause nosocomial pneumonias.[20]

Extension of the first observation to individuals with a normal immune system has required an additional concept—that of microbial translocation. Translocation can be defined as the process by which microbes or microbial products transgress the integrity of the gut lumen, pass through the lamina propria, and subsequently escape the confines of the intestine.

Several routes may exist that are dependent on the microbes or microbial products involved. For example, in some cases direct portal venous invasion by bacteria or bacterial toxins may occur, but in others translocation through lymphatics may be halted at the level of the mesenteric lymph node. Systemic infection may occur after the liver is unable to contain organisms that translocate through the lymphatics or intestinal venules.

One of the principal factors that appears to prevent microbial translocation is colonization resistance, a contention supported by data obtained from experimental models of translocation in which animals are gut decontaminated with antiaerobic and antianaerobic antimicrobial agents and exposed to and colonized with a single aerobic organism. These animals typically exhibit a high degree of microbial translocation to the level of the mesenteric lymph node. Recent studies, however, in which clinical evidence of the occurrence of microbial translocation has been sought have not substantiated this concept, and it remains an intriguing laboratory phenomenon.[21]

The autochthonous microflora of the colon consist of a wide variety of resident Gram-negative and Gram-positive aerobes and anaerobes and yeast.[22] The anaerobic component of the bowel microflora prevents adherence of pathogenic microorganisms, presumably preventing invasion that may lead to bacterial translocation and systemic dissemination. For that reason, selective gut decontamination protocols have used agents that targeted elimination of those pathogenic Gram-negative aerobes and yeast that appear to disseminate while maintaining the anaerobic flora. Although a large number of selective gut decontamination trials have been performed, virtually every trial has demonstrated that, although it is possible to alter outcome with regard to a reduction in both the overall rates of nosocomial infections (particularly nosocomial pneumonia) and the types of nosocomial infections that occur, it has not

been possible to demonstrate a reduction in mortality rate.[23-32]

Two monoclonal antibody preparations (HA-1A, E5) directed against the toxic lipid A component of Gram-negative bacterial endotoxin have shown some degree of efficacy in two recent clinical trials.[33,34] Administration of HA-1A within 24 hours of the onset of symptoms compatible with sepsis was associated with a reduction in mortality rate in patients who subsequently were proved to have developed Gram-negative bacteremia. Unfortunately, these preparations are extremely expensive and probably are most efficacious when administered early after the development of Gram-negative bacteremia is suspected and before the diagnosis has been established. In both studies nearly two thirds of patients who were treated proved to have infection from other types of organisms (Gram-positive bacteria, yeast) against which the antiendotoxin antibody had no effect. The development of rapid, precise diagnostic tests for Gram-negative bacteremia and endotoxemia should significantly improve the clinician's ability to administer these antibodies quickly to those patients who would benefit from therapy.

Because both TNF and IL-1 apparently are causative factors in the development of the deleterious host septic response, current clinical trials are designed to test whether or not anti-TNF monoclonal antibodies or the use of an IL-1 receptor antagonist will improve outcome in severe infection. Since increased TNF and/or IL-1 host production may be caused by Gram-negative or Gram-positive bacterial or fungal pathogens; the use of these preparations is extremely attractive (vide supra) because their efficacy may be less dependent on the type of infecting organism. Although experimental data indicate that these agents may be efficacious for the treatment of the septic state, data from the clinical trials currently being performed are not yet available.

SUMMARY

- Surgical patients develop compromise of various components of their host defense system for many different reasons, which can be grouped into three general categories: (1) underlying disease states, (2) exogenous immunosuppression, and (3) insult associated with a major burn, polytrauma, or a major operative event.
- Intensivists evaluating the immunocompromised patient for infection should immediately consider two observations: (1) this group of patients may not mount a normal response to an infection, and (2) virtually all pathogens (bacterial, fungal, viral, and parasitic) must be considered as potentially causative organisms.
- Any sign of infection mandates institution of diagnostic evaluation to determine whether or not the infection is disseminated while simultaneously attempting to locate a specific nidus of infection and to identify the causative pathogen.
- Diagnostic evaluation should proceed as follows: (1) carefully obtain history of series of events that led up to current illness; (2) obtain a CBC with differential, urine specimen for analysis and culture, and specimen of blood for cultures (culture techniques should allow identification of aerobic, anaerobic, and acid-fast bacterial, fungal, and viral pathogens); (3) attempt to determine if symptoms and signs should direct attention to a particular site; and (4) intensively evaluate suspected site.
- Treatment consists of therapy targeted against one or more identified pathogens or empiric antimicrobial therapy.
- Appropriate empiric therapy must be directed by three factors: (1) knowledge of most common offending pathogens (based on suspected site, type of patient, and time course after operative or immunosuppressive event(s)); (2) willingness to pursue an ongoing diagnostic protocol, coupled with institution of routine supportive measures; and (3) daily reevaluation of effects and side effects of empiric therapy in relation to accumulating microbiologic information and clinical course of the patient.

REFERENCES

1. Dunn DL, Meakins JL. Humoral immunity to infection and the complement system. In Howard RJ, Simmons RL, eds. Surgical Infectious Diseases. East Norwalk, Conn. Appleton & Lange, 1988, p 175.
2. Dunn DL, Barke RA, Knight NB, Humphrey EW, Simmons RL. Role of resident macrophages, peripheral neutrophils, and translymphatic absorption in bacterial clearance from the peritoneal cavity. Infect Immun 49:257, 1985.
3. Christou NV, Rode H, Larsen D, Loose L, Broadhead M, Meakins JL. The walk-in anergic patient. Ann Surg 199:438, 1984.
4. Dunn DL, Najarian JS. Abdominal catastrophes in the immunosuppressed patient. In Najarian JS, Delaney JP, eds. Trauma and Critical Care Surgery. Chicago: Year Book Medical Publishers, 1987, p 271.
5. Dunn DL, Simmons RL. Opportunistic infections after renal transplant. I. Viral and bacterial infections. Infect Surg 8:164, 1989.
6. Dunn SL, Simmons RL. Opportunistic infections after renal transplant. II. Fungal and protozoan infections. Infect Surg 8:277, 1989.
7. Dunn DL, Najarian JS. Infectious complications in transplant surgery. In Shires GT, Davis J, eds. Principles and Management of Surgical Infection. Philadelphia: JB Lippincott, 1990, p 425.
8. Dunn DL. The role of infection and use of antimicrobial agents during multiple system organ failure. In Deitch EA, ed. Multiple Organ Failure. Pathophysiology and Basic Concepts of Therapy. New York: Thieme Medical Publishers, 1990, p 150.
9. Hoy WE, Kissel SM, Freeman RB, Sterling WA. Altered patterns of posttransplant urinary tract infections associated with perioperative antibiotics and curtailed catheterization. Am J Kidney Dis 6:212, 1985.
10. Brooks RG, Hofflin JM, Jamieson SW, Stinson EB, Remington JS. Infectious complications in heart-lung transplant recipients. Am J Med 79:412, 1985.
11. Dunn DL. Immunotherapeutic advances in the treatment of gram-negative bacterial sepsis. World J Surg 11:233, 1987.
12. Cody CS, Dunn DL. Endotoxins in septic shock. In Neugebauer E, Holaday J. CRC Handbook on Mediators in Septic Shock. Boca Raton, Fla.: CRC Press, [in press].

13. Dunn DL, Simmons RL. Rational empiric antibiotic therapy of peritonitis and intraabdominal infection. Infect Surg 2:466, 1983.

14. Burd RS, Raymond CS, Dunn DL. Endotoxin promotes synergistic lethality during concurrent *Escherichia coli* and *Candida albicans* infection. J Surg Res [in press].

15. Balfour HH, Chace BA, Stapleton JT, Simmons SL, Fryd DS. A randomized, placebo-controlled trial of oral acyclovir for the prevention of cytomegalovirus disease in recipients of renal allografts. N Engl J Med 320:1381, 1989.

16. Snydman DR, Werner BG, Heinze-Lacey B, et al. Use of cytomegalovirus immune globulin to prevent cytomegalovirus disease in renal-transplant recipients. N Engl J Med 317:1049, 1987.

17. Dunn DL, Mayoral JL, Gillingham KJ, Loeffler CM, Brayman KL, Kramer MA, Erice A, Balfour HH, Fletcher CV, Bolman RM III, Matas AJ, Payne WD, Sutherland DER, Najarian JS. Treatment of invasive cytomegalovirus disease in solid organ transplant patients with ganciclovir. Transplantation 51:98, 1991.

18. Mayoral JL, Loeffler CM, Fasola CG, Kramer MA, Orrom WJ, Matas AJ, Najarian JS, Dunn DL. Diagnosis and treatment of cytomegalovirus disease in transplant patients based upon gastrointestinal tract manifestations. Arch Surg 126:202, 1991.

19. Tancrede CH, Andremont AO. Bacterial translocation and gram-negative bacteremia in patients with hematological malignancies. J Infect Dis 152:99, 1985.

20. Marshall JC, Christou NV, Horn R, Meakins JL. The microbiology of multiple organ failure: The proximal gastrointestinal tract as an occult reservoir of pathogens. Arch Surg 123:309, 1988.

21. Moore FA, Moore EE, Poggetti R, et al. Gut bacterial translocation via the portal vein: A clinical perspective with major torso trauma. J Trauma 31:629, 1991.

22. Dunn DL. Autochthonous microflora of the gastrointestinal tract. Perspect Colon Rectal Surg 2:105, 1990.

23. Sleijfer DT, Mulder NH, de Vries-Hospers HG, et al. Infection prevention in granulocytopenic patients by selective decontamination of the digestive tract. Eur J Cancer 16:859, 1980.

24. Guiot HFL, van den Broek PJ, van der Meer JWM, van Furth R. Selective antimicrobial modulation of the intestinal flora of patients with acute nonlymphocytic leukemia: A double-blind, placebo-controlled study. J Infect Dis 147:615, 1983.

25. Stoutenbeek CP, van Saene HKF, Miranda DR, Zandstra DF, Binnendijk B. The prevention of superinfection in multiple trauma patients. J Antimicrob Chemother 14:B203, 1984.

26. Guiot HF, Helmig-Schurter AV, van Der Meer JWM, van Furth R. Selective antimicrobial modulation of the intestinal microbial flora for infection prevention in patients with hematologic malignancies. Scand J Infect Dis 8:153, 1986.

27. Ledingham IA, Eastaway AT, McKay IC, Alcock SR, McDonald JC, Ramsay G. Triple regimen selective decontamination of the digestive tract, systemic cefotaxime, and microbiological surveillance for prevention of acquired infection in intensive care. Lancet 1:785, 1988.

28. Ulrich C, Harinck-de Weerd JE, Bakker NC, Jacz K, Doornbos L, de Ridder VA. Selective decontamination of the digestive tract with norfloxacin in the prevention of ICU-acquired infections: A prospective randomized study. Intensive Care Med 15:424, 1989.

29. Tetteroo GWM, Wagenvoort JHT, Castelein A, Tilanus HW, Ince C, Bruining HA. Selective decontamination to reduce gram-negative colonization and infections after oesophageal resection. Lancet 335:704, 1990.

30. Aerdts SJA, Clasener HAL, van Dalen R, Van Lier HJJ, Vollaard EJ, Festen J. Prevention of bacterial colonization of the respiratory tract and stomach of mechanically ventilated patients by a novel regimen of selective decontamination in combination with initial systemic cefotaxime. J Antimicrob Chemother 26:A59, 1990.

31. Goris JA, van Bebber IPT, Mollen RMH, Koopman JP. Does selective decontamination of the gastrointestinal tract prevent multiple organ failure? Arch Surg 126:561, 1991.

32. Cerra FB, Maddaus M, Dunn DL, Wells C, Konstantinides N, Lehmann S, Mann H. Selective gut decontamination does not reduce mortality or organ failure in surgical intensive care unit patients. Arch Surg 127:163, 1992.

33. Ziegler E, Fisher C, Sprung C, Straube R, Sadoff J, Foulke G. Treatment of gram-negative bacteremia and septic shock with HA-1A human monoclonal antibody against endotoxin. N Engl J Med 324:429, 1991.

34. Greenman R, Schein R, Martin M, Wenzel R, MacIntyre N, Emmanuel G, Chmel H, Kohler R, McCarthy M, Plouffe J, Russel J, Xoma Sepsis Study Group. A controlled clincial trial of E5 murine monoclonal IgM antibody to endotoxin in the treatment of gram-negative sepsis. JAMA 266:1097, 1991.

PART FIVE

COMMON SICU PROCEDURES

CHAPTER 48

Bronchoscopy

Marshall I. Hertz · Paul Gustafson

Flexible fiberoptic bronchoscopy (FFB) is an important tool in the diagnostic and therapeutic armamentarium of the critical care practitioner. In this chapter the indications, contraindications, and complications of FFB are discussed. FFB requires specialized training and should be performed only by experienced individuals; therefore a detailed review of the technique of the procedure is beyond the scope of this chapter. A brief description of the method of performing FFB and bronchoalveolar lavage (BAL) in critically ill patients is included to assist critical care physicians in the management of patients during and after these procedures.

OVERVIEW

FFB allows direct visualization of the central airways (i.e., lobar, segmental, and subsegmental bronchi) and biopsy of central and peripheral respiratory tract structures. It is also of therapeutic use in patients with mucous plugging, hemoptysis, and foreign bodies. In the SICU FFB most commonly is used to sample the respiratory tract secretions of patients with suspected pneumonia.[1-3]

Several approaches are used to obtain bronchial secretions through FFB. Sputum may simply be suctioned through the FFB. "Bronchial washings" are obtained by instilling saline solution in small amounts (5 to 10 ml) into the distal bronchi and suctioning through the bronchoscopic channel. "Bronchial brushings" are obtained by use of small plastic bristle brushes passed through the FFB channel. A modified bronchial brush, the "protected brush catheter," uses a telescoping catheter system through which the brush is passed, enabling the bronchoscopist to obtain bronchial secretions uncontaminated by upper respiratory or endotracheal tube microorganisms carried to the lower respiratory tract by the FFB. To increase the specificity of protected brush catheter specimens, quantitative cultures have also been used.[3]

Because FFB usually is performed to evaluate pneumonia in immunocompetent or immunocompromised patients, sampling the alveolar contents is the ultimate goal of the procedure. The initial application of FFB that enabled alveolar sampling was the transbronchial biopsy (TBB). TBB is performed by passing a small forceps through the bronchoscopic channel and obtaining small (approximately 1 mm diameter) biopsies of lung parenchyma under fluoroscopic control. TBB is unique among transbronchoscopic procedures in that it alone can provide specimens for histologic examination. Since some pneumonic processes, particularly granulomatous infections, may not result in shedding of organisms in bronchial or alveolar secretions, TBB remains a useful procedure in selected patients. However, several features of TBB limit its use in most critically ill patients. First, the patient must be transported to the fluoroscopy suite, which entails risks in unstable patients. Further, major complications, including hemorrhage and pneumothorax, occur after TBB in up to 3% of patients.[4] Many immunocompromised patients are thrombocytopenic. They are often not candidates for TBB because they have a prohibitive risk of hemorrhage. Finally, TBB samples only approximately 100 alveoli per biopsy; with a total of 150 million alveoli per lung, the sampling error is very significant.

In recent years BAL has become an important technique for the diagnosis of suspected lower respiratory tract infection.[5,6] This procedure involves instilling relatively large volumes of saline solution (approximately 100 ml) into the alveolar spaces while the bronchoscope is wedged in a segmental or subsegmental bronchus to prevent spillage of the solution throughout the airways. The saline solution, mixed with alveolar and distal bronchial contents, is recovered by suction through the bronchoscope channel and is sent for cultures and analytic studies. BAL avoids many of the drawbacks of other transbronchoscopic procedures, for BAL can be performed at the bedside. The procedure does not result in bleeding or pneumothorax and thus can be offered to many patients in whom TBB is contraindicated. Finally, each lavage samples approximately 1 million alveoli, greatly reducing the magnitude of the sampling error.

INDICATIONS

FFB is used in critically ill patients for both diagnostic and therapeutic indications (Table 48-1).

Suspected pneumonia. The need for bronchoscopically collected lower respiratory tract culture material must be evaluated on a patient-by-patient basis. In general, patients with postoperative pulmonary infiltrates who are producing sputum containing a predominant organism do not require FFB. However, for patients from whose sputum a likely pathogen cannot be obtained or those not producing sputum despite clinical and radiographic deterioration, FFB with protected brush catheter sampling and/or BAL is indicated. In immunocompromised hosts the spectrum of infectious microorganisms causing pneumonia is much broader; BAL and obtaining cultures for detecting bacteria (including *Legionella*), fungi,

TABLE 48-1   Indications for Flexible Fiberoptic Bronchoscopy in Critically Ill Patients

	Diagnostic	Therapeutic
Suspected pneumonia	x	
Atelectasis	x	x
Hemoptysis	x	x
Foreign body	x	x
Suspected tracheobronchial disruption	x	x
Smoke inhalation	x	
Difficult intubation		x

viruses, and mycobacteria are indicated in most of these patients. In patients with suspected fungal pneumonia, TBB may also be helpful.

Atelectasis. FFB is often of therapeutic benefit in patients with postoperative atelectasis. When major atelectasis occurs (e.g., total atelectasis of a lobe or lung), the chest x-ray film should be examined first for improper endotracheal tube placement. Assuming that the tube is properly positioned, FFB can be therapeutic if an endobronchial mucous plug is seen and evacuated. Bronchoscopy is *not* of benefit if mucous obstruction of the bronchus is not present. Therefore the physical examination is of help in determining the need for bronchoscopy; that is, FFB usually is useful only when breath sounds in the atelectatic area are decreased. This is of particular relevance to postcoronary artery bypass patients who frequently develop left lower atelectasis. In most cases this is "open bronchus atelectasis" with preserved breath sounds, and the condition will not be improved by bronchoscopy.

In patients who develop minor degrees of atelectasis without physiologic compromise, chest physical therapy with percussion and postural drainage, encouragement of upright posture, and cough and deep breathing are indicated before FFB and frequently result in radiographic and clinical improvement.[7]

FFB is also indicated in patients who have undergone thoracic surgical procedures, including lobectomy and pneumectomy, and who develop major atelectasis with or without pneumothorax. FFB is used in this setting to identify an endobronchial blood clot and mucous plugging or disruption of the bronchial stump.

Hemoptysis. In SICU patients with normal platelet counts and coagulation tests, hemoptysis is most commonly due to local trauma from the end of the tracheostomy or endotracheal tube or from vigorous suctioning efforts. In such cases FFB allows identification of the bleeding site and leads to appropriate corrective actions. Hemoptysis in patients with tracheostomies may also result from erosion through the trachea into the innominate artery. This complication generally results in massive hemoptysis, and the source is seldom seen with the FFB. Hemoptysis in postoperative patients may also result from other bronchoscopically diagnosable conditions, including endobronchial lesions of the major airways such as bronchogenic carcinoma and less common tumors. In patients with negative bronchoscopic evaluations for hemoptysis, many other causes must be considered, including pulmonary embolization. Pneumonia, especially in patients with coagulopathy, may present with parenchymal bleeding.

FFB is also useful therapeutically in SICU patients with hemoptysis. Hemostatic medications, including epinephrine (3 to 5 ml of 1:10,000 solution), and topically applied thrombin can be applied directly to bleeding endobronchial lesions. When blood is emanating from a distal airway site, these medications can be instilled while the bronchoscope is wedged in a proximal airway. When bleeding is not controlled with medications but can be localized to a bronchopulmonary segment, a 4 Fr or 5 Fr balloon-tipped catheter, passed through the channel of the instrument and inflated in the bronchus, may tamponade the bleeding en route to more definitive diagnostic and therapeutic efforts (e.g., arteriography, bronchial artery embolization, or surgery as indicated; see Chapter 11).

Foreign body. Foreign body aspiration in the SICU is unusual but occasionally occurs. Most aspirated foreign bodies can be visualized with the FFB, and in many cases retrieval of the foreign body with a forceps is possible. Large foreign bodies may require use of a rigid bronchoscope for removal.

Suspected tracheobronchial disruption. In patients who have sustained major chest trauma, particularly when it is associated with first and second rib fractures, partial or complete disruption of the bronchial tree at the level of the trachea or main bronchi is not uncommon.[8] In trauma patients with pneumothorax accompanied by a major air leak after chest tube placement, FFB is indicated to evaluate the integrity of the trachea and main bronchi. Nontraumatic bronchopleural fistulas can also be identified by observing bubbling at the bronchial orifice after saline solution instillation. Successful closure of bronchopleural fistulas has been reported after instillation of "fibrin glue," which consists of fibrinogen and thrombin.[9]

Smoke inhalation. Patients rescued from closed-space fires, particularly those with burns of the nose and mouth, have a very high incidence of laryngeal and tracheal burns.[10] Such patients should be evaluated by FFB immediately to identify laryngeal and tracheal edema and to place an endotracheal tube prophylactically when indicated.

Difficult intubation. FFB can be used for difficult nasotracheal or orotracheal intubations. The endotracheal tube is placed over the FFB, and the tip is visually guided past the glottic aperture. Once the bronchoscope is in the trachea, the endotracheal tube can be advanced through the glottis, using the FFB as a stylette.

CONTRAINDICATIONS

A thorough pre-bronchoscopy evaluation is necessary to identify factors contraindicating the procedure (see box, p. 510). Thrombocytopenic patients (i.e., with a platelet count <80 to 100/mm^3) and those in whom a pneumothorax would not be tolerated, even if recognized and treated immediately, should not undergo transbronchial biopsies.

Less traumatic procedures that are per-

| **Contraindications to FFB** |

Factors mandating endotracheal intubation before bronchoscopy

Severe respiratory distress (e.g., respiratory rate >30/min, use of accessory muscles)

Inability to achieve partial pressure of oxygen in arterial blood (Pao_2) $\geq$70 mm Hg (9.3 kPa) with supplemental oxygen by mask

Abnormal mental status precluding cooperation with the procedure

Factors contraindicating bronchoscopy in intubated patients unless corrected

Cardiovascular instability (e.g., hypotension, significant dysrrhythmias) despite pharmacologic intervention

Inability to achieve Pao_2 >70 mm Hg (9.3 kPa) on fraction of inspired oxygen (Fio_2) of 1

Severe electrolyte or metabolic disturbance (e.g., pH <7.3 potassium level >5.3 mEq/L)

---

formed through the FFB, including BAL, are contraindicated in many critically ill patients unless endotracheal intubation is done before the procedure. Such patients include those with rapidly deteriorating respiratory status, those in whom an arterial partial pressure of oxygen (Pao_2) of at least 70 mm Hg cannot be achieved with supplemental oxygen by mask, and those with abnormal mental status (e.g., agitation, somnolence) that would preclude cooperation with the procedure or contraindicate the administration of sedating medications.

Previously intubated patients are evaluated to identify factors contraindicating FFB unless corrected. These factors include cardiovascular instability despite pharmacologic intervention. Patients whose blood pressure can be maintained above 100 mm Hg systolic with moderate doses of pressor medications and those with non-threatening cardiac dysrhythmias (e.g., with occasional premature ventricular contractions) are not prohibited from undergoing FFB. Patients in whom a Pao_2 >70 mm Hg cannot be achieved despite a fraction of inspired oxygen (Fio_2) of 1 are excluded because the risk of developing refractory hypoxemia during the

procedure is high. Severe electrolyte or metabolic disturbances are corrected before FFB.

BRONCHOSCOPY AND BRONCHOALVEOLAR LAVAGE WITH INTUBATION

Once the need for BAL is established and the pre-bronchoscopy evaluation (including obtaining informed consent) is completed, this protocol is followed:

Supplemental oxygen. Fifteen minutes before the procedure, the Fio_2 is increased to 1, and it is continued at that level throughout the procedure. An Fio_2 of 1 is necessary because even healthy individuals and stable patients undergoing bronchoscopy experience significant decreases in Pao_2 during the procedure.[11,12] After BAL, the Fio_2 gradually is weaned to the lowest Fio_2 required to maintain arterial oxyhemoglobin saturation $\geq$92%.

Bronchoscope. The FFB consists of optical fiber bundles, flexion-extension cables, and a hollow channel for suction and instrument passage, all packaged in a durable plastic sheath. Instruments commonly used in the critical care setting have outside diameters of 4 to 5 mm. The FFB can be passed transnasally or transorally in awake, unintubated patients. In intubated patients an instrument is chosen that can be passed through the endotracheal tube with adequate clearance to allow ventilation. In general, the endotracheal tube's diameter must be at least 2.5 mm larger than the bronchoscope's diameter. Because the pediatric bronchoscope (outside diameter of 4 mm) provides suboptimal BAL fluid returns, an 8 mm or 9 mm endotracheal tube, which will permit passage of a 5 mm diameter instrument, should be placed if possible. When changing to a larger endotracheal tube is not feasible, the smaller bronchoscope is used. A small glottic aperture or a requirement for uninterrupted positive end-expiratory pressure may preclude changing to a larger endotracheal tube.

Ventilator management. The goal is to provide the patient with a minute ventilation during the procedure that is equivalent to that which he/she was receiving before the procedure. The ventilator pressure limit alarm is set at 40 cm H_2O or 10 cm H_2O above the pre-bronchoscopy baseline level, whichever is higher. The tidal volume is decreased by approximately 33%, the respiratory rate is increased by an equal proportion, and the inspiratory flow rate is decreased. In this manner a constant minute ventilation is provided at a lower peak airway pressure to avoid repeatedly exceeding the preset pressure limit of the ventilator. After the bronchoscope has been inserted into the airway, the exhaled minute volume is monitored. The inspired tidal volume is increased to compensate for the volume lost when air leak occurs at the site of bronchoscopic insertion.

Monitors. All patients are monitored with continuous ECG and continuous pulse oximetery. Many patients have indwelling arterial catheters for blood pressure monitoring. Intermittent automated blood pressure monitoring is generally used for patients who do not have indwelling arterial catheters.

Medications. Analgesics and tranquilizers (opiates and benzodiazepines, respectively) are used to ensure patient comfort during the procedure. In most cases a nondepolarizing muscle relaxant is required to maintain optimal control of the procedure (i.e., to eliminate cough and agitation). In patients judged not to require muscle relaxation, 1% lidocaine (Xylocaine) is applied topically to the airways as needed to control cough.

Bronchoalveolar lavage technique. After the administration of medications, the bronchoscope is passed into the endotracheal tube through a plastic adapter with a rubber diaphragm designed to minimize air leakage. The bronchoscope is attached to tubing with a three-way stopcock between the suction port and the collection traps (Fig. 48-1). The bronchoscopist wedges the bronchoscope in the optimal position while an assistant performs the lavage. Use of two persons minimizes the likelihood of dislodging the bronchoscope and spilling saline solution throughout the airways. The bronchoscopic channel is flushed with saline solution and gently wedged in a segmental or subsegmental bronchus in the area of abnormality observed on chest x-ray film. In patients with diffuse pulmonary infiltrates, two to three nondependent segments, usually the

right middle lobe and the lingula of the left upper lobe, are lavaged because lavage of nondependent segments results in a higher percent recovery of the instilled fluid. Lavage is carried out in each anatomic location by instilling 100 ml of sterile isotonic saline solution (at 37° C) in five 20 ml aliquots, with each aliquot gently suctioned (wall suction <150 mm Hg) before adminsitration of the next aliquot. In general, 50% to 75% of the instilled saline solution is recovered in the lavage effluent. A lavage is considered acceptable after ≥40% of the volume of instilled saline solution is returned. The lavage effluent from all sites is usually pooled and treated as a single specimen.

At our institution, lavage effluent from all SICU patients is sent for the following studies: RBC and WBC counts and WBC differential; cytologic examination; cultures for bacteria, mycobacteria, *Legionella,* fungi, and viruses; and direct fluorescent antibody for *Legionella.* In immunocompromised patients additional rapid viral detection modalities are used, including shell vial culture with monoclonal antibody staining to identify cytomegalovirus ("rapid antigen") and respiratory syncytial virus antigen detection by enzyme-linked immunosorbent assay (ELISA).

COMPLICATIONS

Complications are unusual during FFB performed to visualize the airways, but laryngospasm (in unintubated patients) and bronchospasm may occur, particularly in asthmatic patients. Arterial oxygen tension regularly falls during FFB.[11,12] Administering supplemental oxygen will correct hypoxemia. When additional procedures such as transbronchial biopsy and BAL are performed, additional complications may ensue (Table 48-2). Transbronchial biopsy poses a 1% to 3% risk of pneumothorax, and there is a similar incidence of severe bleeding, even in patients with normal platelet count and coagulation parameters. In patients who are uremic, thrombocytopenic, or coagulopathic, the risk of major bleeding increases dramatically.[4]

Complications of BAL include hypoxemia, fever, and pneumonia. Hypoxemia begins during or soon after the procedure and persists until

TABLE 48-2 Complications of Transbronchoscopic Procedures*

	Transbronchial Biopsy	Bronchoalveolar Lavage
Major hemorrhage	<1%†	
Pneumothorax	1%-3%	
Decreased arterial oxygenation	Common	Common
Fever		~5%
Pneumonia		~1%

*Modified from Fulkerson WJ. Current concepts: Fiberoptic bronchoscopy. N Engl J Med 311:511-516, 1984.
†Risk markedly increased in patients with uremia, thrombocytopenia, or other coagulopathy.

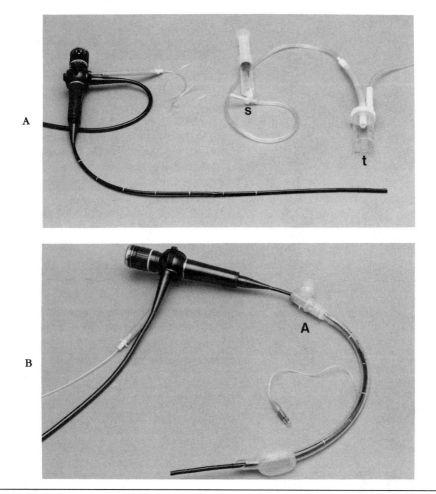

FIG. 48-1 **A,** Bronchoscope is modified by interposition of three-way stopcock *(s)* in suction tubing to allow instillation and withdrawal of lavage fluid by an assistant, leaving both hands of bronchoscopist free to manipulate bronchoscope. Collection traps *(t)* are introduced into suction tubing circuit after local anesthetic has been administered, upper airway secretions are cleared, and bronchoscope is wedged in segmental or subsegmental bronchus. **B,** Bronchoscope is passed into endotracheal tube through plastic adapter *(A)* with a rubber diaphragm. (From Hertz M, Woodward ME, Gross CR, et al. Safety of bronchoalveolar lavage in the critically ill, mechanically ventilated patient. Crit Care Med 19:1526-1532, 1991.)

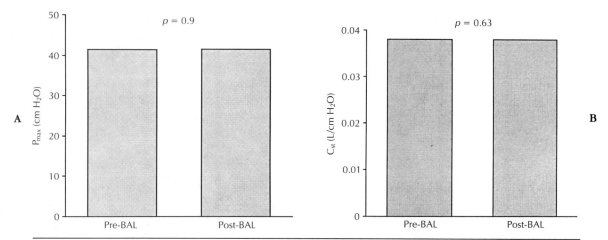

FIG. 48-2   Variables reflecting lung mechanics before and after bronchoalveolar lavage. **A,** No significant change occurred in maximal inspiratory airway pressure (P_{max}) after BAL (41.45 ± 2.98 cm H_2O pre-BAL vs. 41.58 ± 2.76 cm H_2O post-BAL; $p = 0.90$). **B,** No significant change occurred in static lung compliance (C_{st}) after BAL (0.0378 ± 0.004 L/cm H_2O pre-BAL vs. 0.0384 ± 0.004 L/cm H_2O post-BAL; $p = 0.63$).

residual fluid is absorbed from the alveoli into the vascular space. Therefore patients are given supplemental oxygen for 2 hours after BAL. Approximately 5% of patients develop fever after BAL. Although shaking chills may accompany the fever, blood cultures are usually sterile, and the fever resolves promptly with symptomatic treatment. Prolonged fever should raise the suspicion of BAL-induced pneumonia, which occurs after less than 1% of such procedures. Pneumonia as a result of BAL may be difficult to diagnose since the procedure usually is performed in patients who already have pulmonary infiltrates. In addition, the BAL itself will cause a pulmonary infiltrate that may not resolve for 24 hours, even when pneumonia is not present. Therefore our practice has been to administer antibiotics empirically if post-BAL fever has not resolved within 12 to 24 hours.

In addition to fever and pneumonia, BAL can adversely affect respiratory function in critically ill mechanically ventilated patients. We recently analyzed 99 consecutive BAL procedures performed in 81 such patients,[13] including 46 men and 35 women, with ages ranging from 18 to 80 years (median, 47 years). All BAL procedures were performed to evaluate suspected lower respiratory tract infection. Both immunocompromised (n = 44) and nonimmunocompromised (n = 37) patients underwent BAL. Vari-

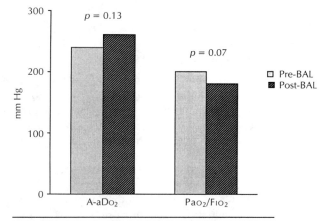

FIG. 48-3   Comparison of A-aDo_2 and Pao_2/Fio_2 before and after BAL. No significant change occurred in A-aDo_2 (240.55 ± 36.68 mm Hg pre-BAL vs. 261.63 ± 31.29 mm Hg post-BAL; $p = 0.13$) or Pao_2/Fio_2 ratio (201.08 ± 26.49 pre-BAL vs. 180.77 ± 20.20 post-BAL; $p = 0.07$).

ables of airflow resistance (peak inspiratory airway pressure) and lung mechanics (static lung compliance) showed no significant change after BAL (Fig. 48-2). Two variables reflecting the efficiency of arterial oxygenation were examined: the alveolar to arterial oxygen gradient (A-aDo_2) and the Pao_2 to Fio_2 ratio (Pao_2/Fio_2) (Fig. 48-3). For the patient group as a whole, no statistically significant change in these variables occurred after BAL. However, 13 of 67 patients (19%) experienced widening of the A-aDo$_2$ by more than 100 mm Hg. On review of the medical charts, the deterioration seen in these patients could not have been predicted by assessment of readily available clinical characteristics, including sex, age, and number of days on the ventilator before BAL. Therefore the oxygenation status of all patients must be carefully monitored after BAL to identify those who deteriorate after the procedure.

SUMMARY

- FFB allows direct visualization of central airways, biopsy of respiratory tract structures, and supplying of bronchial secretions.
- FFB permits treatment of mucous plugging, hemoptysis, and foreign bodies.
- Indications for FFB include suspected pneumonia, atelectasis, hemoptysis, presence of foreign bodies, suspected tracheobronchial disruption, smoke inhalation, and difficult intubation.

- FFB must not be performed in hemodynamically unstable patients, severely hypoxemic patients (Pao$_2$ <70 mm Hg or Fio$_2$ of 1), or patients with severe metabolic disturbances.
- The use of diagnostic FFB should be considered when sputum culture fails to reveal a pathogen and for immunocompromised patients.

REFERENCES

1. Olopade CO, Prakash UBS. Bronchoscopy in the critical-care unit. Mayo Clin Proc 64:1255, 1989.
2. Saito H, Anaissie EJ, Morice RC, et al. Bronchoalveolar lavage in the diagnosis of pulmonary infiltrates in patients with acute leukemia. Chest 94:745, 1988.
3. Ognibene FP, Shelhamer J, Gill V, et al. The diagnosis of *Pneumocystis carinii* pneumonia in patients with the acquired immunodeficiency syndrome using subsegmental bronchoalveolar lavage. Am Rev Respir Dis 129:929, 1984.
4. Fulkerson WJ. Current concepts: Fiberoptic bronchoscopy. N Engl J Med 311:511-516, 1984.
5. Chastre J, Fagon J-Y, Soler P, et al. Diagnosis of nosocomial bacterial pneumonia in intubated patients undergoing ventilation: Comparison of the usefulness of bronchoalveolar lavage and the protected specimen brush. Am J Med 85:499, 1988.
6. Torres A, de la Bellacasa JP, Xaubet A, et al. Diagnostic value of quantitative cultures of bronchoalveolar lavage and telescoping plugged catheters in mechanically ventilated patients with bacterial pneumonia. Am Rev Respir Dis 140:306, 1989.
7. Kirilloff LF, Owens GR, Rogers RM, Mazzocco MC. Does chest physical therapy work? Chest 88:436, 1985.
8. Hood RM. Injury to the trachea and major bronchi. In Hood RM, Boyd AD, Culliford AT, eds. Thoracic trauma. Philadelphia: WB Saunders, 1989.
9. Baumann MH, Sahn SA. Techniques for managing bronchopleural fistulas: How to maximize ventilation and resolve fistulas medically. J Crit Illness 5:627, 1990.
10. Crapo RO. Smoke-inhalation injuries. JAMA 246:1694, 1981.
11. Albertini RE, Harrell JH, Kurihara N, et al. Arterial hypoxemia induced by fiberoptic bronchoscopy. JAMA 230:1666, 1974.
12. Karetsky MS, Garvey JW, Brandstetter RD. Effect of fiberoptic bronchoscopy of arterial oxygen tension. NY State J Med 1:62, 1974.
13. Hertz M, Woodward ME, Gross CR, Swart M, Marcy TW, Bitterman PB. Safety of bronchoalveolar lavage in the critically ill, mechanically ventilated patient. Crit Care Med 19:1526-1532, 1991.

CHAPTER 49

Care of Central Lines

Steven D. Eyer

Central lines are important in the management of many surgical patients with complications. They reduce patient discomfort and interventions when long-term or multiple IV access is needed. They are essential for hemodynamic monitoring, parenteral nutrition, and acute dialysis. Two principal complications of their use relating to line care are thrombosis and infection. The purpose of this chapter is to provide an understanding of and to prevent central line thrombosis, colonization, and sepsis.

CATHETER-RELATED SEPSIS
Incidence

The incidence of infectious complications from central lines varies with patient population. It is near 0% in nonstressed patients requiring central catheters for less than 72 hours, 1.5% to 5% in mixed SICU patients, 3% to 15% in various parenteral nutrition groups, and as high as 23% in patients receiving parenteral nutrition in bone marrow transplant units. Because catheters are used so frequently, catheter-related sepsis affects thousands of patients annually and increases their length of stay and hospital costs.

Causes

The accepted causes of catheter infection are multiple. Implicated causes are infusate contamination, endogenous seeding, hub colonization with internal migration down the catheter, and skin colonization with external migration to the subcutaneous tract followed by migration down the catheter. Infusate contamination is uncommon and of such small inoc-

ulum that when it does occur, it rarely produces clinical infection. It is least likely to occur when IV medications are formulated by pharmacists under sterile conditions and in laminar flow hoods. To minimize this complication, parenteral nutrition formulas should be prepared under similar conditions and discarded after 24 hours.

Endogenous infection preceding catheter colonization or sepsis is of particular concern in surgical patients with complications. A distant abscess or recurrent isolation of a sputum pathogen from a patient with pneumonia may be followed by bacteremia and secondary growth on the catheter. Although unsupported by data, a reasonable assumption is that patients with recurrent bacteremia from other sources are at higher risk for catheter colonization and sepsis.

Hub colonization has been well documented. This source is correlated to the number of infusions through the hub for multiple interventions and poor adherence to aseptic technique. The importance of swabbing hubs before disconnecting and reconnecting cannot be overemphasized.

The skin site is the most common source of catheter colonization in nearly all study populations reported, and *Staphylococcus epidermidis* is the most common organism. Antiseptic skin preparation at the time of line placement, use of antibiotic ointment or an impregnated cuff, provision of an antiseptic dressing change every 48 hours, and prompt line removal when skin site infection is suspected are clinically important aspects of care. Infrequent catheter ma-

515

nipulation may minimize subcutaneous tract colonization.

A number of factors have been recognized that affect the incidence of catheter-related sepsis, including aseptic technique, frequent line manipulations, number of lumens, insertion site, catheter longevity, severity of underlying disease, type of catheter material used, and physician experience. Frequency of line manipulations and use of multilumen catheters are factors associated with the severity of underlying disease and need for interventions. Triple-lumen catheters clearly are more likely to become colonized and develop subsequent sepsis than single-lumen central lines, but less clear is whether this observation is a result of increased portals of entry, manipulations, or patient illness. Studies of insertion site as the primary outcome variable do not support any particular site as protective.

Although steel is the least infectious prone material, it is impractical for central line construction. Many other synthetic catheters are available for clinical use. Although there are differences between nonsteel catheters, thrombus and fibrin sheath formation commonly occur with all synthetic catheters, including Teflon, silicone, and polyvinyl chloride. The perfect material is still being sought. Physician experience is more important in regard to mechanical complications than to infections. Catheter sepsis rates are directly related to catheter longevity but not to frequency of catheter changes. Careful consideration should be given before placing central lines, and reconsideration of their continued use should be made on a daily basis. Pulmonary artery catheters and dialysis access catheters have the highest risk of colonization and sepsis. They should be removed at the earliest possible time when no longer needed. Pulmonary artery catheter sepsis is particularly hazardous because increased risk exists for endocarditis of the right side of the heart and for pulmonary arteritis. Maintenance of stringent asepsis is the most important and the easiest way of reducing risk of infection.

ASEPTIC TECHNIQUE

All central lines should be placed under strict aseptic technique. The operator should wear a mask, sterile gown, and sterile gloves. The placement site should be widely prepared with an antiseptic (povidone-iodine or chlorhexidine) scrub and solution. The use of large sterile drapes minimizes catheter contamination during placement. A full-time nurse epidemiologist, central line team, or monitoring service should supervise all catheter placements. This surveillance not only helps ensure preparation according to protocol and adherence to sterile technique but is of proven effectiveness in reducing catheter sepsis. Because asepsis is less stringent under emergency conditions, lines placed for emergency resuscitation should be replaced electively by guidewire exchange as soon as patient stability permits.

Adherence to aseptic principles extends the life of the catheter. Further infectious-free use of the central catheter requires protocols for catheter care. Occlusive dressings and IV tubing should be changed routinely; every 48 hours is recommended. Soiled dressings should be changed immediately. Sterile gloves are used to remove old dressings. The skin puncture site is inspected for local infection. If none is present, the nurse should reglove; apply antiseptic solution to the skin site and catheter; cleanse, disconnect, and swab the hub with antiseptic solution; and perform the tubing change. Antiseptic ointment is applied to the line entrance site, and a new sterile occlusive dressing is placed. Any suspected skin site infection is called to the attention of the responsible physician. Injection sites are swabbed with an antiseptic before use. Hyperalimentation should be administered only through dedicated catheter ports.

Antibiotic prophylaxis is of no proven benefit. Antibiotic-impregnated cuffs can reduce catheter sepsis rates by preventing cutaneous migration of bacteria, but their use may not be necessary to decrease infection complications. In my experience skin overgrowth of bacteria is not a significant problem with good skin site aseptic protocols. The cuffed lines are expensive and present their own complications.

The site of percutaneous puncture is considered infected if purulent drainage from the site, expanding erythema and cellulitis (tenderness and edema), or erythema and a positive qualitative skin culture from a moist swab of the site after 24 hours are present. The nursing staff should contact the physician if a skin site infection is suspected. In all cases a saline solution–moistened sterile swab is applied to the site using sterile gloves. With purulence or cellulitis, the catheter should be removed and replaced at a new site by percutaneous technique. For erythema alone, the catheter may be left in place. If after 24 hours the skin culture is positive, the catheter should be removed and a new line placed at a different site.

CATHETER REMOVAL OR EXCHANGE
Central Venous Catheters

Central venous catheters and the surrounding skin should be prepared thoroughly with antiseptic scrub and solution. This preparation should include the entire catheter, including the hub and a portion of the attached IV tubing. The field is defined with sterile drapes, and the tubing is disconnected and the hub wiped with antiseptic solution. If desired, a drawback blood culture may be obtained. If the line is to be exchanged, a sterile guidewire is threaded through the indwelling catheter. The catheter then is removed and suspended over a sterile towel, and, 3 cm from its end, the tip is cut sharply onto the towel. If a tunnel segment is also desired, the originally suspended line, once withdrawn, is cut 0.5 cm distal to the junction of antiseptic staining (brown) and catheter slime (clear). With sterile scissors, 3 cm segments are cut from the tunnel and catheter tip ends, placed in sterile containers, labeled appropriately (*catheter tip* or *catheter tunnel*), and sent immediately to the microbiology laboratory for culture. Some centers prefer one culture site over the other, but both sites are not always synchronously involved in documented catheter sepsis. I personally recommend culturing tips only. Concomitant tunnel cultures increase the positive culture yield only slightly but at considerable increase in expense. If there is no clinical suspicion of catheter infection and another line will not be exchanged through the guidewire at the same site, no culture of the catheter is necessary.

Pulmonary Artery Catheters

Pulmonary artery catheters must be managed in a different manner. Because of their length and attached contamination shield, the latter must be disconnected and retracted and a sufficient length of exposed catheter prepared with antiseptic scrub and solution. Specific attention should be paid to antiseptic preparation of the introducer valve where the pulmonary artery catheter enters. The catheter is withdrawn to the 10 cm distance marker and grasped firmly to prevent whipping while it is completely withdrawn. The tip is then cut as for a central venous line. Pulmonary artery catheters are inserted through introducers. If a tunnel segment is desired, it should be taken from the introducer on its subsequent removal and not from the pulmonary artery catheter.

Samples for Culture

Catheter samples for culture should be transferred to the microbiology laboratory as quickly as possible. The catheters are first rolled onto blood agar plates. The tip is implanted but not completely submerged into the agar itself. This procedure should expose the interior of the catheter to the culture media. The plates are incubated at 35° C in 5% carbon dioxide and are examined for 72 hours. Positive cultures are reported when more than 15 colony-forming units are detected during this period of time.

Replacement of Lines

The replacement of indwelling central lines with new ones (i.e., line change frequency) and the method of changing them are other areas with widely varying national standards. The only universally agreed upon tenet is removal of central lines at the earliest possible time. Many protocols call for changes every 3 days, others every 7 days, and some no change at all. Some protocols allow one change by guidewire technique; others never allow use of a guidewire; whereas others change by guidewire even with known line colonization. Policies requiring 3-day change intervals evolved from peripheral line data that demonstrated a marked increase in thrombophlebitis after 72 hours and central and arterial line data showing a near-zero infection rate for catheters with longevities <3 days. Phlebitis is an infrequent problem with central lines. Data about phlebitis are from elective, nonstressed patients and do not necessarily relate to patients requiring long-term catheterization. In children calculated probability density function shows no relationship between catheter longevity and the daily risk of line infectious complications.

In a prospective, randomized comparison of long-term maintenance techniques in critically ill surgical patients, the investigators demonstrated no significant difference in catheter-related sepsis rates between line change every 7 days to a new site, 7-day change by guidewire technique, or no change at all.[1] The probability of line sepsis was 0.3% to 0.5% per line per day, independent of the method of management. Not changing the line without clear clinical indications reduces both the expense and the chance for placement complications. An additional benefit in the study cited was a lower colonization rate of the catheter tip.

Clinical Reasons for Replacement

Catheters do require changing under certain clinical circumstances (see box). Lines should be removed and replaced at a new site in the presence of skin site infection. The site is considered infected if purulent drainage from the site or expanding erythema and cellulitis (tenderness and edema) are present. For erythema alone, any positive qualitative skin culture from a moist swab of the site should be considered infected. Lines placed under emergency conditions for the purpose of resuscitation should be replaced under strict aseptic conditions once the patient is stable and time allows. Less stringent attention is paid to sterile technique when placing vascular catheters under emergency conditions, and an increased catheter infection rate has been observed in these situations. Leaking, malpositioned, and thrombosed catheters usually must be replaced, although there may be a role for thrombolytic infusion in some cases of catheter thrombosis.

If the ports of a triple-lumen catheter or pulmonary artery catheter are needed for patient care, discontinuing or adding a pulmonary artery catheter requires either changing one for the other (interconversion) or adding an extra catheter. Interconversion is preferable to reduce mechanical and infectious risks.

Positive blood cultures necessitate central

Catheter Management Guidelines

- Lines will be left in place and not changed unless otherwise indicated.
- Lines will be changed by guidewire exchange for the following:
  1. All central lines placed under emergency conditions within 24 hours of admission to the SICU
  2. Line malfunction
  3. Central lines exchanged for pulmonary artery catheters and vice versa
  4. Any positive blood culture obtained since the line was last changed
  5. For a septic clinical pattern when there is no other likely source of sepsis
  6. To provide an unused port for delivery of hyperalimentation
- Lines will be removed and replaced at a new site when:
  1. Skin site infection is determined by the following criteria:
     a. Purulent drainage at the skin puncture site (culture site)
     b. Cellulitis (erythema, tenderness, and edema) at the skin puncture site (culture site)
     c. Erythema at the skin puncture site and a skin organism at 24 hours by qualitative culture
  2. Patient has persistent clinical sepsis (without positive blood culture) and no obvious source and previous positive guidewire-exchanged catheter culture

---

line changes. Because the positive blood culture could be secondary to a catheter source, removal of the catheter is the only way to determine catheter sepsis (positive blood culture and catheter segment culture with the same organism). All indwelling venous and arterial lines should be changed and sent for culture, the only exception being lines that have been changed in the interval between the time of obtaining the blood specimen that now demonstrates organisms and its reporting.

Hyperalimentation should be administered through dedicated lumens not previously used for other purposes. No medications should be administered through this lumen, nor should blood be drawn from it. When central lines are placed and hyperalimentation is anticipated, a port should be capped and labeled "for total parenteral nutrition (TPN) only."

Although all patients with a fever do not have line sepsis, an appropriate strategy is catheter replacement to rule out a catheter source for any septic clinical pattern when no other obvious cause is identified. However, the patient with an isolated head injury who has a persistent high fever and extensive but nondiagnostic evaluation for infection, including line change and culture, does not need repeated line changes. Similarly, the newly septic patient with clinical and x-ray film evidence of acute pneumonia does not need line change and culture unless the process does not respond to appropriate therapy.

Guidewire Exchange

When catheters do require change, available data are less clear on the practice of guidewire exchange. The advantage of this practice is minimal placement complications, ease, and patient comfort. Microorganisms can reside in the subcutaneous portion of the catheter tract, and guidewire exchange of culture-positive catheters has the theoretic disadvantage of transferring microbes to the new catheter and increasing the risk of sepsis. Bozzetti et al.[2] have shown that repeated guidewire exchanges eventually result in sterile catheters. This observation has not been tested widely. Culture-negative guidewire exchange can be repeated indefinitely. My practice is to follow guidewire exchanged lines clinically when the prior catheter culture returns positive (catheter colonization). Any evidence for infection in these patients is managed by line removal, catheter culture, and replacement at a new site.

CATHETER-RELATED THROMBOSIS

Catheter-related thrombosis has been studied far less than catheter infection. Indwelling catheters develop a thrombus sheath within hours of their placement. Heparin bonding effectively averts this problem for at least 15 to 30 hours but at considerable increased cost. At this time no prospective, randomized data on the effectiveness of heparin flushing of central lines in preventing line thrombosis exists, although unpublished data on radial artery lines suggest this practice might be helpful. Peripheral lines used for 48 to 72 hours have equal patency rates with heparin and saline solution flushes. Until more convincing evidence is available, I currently recommend saline solution flushing of central lines to avoid the problem of heparin antibody–induced thrombocytopenia.

SUMMARY

- Major complications of central venous catheter use are thrombosis and infection.
- Sources of catheter infections include skin colonization with migration of organisms to the catheter, catheter hub colonization from frequent use, endogenous seeding from distant sites of infection, or infusate contamination.
- Poor adherence to aseptic technique, increased number of catheter manipulations, increased number of lumens per catheter, increased time of use, increased severity of underlying disease, inappropriate catheter material, and physician inexperience are associated with increased infectious or mechanical complications.

- Site of percutaneous catheter puncture is infected if purulent drainage from the site, expanding erythema and cellulitis (tenderness and edema), or erythema and a positive qualitative skin culture are present.
- Guidelines for changing central venous catheters are listed in the box on p. 518.
- Hyperalimentation (TPN) should be administered through a dedicated port not previously used. The TPN port should not subsequently be used for other IV infusion.
- Saline solution flushes of central venous catheters achieve comparable patency of ports as heparin flushes without the risk of heparin-induced thrombocytopenia.

REFERENCES

1. Eyer SD, Brummitt C, Crossley K, Siegel R, Cerra FB. Catheter-related sepsis: Prospective, randomized study of three methods of long-term catheter maintenance. Crit Care Med 18:1073, 1990.
2. Bozzetti F, Terno G, Bonfanti G, et al. Prevention and treatment of central venous catheter sepsis by exchange via a guidewire. Ann Surg 198:48, 1982.

BIBLIOGRAPHY

Cobb DK, High PH, Sable CA, et al. A randomized controlled trial of scheduled central venous catheter replacement [abstract]. Presented at Twenty-ninth Interscience Conference on Antimicrobial Agents and Chemotherapy, Houston, Tex., Sept. 17-20, 1989. Washington D.C.: American Society for Microbiology, 1989.

Damen J. The microbiologic risk of invasive haemodynamic monitoring in open-heart patients requiring prolonged ICU treatment. Intensive Care Med 14:156, 1988.

Hoar PF, Stone JG, Wicks AE, Edie RN, Scholes JV. Thrombogenesis associated with Swan-Ganz catheters. Anesthesiology 48:445, 1978.

Keohane PP, Jones BSH, Attril H, et al. Effect of catheter tunnelling and a nutrition nurse on catheter sepsis during parenteral nutrition: A controlled trial. Lancet 2:1388-1390, 1983.

Maki DG, Cobb L, Garman JK, Schapiro JM, Ringer M, Helgerson RB. An attachable silver-impregnated cuff for the prevention of infection with central venous catheters: A prospective randomized multicenter trial. Am J Med 85:307, 1988.

Maki DG, Weise CE, Sarafin HW. A semiquantitative culture method for identifying intravenous catheter-related infection. N Engl J Med 296:1305, 1977.

Mangano DT. Heparin bonding and long-term protection against thrombogenesis [letter]. N Engl J Med 307:894, 1982.

Rowley KM, Clubb KS, Smith JW, Cabin HS. Right-sided infective endocarditis as a consequence of flow-directed pulmonary artery catheterization. N Engl J Med 311:1152, 1984.

Senagore A, Waller JD, Bonnell BW, et al. Pulmonary artery catheterization: A prospective study of internal jugular versus subclavian approaches. Crit Care Med 13:264, 1985.

Snyder RH, Archer FJ, Endy T, et al. Catheter infection. Ann Surg 208:651, 1988.

Stenzel JP, Green TP, Fuhrman BP, Carlson PE, Marchessault BS. Percutaneous central venous catheterization in a pediatric intensive care unit: A survival analysis of complications. Crit Care Med 17:984, 1989.

CHAPTER 50

Vascular Access

Thomas Wozniak · Larry Micon

Access to the central venous and arterial circulation is frequently required in surgical patients. Numerous methods and routes for central venipuncture exist, each with inherent advantages and risks. The most frequently used sites are the subclavian, internal jugular, and femoral veins. However, central venous access may be achieved via the axillary, external jugular, and antecubital veins as well. Potential sites for arterial access include radial, femoral, dorsalis pedis, axillary, and brachial arteries. This chapter discusses the indications, contraindications, placement techniques, and complications of vascular access procedures.

CENTRAL VENOUS ACCESS
Indications for Catheterization

Indications for central venous catheterization can be grouped into four major categories: hemodynamic monitoring, fluid or medication infusion, parenteral nutrition, and other invasive maneuvers (see box). Many SICU patients require careful assessment and ongoing monitoring of the circulation, aided by a pulmonary artery or central venous catheter. Some medications require central administration. Patients needing early nutrition or metabolic support because of an impaired gastrointestinal tract also require central venous access.

A number of less commonly performed procedures, including hemodialysis, plasmapheresis, transvenous cardiac pacing, vena caval filter placement, and transvenous pulmonary embolectomy, necessitate central venipuncture. Once the need for such access is established,

a consideration of available sites should follow.

Maintenance of a sterile field is essential. An adequate area including and surrounding the venipuncture location should be clipped or shaved, scrubbed with antiseptic, and isolated

---

Indications for Central Venous Catheterization*

Hemodynamic

Hemodynamic assessment
Central venous pressure monitoring
Pulmonary artery pressure monitoring
Thermodilution cardiac output monitoring

Fluid or medication administration

Intravenous fluid administration (when peripheral access is unavailable)
Continuous vasoactive medication administration
Administration of sclerosing medications (e.g., KCL, amphotericin B)
Chronic medication administration and blood sampling (e.g., chemotherapy, opiates)

Parenteral nutrition

Other procedures

Acute hemodialysis
Plasmapheresis
Transvenous cardiac pacing
Diagnostic radiology
Vena caval filter placement
Transvenous pulmonary embolectomy

---

*From Micon LT. Internal jugular venous cannulation. Perspect Crit Care 3(2):75, 1990.

with sterile drapes. We use sterile gloves and sterile gowns. Institutions variably require masks, head and shoe covers, and protective eyeware. Sufficient personnel to aid in line placement should be present before beginning the procedure.

Subclavian Vein Catheterization

Successful cannulation of the subclavian vein occurs in over 95% of attempts. The only absolute contraindication to this approach is known preexisting thrombosis of the vessel. Relative contraindications are listed in the box.

Proper positioning of the patient is important to ensure successful venipuncture. The patient should be supine with the head turned to the contralateral side. The bed is then placed in the Trendelenburg (head-down) position, distending the upper central venous system. A

Contraindications to Subclavian Vein Catheterization

Absolute
  Thrombosed vessel
Relative
  Coagulopathy
  Transvenous pacemaker
  Axillary-femoral bypass
  Mastectomy
  Distal hemodialysis access
  Tenuous pulmonary reserve

---

rolled-up towel or sheet may be placed longitudinally between the scapulae to abduct the shoulders. After preparation and draping, the skin puncture site is anesthetized. The subcutaneous tissue and, most important, the periosteum of the clavicle are infiltrated with local anesthetic. The skin puncture site is placed 1 cm below the clavicle, at the point of maximal "bend" as the clavicle passes laterally from the sternoclavicular joint (Fig. 50-1). This site is in proximity to the junction of the medial and middle thirds of the clavicle, which may also be used to identify an appropriate site. The needle is directed toward the sternal notch at approximately a 30-degree posterior angle to the skin until it contacts the clavicle. The clavicle should be "walked down" by carefully redirecting the needle to a steeper angle of entry. As the needle passes under the clavicle, constant subatmospheric pressure is maintained on the attached syringe. Abrupt return of blood into the syringe signals successful venipuncture. To prevent an air embolus, a finger should be placed over the open end of the introducer needle when inserting the guidewire. Catheterization is then completed by passing first a guidewire, then the catheter into the vein. The catheter tip should come to rest in the superior vena cava, approximately 15 cm from a skin puncture on the right side or 17 cm from the left side in the average-size adult. Intravenous placement is confirmed by aspiration of blood from the catheter. The procedure is completed by securing the catheter with sutures and ap-

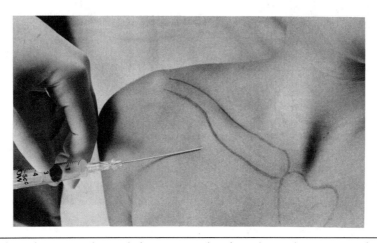

FIG. 50-1 Infraclavicular approach to subclavian vein. Clavicle and manubrium are outlined.

plying a sterile dressing. A CXR should be obtained promptly to verify appropriate positioning and to exclude a pneumothorax.

The most frequently encountered complications with subclavian venipuncture are pneumothorax, arterial puncture, and malpositioning of the catheter tip.[1-6] Other less frequently encountered complications are listed in the upper box.

Internal Jugular Approach

Internal jugular vein cannulation is a second means of accessing central venous circulation. Absolute contraindications are known thrombosis or absence (from previous surgery) of the vessel. Relative contraindications are few (see lower box). Advantages of the internal jugular route include decreased likelihood of pneumothorax and only local hematoma (rather than hemothorax) should bleeding occur.

Proper positioning for internal jugular line placement includes rotation of the head away from the side of cannulation and the Trendelenburg position. The neck is prepared with antiseptic and the field isolated with sterile drapes. The anterior and posterior borders of the sternal and clavicular heads of the sternocleidomastoid muscle are carefully delineated. Anterior, central, and posterior approaches to internal jugular venipuncture have been described. The right side is preferable, since the internal jugular and innominate veins are more directly aligned with the right atrium. In addition, the left side carries a greater risk of potential for thoracic duct injury.

In the anterior approach, the skin is punctured along the anterior border of the sternocleidomastoid muscle approximately 5 cm above the clavicle (Fig. 50-2). The needle is advanced toward the ipsilateral nipple with a 45-degree posterior angle to the skin. Suction is maintained on the attached syringe, and prompt venous return signals successful venipuncture. The guidewire and then the catheter are introduced. Intravascular placement is confirmed by aspiration of blood from the catheter.

Complications of Percutaneous Central Venous Catheterization	
Pneumothorax	Subclavian artery pseudoaneurysm
Hemothorax	
Arterial puncture	Vertebral artery pseudoaneurysm
Chylothorax	
Air embolus	Guidewire embolus
Catheter embolus	Thoracic duct injury
Brachial plexus injury	Dysrhythmia
Horner's syndrome	Cardiac tamponade
Catheter tip malposition	Thromboembolism
	Tracheal perforation
	Right atrial perforation

Contraindications to Internal Jugular Vein Catheterization

Absolute
  Thrombosed vessel
  Surgical absence of vessel
Relative
  Coagulopathy
  Carotid-subclavian artery bypass

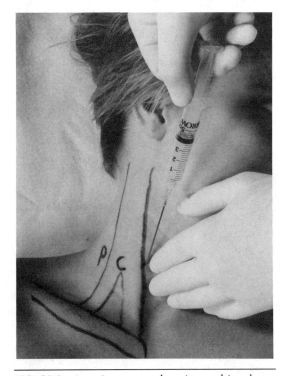

FIG. 50-2 Anterior approach to internal jugular vein. Sternocleidomastoid muscle and clavicle are outlined. Central *(C)* and posterior *(P)* puncture sites are shown.

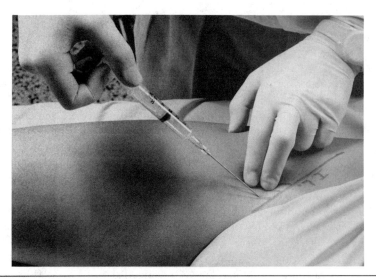

FIG. 50-3   Femoral vein cannulation. Femoral artery (physician's fingers) and vein (introducer needle) are outlined. *IL,* Inguinal ligament.

The procedure is completed by securing the catheter with sutures and applying a sterile dressing. Correct catheter tip position is in the superior vena cava and should be verified by CXR examination before use. The atriocaval junction is approximately 15 cm from a right-sided venipuncture in an average adult (slightly further from the left).

The central technique uses a puncture site at the apex of the triangle created by the sternal and clavicular heads of the sternocleidomastoid muscle and the clavicle (see Fig. 50-2). The needle is introduced at a 30- to 45-degree posterior angle to the skin and directed toward the ipsilateral nipple. The posterior technique is performed by inserting the needle along the posterior border of the sternocleidomastoid muscle, 5 cm above the clavicle, and directing the needle toward the suprasternal notch (see Fig. 50-2). Similar success rates (approximately 85%) will be achieved for all three methods.

Complications of internal jugular catheterization are similar to subclavian line placement.[7] Pneumothorax is still possible but should occur less frequently with the internal jugular approach. Arterial puncture and catheter tip malpositioning occur with similar frequency. The less common complications listed in the upper box on p. 523 apply to both routes. Hemothorax and hydrothorax should occur

less frequently with internal jugular lines.[8] Horner's syndrome resulting from stellate ganglion injury or compression and phrenic nerve paralysis have been reported after catheterization.[9]

Femoral Vein Cannulation

The femoral vein is another commonly used portal to the central venous circulation. Femoral vein cannulation may be necessary if the other sites are thrombosed, already cannulated, or difficult to access, as during closed cardiac massage.

The technique for femoral vein cannulation relies on the ability to palpate the femoral artery just below the inguinal ligament. The site of venipuncture is then just medial to the physician's fingers on the femoral artery.

After infiltration of the skin and deeper tissues with local anesthetic at the selected site, the needle is introduced at approximately a 30-degree posterior angle to the skin (Fig. 50-3). Suction is maintained on the attached syringe. Successful venipuncture is indicated by prompt return of venous blood. A guidewire is passed into the femoral vein. The catheter is then fully inserted (20 cm) and sutured in place.

Femoral line placement does not entail many of the hazards associated with subclavian or internal jugular venipuncture, such as pneumothorax or hemothorax. It still, however, carries risks of arterial puncture, nerve injury, and catheter or guidewire embolus.

A common belief is that femoral lines are at higher risk for line-related sepsis. However, with careful preparation, strict sterile insertion technique, and proper line care, the infection rate is acceptable and, in many studies, is no higher than for other routes of central venous access.[10,11] The main drawback to femoral catheters is that of impaired mobility in otherwise ambulatory patients.

ARTERIAL ACCESS
Pulmonary Artery Catheterization

Ensuring that oxygen delivery meets or exceeds oxygen demand is central to the care of the critically ill. Bedside catheterization of the right side of the heart has allowed a window through which the clinician can objectively monitor the balance of oxygen supply and demand over time.[12,13]

Pulmonary artery (PA) catheterization is indicated in any patient with uncertain or insufficient cardiopulmonary function (see upper box). Examples include patients suffering from significant hemorrhage, necrotizing pancreatitis, sepsis, and trauma who have elevated oxygen requirements and uncertain hemodynamic compensation. Patients with impaired cardiac function after myocardial infarction or valvular disease may need right-side heart catheterization for optimal management. Evidence of end organ insufficiency, end organ failure, or lactic acidosis during acute illness reflects an imbalance in oxygen economy, requiring further investigation and therapy aided by PA catheterization.

Similarly, the differentiation of cardiogenic from noncardiogenic pulmonary edema may require PA pressure measurement. Respiratory failure mandating high levels of positive end-expiratory pressure for management requires a PA line to assess the hemodynamic consequences.[14] Finally, surgical patients with other morbid illnesses or even healthy patients requiring major surgical interventions may need invasive hemodynamic assessment and monitoring in the perioperative period. The lower box lists variables that can be obtained from a PA catheter.

Indications for PA Catheterization

Restoration of oxygen transport
Cardiogenic shock
Hypovolemic shock
Sepsis
Multiple organ insufficiency
Inflammation (e.g., pancreatitis)
Respiratory failure

Commonly Obtained Variables From PA Catheterization*

Central venous pressure
Pulmonary artery pressure
Pulmonary capillary wedge pressure
Cardiac output/index
Systemic vascular resistance/index
Pulmonary vascular resistance/index
Mixed venous oxygen saturation
Oxygen delivery
Oxygen consumption

---

*Data from Grabenkort RW. A cardiopulmonary physiologic profile for use with the Swan-Ganz catheter. Res Staff Phys 29(7):80, 1983.

A unique relative contraindication to PA catheter placement is a preexisting left bundle branch block (LBBB). The development of a new right bundle branch block (RBBB) has been described with PA catheterization, and in patients with an existing LBBB, complete heart block can result. Although it is a potentially hazardous complication, the incidence of complete heart block is low. Nonetheless, external or transvenous cardiac pacing should be ready before attempting right-side heart catheterization.[15]

Technique

PA catheters are passed through introducer sheaths placed in a central vein (usually the subclavian or internal jugular vein) using the methods previously described. Once the sheath has been sutured in place, the PA catheter is brought into the sterile field and calibrated at the patient's fourth intercostal space in the midaxillary line.[16,17] The balloon is tested, and if an eccentric (asymmetric) balloon is noted, a new catheter should be used. Eccentric balloon tips have a higher incidence of PA perforation. The catheter is threaded through the introducer sheath to a distance of 20 cm, and the balloon is inflated. To decrease the risk of atrial, ventricular, or PA perforation, the catheter should not be advanced without the balloon inflated. Conversely, the catheter should never be withdrawn with the balloon inflated. The catheter is then advanced or "floated" through the right side of the heart into the pulmonary artery with the aid of waveform monitoring. Fluoroscopy may occasionally be necessary in cases of anomalous venous anatomy or low output states. As the catheter tip passes through the right atrium, right ventricle, and pulmonary artery and ultimately into the wedge position, the monitor displays the respective pressures. A characteristic waveform is illustrated in Fig. 50-4. The normal right-sided heart pressures (mm Hg) for each location are:

Right atrium, 0-8
Right ventricle, 20-30/0-7
Pulmonary artery, 15-30/5-15
Pulmonary capillary wedge, 5-12

The approximate distances (cm) from the insertion site to each location are:

Right atrium, 20
Right ventricle, 30-40
Pulmonary capillary wedge, 45-60

Once the catheter is "wedged," the balloon is deflated to display the PA waveform. If a "wedge" waveform persists, the catheter has been advanced too far and should be withdrawn (with the balloon deflated) until a PA waveform is observed.

Complications

The complications associated with PA catheter placement may be considered the same as those from accessing the central venous circulation and those unique to the longer, balloon-tipped device. The former have already been discussed in this chapter. Other complications directly related to PA catheterization are listed in the box. Preexisting LBBB entails a risk of complete heart block and necessitates immediate availability of cardiac pacing. Ventricular dysrhythmias are common but only occasionally require treatment. Patients with preexisting ventricular dysrhythmia may be given prophylactic lidocaine.

Puncture of the right ventricle can occur if the catheter tip lodges in the trabeculae during insertion. The resulting cardiac tamponade is

---

Complications of PA Catheterization*

1. Complications of central venipuncture
2. Complications unique to PA catheter
   a. Dysrhythmia
   b. Heart block
   c. Catheter knotting
   d. Catheter tip malposition
   e. Cardiac tamponade
   f. Valvular injury
   g. PA perforation
   h. Pulmonary infarction

---

*Data from Horst MH, et al. The risks of pulmonary arterial catheterization. Surg Gynecol Obstet 159:229-232, 1984; Elliot C, et al. Complications of pulmonary artery catheterization in the care of critically ill patients. Chest 76:647-652, 1979.

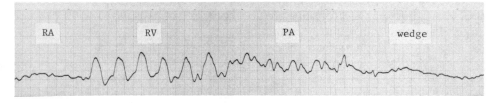

FIG. 50-4   Actual PA catheter waveform as balloon tip passes from right atrium to wedge position in pulmonary vasculature. Note differences in right atrial *(RA)*, right ventricular *(RV)*, pulmonary artery *(PA)*, and wedge waveforms.

indicated by PA catheter readings. Prompt evacuation of the pericardial sac and surgical closure of the puncture are required for successful management.

Pulmonary infarction results from excessively distal placement or migration of the catheter tip and can be recognized by bloody sputum, changes in oxygenation, or a wedge-shaped deformity on chest x-ray examination. PA perforation can be recognized by the abrupt onset of hemoptysis or suctioning of blood from the lungs. It can be caused by migration of the tip, overinflation of the balloon, or the use of an eccentric balloon.[18-20] The catheter should be pulled back immediately and the balloon reinflated; if the hemorrhage does not subside, prompt surgical therapy may be required.

Cardiac valvular injury is rare but results from traumatic passage or withdrawal of the catheter through the pulmonic or tricuspid valve with the balloon inflated. Intracardiac knotting is likewise rare and usually occurs during insertion. Manipulation under fluoroscopy, occasionally with a guidewire, may resolve the problem. If not, surgical cutdown is necessary for withdrawal.

"Wedge" pressure interpretation

The pulmonary capillary wedge pressure (PCWP) is used to estimate left ventricular preload. A fundamental assumption is that PCWP, left atrial pressure (LAP), and left ventricular end-diastolic pressure (LVEDP) are equivalent and accurately reflect left ventricular end-diastolic volume (LVEDV), the most reliable clinical measure of the left ventricular preload.

Circumstances in which these assumptions are not true are relatively common, making accurate interpretation of the wedge pressure difficult. The wedge pressure will not correlate with the LAP if the catheter is malpositioned or the monitoring system is not properly calibrated, contains air bubbles, or is excessively affected by overdamping or underdamping.[21,22] Other situations in which pulmonary artery diastolic (PAD) pressure may not equal PCWP include chronic obstructive pulmonary disease, increased pulmonary arteriolar resistance, a heart rate greater than 125 beats/min, wedge position other than a zone III portion of the lung, increased pulmonary interstitial pressure, and constriction of pulmonary veins. In addition, overwedging or an eccentric balloon may affect the accuracy with which the PCWP correlates with the LAP.[23]

The PCWP and the LAP may not reflect the LVEDP in instances of aortic or mitral valvular disease or altered left ventricular compliance. Finally, the relationship between LVEDP and LVEDV may be distorted. Alterations of pericardial pressure, right ventricle volume, and ventricular stiffness have significant influence on the pressure-volume relationship of the left ventricle.

Thus a measure of clinical expertise is required to assess the accuracy of the PCWP value and to interpret its clinical significance. In combination with other data obtained from the PA catheter (e.g., cardiac output, oxygen delivery, oxygen consumption), the wedge pressure provides essential information about the hemodynamic state of a critically ill patient.

Arterial Catheterization

Indications for arterial catheterization include continuous blood pressure monitoring, frequent sampling of blood, especially for arterial blood gas determination, and blood pressure monitoring of patients in shock when indirect methods are unreliable. The usual sites of catheterization in order of preference are the (1) radial, (2) dorsalis pedis, (3) femoral, and (4) axillary arteries. Note that brachial artery lines are rarely used. In some patients, a brachial arterial line may cause ischemic injury to the hand and resulting loss of tissue and function. Patients at risk include those with small-vessel disease of the upper extremity, such as those with diabetes mellitus.

In summary, the radial artery is the most commonly cannulated artery and consequently the most familiar. It is in a superficial location, which makes it easier to cannulate. The ulnar artery usually provides abundant collateral circulation. The modified Allen's test is designed to assess the collateral circulation of the hand and should be done on all patients before insertion of a radial artery catheter. The patient elevates his/her hand, and the examiner occludes both the radial and ulnar arteries. The patient is asked to make a fist, emptying the hand of blood. The hand is lowered and opened. The wrist should not be hyperextended to prevent a false positive interpretation. Pressure over the ulnar artery is then released and the time to return of flush to the hand noted. The flush should occur in fewer than 6 seconds. Both ulnar and radial arteries should be tested. Doppler flow studies should be added in cases of questionable flow.[24]

Some problems exist with radial catheterization. Catheter malfunction occurs in 13% to 38% of the cases, which may be related to the length and caliber of the catheter.[25] Arterial flow can be obstructed and again relates to catheter size. Ischemia and tissue loss occur far less frequently than thrombosis.[26] Inaccurate blood pressure readings may be produced when vessels lose elasticity or are involved with atherosclerosis. Additional information about arterial blood pressure measurement is found in Chapter 52.

Dorsalis pedis artery

Like the hand, the foot has good collateral circulation. In the foot, collateral blood flow arises from the posterior tibial artery. A similar test of collateral flow can be performed. The dorsalis pedis and the posterior tibial arteries are occluded, producing blanching in the great toe. The posterior tibial artery is released and flow should return to the toe within 5 seconds.

Again blood pressure accuracy may be a problem in the face of atherosclerotic vascular disease. This artery is congenitally absent in 12% of the population.[26]

Femoral artery

The femoral artery is often the only palpable pulse in a patient with shock. Larger vessels have a lower incidence of thrombosis and embolism. The femoral artery provides reliable blood pressure monitoring. Care should be exercised when using this vessel in patients with peripheral vascular disease. The overall catheter complication rate for this location is 8%.[27]

Axillary artery

As with the femoral artery, the axillary artery is a large blood vessel that has a lower incidence

of thrombosis and provides reliable blood pressure monitoring. It is deeper, however, and therefore more difficult to cannulate. If the right side is chosen, a risk of air embolus to the cerebral circulation exists.[28]

Brachial artery

The brachial artery is often easier to palpate than the radial artery. It does not have collateral circulation, so that thrombosis or embolization results in greater ischemia and tissue loss. Safe short-term use has been documented, but this artery is not recommended if other sites are available.[29]

Technique

1. The skin of the chosen site is cleansed with antiseptic solution and a sterile field prepared.
2. Sterile gloves are worn and the pulse palpated. The areas overlying and on either side of the artery are infiltrated with 1% lidocaine.
3. For small vessels a 20-gauge catheter should be used. Larger vessels will accommodate an 18- or 16-gauge catheter.
4. If the radial site is chosen, the wrist should be hyperextended with the thumb abducted. If the dorsalis pedis artery is chosen, the ankle should be extended as much as possible. When the axillary artery is chosen, the arm is abducted and the elbow flexed.
5. The artery is punctured at a 45-degree angle. When blood return is seen, the catheter and needle are inserted a few millimeters further and the wire slid into the vessel. The catheter is advanced into the vessel using a twisting motion. The needle/wire complex is removed and the free return of blood noted. The catheter can be capped to prevent further blood spillage and the catheter secured with 2-0 or 3-0 suture. The cap is then removed and the transducer connected.

Complications

1. *Thrombosis.* The incidence of thrombosis is increased with multiple arterial punctures, atherosclerosis, increased duration of catheterization, and low cardiac output. Catheters larger than 20 gauge and those made of

polypropylene have a higher incidence of thrombosis. Catheters left longer than 4 days have a higher incidence of thrombosis. Rates vary from 11% to 29%.[30] Distal embolization may occur and produce ischemic necrosis. Examination of the patient for blanching when the artery is flushed may identify patients at risk and allow intervention before thrombosis.

2. *Infection.* The risk of infection is increased for catheters left longer than 4 days. There may be no local signs of inflammation. The reported incidence of infection is 1% to 2%.[31]

3. *Other complications.* Neuropathies second-ary to prolonged hyperextension, median nerve injury, or hematomas around the brachial artery are other complications of arterial catheterization. Pseudoaneurysms can occur in any location.

Doppler-Guided Catheterization

A needle is now available that contains an internal Doppler probe. This device can be helpful in patients who have poorly palpable pulses (edematous patients or patients who have had multiple catheters). Once the vessel has been located with needle and probe, the probe is withdrawn, a wire is inserted, and a catheter is threaded over the wire.

SUMMARY

- Use central venous catheterization for hemodynamic monitoring of fluid or medication infusion, parenteral nutrition, acute hemodialysis, plasmapheresis, transvenous cardiac pacing, and vena caval filter placement.
- Strict sterile technique or insertion reduces incidence of catheter infection.
- Common access sites include the subclavian, internal jugular, and femoral veins. Similar complications occur for subclavian and internal jugular approaches. With proper line care, femoral catheterization does not have a higher infection rate.

- When placing a PA catheter in patients with LBBB, have external or transvenous cardiac pacing devices ready.
- Use external catheterization for continuous blood pressure monitoring, frequent sampling of ABGs, monitoring for patients in shock, and when other methods are unreliable.
- Arterial cannulation sites in order of preference are radial, dorsalis pedis, femoral, and axillary.
- Perform Allen's test before attempting radial artery cannulation.

REFERENCES

1. Feliciano DV, Mattox KL, Graham JM, et al. Major complications of percutaneous subclavian vein catheters. Am J Surg 138:869-874, 1979.

2. Edwards H, King T. Cardiac tamponade from central venous catheters. Arch Surg 117:965-967, 1982.

3. Maschke S, Rogove H. Cardiac tamponade associated with a multilumen central venous catheter. Crit Care Med 12:611-613, 1984.

4. Conces D, Holden R. Aberrant locations and complications in initial placement of subclavian vein catheters. Arch Surg 119:293-295, 1984.

5. Zavall J, Taha A, Thomford N. Cardiac tamponade from central venous catheterization. Hosp Phys 25(12):16-19, 1989.

6. Amaral JF, Grigoriev VE, Dorfman GS, et al. Vertebral artery pseudoaneurysm. A rare complication of subclavian artery catheterization. Arch Surg 125:546-547, 1990.

7. Krespi YP, Komisar A, Lucente FE. Complications of internal jugular vein catheterization. Arch Otolaryngol 107:310-312, 1981.

8. Khalil KG, Parker FB Jr, Mukherjee N, et al. Thoracic duct injury: A complication of internal jugular vein catheterization. JAMA 221:908-909, 1972.

9. Parikh RK. Horner's syndrome. A complication of percutaneous catheterization of the internal jugular vein. Anesthesia 27:327-329, 1972.

10. Williams JF, Seneff MG, Friedman BC, et al. Use of femoral venous catheters in critically ill adults: Prospective study. Crit Care Med 19:550-553, 1991.

11. Getzen LC, Pollak EW. Short-term femoral vein catheterization: A safe alternative venous access? Am J Surg 138:875-878, 1979.

12. Nelson LD. Continuous venous oximetry in surgical patients. Ann Surg 20:329-333, 1986.

13. Vaughn S. Puri V. Cardiac output changes and continuous mixed venous oxygen saturation measurement in the critically ill. Crit Care Med 16:495-498, 1988.

14. Rajacich N, Burchard KW, Hasan FM, et al. Central venous pressure and pulmonary capillary wedge pressure as estimates of left artrial pressure: Effects of positive end-expiratory pressure and catheter tip malposition. Crit Care Med 17:7-11, 1989.

15. Sprung CL, Elser B, Schein RM, et al. Risk of right bundle-branch block and complete heart block during pulmonary artery catheterization. Crit Care Med 17:1-3, 1989.

16. Amin DK, Shah PK, Swan HJC. The Swan-Ganz catheter: Tips on interpreting results. J Crit Ill 1(4):24-25, 1986.

17. Swan HBL, Shah PK. The rationale for bedside hemodynamic monitoring. J Crit Ill 1(5):40-61, 1986.

18. Khan AH, Taha AM, Thomford NR, et al. Perforation of the pulmonary artery secondary to Swan-Ganz catheters. Contemp Surg 34:53-56, 1989.

19. Barash PG, Nardi D, Hammond G, et al. Catheter-induced pulmonary artery perforation. Mechanisms, management, and modifications. J Thorac Cardiovasc Surg 82:5-12, 1981.

20. Pape LA, Nardi D, Hammond G, et al. Fatal pulmonary hemorrhage after use of the flow-directed balloon-tipped catheter. Ann Intern Med 90:344-347, 1979.

21. Raper R, Sibbald WJ. Misled by the wedge? The Swan-Ganz catheter and left ventricular preload. Chest 89:427-434, 1986.

22. Abrams JH, Olson ML, Marino JA, et al. Use of a needle valve variable resistor to improve invasive blood pressure monitoring. Crit Care Med 12:978-982, 1984.

23. Calvin JE, Driedger AA, Sibbald WJ. Does the pulmonary capillary wedge pressure predict left ventricular preload in critically ill patients? Crit Care Med 9:437-443, 1981.

24. Ejrup B, Fischer B, Wright IS, et al. Clinical evaluation of blood flow to the hand: The false positive Allen test. Circulation 33:778-780, 1966.

25. Weis BM, Gattiker RI. Complications during and following radial artery cannulation: A prospective study. Intensive Care Med 12:424-428, 1986.

26. Clark CA, Harman EM. Hemodynamic monitoring: Arterial catheters. In Taylor RW, Civetta JM, Kirby RR, eds. Techniques and Procedures in Critical Care. Philadelphia: JB Lippincott, 1990, pp 218-231.

27. Gurman GM, Kriermerman S. Cannulation of big arteries in critically ill patients. Crit Care Med 13:217-220, 1985.

28. Bryan-Brown CW, Kwun KB, Lumb PD, et al. The axillary artery catheter. Heart Lung 12:492-497, 1983.

29. Barnes RW, Foster EJ, Janssen GA, et al. Safety of brachial artery catheters as monitors in the intensive care unit—Prospective evaluation with the Doppler ultrasonic velocity detector. Anesthesiology 44:260-264, 1976.

30. Sladen A. Complications of invasive hemodynamic monitoring in the intensive care unit. Curr Probl Surg 25(2):75-145, 1988.

31. Band JD, Maki DG. Infections caused by arterial catheters used for hemodynamic monitoring. Am J Med 67:735-741, 1979.

CHAPTER 51

Lumbar Puncture, Thoracentesis, Thoracostomy, and Paracentesis

Sharon Henry

LUMBAR PUNCTURE

The usual indications for lumbar puncture, that is, tapping of the subarachnoid space in the lumbar region, include the following: to diagnose suspected CNS infection; to diagnose subarachnoid hemorrhage (if CT scan is normal); to diagnose certain demyelination neurologic diseases (e.g., multiple sclerosis); to treat pseudotumor cerebri; and to administer antibiotics, analgesics, and chemotherapy.

The major contraindication to lumbar puncture is increased intracranial pressure (ICP). Decreasing lumbar pressure with the removal of CSF can result in tonsillar herniation. Coagulopathy or thrombocytopenia increases the risk of intraspinal hemorrhage, and local skin infections increase the risk of secondary CSF infection.

Anatomy. In the adult's spinal column, the spinal cord terminates between L1 and L2. Each vertebra is composed of the body, laminae, pedicles, and transverse and spinous processes. The vertebral ligaments include the supraspinous, the interspinous, and the ligamentum flavum[1] (Fig. 51-1).

Positioning. The patient is placed in the lateral decubitus position with knees and hips flexed while attempting to touch his/her chin to the knees. The back should be at right angles to the bed. In critically ill patients the position indicated in Fig. 51-2, *A,* is normally the only possible approach. Alternatively, the patient is seated and leans forward against a table or an assistant, with his/her feet supported on a stool (Fig. 51-2, *B*).

Procedure

An imaginary line is drawn between the iliac crests. This line represents the L3-4 interspace. (The L4-5 interspace may also be used.) The area is prepared with antiseptic solution and is draped. Sterile gloves are worn by the clinician. The landmarks are reestablished and the spinous process of L3-4 palpated with the thumb. Using 1% lidocaine and a 25-gauge needle, the clinician anesthetizes the skin overlying the site. Then a 20-gauge or smaller spinal needle with stylet in place is advanced perpendicular to the axis of the spine, with the bevel oriented horizontally. Once through the skin, the needle is advanced with a firm steady pressure to allow the needle to pass beneath the spinous process.[2] A sensation of a "give" or "pop" is ex-

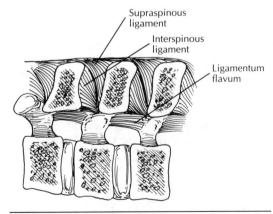

Supraspinous ligament

Interspinous ligament

Ligamentum flavum

FIG. 51-1 Vertebral ligaments. (Redrawn from Taylor RW, Civetta JM, Kirby RR, eds. Techniques and Procedures in Critical Care. Philadelphia: JB Lippincott, 1990, p 390.)

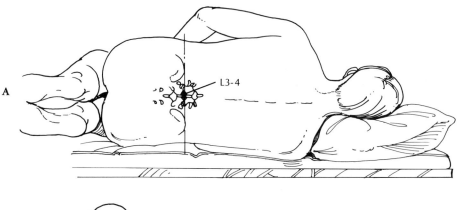

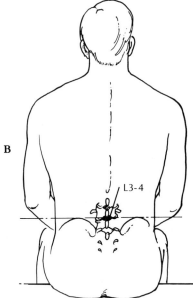

FIG. 51-2 Lumbar puncture positions.
A, Usual position, especially for critically ill
patients. **B,** Alternate position. (Redrawn
from Taylor RW, Civetta JM, Kirby RR, eds.
Techniques and Procedures in Critical
Care. Philadelphia: JB Lippincott, 1990, p
391.)

perienced once the ligamentum flavum is passed. The obturator is removed, and the clinician checks for flow of fluid. The needle may be rotated 90 or 180 degrees if no fluid flow occurs. The obturator is replaced before further repositioning of the needle. If hard resistance is met, bone most likely has been encountered, and the needle should be repositioned. Once spinal fluid has returned, pressures can be measured. A manometer is attached to the needle by way of a stopcock. Readings in excess of 20 cm H_2O are abnormal. Measurements made with the patient in the upright position are less reliable.[2]

PARAMEDIAN APPROACH. The paramedian approach is used on patients who are unable to flex the lumbar spine adequately or who have ligamentous calcification. The skin is infiltrated slightly lateral to and below the spinous process. The needle is advanced to the lamina. The needle is removed and then reinserted after being angled medially. The needle can then be slipped into the ligamentum flavum.[1]

Cerebral Spinal Fluid Analysis

A cell count of the CSF >5 WBC/mm^3 is abnormal. Normal glucose level is 50 to 75 mg/dl, whereas the normal protein level is 15 to

45 mg/dl. CSF to serum glucose concentration ratios range from 0.6 to 0.7. Protein electrophoresis is performed on the CSF, as are assays for bacterial antigens and for myelin base protein. Bacterial, fungal, viral, and tuberculin cultures are obtained as are Gram's, acid-fast bacillus, and cytologic stains. Cytology is performed. Any xanthochromic appearance is noted. India ink is used to evaluate the possibility of cryptococcal infection.

Complications

Headache occurs as a complication of lumbar puncture in 10% to 25% of patients.[2] This incidence is decreased by using a smaller gauge needle and possibly by having the patient lie prone after the procedure.

Painful and persistent paresthesias that resolved within 1 year occurred in 0.2% to 0.7% of patients. Persistent or disabling complications occurred in 0.19% to 0.43% of patients undergoing spinal anesthesia.[3]

Local bleeding as a result of a traumatic tap occurs in up to 20% of patients. Coagulopathic or thrombocytopenic patients are at increased risk and may develop spinal epidural or subdural hematomas.[4] Spinal subdural or epidural hematomas are rarely reported but are more common in patients with coagulopathy.[4]

Infection occurs uncommonly, even in bacteremic patients, and tonsillar herniation may occur in patients with increased ICP.

THORACENTESIS

Thoracentesis, puncture of the chest wall to enter the parietal cavity to aspirate fluids, is indicated either to diagnose or to treat pleural effusion. Localization with CT scan or ultrasound may be necessary if loculated effusions are present.

Procedure

The patient may be supine or in the lateral decubitus position. Alternatively, the patient may be seated, leaning over a stand or table (Fig. 51-3). The level of the fluid is identified by percussion; if indicated, ultrasound or CT localization is used. One or two interspaces be-

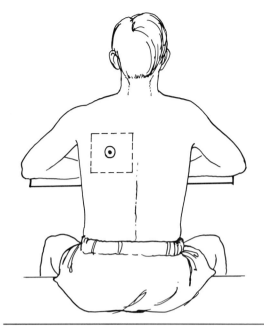

FIG. 51-3 Seated position for thoracentesis. (Redrawn from Taylor RW, Civetta JM, Kirby RR, eds. Techniques and Procedures in Critical Care. Philadelphia: JB Lippincott, 1990, p 296.)

low the fluid location is chosen as the site for the thoracentesis, but it should generally be performed at or above the eighth intercostal space.

The skin is prepared with antiseptic solution and sterilely draped. At the midportion of the rib, 1% to 2% lidocaine is infiltrated to the skin and subcutaneous tissue. A 20-gauge or larger angiocatheter, with syringe attached, is used to enter the skin at the midportion of the rib and then is "walked" up the rib. The syringe is used for aspiration, and the angiocatheter is advanced. The pleural cavity is entered above the rib. The pleural cavity must not be entered at the inferior edge of the next superior rib. Risk of injury to intercostal vessels is high.

When fluid returns, the catheter is advanced into the pleural cavity. A stopcock can be attached. It is connected to a drainage bag with extension tubing. With the use of a stopcock, risk of introducing air into the thoracic cavity is reduced, and there is little chance for spillage of the fluid. Specimens for analysis are taken. Then the needle is removed and a dressing is applied.

Complications

Complications of thoracentesis include pneumothorax, bleeding, and visceral punctures.

Fluid Analysis

Analysis of fluids aspirated from the parietal cavity reveals the following: cell count; protein content; lactate dehydrogenase (LDH) values; pH; cultures (bacterial and fungal); and stains (Gram's and acid-fast bacillus).

THORACOSTOMY

Thoracostomy, the creation of an opening in the chest wall to allow drainage, is done because of trauma (i.e., for pneumothorax, hemothorax, pneumohemothorax, or chylothorax) or in patients with certain nontraumatic conditions (i.e., spontaneous pneumothorax, pleural effusion, empyema, or chylothorax).

Precautions must be observed in patients with a previous thoracotomy, multiple adhesions, clotting disorders, or a massive hemothorax with hypovolemia.

Procedure

The procedure begins with tube selection. Small-caliber tubes (18 to 22 Fr) are used to remove air, and large-caliber tubes (36 to 40 Fr) are used to drain fluid. An anterior site (the second intercostal space, midclavicular line) or a posterolateral site (intercostal space 4-8) is used. Standard practice when selecting a posterolateral site is to use the fifth or sixth intercostal space between the anterior and midaxillary lines. The patient is either supine or in the lateral decubitus position with the elbow bent. Except for emergencies, the procedure must be explained to the patient and his/her informed consent obtained. The area for the thoracostomy is prepared with antiseptic solution and is draped with sterile towels. Many institutions provide thoracostomy trays, which contain two large Kelly clamps, a scalpel, a needle holder, forceps, 0 sutures, a cup for local anesthetic, 22- and 18-gauge needles, 10 and 20 ml syringes, and gauze pads. Adequate local

anesthetic must be administered. The proposed area of insertion and an interspace above and below it should be liberally injected with 1% or 2% lidocaine (20 to 25 ml).

The skin incision is made parallel to the long axis of the rib, overlying the rib an interspace below the proposed site of insertion (Fig. 51-4, *A*). A large Kelly clamp is used to dissect the area for a tunnel up to the superior border of the rib (Fig. 51-4, *B*). The intercostal muscles are bluntly dissected at the superior margin of the rib. Entering the pleural space at the superior margin of the rib avoids injury to the intercostal neurovascular bundle. The jaws of the clamp then are closed and placed over the superior margin of the rib, and the pleural space is entered. A finger is inserted into the pleural space and rotated 360 degrees to ensure that the lung is not adherent to the chest wall (Fig. 51-4, *C*).

The chest tube is then inserted, using a Kelly clamp to guide it into the apex, if air is being drained, or it is inserted posteriorly if fluid is being drained. A second clamp should be placed on the end of the tube if fluid is being drained to prevent spillage. A 0 silk purse-string suture is placed in the skin surrounding the tube. A single knot is thrown, and the remaining length of the suture is wrapped around the tube and tied. This suture can be used to close the skin opening when the tube is removed. Another suture can be used to close the skin around the tube if a large incision has been made. The tube is connected to a closed drainage system.

Petrolatum gauze and a dressing are applied and securely taped. All connections should be secured with tape or chest tube bands. If the patient is in extremis with a tension pneumothorax, a 14-gauge IV catheter should be placed in the second intercostal space at the midclavicular line. This maneuver relieves the tension and allows more controlled placement of the chest tube.

Complications

Malpositioning of tube. A tube inserted too far can injure mediastinal structures. One not inserted far enough can lead to persistent air leak or incomplete drainage of the pneumo-

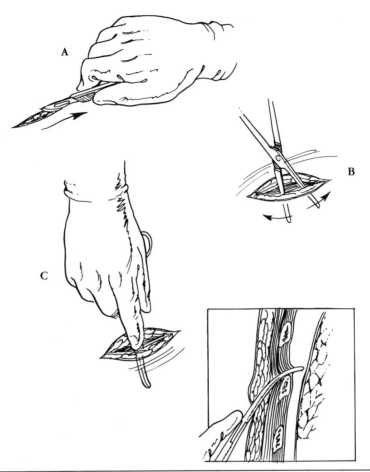

FIG. 51-4 Thoracostomy. **A,** Skin incision. **B,** Kelly clamp used for dissection. **C,** Insertion of finger into pleural space. Inset: Insertion of clamp into pleural space. (Redrawn from Taylor RW, Civetta JM, Kirby RR, eds. Techniques and Procedures in Critical Care. Philadelphia: JB Lippincott, 1990, p 303.)

thorax. The tube may also be positioned completely outside the thoracic cavity. Intra-abdominal insertions may occur if too low an interspace is chosen. The insertion site should be carefully chosen in patients with elevated diaphragms. Malpositioned tubes should be removed, and a new tube inserted through a new incision.[5]

Bleeding. Intercostal vascular injury may occur during insertion. Pulmonary vessels may be injured when the trocar technique is used (use of a trocar is not recommended). Adhesions can be very vascular and, if disrupted, can cause bleeding. If digital examination reveals extensive adhesions, an alternate site is chosen.

Abdominal visceral injury. Such an injury can occur during this procedure, especially if too low an insertion site is chosen. The liver and spleen are at greatest risk. Extreme caution must be used in patients with elevated hemidiaphragms in order to avoid this complication.

Mechanical problems associated with collection system. Such problems include tubing constrictions; clotting of the tube (if an air leak persists, the patient could develop a tension pneumothorax); and disconnection of the chest tube from the collecting system.

Reexpansion pulmonary edema. Reexpansion pulmonary edema usually occurs hours after reexpansion of the lung after evacuation of a long-standing pneumothorax or drainage of a massive effusion. The mechanism is thought to involve increased capillary permeability in the collapsed lung. This phenomenon can be avoided by using gradual reexpansion of drainage. Large collections should be allowed to drain to a water seal, rather than being placed initially to suction.

Infection. Local infections at the insertion site can occur. Attention to skin care can prevent this complication. Pneumonias and empyemas are rarer events (3%).[6]

Lung injury. Lung injury occurs more often when the trocar technique is used or when patients have decreased lung compliance or adhesions.[7]

Drainage Systems

Modern drainage systems use a variation of the three-bottle system (Fig. 51-5). The chest tube is connected to the apparatus by rubber tubing that is usually ½ inch in internal diameter, allows flow of 50 to 60 ml/min, and is 6 feet in length.[8] The tubing from the patient is connected to the collection chamber or bottle, which is in turn connected to the water seal bottle. In the water seal bottle, the water level will move in synchrony with respiration if the tube is not occluded. If an air leak is present, air will bubble through this chamber. Connected to this bottle is the suction control bottle, which is connected to a vacuum. The amount of water in the vacuum bottle determines the amount of subatmospheric pressure exerted on the pleural cavity; 20 cm of H_2O is standard.

Chest Tube Removal

The tube is removed when no air leak is noted for 24 hours. A CXR with the patient on water seal alone ("clamped"), without suction, is usually obtained. If no pneumothorax is observed, the chest tube can be removed. If the tube has been placed to drain fluid, it can be removed when the drainage is <100 ml/day.

Procedure. To perform chest tube removal, the dressings are removed and sutures cut. The patient is asked to inspire deeply and perform a Valsalva maneuver,[9] which increases intrathoracic pressure and discourages air from entering the thorax. The tube is removed rapidly, and the sutures are tied. Petrolatum gauze and gauze pads are applied.

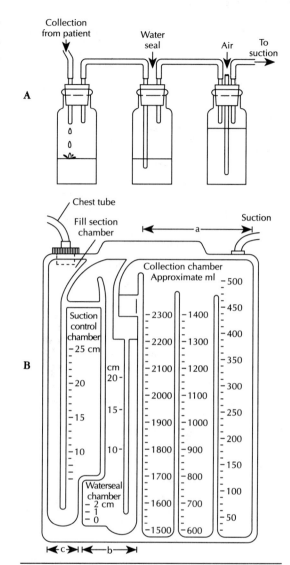

FIG. 51-5 Drainage systems. **A,** Three-bottle system. **B,** Variation of three-bottle system; *a,* collection chamber; *b,* water seal chamber; *c,* suction control chamber. (Redrawn from Taylor RW, Civetta JM, Kirby RR, eds. Techniques and Procedures in Critical Care. Philadelphia: JB Lippincott, 1990, p 311.)

Sclerosis

Pleural sclerosis can be used to treat recurrent effusion or malignant effusions. When the lung is completely reexpanded, no air leak persists, and fluid drainage is <100 ml/day, the following procedure is used:

- 1 g of tetracycline is instilled into the thorax through the chest tube.

- The tube is clamped for 4 to 6 hours (procedure is painful, and adequate analgesia must be provided).

These collections may require tube placement under ultrasonic or CT scan guidance. The effusions occur in patients who have had multiple chest tubes or have had empyemas. Care should be exercised in draining pneumothoraxes in patients with extensive bullous disease. It is sometimes necessary to obtain a CT scan to determine if an air collection is a large bleb or a loculated pneumothorax. Placement of a tube into a bleb can result in bronchopleural fistula and/or bleeding.

Maintaining Chest Tube Patency

Chest tube patency is maintained by using the following methods: (1) stripping; (2) irrigation; (3) instillation of urokinase; or (4) mechanical dislodgment of obstructing matter using an endotracheal suction catheter.[10]

PARACENTESIS

Paracentesis, puncture of the abdominal cavity to aspirate peritoneal fluid, is used for the diagnostic evaluation of ascites, treatment of disabling ascites, and diagnosis of intra-abdominal sepsis. Its use is contraindicated in patients who have had multiple previous abdominal operations, those who currently have massive bowel distention or abdominal wall cellulitis, or women who are pregnant.

Procedure

A useful site for performing paracentesis is lateral to the rectus muscle at the level of the umbilicus or 1 cm below or above the umbilicus (Fig. 51-6). Sonography or a CT scan can be used to guide the appropriate choice of site.

The skin is prepared with antiseptic solution, and the sterile field is draped. A 25-gauge needle is used to administer local anesthetic with epinephrine. A 21-gauge IV catheter (larger gauge may be used) with syringe attached is passed through the skin perpendicularly and then is angled to create a Z tract. As the needle is advanced, the syringe is aspirated. A pop or give is felt as the needle passes through the fascia and peritoneum. When fluid is aspirated, the catheter is advanced, and the needle is re-

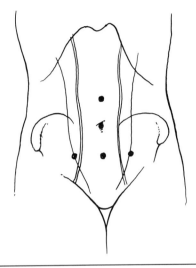

FIG. 51-6 Sites for paracentesis. (Redrawn from Taylor RW, Civetta JM, Kirby RR, eds. Techniques and Procedures in Critical Care. Philadelphia: JB Lippincott, 1990, p 312.)

moved. A larger syringe then is attached to collect fluid for diagnostic study. Alternatively, a stopcock can be attached to the catheter, which is connected to extension tubing and a drainage bag, and the desired amount of fluid removed through a closed system. The catheter is removed and the area covered with a dressing.

Diagnostic Tests

Diagnostic tests of the peritoneal fluid include those for the following:

- Specific gravity
- Protein content
- Cell count
- Cytology
- Gram's stain
- Bacterial and fungal cultures
- Acid-fast bacillus stain
- Amylase
- Bilirubin

Complications

Complications of paracentesis include bowel or bladder perforation, infection, persistent ascitic leak, and hypotension if too much volume is removed.[6]

OPEN AND CLOSED PERITONEAL TAP AND LAVAGE

Diagnostic peritoneal lavage (DPL) is used to evaluate both blunt and penetrating trauma. It is also useful for evaluating peritonitis in patients with altered mental status, in patients with altered sensation, and in critically ill patients in whom transport represents a major risk.[11]

Caution must be used in performing this procedure in a patient with multiple abdominal scars. The procedure is absolutely contraindicated only if there is a definite indication for laparotomy.

Closed Procedure

The closed peritoneal tap (Fig. 51-7) is usually performed at the infraumbilical midline. If the patient has pelvic fractures, the supraumbilical midline is used. The area is prepared with antiseptic solution and is sterilely draped. The skin is punctured with a No. 11 blade, and pressure is held with a gauze pad until the bleeding stops. Kits are available that contain an 18-gauge needle, a guidewire, and a 14 Fr catheter with multiple side holes. The needle is passed through the rectus fascia and peritoneum. A characteristic pop or give is felt, the guidewire is passed through the needle, and the needle is withdrawn. The catheter is passed over the

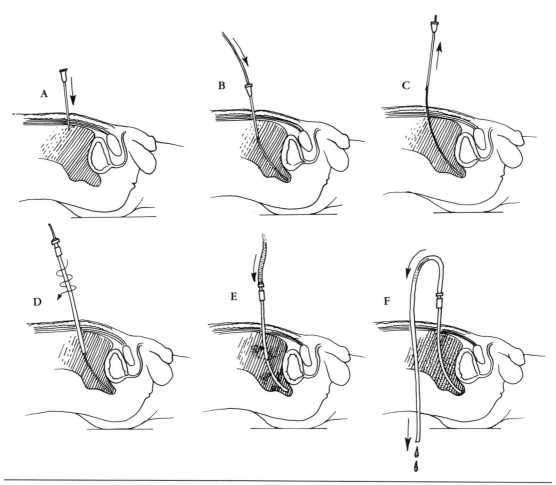

FIG. 51-7 Closed peritoneal tap and lavage. **A,** Needle is inserted into peritoneal cavity. **B,** Flexible guidewire is passed through needle. **C,** Needle is withdrawn with guidewire left in place. **D,** Teflon catheter is advanced over wire. **E,** Wire is withdrawn and salt solution is infused through catheter. **F,** Seal on intravenous solution is broken and fluid is allowed to drain into infusion container. (Redrawn from Danto L. Paracentesis and diagnostic peritoneal lavage. In Blaisdell FW, Traukey DD, eds. Trauma Management, vol 1. Abdominal Trauma. New York: Thieme Medical, 1982, pp 45-57.)

wire into the peritoneal cavity. A 10 ml syringe is used to aspirate the catheter. If ≤5 ml of blood is obtained, lavage is performed, and 1 L of normal saline solution or lactated Ringer's solution is infused and allowed to return by gravity. At least 200 ml should return. The fluid is sent for cell count and amylase and bilirubin concentrations.

Open Procedure

After the patient has been scrubbed with antiseptic solution, draped, and anesthetized, an incision is made in the skin. The soft tissues are dissected and the rectus fascia identified. Rectus fascia is divided in the midline, and stay sutures are placed on either side. The peritoneum is grasped, and a purse-string suture is placed. The peritoneum is then incised, and a dialysis catheter is inserted and directed to the pelvis. If ≤5 ml of blood are aspirated, lavage is performed. The catheter is removed after the fluid is recovered, and the purse-string suture is tied. The rectus fascia is repaired with No. 0 or 1

suture and the skin is closed with 3-0 or 4-0 nylon.

Semi-open Procedure

This procedure involves visualizing the fascia and then passing a peritoneal lavage catheter through the fascia blindly. The procedure is useful in the obese patient.

Results

Results of peritoneal tap and lavage are 97% accurate, with a false positive rate of 1%.[12] The red cell count in a patient with blunt trauma is considered positive with >100,000 RBC/mm^3 and equivocal with 50,000 to 100,000 RBC/mm^3. In a patient with penetrating trauma >20,000 RBC/mm^3 is considered positive, whereas 10,000 to 20,000 RBC/mm^3 is considered equivocal. A WBC count >500 WBC/mm^3 is positive, and one of 100 to 500 WBC/mm^3 is equivocal. A positive DPL is indicated by the presence of stool or particulate matter, bile, bacteria on a Gram's stain, or an amylase concentration >175 U/dl.[13]

SUMMARY

- Use lumbar puncture to diagnose CNS infection, subarachnoid hemorrhage, or demyelination.
- Use lumbar puncture to administer antibiotics, analgesics, or chemotherapy.
- Do not perform lumbar puncture in patients with elevated ICP, coagulopathy, or local skin infection.
- Perform lumbar puncture at the L3-4 or the L4-5 interspace.
- Perform thoracentesis for diagnosis or treatment of pleural effusion. Loculated effusions may require ultrasound or CT localization.
- When performing thoracentesis or thoracostomy, enter the pleural cavity over the superior edge of the rib that defines the lower border of the selected intercostal space.
- Perform thoracostomy for pneumothorax, hemothorax, pneumohemothorax, chylothorax, or empyema.

- Use large-caliber tubes (36 to 40 Fr) for drainage of hemothorax.
- Perform paracentesis for diagnosis of ascites, diagnosis of abdominal sepsis, or treatment of refractory ascites.
- Avoid performing paracentesis in patients with multiple previous operations, massive bowel distention, abdominal wall cellulitis, or pregnancy.
- Perform peritoneal lavage in evaluation of blunt trauma or penetrating trauma. Consider peritoneal lavage in diagnosing abdominal pathology in high-risk patients with equivocal signs and symptoms.
- Use caution in patients with previous abdominal surgery.
- Do not perform peritoneal lavage in patients with a definite indication for laparotomy.

REFERENCES

1. Brown DL, Flynn JF. Lumbar puncture and epidural analgesia in the ICU. In Taylor RW, Civetta JM, Kirby RR, eds. Techniques and Procedures in Critical Care. Philadelphia: JB Lippincott, 1990, pp 388-399.

2. Gorelick PE, Biller J. Lumbar puncture: Technique, indications, and complications. Postgrad Med 79(8):257-266, 1986.

3. Marton KI, Gean AD. The spinal tap: A new look at an old test. Ann Intern Med 104:840-848, 1986.

4. Edelson RN, Chernick NL, Posnen JB, et al. Spinal subdural hematomas complicating lumbar puncture: Occurrence in thrombocytopenic patients. Arch Neurol 31:134-137, 1974.

5. Dalbec DL, Krome RL. Thoracostomy. Emerg Med Clin North Am 4:441-457, 1986.

6. Yeston NS, Niehoff JM. Important procedures in the intensive care unit. In Taylor RW, Civetta JM, Kirby RR, eds. Techniques and Procedures in Critical Care. Philadelphia: JB Lippincott, 1990, pp 295-345.

7. Fraser RS. Lung perforation complicating tube thoracostomy: Pathologic description of three cases. Hum Pathol 19:518-523, 1988.

8. Miller KS, Sahn S. Chest tubes: Indications, techniques, management and complications. Chest 91:258-264, 1987.

9. Daly RC, Mucha P, Pairolero PC, et al. The risk of percutaneous chest tube thoracostomy of blunt thoracic trauma. Ann Emerg Med 14:865-870, 1985.

10. Halejian BA, Badach MJ, Trilles F, et al. Maintaining chest tube patency. Surg Gynecol Obstet 167:521-522, 1988.

11. Richardson JD, Flint LM, Polk HC, et al. Peritoneal lavage: A useful diagnostic adjunct for peritonitis. Surgery 94:826-829, 1983.

12. Powell DC, Bivins BA, Bell RM, et al. Diagnostic peritoneal lavage. Surg Gynecol Obstet 155:257-264, 1982.

13. Danto L. Paracentesis and diagnostic peritoneal lavage. In Blaisdell FW, Traukey DD, eds. Trauma Management, vol 1. Abdominal Trauma. New York: Thieme-Medical, 1982, pp 45-57.

PART SIX

MEASUREMENT AND INTERPRETATION OF DATA

CHAPTER 52

Blood Pressure Monitoring

Jerome H. Abrams

The use of indwelling pressure monitoring catheters is widespread in the SICU. Clinicians rely on accurate blood pressure measurements from the arteries and the heart to support oxygen delivery and organ function. Although pressure measurements alone do not provide information about blood flow, optimum outcome requires combined blood pressure and blood flow information.[1-3]

Invasive pressure monitoring presents certain problems to the clinician. Most clinicians can recall instances when the blood pressure measured by the arterial line disagreed by 15 mm Hg or more with the value obtained by a blood pressure cuff. Which is the correct value? Are all indwelling catheters accurate? The answers to these questions require familiarity with resonance and damping.

DAMPED OSCILLATING SYSTEMS: RESONANCE

The phenomenon of resonance can be very important: one need only ask the designers of the Tacoma Narrows Bridge, which was destroyed when the wind excited its resonance frequencies and caused high-amplitude vibrations of the bridge roadway[4,5] (Fig. 52-1). Any damped system that oscillates can demonstrate resonance, the production of large-amplitude vibrations in response to a succession of small impulses applied at the proper time. The frequency at which the forced oscillations have their maximum amplitude is termed the resonance frequency (Fig. 52-2). Resonance can occur in clinical practice, for example, in peripheral and pulmonary artery blood pressure monitoring systems. In such situations, resonance can produce artificially high blood pressure peaks. Commercial electronic monitors cannot detect the presence of resonance and may give elevated readings, 15 mm Hg or above correct reading.[6]

The peripheral and pulmonary arterial pressure measuring systems may be described as a damped harmonic oscillator. An oscillating system of mass (m) with a sinusoidal driving force [F(t)], a linear restoring force (kx), or spring constant, and a damping force (cx) conforms to the following equation[7]:

$$m\ddot{x} + c\dot{x} + kx = F(t)$$

From this relationship, a plot of amplitude ratio vs. frequency ratio may be obtained. The amplitude ratio is the amplitude of the damped system divided by that of an undamped reference system, and the frequency ratio is the driving frequency divided by the resonance frequency of the system. The family of curves obtained, which can be verified experimentally,[8] is shown in Fig. 52-3. Several features should be noted. First, the damping coefficient (h) can be determined by varying the frequency over a sufficiently wide range and examining the amplitude of a test system compared to a reference system. Second, if the resonance frequency is sufficiently large, its effect on the system may be small. In other words, if the resonance frequency is far from the frequency to be mea-

543

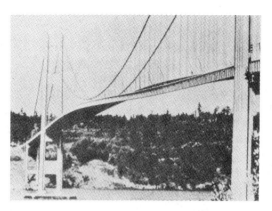
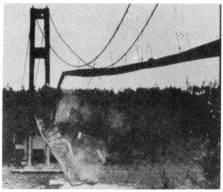

FIG. 52-1 On July 1, 1940, the Tacoma Narrows Bridge at Puget Sound, Washington, was completed and opened to traffic. Just 4 months later a mild gale set the bridge oscillating until the main span broke up, ripping loose from the cables and crashing into the water below. The wind produced a fluctuating resultant force in resonance with a natural frequency of the structure. This caused a steady increase in amplitude until the bridge was destroyed. Many other bridges were later redesigned to make the aerodynamically stable. (From Resnick R, Halliday D. Physics, Part I. New York: John Wiley, 1967.)

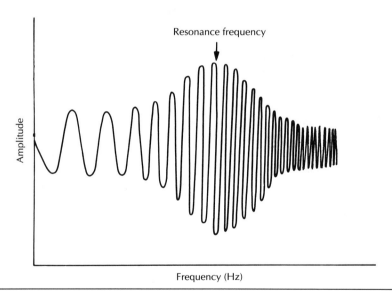

FIG. 52-2 Amplitude vs. frequency of driving force. (From Abrams JH, Olson ML, Marino JA, Cerra FB. Use of a needle valve variable resistor to improve invasive blood pressure monitoring. Crit Care Med 12:978-982, 1984. © Williams & Wilkins.)

sured, little effect of resonance will be seen. Third, no increase in the amplitude ratio will occur at any frequency if the value of the damping coefficient is 0.707, $1/\sqrt{2}$, or greater. With these considerations, if one wishes to measure a quantity whose frequency falls in the range of the resonance frequency of the measuring system, the situation can be improved by in-creasing the damping of the measuring system. The resonance frequency of the patient's catheter monitoring system is fixed by the length, diameter, and compliance of the connecting tubing and by the nature of the pressure transducer. Do the commonly found pressure measuring systems in clinical use have favorable frequency characteristics? To answer this ques-

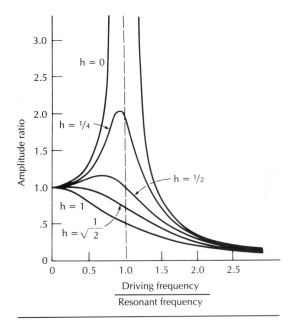

FIG. 52-3 Amplitude ratio vs. frequency ratio. (From Abrams JH, Olson ML, Marino JA, Cerra FB. Use of a needle valve variable resistor to improve invasive blood pressure monitoring. Crit Care Med 12:978-982, 1984. © Williams & Wilkins.)

tion, one needs to know both their resonant frequencies and their damping coefficients.

MEASURING DAMPING COEFFICIENTS: THEORY

How might the resonant frequencies and the damping coefficients be obtained? The frequency-amplitude response curves in Fig. 52-3 show one method of evaluating these two variables. The resonance frequency can be determined from the amplitude maximum as the system is driven over an appropriate frequency range. A damping coefficient (h) can be obtained from:

$$h = [(1 - w_r^2/w_u^2)/2]^{1/2}$$

where w_r is the resonance frequency of the damped system and w_u is the frequency at which the phase lag is 90 degrees. Generally, a frequency range of 10 times the fundamental frequency allows for reasonable approximations of the blood pressure waveform.[9] Since the fundamental frequency is heart rate, approximately 2 Hz, a frequency range of 0 to 20

Hz should be adequate. Another method is the decay of the step impulse or the square-wave impulse,[10] the clinical analog of which is the snap test (Fig. 52-4). It can be noted the rate of decay of the impulse falls within an envelope that may be modeled as an exponential. The damping coefficient (h) may be obtained from:

$$h = \left[\frac{[\ln(x_2/x_1)]^2}{\pi^2 + [\ln(x_2/x_1)]^2} \right]^{1/2}$$

where x_1 is the amplitude of the first peak above the amplitude of the square-wave impulse and x_2 is the amplitude of the second peak above the amplitude of the square-wave impulse.

MEASURING DAMPING COEFFICIENT: CLINICAL APPLICATION

Do the usual blood pressure monitoring configurations in common use have adequate frequency characteristics? If not, can their measuring performance be improved? Damping coefficients have been measured by the two methods described here in systems used in actual clinical practice for blood pressure measurement.[11] A snap test was used to adjust damping. In the snap test, a shunt positioned around the capillary device that allows for continuous flushing of the arterial line is quickly opened and suddenly occluded. A variable-resistance damping device (Fig. 52-5), one method for adding damping, was then manipulated to allow approximately 5% to 7% overshoot with respect to the steady-state response to the step impulse. The variable resistor was adjusted without any knowledge of the patient's blood pressure. This device can be easily placed in the monitoring system and readily adjusted to produce a satisfactory step-impulse response, or square-wave test (Fig. 52-6), of the pressure monitoring system. Measurement of the damping coefficient and the resonance frequency both before and after adding auxiliary clamping allowed evaluation of the increase in damping that was caused by the variable resistance.

In commonly used arterial blood pressure monitoring systems without additional damping, arterial line pressure was often higher than cuff blood pressure. After adjustment of the variable resistor to more closely approximate

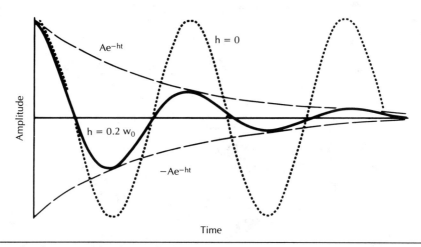

FIG. 52-4 Amplitude vs. time for decay of a free vibration. h, Damping coefficient; w_0, natural frequency in absence of damping. (From Abrams JH, Olson ML, Marino JA, Cerra FB. Use of a needle valve variable resistor to improve invasive blood pressure monitoring. Crit Care Med 12:978-982, 1984. © Williams & Wilkins.)

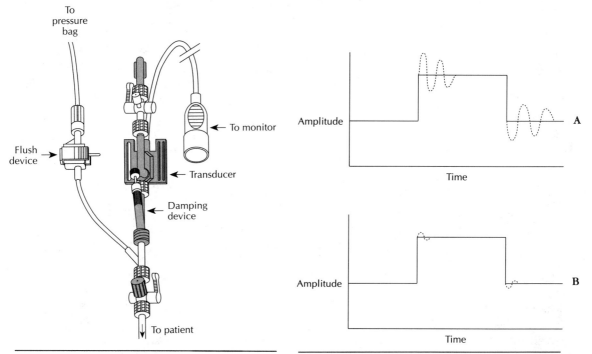

FIG. 52-5 Location of variable resistor in monitoring system. (Courtesy Cardiorespiratory Services, University of Minnesota, Minneapolis.)

FIG. 52-6 Square-wave test. **A**, no auxiliary damping; **B**, auxiliary damping added.

a square wave without knowledge of the patient's blood pressure, the arterial line and cuff blood pressures agreed well. Without additional damping, the resonance frequency of the measuring system was in some cases only twice the fundamental frequency, the heart rate. In nearly all cases an increase in damping was required to approximate a square wave without excessive ringing. An example of a pressure waveform from the pulmonary artery, before and after the addition of damping, is shown in Fig. 52-7. An example of a radial artery pressure

waveform, also before and after additional clamping, is shown in Fig. 52-8.

What should a damping coefficient be in clinical practice? Probably everyone agrees that a pressure measuring system is functioning properly if the input of a square wave results in the output, by the measuring system, of an identical square wave. Such a result is impossible in a damped oscillator. If the system is underdamped, the amount of overshoot will be unacceptably high. If the system is overdamped, it will take an unacceptably long time to reach

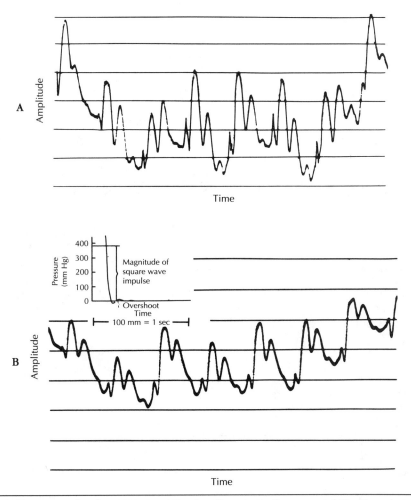

FIG. 52-7 **A,** Uncorrected pulmonary artery tracing. Resonance frequency, 5 Hz; damping coefficient, 0.38. **B,** Corrected pulmonary artery tracing. Damping coefficient, 0.67. Inset shows bedside snap test. (From Abrams JH, Olson ML, Marino JA, Cerra FB. Use of a needle valve variable resistor to improve invasive blood pressure monitoring. Crit Care Med 12:978-982, 1984.)

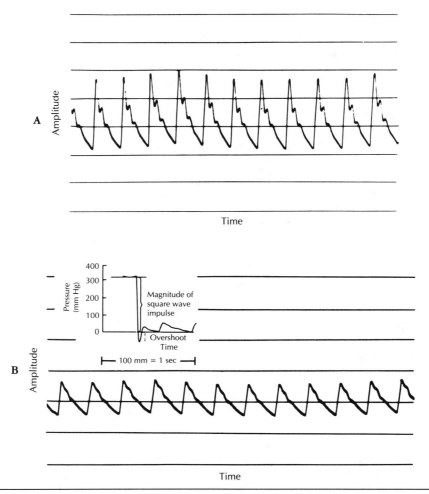

FIG. 52-8 **A,** Uncorrected radial artery tracing. Resonance frequency, 12.7 Hz; damping coefficient, 0.15. **B,** Corrected radial artery tracing. Damping coefficient, 0.49. Inset shows bedside snap test. (From Abrams JH, Olson ML, Marino JA, Cerra FB. Use of a needle valve variable resistor to improve invasive blood pressure monitoring. Crit Care Med 12:978-982, 1984. © Williams & Wilkins.)

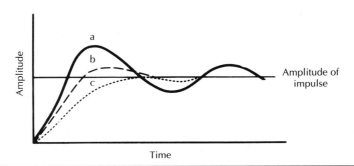

FIG. 52-9 Amplitude vs. time. Damping coefficient is such that damping for system a < b < c. (From Abrams JH, Olson ML, Marino JA, Cerra FB. Use of a needle valve variable resistor to improve invasive blood pressure monitoring. Crit Care Med 12:978-982, 1984. © Williams & Wilkins.)

the amplitude of the input pressure. Therefore a compromise must be reached.

As the damping coefficient is increased, the time response also increases (Fig. 52-9). The optimum compromise between damping and time response depends on the context. In clinical practice, decisions are nearly always made on the basis of the pressure magnitude averaged over several hundred heartbeats. Few decisions are made based on fractional-second time response. It therefore seems reasonable to minimize overshoot rather than to minimize response time. A damping coefficient in the range of 0.5 to 0.75 has proved satisfactory at our institution. This seemingly wide range is related to the wide range of resonance frequency in the tubing configurations in common use: the higher the resonance frequency of the tubing configuration, the lower the damping coefficient may be.

SUMMARY

- Many commonly used pressure measurement systems are underdamped; as a result, pressure values may be artifically high.
- Resonance frequency of these pressure monitoring systems is often in the range of physiologic interest.
- A variable resistor or other damping device improves invasive blood pressure monitoring systems as measured by damping coefficients.

- Improved amplitude transmission is obtained at the expense of minimum time response, but the results are clinically useful.
- Damping may be successfully added in actual clinical practice under widely different conditions.
- Calibration of the pressure monitoring system using a step-impulse test can be done easily at the patient's bedside.

REFERENCES

1. Shoemaker WC, Appel PL, Blaid RD. Use of physiologic monitoring to predict outcome and to assist in clinical decisions in critically ill postoperative patients. Am J Surg 146:43, 1983.
2. Shoemaker WC. Hemodynamic and oxygen transport patterns in septic shock: Physiologic mechanisms and therapeutic implications. In Sibbald WJ, Sprung CL, eds. Perspectives on Sepsis and Septic Shock. Fullerton, Calif.: Society of Critical Care Medicine, 1986, pp 203-234.
3. Abrams JH, Barke RA, Cerra FB. Quantitative evaluation of the clinical course of septic patients: The data conform to catastrophe theory. J Trauma 24:1028-1037, 1984.
4. Resnick R, Halliday D. Physics, Part I. New York: John Wiley, 1967, p 372.
5. Braun M. Differential Equations and Their Applications, 3rd ed. New York: Springer-Verlag, 1983, pp 167-173.
6. Gardner RM. Direct blood pressure measurement—Dynamic response requirements. Anesthesiology 54:227, 1981.
7. Fry DL. Physiologic recordings by modern instruments with particular reference to pressure recording. Physiol Rev 40:753, 1960.
8. Wylie CR. Advanced Engineering Mathematics. New York: McGraw-Hill, 1975, p 186.
9. Shinozaki T, Deane RS, Mazuzan JE. The dynamic responses of liquid-filled catheter systems for direct measurement of blood pressure. Anesthesiology 53:498, 1980.
10. Marion JB. Classical Dynamics of Particles and Systems. New York: Academic Press, 1970, p 287.
11. Abrams JH, Olson ML, Marino JA, Cerra FB. Use of a needle valve variable resistor to improve invasive blood pressure monitoring. Crit Care Med 12:978-982, 1984.

CHAPTER 53

Cardiac Output

Jerome H. Abrams

The use of invasive hemodynamic monitoring in the SICU can be divided into three general categories: restoration of oxygen transport, optimization of specific organ function, and preoperative cardiac evaluation. Restoration of oxygen transport, described in Chapter 2, requires measurement of cardiac output (CO) to determine both oxygen consumption and oxygen delivery. (Optimization of specific organ function is a theme of several chapters in this book.) Knowledge of ventricular function, especially left ventricular function, is refined by measuring CO and correlating it with the pressure necessary to produce that flow. Information about systolic function, diastolic function, and systemic response to stress is obtainable, in part, through measurement of CO. Optimization of renal function, by identification and treatment of pre-renal components of dysfunction, can be achieved with measurement of CO. Chapter 6 describes preoperative optimization of cardiac function and restoration of oxygen transport to reduce perioperative cardiac risk.

It is clear that a need for measuring CO exists in an SICU, where patients have complex clinical courses and simultaneous compromise of all major organ systems. In the SICU the most commonly used procedure for clinical measurement of CO is thermodilution. Thermodilution measurements are an extension of the Fick principle. This chapter considers the Fick principle, thermodilution CO, and ultrasonic procedures, which may enjoy wider use in the future. Since thermodilution measurements are an extension of the Fick principle, an understanding of this principle is important for a better appreciation of the foundations of thermodilution measurements.

THE FICK PRINCIPLE

The Fick principle states that total uptake or release of a substance by an organ is the product of blood flow to the organ and the arteriovenous concentration difference of the substance.[1]

In the direct Fick method, oxygen consumption ($\dot{V}O_2$) and the arteriovenous oxygen content difference ($C_aO_2 - C\bar{v}O_2$) determine CO from the relation[2]:

$$CO = \frac{\dot{V}O_2}{(C_aO_2 - C\bar{v}O_2)} \times 10$$

The factor of 10 is necessary to maintain consistent units.

In the absence of intracardiac shunt, and if pulmonary blood flow equals systemic blood flow, the direct Fick method can be used to measure CO. The measurement requires determination of oxygen consumption, arterial oxygen content, and venous oxygen content. Commonly used methods for determining oxygen consumption are collection of expired gas in a Douglas bag and analysis of expired gas by the metabolic rate cart. Arterial oxygen content measurement is routinely done in most hospitals, and catheterization of the pulmonary artery is a routine procedure in the SICU. From pulmonary artery blood, mixed venous oxygen is determined. Under steady-state conditions, the Fick method provides reproducible COs with a standard error of approximately 7% of the average value.[3-5]

Sources of error are largely a result of technical problems in expired gas sampling or collection or the inability to achieve a steady state. If the Douglas bag method of expired gas sampling is used, incomplete collection will produce a measured CO that is lower than the actual CO. Another source of error arises from the absence of stable pulmonary volume during the measurement interval. Both the Douglas bag and the metabolic rate cart measure uptake of oxygen by the lungs. If the lung, acting as a reservoir, were to trap gas during the measurement, uptake of oxygen by the circulation might not equal that of the lung. Another source of error arises from the respiratory quotient. Since the volume of expired carbon dioxide does not equal the volume of oxygen consumed in the same interval, failure to use the respiratory quotient introduces some error into the CO determination.[1]

An extension of the Fick principle is the indicator dilution procedure. In the direct Fick method, the indicator is oxygen and the injection site is the lung. A continuous infusion of oxygen is the injection procedure. In indicator dilution methods, an appropriate indicator is chosen, the injection site is usually a proximal vessel or chamber of the heart, and either continuous or bolus injection is done.

The most widely used indicator in clinical practice is temperature, and a bolus injection procedure is the norm. The use of indocyanine green, another indicator, involves a continuous infusion procedure. For indicator dilution procedures to be successful, certain requirements must be met[1]:

1. The indicator is nontoxic, mixes completely with blood, and can be measured with sufficient accuracy.
2. The indicator substance, once injected, is not lost or metabolized before it reaches the detector.

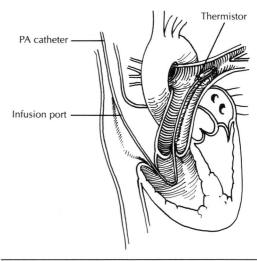

FIG. 53-1 Position of pulmonary artery catheter for measurement of cardiac output.

3. The indicator flows past the detector before recirculation begins.
4. The indicator substance mixes thoroughly.

To perform thermodilution measurements, the clinician most commonly places a thermistor-equipped pulmonary artery catheter (Fig. 53-1). A thermal indicator, usually iced or room temperature saline, is injected into the right atrial port. The thermal indicator mixes and is detected downstream by the thermistor.

Hamilton et al.[6] observed that the amount of an appropriate indicator detected downstream from the site of injection is equal to the product of CO and the integrated change in concentration for the duration of the measurement. CO then can be calculated from:

$$I = CO \int_0^\infty C(t)\, dt$$

Rearranging as:

$$CO = \frac{I}{\int_0^\infty C(t)\, dt}$$

where:

CO = Cardiac output
I = Amount of indicator
C(t) = Concentration of indicator as a function of time

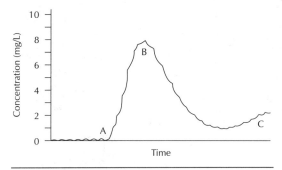

FIG. 53-2   Indicator dilution concentration curve in a patient with normal cardiac output: 1 ml of indocyanine green dye solution (5.0 mg/ml) was injected into pulmonary artery at time zero. Blood was withdrawn continuously from brachial artery through a densitometer cuvette, and time-concentration curve from densitometer was recorded. First appearance *(A)* is followed by a steep rise to peak concentration *(B)*, and subsequent gradual decline of indicator curve, which is interrupted by a secondary rise *(C)* due to recirculation of indicator substance. (From Grossman W. Cardiac Catheterization and Angiography, 3rd ed. Philadelphia: Lea & Febiger, 1986, p 114. Reprinted with permission.)

An example of an indicator dilution curve is shown in Fig. 53-2.

A bolus of cold solution produces a time-temperature curve that is similar to the time-concentration curve of, for example, indocyanine green dye.[7] For measurement of CO by thermodilution, the relation described by Hamilton and colleagues needs modification. Since a thermal indicator is used, the volume of injectate (V), the initial blood temperature (T_B), the initial injectate temperature (T_I), a density factor (K_1), and a computation constant (K_2) are used. The CO then may be calculated as:

$$CO = \frac{V(T_B - T_I) \times K_1 \times K_2}{\displaystyle\int_0^\infty \Delta T_B (t)\, dt}$$

The denominator is the integral of temperature change of the blood.[2] Accuracy of thermodilution, when compared to that of calibrated me-

chanical pumps, is 7% to 13%.[8,9] For single injections of thermal indicators, differences from calibrated flow were as high as 15% to 25%.[9] Correlation coefficients of 0.96 and 0.91 have been obtained for thermodilution COs compared to the direct Fick and indocyanine green methods, respectively.[10]

In clinical practice, the error of measurement, when commercially available equipment is used, makes a 12% to 15% change in CO necessary to be of clinical significance.[11] Other clinical variables may affect CO determination by thermodilution. Injection of the thermal indicator at different phases of the respiratory cycle can result in significant variation of the CO.[12,13] Errors in CO determination during rapid intravenous volume infusion have been reported.[14] Slowing of the heart rate after injection of iced saline as a thermal indicator also has been reported.[15,16]

Careful technique is necessary for minimizing error with thermodilution. The commercially available CO computers use carefully specified volumes and temperatures of thermal indicator. If the amount of indicator injected is less than that programmed, the CO value will be falsely elevated. Further, if the temperature of the indicator is higher than that programmed, the amount of indicator will appear to the CO computer to be less than that expected. The calculated CO will be similarly elevated. Use of iced saline is more likely to produce the latter type of error. Underestimation of CO occurs when a greater volume of indicator is injected than was programmed.[2] In view of these considerations, multiple injections of thermal indicator should be used. With three injections, the probability that the thermodilution CO is within 10% of the true value is 89%. With five injections, a 98% probability exists that the CO is within 10% of the true value.[17]

OTHER METHODS OF MEASUREMENT

The error in measurement and the capability of obtaining only intermittent CO measurements with thermal dilution present limitations on both observing CO and improving understanding of ventricular function in clinical settings. Other methods for measuring CO attempt to address these limitations. Thoracic electrical impedance has been used for clinical determination of CO.[18,19] Ultrasound methods have the potential to provide continuous (beat-to-beat) COs and are noninvasive. CO is the product of blood velocity ($\bar{v}$) and aortic cross-sectional area (A):

$$CO = \bar{v}A$$

Both $\bar{v}$ and A may be obtained from ultrasound by using both the Doppler principle and ultrasound range gating, respectively. The Doppler principle can evaluate blood velocity ($\bar{v}$) from the velocity of ultrasound in tissue (c), the Doppler shift (Δf), the ultrasound carrier frequency (f_0), and the angle of the ultrasound beam with respect to flow (ϑ)[20–22]:

$$\bar{v} = \frac{c\Delta f}{2f_0 \cos \vartheta}$$

Ultrasound range gating can provide a blood vessel diameter. If a circular cross section (A) is assumed, the cross-sectional area required for calculation of CO can be found. Different anatomic windows have been used for ultrasound measurements. COs have been obtained from esophageal ultrasound probes.[23] A procedure under development is the transtracheal Doppler approach. By combining ultrasound technology with endotracheal intubation, the transtracheal Doppler procedure measures aortic diameter and blood velocity in the ascending aorta proximal to the origin of the arch vessels.[24,25] In endotracheally intubated patients, the transtracheal Doppler approach allows measurement of continuous CO without the need for additional invasive procedures. Other potential advantages of the transtracheal Doppler procedure include (1) accuracy over a wide range of COs, (2) ability to detect changes in flow sensitively, (3) absence of effect on CO during measurement source, (4) ability to measure continuous CO, and (5) absence of additional risk to the endotracheally intubated patient.

SUMMARY

- CO measurements are necessary for restoration of oxygen transport, optimization of specific organ function, and preoperative cardiac evaluation.
- Thermodilution is the most widely used clinical method of determining CO.
- Thermodilution evolved from the Fick principle. Indicator dilution methods estimate CO from the general relationship:

$$CO = \frac{I}{\int_0^\infty C(t)\, dt}$$

- For accurate thermodilution measurements, careful technique, with precise volume and temperature of injectate, is necessary. Five injections per CO determination produce a 90% chance of being within 10% of the true CO value.
- A 12% to 15% change in CO is necessary to have clinical significance when thermodilution is used in clinical settings.
- Variations in respiration or intravenous volume infusion can introduce error in thermal dilution CO determination.
- Ultrasonic methods show promise for use in continuous noninvasive CO determination.

REFERENCES

1. Grossman W. Blood flow measurement: The cardiac output. In Grossman W, ed. Cardiac Catheterization and Angiography. Philadelphia: Lea & Febiger, 1986, pp 101-117.
2. Thys DM. Cardiac output. Anesthesiol Clin North Am 6:803-824, 1988.
3. Selzer A, Sudrann RB. Reliability of the determination of cardiac output in man by means of the Fick principle. Circ Res 6:485-490, 1958.
4. Thomasson B. Cardiac output in normal subjects under standard basal conditions. Scand J Clin Lab Invest 9:365-376, 1957.
5. Howell CD, Horvath SM. Reproducibility of cardiac output measurements in the dog. J Appl Physiol 14:421-423, 1959.
6. Hamilton WF, Moore JW, Kinsman JM. Studies on the circulation IV. Further analysis of the injection method, and changes in hemodynamics under physiological and pathological conditions. Am J Physiol 99:534, 1932.
7. Fegler G. Measurement of cardiac output in anesthetized animals by a thermodilution method. Q J Exp Physiol 39:153, 1954.
8. Salgado CR, Galleti PM. In vitro evaluation of the thermodilution technique for the measurement of ventricular stroke volume and end-diastolic volume. Cardiologia 49:65-78, 1966.
9. Bilfinger TV, Lin C-Y, Anagnostopoulos CE. In vitro determination of accuracy of cardiac output measurements by thermal dilution. J Surg Res 33:409-414, 1982.
10. Goodyer AVN, Huvos A, Eckhardt WF. Thermodilution curves in the intact animal. Circ Res 7:432-441, 1959.
11. Stetz CW, Miller RG, Kelly GE. Reliability of the thermodilution method in the determination of cardiac output in clinical practice. Am Rev Respir Dis 126:1001-1004, 1982.
12. Snyder JF, Powner DJ. Effects of mechanical ventilation on the measurement of cardiac output by thermodilution. Crit Care Med 10:677-682, 1982.
13. Stevens JH, Raffin TA, Mihm FG. Thermodilution cardiac output measurement. JAMA 253:2240-2242, 1985.
14. Wetzel RC, Latson TW. Major errors in thermodilution cardiac output measurement during rapid volume infusion. Anesthesiology 62:684-687, 1985.
15. Nisikawa T, Dohi S. Slowing of heart rate during cardiac output measurement by thermodilution. Anesthesiology 57:538-539, 1982.
16. Harris AP, Miller CF, Battie C. The slowing of sinus rhythm during thermodilution cardiac output determination and the effect of altering injectate temperature. Anesthesiology 63:540-541, 1985.
17. Hoel BL. Some aspects of the clinical use of thermodilution in measuring cardiac output. Scand J Clin Invest 38:383, 1978.
18. Kubicek WG, Karegis JN, Patterson RP. Development and evaluation of an impedence cardiac output system. Aerospace Med 37:1208, 1966.
19. Bernstein DP. Continuous non-invasive real-time monitoring of stroke volume and cardiac output by thoracic electrical bio-impedance. Crit Care Med 14:898-901, 1986.
20. Baker DW. Pulsed ultrasonic Doppler blood-flow sensing. IEEE Transactions on Sonic and Ultrasonics. SU 17:170-185, 1970.
21. Hartley CJ, Cole JS. An ultrasonic pulsed Doppler system for measuring blood flow in small vessels. J Appl Physiol 37:626-629, 1974.
22. Blair AK, Lucas CL, Hsia HS. A removable ultrasound Doppler probe for continuous monitoring of changes in cardiac output. J Ultrasound Med 2:357-362, 1983.
23. Kamal GD, Symreng T, Stan J. Inconsistent esophageal Doppler cardiac output during acute blood loss. Anesthesiology 72:95-99, 1990.
24. Abrams JH, Weber RE, Holmen KD. Transtracheal Doppler: A new procedure for continuous cardiac output measurement. Anesthesiology 70:134-138, 1989.
25. Abrams JH, Weber RE, Holmen KD. Continuous cardiac output determination using transtracheal Doppler: Initial results in humans. Anesthesiology 71:11-15, 1989.

CHAPTER 54

Respiratory Monitoring

Ian J. Gilmour

In the SICU gas movement and gas exchange are the determinants of respiratory function. Although performing formal pulmonary function tests before the onset of acute lung injury might be valuable, formal pulmonary function testing is generally not possible in the SICU. Since optimal patient management requires information about current lung function, the remaining discussion considers monitoring of gas flow and then gas exchange in the SICU patient. Table 54-1 lists definitions and gives explanation of acronyms.

Pressure (P), gas flow, and lung volumes are all related. For example, an inverse relationship between lung volume (V) and resistance to flow has been identified (Fig. 54-1). For constant flow, airway resistance is a hyperbolic function of lung volume.

Inspiratory airway resistance to flow in mechanically ventilated patients can be assessed by the following relationship:

EQUATION 1

$$R = \triangle P/V$$

where

R = Resistance
$\triangle P = P_{AO} - P_{ALV}$
V = Flow

Direct measurement of R requires measurement of both pressure gradient and gas flow. Measurement of both P_{ALV} and gas flow are extremely difficult. P_{ALV} is usually estimated by interrupting flow and measuring airway pressure at zero flow; if flow is truly zero, airway pressure will be the same as P_{ALV}.

In patients with severe obstructive lung disease (OLD) the zero flow requirement probably will not be met, and airway pressure does not really represent P_{ALV}. Because of these limitations, calculation of actual inspiratory resistance is not commonly undertaken in clinical medicine. Measurement of expiratory resistance is even more difficult because flow rate during expiration is not constant: lung elastic

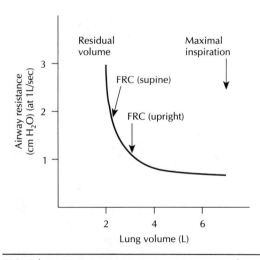

FIG. 54-1 Airway resistance is an increasing hyperbolic function of decreasing lung volume. Functional residual capacity (FRC) decreases with changing from upright to supine position. (From Nunn JF. Applied Respiratory Physiology, 3rd ed. London: Butterworth-Heinemann Limited, 1987, p 64.)

TABLE 54-1 Glossary of Respiratory Terms

Term or Abbreviation	Definition
Restrictive lung disease (RLD)	Abnormality of lung parenchyma or chest wall that results in a decrease in TLC
Obstructive lung disease (OLD)	Lung disease resulting from increased resistance to flow in the tracheo-bronchial tree
Static lung volume	Lung volume that does not change during ventilation, (e.g., functional residual capacity, residual volume)
Dynamic lung volume	Lung volume that changes with ventilation (e.g., IC, VT, VC)
Resistance (R)	Application of Ohm's law; pressure drop per unit flow
Compliance (C)	Change in volume per unit change in pressure
P_{max}	Peak airway pressure achieved on inspiration during positive pressure ventilation; reflects both resistance and compliance
P_{ei}	End-inspiratory pressure; pressure at end inspiration with no gas flow; reflects elastic recoil of the respiratory system (i.e., compliance); also called plateau pressure
Auto-PEEP	Intrinsic positive end-expiratory pressure (PEEP); an increase in airway pressure that occurs because emptying of the lung is incomplete; thought to reflect P_{ALV}
P_{ALV}	Alveolar pressure: driving pressure for exhalation
P_{PL}	Pleural pressure; most commonly measured indirectly by esophogeal balloon
C_{CO_2}	Oxygen content of blood in pulmonary capillaries
Ca_{O_2}	Oxygen content of arterial blood
$C\bar{v}_{O_2}$	Oxygen content of mixed venous blood
P_{AO}	Pressure at the airway opening (i.e., endotracheal tube, mouth)
V_T	Tidal volume (see Fig. 54-4)
IC	Inspiratory capacity (see Fig. 54-4)
VC	Vital capacity (see Fig. 54-4)
TLC	Total lung capacity (see Fig. 54-4)
C_L	Lung compliance
C_{cw}	Chest wall compliance
C_{rs}	Compliance of respiratory system
$\dot{V}$	Flow
$\dot{V}_A$	Alveolar ventilation per minute
$\dot{V}_E$	Total minute ventilation (respiratory rate × VT)
$A\text{-}aD_{O_2}$	Difference between alveolar oxygen tension (PA_{O_2}) and arterial oxygen tension (Pa_{O_2})
FI_{O_2}	Fraction of inspired oxygen
PI_{O_2}	Partial pressure of inspired oxygen

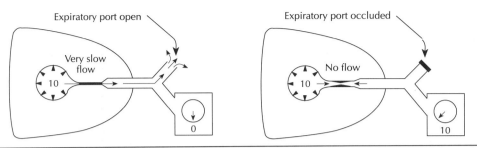

FIG. 54-2 Auto-PEEP effect and its measurement. In presence of severe airflow obstruction and high ventilation requirements, alveolar pressure at end exhalation remains elevated as flow continues throughout expiration, driven by recoil pressure of hyperexpanded lung (left). Transiently stopping flow at end exhalation allows equilibration of pressure throughout circuit. Occult alveolar pressure is then detectable on ventilator manometer. (From Marini JJ, Wheeler AD. Respiratory Monitoring in Critical Care Medicine: The Essentials. Baltimore: Williams & Wilkins, 1989, pp 47-60.)

recoil, the driving force, is a nonlinear function of lung volume.

If it is assumed that flow is constant during inspiration, R can be estimated by using pressures easily obtained from the ventilator's manometer. Two of these pressures are the pressure at which inspiration is initiated (positive end-expiratory pressure [PEEP]) and P_{max}. The difference between P_{max} and PEEP is the pressure required to overcome resistance in the airway and to inflate the lungs. End-inspiratory pressure (P_{ei}) can also be obtained easily. The difference between P_{max} and P_{ei} (ΔP) approximates the pressure required to overcome resistance in the system (i.e., ventilator circuit, endotracheal tube, and tracheobronchial tree). Although not identical to $P_{AO} - P_{ALV}$ (Equation 1), ΔP is suitable for clinical use. As the contribution of the ventilator circuit and the endotracheal tube remains constant, changes in ΔP *at constant inspiratory flow and volume* represent changes in R within the tracheobronchial tree; thus ΔP can be used as an approximation of resistance, and changes in P represent changes in R. For example, the effect of bronchodilators can be assessed by noting ΔP before and after their administration. For these comparisons to be meaningful, inspiratory flow rate must be kept constant because flow changes will affect ΔP.[1]

Most modern ventilators offer a choice of flow patterns, including a square wave or constant flow. Assuming that flow actually is constant for a square-wave flow pattern, square-wave flow patterns, if available, should be used for R estimates. With a square-wave flow of 40 to 60 L/min in patients with endotracheal tubes of reasonable size (7 to 7.5 mm in adult females; 8 to 8.5 mm in adult males), a ΔP of <5 cm H_2O can be expected. ΔP greater than this suggests that resistance to flow is increased. If a square-wave flow pattern is not available, ΔP will not correlate well with R, but changes in ΔP from one situation to the next, assuming constant flow and volume, will correspond to changes in R. Since P_{max} represents all the work required to inflate the lung, ventilatory efforts by the patient may either exaggerate or cause underestimation of ΔP.

Auto-PEEP is usually defined as airway pressure higher than preset machine PEEP at end expiration and is thought to reflect an elevated P_{ALV} caused by incomplete emptying of the lung (Fig. 54-2). The presence of intrinsic PEEP or auto-PEEP is thought to reflect increased resistance.[2] Auto-PEEP is most often seen in patients with OLD but can be caused by anything that increases resistance such as a pinched or obstructed endotracheal tube or by an excessive respiratory rate.

A capnograph, if available, may indicate abnormal airway resistance. An increased slope, coupled with a large gradient between partial pressure of end-tidal carbon dioxide ($Petco_2$) and partial pressure of carbon dioxide ($Paco_2$) is often seen with OLD[3] (Fig. 54-3).

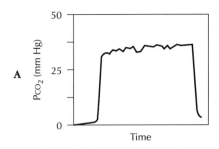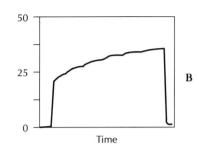

FIG. 54-3 Examples of capnograph waveforms. **A,** Normal tracing. **B,** Increased slope of phase III, usually representing uneven gas mixing within lung. See also Fig. 54-8. (From Moon RE, Camporesi EM. Respiratory monitoring in anesthesia. In Miller RD, ed. Anesthesia, 3rd ed. New York: Churchill Livingstone, 1990, p 1146.)

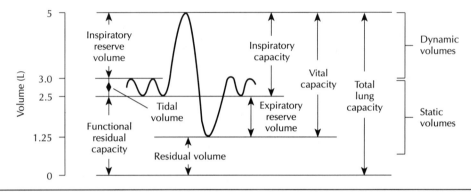

FIG. 54-4 Dynamic lung volumes that can be measured by simple spirometry are tidal volume, inspiratory reserve volume, expiratory reserve volume, inspiratory capacity, and vital capacity. Static lung volumes are residual volume, functional residual capacity, and total lung capacity. Static lung volumes cannot be measured by observation of a spirometer trace and require separate methods of measurement. (From Benumof JL. Respiratory physiology and respiratory function during anesthesia. In Miller RD, ed. Anesthesia, 3rd ed. New York: Churchill Livingstone, 1990, p 519.)

Pressure measurements can also be useful during weaning. Maximum inspiratory pressure (MIP) (also called *negative inspiratory force)* has long been used to assess the instantaneous strength of inspiratory muscles. To determine MIP the airway is occluded for 20 to 25 seconds at end expiration to insure maximal effort. A pressure more negative than -30 cm H_2O (in this case the more negative, the better) is a favorable indication for weaning. Note that a satisfactory MIP does not guarantee that the patient will be able to sustain adequate ventilation.

MONITORING LUNG VOLUMES

Most acute pulmonary dysfunction is restrictive, usually associated with decreases of both static

and dynamic lung volumes (Fig. 54-4). In most instances restrictive lung disease (RLD) is caused by lung parenchymal disease (adult respiratory distress syndrome [ARDS], atelectasis). RLD may also arise from problems in the pleural space (hemothorax, pneumothorax), the chest wall (ascites, obesity), or neuromuscular disease (Guillain-Barré). Preexisting pulmonary disease compounds and confuses the problem.

Inspiratory capacity (IC) or vital capacity (VC) cannot be measured in the sedated, unconscious, or paralyzed SICU patient, and attempts to do so are potentially dangerous. Ventilator spirometers can be used to measure spontaneous IC or VC, measurements that are useful in weaning. Ventilator spirometers can also provide a reasonably accurate estimate of tidal volume (V_T) which may be used to calculate total minute ventilation ($\dot{V}_E$). $\dot{V}_E$ is affected by both metabolic rate and lung function: increases in either metabolic rate or dead space demand a greater $\dot{V}_E$ to maintain normal $Paco_2$. $\dot{V}_E$ can also be used to assess the probability of weaning a patient from mechanical ventilation. Many patients are unable to maintain the level of respiratory work required when spontaneous $\dot{V}_E > 10$ L/min.

Ventilator-recorded V_T can also be used for compliance measurements. Compliance measures the stiffness of the lung and/or chest wall. Generally speaking, the lower the lung compliance (C_L) the more severe is the degree of dysfunction.

EQUATION 2

$$C_{rs} = \Delta V/\Delta P$$

where C_{rs} is compliance of the respiratory system, ΔV is V_T, and ΔP is P_{ei} minus PEEP.

Compliance is usually measured in L/cm H_2O (or ml/cm H_2O). When C_{rs} is <40 ml/cm H_2O, respiratory work is markedly increased, and mechanical ventilation is often required. To use V_T in compliance measurements, it must be recalled that a portion of each V_T distends and is compressed within the ventilator circuitry. Although this volume is measured by the spirometer, it is not delivered to the patient. Volume lost this way is called *machine compliance volume* (MCV). MCV is a function of both the ventilator circuit and the pressures achieved; therefore Equation 2 should be modified as follows:

EQUATION 3

$$C_{eff} = \frac{V_T - C_{cf}[\Delta P]}{\Delta P}$$

where C_{cf} is the compliance factor of the ventilator and ΔP is the pressure change.

Dynamic compliance (C_{dyn}) considers the volume change resulting from the total pressure change ($P_{max} - $ PEEP) and includes the pressure necessary to overcome airway resistance (see discussion on resistance at beginning of chapter). Static compliance (C_{st}) takes into account only the pressure required to inflate the lung and chest wall (i.e., $P_{ei} - $ PEEP). In this section static lung compliance is discussed:

EQUATION 4

$$C_{st} = \frac{V_T - C_{cf}(P_{ei} - PEEP)}{P_{ei} - PEEP}$$

As shown in Fig. 54-5, the compliance curves of the lung and chest wall do not coincide.[3] In clinical practice compliance is commonly calculated for the respiratory system as a whole because chest wall compliance (C_{cw}) is usually linear. In the presence of massive ascites or other chest wall diseases, the shape and slope of the chest wall compliance curve may change enough that it would be necessary to consider chest wall mechanics separately.[2]

EQUATION 5

$$C_L = \Delta V/\Delta(P_{ALV} - P_{PL})$$

EQUATION 6

$$C_{cw} = \Delta V/\Delta P_{PL}$$

To separate C_L or C_{cw} from C_{rs}, one must be able to measure pleural pressure (P_{PL}). Direct measurement of P_{PL} is technically difficult and seldom performed. Indirect measurement, using esophageal balloon manometry, is more readily available, but accuracy is questionable except in knowledgeable and experienced hands. Although gas exchange frequently improves as lung volumes (and compliance) improve, the relationship between C_L and gas exchange is complex. The interaction between intrathoracic pressure and cardiorespiratory function is not fully explained by compliance.

Static lung volumes (most commonly functional residual capacity [FRC]) can be measured by a variety of techniques in mechanically ventilated patients, including open and closed circuit techniques and planimetry of CXRs or CT scans. Body plethysmography is not possible in mechanically ventilated patients. These methods share technical problems, require sophisticated technology, and are difficult to perform. Their usefulness in clinical care is limited. Respiratory impedance (inductance) plethysmography can be used to detect changes in FRC that result from various therapeutic maneuvers. It

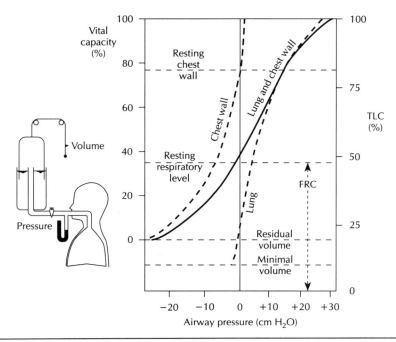

FIG. 54-5   Relaxation pressure-volume curve of lung and chest wall. Patient inspires (or expires) to a certain volume from spirometer, tap is closed, and he/she relaxes respiratory muscles. Curve for lung and chest wall can be explained by addition of individual lung and chest wall curves. (Modified from West JB. Respiratory Physiology—The Essentials, 4th ed. Baltimore: Williams & Wilkins, 1990, p 100.)

has become a popular clinical tool for measuring volume and breathing pattern. Wide elastic bands enclosing Teflon-insulated electrical coils are placed around the chest and abdomen. Expansion of the rib cage and abdomen alters inductance, changing the oscillator-generated frequency of the electrical current coursing through the coils. Of the available non–airway-dependent monitoring methods, respiratory impedance plethysmography is least affected by changes in body position, provided that the bands fit snugly and are not displaced.[1] Although generally available, this type of plethysmography requires training and experience before it is useful.[4]

MONITORING GAS EXCHANGE

Over the last decade, intensivists have been assessing partial pressure of oxygen, (Pao_2) in the light of tissue oxygen delivery (see Chapter 2). In this chapter, however, the use of arterial blood gas (ABG) data to estimate lung efficiency is emphasized.

A common method of assessing the efficiency of oxygenation is by calculating the shunt fraction (Qs/Qt):

EQUATION 7

$$Qs/Qt = \frac{Cco_2 - Cao_2}{Cco_2 - C\bar{v}o_2}$$

where Cco_2 is oxygen content of blood in pulmonary capillaries, Cao_2 is oxygen content of arterial blood, and $C\bar{v}o_2$ is oxygen content of mixed venous blood.

This equation assumes the three-compartment lung model (i.e., all alveoli are either ideal [functioning perfectly], shunting [$\dot{V}a/Qt = 0$], or functioning as dead space [$\dot{V}a/Qt = \infty$]).[5] The normal Qs/Qt <5% is caused by anatomic shunts (e.g., thebesian veins).[2] Using Qs/Qt to assess oxygenation is cumbersome, requires extensive laboratory data and calculations for each measurement, and is an oversimplification of ventilation/perfusion relationships. Abnormalities in the average SICU patient occur at

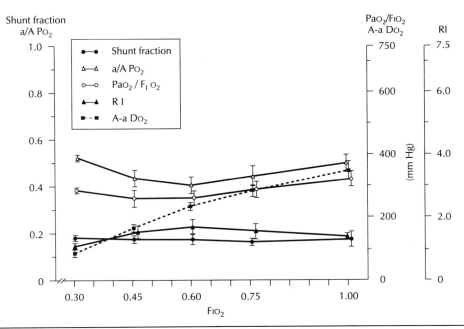

FIG. 54-6 Mean value for each index and for shunt fraction at each level of FIO_2. Bars represent standard error of mean (n = 8 at FIO_2 = 0.30; n = 10 at all other levels of FIO_2). For visual clarity, some data points have been adjusted laterally at each level of FIO_2. (From Herrick IA, Champion LK, Froese AB. A clinical comparison of indices of pulmonary gas exchange with changes in inspired oxygen concentration. Can J Anaesth 37:69-76, 1990.)

many points on the continuum between shunt and dead space.

For these reasons several other methods of assessing the efficiency of oxygenation have been used, most commonly the difference between alveolar oxygen tension (PAO_2) and arterial oxygen tension ($A-aDO_2$). PAO_2 is calculated using the alveolar gas equation:

EQUATION 8

$$PAO_2 = (PB - PH_2O)\, FIO_2 - PACO_2/R + F$$

where

$$F = (PACO_2)\,(FIO_2)\,[(1 - R)/R]$$
$$R = \text{Respiratory quotient}$$
$$PB = \text{Barometric pressure}$$
$$PH_2O = \text{Water vapor pressure}$$

For clinical purposes this equation can be simplified to:

EQUATION 9

$$PAO_2 = PIO_2 - 1.25\,(PACO_2)$$

The $A-aDO_2$ is limited by its dependence on the fraction of inspired oxygen (FIO_2). In other words, an $A-aDO_2$ of 100 is not necessarily worse than an $A-aDO_2$ of 50 (Fig. 54-6). The discrepancy results from the dependence of this type of index on changes in PaO_2, whereas shunt fraction depends on changes in oxygen content, a much more accurate reflection of how efficiently the lungs are oxygenating blood.[6] Shunt (or $A-aDO_2$) is not necessarily increased in patients whose hypoxia arises from alveolar hypoventilation; in these patients PaO_2 falls as partial pressure of carbon dioxide in the alveoli ($PACO_2$) rises. To make this clear, the alveolar gas equation is used to calculate PAO_2 in a patient breathing room air, assuming a $PACO_2$ of 80 mm Hg:

$$
\begin{aligned}
PAO_2 &= (P_B - PH_2O)FIO_2 - PACO_2/R + F \\
&= (760 - 47)(0.21) - 80/0.8 + \\
&\quad (80)(0.21)(1 - 0.8/0.8) \\
&= 150 - 100 + 4.2 \\
&= 54.2 \text{ mm Hg}
\end{aligned}
$$

Alternatives to using intermittent ABG values for monitoring oxygenation have important limitations. Transcutaneous oximetery and pulse oximetry do not allow differentiation between ischemic hypoxia (tissue hypoxia resulting from inadequate blood flow) and hypoxemic hypoxia (tissue hypoxia from inadequate arterial oxygen content).[7] Nonetheless, these techniques are available and can provide very useful information if their limitations are recognized. Pulse oximetry has become a very popular tool to monitor changes in oxygenation. Because of its limitations, transcutaneous monitoring is seldom used in adults; accordingly, it is not discussed.

PULSE OXIMETRY

For details of pulse oximetry design and function, see the articles by Kemper[7] and Kemper and Barker.[8] Pulse oximeters have become popular because they are easy to use: no calibration is necessary, and probes are easily placed and are noninvasive. They were designed to assess oxygenation during airway procedures (e.g., intubation, bronchoscopy), to monitor unstable patients (e.g., those with changing FiO_2, respiratory distress), or for use in any situation in which trending information is useful to alleviate patient safety concerns.

However, pulse oximeters do have several drawbacks that limit their usefulness as diagnostic tools:

- Pulse oximeters reveal nothing about alveolar ventilation. It is quite possible for a patient with perfectly acceptable pulmonary oxygen saturation (SpO_2) and percent oxygen saturation in arterial blood (SaO_2) to have a severe respiratory acidosis.
- Pulse oximeters are unreliable in vasoconstricted patients because they depend on pulsatile flow to calculate saturation. Data from a pulse oximeter in which the pulse rate is inaccurate should be viewed with suspicion.
- Pulse oximeters are accurate only to within ± 2% to 3% and only at SpO_2 >85%.[7] There is a wide variation in PaO_2 within the range of ± 3% saturation on the steep part of the oxyhemoglobin dissociation curve (Fig. 54-

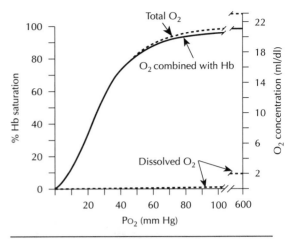

FIG. 54-7 Oxygen dissociation curve (solid line) for pH 7.4, PcO_2, 40 mm Hg, and 37° C. Total blood oxygen concentration also is shown for hemoglobin concentration of 15 g/dl of blood. (From West JB. Respiratory Physiology—The Essentials, 4th ed. Baltimore: Williams & Wilkins, 1990, p 70.)

7). Since diffusion of oxygen to the tissues depends on PaO_2, a low PaO_2 may have an adverse effect on tissue oxygenation. Thus pulse oximetery data should be confirmed by obtaining blood gas values at low saturations ($SpO_2 \leq 93\%$), and the SpO_2 should be used only as trending data.

- Substances such as methylene blue, indocyanine green, methemoglobin, and carboxyhemoglobin, which interfere with light absorption at red and infrared frequencies, will cause erroneous readings.[7,9] Normal tissue pigments or hyperbilirubinemia does not appear to cause clinically significant variability.
- Other sources of light, particularly fluorescent light, can interfere with the photodiode and cause inaccurate readings. For this reason, pulse oximetric probes usually should be covered with an opaque dressing.
- Long-term placement of probes, particularly if the probe is from a manufacturer different from that of the electronic monitor, can result in patient burns.[10]
- Pulse oximeters cannot detect changes in ox-

ygenation reliably until saturation drops below 97% ($PaO_2 \approx 80$ mm Hg) because hemoglobin (Hb) is 100% saturated as long as PaO_2 is above 154 mm Hg (see Fig. 54-7) and pulse oximeters are only accurate to $\pm 3\%$. The pulse oximeter cannot be used to detect endobronchial intubation reliably. With endobronchial intubation, enough desaturation may not occur.[7]

- SpO_2 reflects events in the pulmonary circulation at a place in the peripheral circulation. The inherent delay must be recognized during intubations and ventilator changes.

MONITORING CARBON DIOXIDE REMOVAL

Most of the carbon dioxide produced by normal metabolic processes ($\dot{V}CO_2$) is excreted through the lungs. The efficiency of that process is usually assessed intermittently by measuring partial pressure of carbon dioxide (PCO_2) in a sample of arterial blood with a Severinghaus electrode. The clinician obtains "snapshots" of carbon dioxide excretion. In critical situations continuous on-line measurement of partial pressure of carbon dioxide ($PaCO_2$) would be preferred. Although this is still in the experimental stage, the use of end-tidal PCO_2 ($PetCO_2$) as a reflection of $PaCO_2$ has been practical for several years.

The amount of carbon dioxide in arterial blood, as reflected by $PaCO_2$, is inversely proportional to alveolar ventilation ($\dot{V}A$). The lower the $\dot{V}A$, the higher $PaCO_2$ will be:

EQUATION 10

$$PaCO_2 = (\dot{V}CO_2/\dot{V}A)\ K$$

where K is a constant.

Equation 10 is valid for any reason that causes a change in $\dot{V}A$. $\dot{V}A$ may fall because of a decrease in total minute ventilation ($\dot{V}E$) such as might occur after administration of morphine sulfate or if the dead space (VD) increases, as in emphysema.

To understand the limitations of capnometry, as the measurement of expired carbon dioxide is called, it is necessary to review the concept of VD. The portion of VT that does not participate in gas exchange is referred to as VD.

In healthy people VD approximates the volume of the tracheobronchial tree and is called *anatomic dead space*. In pathologic high V/Q situations when perfusion to ventilated alveoli is relatively diminished, VD will consume an increasing portion of each VT, and VA will fall unless $\dot{V}E$ increases. Using the Bohr equation, VD relative to VT can be calculated if it is assumed that all alveoli are "ideal," "shunt," or "dead space."

EQUATION 11

$$VD/VT = \frac{PaCO_2 - PetCO_2}{PaCO_2}$$

High VD/VT supports V/Q mismatch as the cause of elevated $PaCO_2$ as opposed to problems such as hypoventilation (caused by an excess of narcotics) or increased carbon dioxide production (e.g., caused by an abnormal respiratory quotient or increased metabolic rate). In healthy people there is little VD apart from anatomic dead space and $PaCO_2 \approx PetCO_2$. In patients with pulmonary dysfunction, expired gas comes from alveoli with a myriad of V/Qs so that $PetCO_2$ will be significantly lower than $PaCO_2$; the difference between the two is an indirect measure of the increase in VD because of V/Q mismatch (Table 54-2).

Most commonly, capnometers use infrared technology, but other systems are available. Regardless of the technology used, expired gas is sampled as close to the patient as possible, and expired carbon dioxide is plotted as a function of time to provide a waveform or capnogram. A normal capnogram can be seen in Fig. 54-8. Causes of variation from the normal capnogram can be found in Table 54-3.

Most currently used capnometers are sidestream samplers, which means they sample only a portion of the expired gas. Some infrared spectrometers, however, are capable of mainstream sampling (see box, p. 564).

Although capnometry is a useful monitor of $\dot{V}A$, several simple rules must be followed[11]:

- Rely on the capnogram rather than digitally reported $PetCO_2$.
- Consider the possibility of equipment malfunction such as sampling leaks.

- Remember that changes in $Petco_2$ often do not parallel changes in $Paco_2$.

After a pulmonary embolism, although $Petco_2$ has decreased precipitously, $Paco_2$ may well be rising unless $\dot{V}A$ is increased. $Petco_2$ and $Paco_2$ may diverge without any obvious clinical signs. For this reason, $Petco_2$ alone is an unreliable monitor for such purposes as weaning from mechanical ventilation, and $Petco_2$ data should periodically be confirmed by ABG values.[12,13]

Comparison of Mainstream vs. Sidestream Capnometers

Mainstream	Sidestream
Fast	Sampling delay
No problem with condensation	Apparatus dead space
	Limited sampling rate
Very heavy	Problems with condensation
High cost	
	Potential for multiple gas analysis

TABLE 54-2 Arterial End-Tidal Carbon Dioxide Tension ($Paco_2$ − $Petco_2$) Gradient During General Anesthesia*

Investigator	Year	$Paco_2$ − $Petco_2$ (mm Hg)		Comments
		Mean	Range	
Nunn	1960			No cardiac or pulmonary disease
		4.5 ± 2.5	−0.4-7.7	Spontaneous respiration
		4.7 ± 2.5	1.7-9.1	Artificial respiration
Askrog	1964	3.6	1.5-6.1	After induction (halothane group)
		5.5	2.6-10	After 90-150 min of halothane anesthesia
		0.9	0.6-1.9	Unanesthetized controls
Takki	1972	3.5 ± 0.5		
Whitesell	1981	0.8 ± 0.3		No lung disease
		3.3 ± 0.6		Lung disease
				Stable gradient on repeated measurements
Valentin	1982	5	−4-13	Pediatric patients Spontaneous respiration
Raemer	1983	4.1	0.8-13	Varying gradient on repeated measurements
Fletcher	1984	4.6	1.5-10.1	Small tidal volumes
		2.3	−0.8-8.5	Large tidal volumes
Shanker	1986	5.3 ± 2.9	3.5-7.1	Nonpregnant patients
		0.8 ± 0.7	−4-6.8	Pregnant patients; 50% had negative gradients

*From Good ML. Capnography: Uses, interpretations, and pitfalls. In Barash PG. Refresher Courses in Anesthesiology. Philadelphia: JB Lippincott, 1990, p 184.

TABLE 54-3   Untoward Situations Detected With Capnography*

Problem	Causes
No (or little) exhaled carbon dioxide	Esophageal intubation, tracheal extubation, disconnection, complete obstruction, apnea, cardiac arrest, pulmonary embolism
Elevated inspiratory baseline (phase I)	Incompetent expiratory valve
Prolonged expiratory upstroke (phase II)	Obstruction (equipment, pulmonary disease), slow gas sampling or instrument response time
Upward sloping expiratory plateau (phase III)	Obstruction (equipment, pulmonary disease)
Prolonged inspiratory downstroke (phase IV)	Incompetent inspiratory valve, slow gas sampling or instrument response time
Elevated $Petco_2$	Hypoventilation (leak, obstruction, inadequate ventilator settings), carbon dioxide rebreathing, increased carbon dioxide production or delivery (malignant hyperthermia, febrile illness, carbon dioxide insufflation, bicarbonate administration)
Decreased $Petco_2$	Hyperventilation, decreased carbon dioxide production or delivery (hypothermia, decreased cardiac output), increased arterial to end-tidal carbon dioxide gradient (ventilation/perfusion mismatching, hypotension, endobronchial intubation, pulmonary embolism [air, fat, thrombus, amniotic fluid], shallow or rapid breathing, instrument or sampling problems, sampling leak, miscalibration)

*Modified from Good ML. Capnography: Uses, interpretations, and pitfalls. In Barash PG. Refresher Courses in Anesthesiology. Philadelphia: JB Lippincott, 1990, p 190.

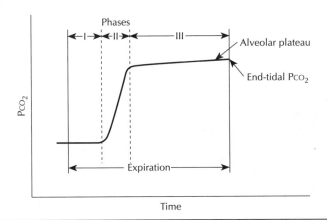

FIG. 54-8   Three phases of normal capnogram. Phase I is series dead space, length of which depends on amount of apparatus and anatomic dead space. Phase II is mixture of anatomic series and alveolar parallel gas. Phase III (alveolar plateau) is produced by mixture of ideal alveolar gas from well-perfused alveoli and alveolar dead space gas from unperfused alveoli. (From Kemper KK. Interpretation of noninvasive oxygen and carbon dioxide data. Can J Anaesth 37:S27-S32, 1990.)

SUMMARY

- P_{max} minus PEEP is pressure required to overcome airway resistance and to inflate the lungs.
- P_{max} minus P_{ei} is pressure required to overcome total airway resistance.
- Changes in P_{max} minus P_{ei} at constant flow and volume approximate changes in tracheobronchial resistance.
- Auto-PEEP is increase in airway pressure above preset PEEP at end expiration.
- Most acute pulmonary dysfunction is restrictive.

- Static lung compliance:

$$C_{st} = \frac{V_T - C_{cf}(P_{ei} - PEEP)}{P_{ei} - PEEP}$$

- $Qs/Q_T = \dfrac{Cco_2 - Cao_2}{Cco_2 - C\overline{v}o_2}$
- For clinical use: $Pao_2 = Pio_2 - 1.25\,(Paco_2)$
- $Paco_2$ varies inversely with alveolar ventilation.
- Capnometry, despite limitations, has clinical use in monitoring carbon dioxide excretion.

REFERENCES

1. Marini JJ. Lung mechanics determinations at the bedside: Instrumentation and clinical application. Respir Care 35:669-693, 1990.
2. Marini JJ, Wheeler AD. Respiratory Monitoring in Critical Care Medicine: The Essentials. Baltimore: Williams & Wilkins, 1989, pp 47-60.
3. Moon RE, Camporesi EM. Respiratory monitoring in anesthesia. In Miller RD. Anesthesia, 3rd ed. 1989, pp 1129-1165.
4. Pearson DJ. Measuring and monitoring lung volume outside the pulmonary function laboratory. Respir Care 35:660-667, 1990.
5. West JB. Respiratory Physiology—The Essentials, 4th ed. Baltimore: Williams & Wilkins, 1990, p 100.
6. Herrick IA, Champion LK, Froese AB. A clinical comparison of indices of pulmonary gas exchange with changes in the inspired oxygen concentration. Can J Anaesth 37:69-76, 1990.
7. Kemper KK. Interpretation of noninvasive oxygen and carbon dioxide data. Can J Anaesth 37:S27-S32, 1990.
8. Kemper KK, Barker SJ. Fundamental principles of monitoring instrumentation. In Miller RD. Anesthesia, 3rd ed. 1989, pp 957-999.
9. Schweitzer SA. Spurious pulse oximeter desaturation due to methemeglobinemia. Anaesth Intensive Care 19:269-271, 1991.
10. Murphy KG, Secunda JA, Rockoff MA. Severe burns from a pulse oximeter. Anesthesiology 76:350-352, 1990.
11. Good ML. Capnography: Uses, interpretations and pitfalls. In Barash PG. Refresher Courses in Anesthesiology. Philadelphia: JB Lippincott, 1990, pp 175-193.
12. Russell GB, Graybeal JM, Strout JC. Stability of arterial to end tidal carbon dioxide gradients during postoperative cardiorespiratory support. Can J Anaesth 37:560-566, 1990.
13. Hess D, Schlottag A, Levon B, et al. An evaluation of the usefulness of end tidal Pco_2 to aid weaning from mechanical ventilation following cardiac surgery. Respir Care 36:837-843, 1991.

SUGGESTED READINGS

Gravenstein JS. Gas monitoring and pulse oximetry. London: Butterworth-Heinemann, 1990.

Kemper KK, Barker SJ. Pulse oximetry. Anesthesiology 20:98-108, 1989.

Szaflarski NL, Cohen NH. Use of capnography in critically ill adults. Heart Lung 20:363-374, 1991.

Tobin MJ. Respiratory monitoring in the intensive care unit. Am Rev Respir Dis 138:1625-1642, 1988.

Truwit JD, Marini JJ. Evaluation of thoracic mechanics in the ventilated patient. Part I: Primary measurements. J Crit Care 3:133-150, 1988.

Truwit JD, Marini JJ. Evaluation of thoracic mechanics in the ventilated patient. Part II: Applied mechanics. J Crit Care 3:199-213, 1988.

PART SEVEN

THE ART OF PRACTICE

CHAPTER 55

Other Aspects of Patient Care

Frank B. Cerra

Several other aspects of care of the SICU patient are presented in this section. The topics include chart notes, advanced directives, "do not resuscitate" orders, and the decision to forego life-sustaining treatment.

CHART NOTES

Writing notes in the patient's chart is one of the aspects of patient care least liked by physicians. Yet it is one of the most important functions that can be performed on behalf of the patient, particularly with regulated care and with managed care providers assuming an increasing proportion of the financial responsibility of patient care.

The chart note is meant to communicate information about the patient to a variety of audiences that provide, purchase, evaluate, and regulate the delivery and outcomes of the health care provided. *This is a fact of life.* The patient's chart is the written record of the care delivered and received at the time of the illness. As such, it is perceived as the most accurate and reliable record of those events. With better health care information communicated in the chart, fewer issues are likely to arise during the review processes. Poor record keeping will not protect anyone from inquiries, claims reviews, malpractice actions, or any other actions by appropriate individuals and agencies.

A variety of individuals and agencies will use the patient's chart: other physicians, other health care providers, purchasers of health care, quality management personnel, and legal personnel. Other physicians and health care providers who administer to the patient need accurate and complete chart notes to understand the medical condition and care plan of the patient, especially if the attending physician is not present to talk to them. Other inquiries related to quality of services, appropriateness of services, worker's compensation, reimbursement, other regulatory issues, and legal proceedings also are facilitated by accurate chart notes that communicate the interaction among the patient, physicians, and other health care providers.

The chart note is meant to communicate information relevant to patient care. It is not a place to reproduce indiscriminately the information contained in the radiology and laboratory reports. The chart notes must include relevant information about the following:

- Preexisting disease, medications, allergy status, surgical procedures, and relevant portions of history and physical examination
- Reason for admission and current medical status
- Summary of the care plan or changes in the care plan, along with a reasonable explanation for the components or changes
- Statement about patient competency for decision-making
- Status of advanced directives for care and an explanation of the informed consent process and patient agreement with and participation in the care plan
- Description of complications that have oc-

curred and whether they have been discussed with the patient
- Statement concerning prognosis
- Summary of any care conferences that are held, including who attended, what information was communicated, what decisions were made, and what actions are to be taken
- Clear description of the physician services provided, including procedure notes, and adequate documentation of the intensity and time of services (*Intensity* describes the judgment complexity, mental and physical effort, and stress involved in the work performed)

A variety of formats can be used in this communication.

ADVANCED DIRECTIVES

Advanced directives, or "living wills," are an important source of information about a patient's wishes for treatment or limitations on treatment in settings in which patients no longer have adequate mental competence to make those decisions for themselves. These documents usually are prepared before hospitalization under guidelines and directives that vary by state. When a patient is admitted to the SICU, a specific inquiry should be made about such a document from the patient or someone who is next in line in decision-making.

Whether or not an advanced directive exists, a determination should be made about the treatment status of the patient, including whether or not resuscitation is desired or indicated, when a patient enters the SICU. When this status is not clear, a care conference should be held with the patient or the next responsible person to discuss and clarify the patient's wishes. Care conferences should also be held on a periodic basis to communicate patient status and to define and to clarify the patient's treatment plan.

DO NOT RESUSCITATE

"Do not resuscitate" is an expression used to describe the withholding of cardiopulmonary resuscitation (CPR) in the circumstance in which cardiac or respiratory arrest occurs. The interval between cardiac or pulmonary arrest

and initiation of CPR is a major determinant of outcome. For that reason, CPR is always initiated unless a written order preventing it is present in the chart. Because of terminology confusion in the area, a few definitions are necessary.

These definitions and the process and procedure of communicating a preference for no CPR vary from hospital to hospital; thus the policies and procedures of each institution should be consulted and followed.

Cardiopulmonary resuscitation. *CPR* is a treatment instituted to attempt to restore cardiac or respiratory function when cardiac or respiratory arrest has occurred. Three major components can be used: electric defibrillation, closed-chest cardiac compression, and manually or mechanically assisted ventilation.

No CPR. *No CPR* is a written order placed in the patient's chart when a determination has been made that CPR as defined will not be undertaken. This order does not preclude any other therapeutic intervention, including surgery, SICU care, or intubation outside the situation of cardiac or respiratory arrest.

Competency. *Competence* is a functional, legal concept relating to the patient's ability to understand, reflect on, and reiterate the medical situation, including the consequences of not receiving CPR. Competence is usually determined by the patient's physician.

Patient representative. A *patient representative* is a person who acts on behalf of the incompetent patient (sometimes referred to as a *surrogate decision-maker*). For a child, the patient representative is the child's parents or legal guardian. For adult patients, the usual order of priority is the proxy defined in the valid living will, the legal guardian, the spouse, an adult son or daughter, a parent, a sibling, a close family member, or a close personal friend. Variations in ranking may occur according to locality. The institutional attorney should be consulted whenever questions arise or clarification of the patient representative is necessary.

■　■　■

As with any patient intervention, the physician must determine whether CPR is medically indicated for a patient. The following are reasons to write a No-CPR order: (1) a competent patient gives explicit refusal; (2) for an incompetent patient, the patient representative gives explicit refusal; and (3) the attending physician determines that CPR is not medically indicated. This complex medical judgment should be communicated to other members of the health care team and, many physicians believe, to the patient's family at the time of informing the patient of the decision. Factors included in the assessment of this decision include long-term survival potential if CPR were administered, survival potential if CPR were administered and the patient survived the acute event, and the duration of cardiac arrest before initiation of CPR.

Once a determination of No-CPR status has been made, an order should be written in the chart along with a chart note describing the process, rationale, and decision-making. The note should be signed by the attending physician.

DECISIONS TO FOREGO LIFE-SUSTAINING TREATMENT

In some clinical situations the decision to forego life-sustaining treatment is appropriate. In this context no distinction is made between care withdrawal and the withholding of care. The process varies from institution to institution, and each physician should consult his/her own institution's policy or guidelines for this process. Several principles apply:

- The patient has the legal and ethical right of self-determination.
- When a patient is incompetent, decisions to forego life-sustaining treatments are made by the patient's representative.
- After a decision has been made to forego life-sustaining treatment, the patient shall continue to receive care that maintains dignity, comfort, and hygiene.
- Periodic review of the decision to forego life-sustaining treatment should be done to ensure that the decision remains consistent with the patient's status and wishes.
- If questions or concerns remain after a decision to forego life-sustaining treatment has been made, a mechanism should be available to discuss and resolve these concerns.
- Consideration should be given to the No-CPR status of the patient.

The primary decision-makers in this process are the patient, or patient representative if the patient is incompetent, and the attending physician. Throughout the process, communication and dialogue with health care personnel and family members are encouraged. When a decision has been reached concerning what treatments the patient will forego, documentation should be made in the patient's chart and clear orders written for the care plan. The documentation should include who the decision-makers were, the rationale for mental incompetence if it exists, what information was presented, and a summary of the specific decisions reached.

The care plan must be presented clearly in the care orders for the patient. These orders should itemize specifically what treatments will be withheld and/or discontinued and what medications will be administered. During the withdrawal or withholding process, the goal of treatment is to relieve pain and suffering to the extent consistent with the patient's wishes. Neuromuscular blocking agents are excluded from these medications. They are not analgesics, and their use precludes an assessment of the amount of pain and suffering that is present. Adequate doses of analgesics and sedatives should be used. Vital signs may be obtained to assess the patient's status in the dying process but should not influence decisions about administering medications in the presence of continued pain or other distressing symptoms for which the medication is an accepted treatment. The attending physician must document clearly in the patient's chart all clinical indications for administration of medication, including all dosage changes.

Because a wide variation exists from institution to institution in the policy to forego life-sustaining treatment, the physician must consult his/her own institution's policy and guidelines for this process.

SUMMARY

- Complete and accurate chart notes provide vital information to everyone concerned with a patient's care.
- Chart notes should reflect the thought behind a patient care plan and include information about preexisting disease, admitting reason, current medical status, a summary of the care plan, a statement of patient competency, complications, prognosis, a summary of care conference, and a clear description of physician services provided.
- Physician should ask whether patients have an advanced directive, a living will, at the earliest possible time.

- CPR includes manually or mechanically assisted ventilation, closed-chest cardiac compression, and electrical defibrillation. A No-CPR order means that these components will not be done. A No-CPR order does not preclude other medical care.
- A patient representative is a person who acts on behalf of the incompetent patient.
- In some clinical situations a decision to forego late sustaining treatment is appropriate under the circumstances, and no distinction is made between care withdrawal and withholding care.

BIBLIOGRAPHY

University of Minnesota Hospital and Clinic Policy 16.4. Making Decisions to Forego Cardiopulmonary Resuscitation. Minneapolis, 1992.

University of Minnesota Hospital and Clinic Policy 4.7. Making Patient Care Decisions to Forego Life-Sustaining Treatment. Minneapolis, 1992.

INDEX

A

A-aDo$_2$; *see* Alveolar-arterial oxygen tension difference
A blood group, 473-474
AB blood group, 473-474
Abdomen
  acute, 374-383
  injured patient and, 42-43
Abdominal cavity
  anatomy and physiology of, 419
  paracentesis and, 537
Abdominal injury, 45-46
Abdominal pain
  acute abdomen and, 374-375
  adrenal insufficiency and, 398
  nonsurgical causes of, 381
  pancreatitis and, 366
  surgically treatable causes of, 380
Abdominal radiography
  acute abdomen and, 378
  secondary peritonitis and, 421
Abdominal surgery
  peritoneal dialysis patient and, 85
  pulmonary embolism and, 114
    prophylaxis for, 123
  pulmonary risk and, 92
Abdominal thrust, 60
Abdominal visceral injury, thoracostomy and, 535
Abductor pollicis brevis muscle, spinal cord injuries and, 205
ABG analysis; *see* Arterial blood gas analysis
ABO blood groups
  hemolytic transfusion reaction and, 476
  transfusions and, 473-474
Abscess
  airway management in, 102
  intra-abdominal, 422-424
  multiple system organ failure and, 7
Absence seizures, 181
Absence status epilepticus, 184
Absorption atelectasis, 213
Absorption of drugs, 146-147
Acalculous cholecystitis, 381-382

ACE inhibitors; *see* Angiotensin-converting enzyme inhibitors
Acetabulum fracture, 391-394
Acetazolamide, hyperphosphatemia and, 414
Acetyl-CoA, hyperlactatemia and, 30
Acetylcysteine, bronchospasm and, 296
Acid-base homeostasis, 317-329
  arterial blood gas analysis and, 317-320
  metabolic acid-base disorders and, 320-325
  respiratory acid-base disorders and, 325-329
Acidemia
  hyperlactatemia and, 31
  sodium bicarbonate and, 63
Acidosis
  acute renal failure and, 337
  calcium and, 405
  definition of, 318
  lactic, 30-33
  metabolic, 320-323
  respiratory, 326, 328
    sodium bicarbonate and, 63
Acquired immunodeficiency syndrome, 427-436
  transfusions and, 477
Acromegaly, airway management in, 103
ACTH; *see* Adrenocorticotropic hormone
Actinomyces israelii, immunocompromised patient and, 495
Activated complement, anaphylaxis and, 448, 449
Active range of motion, 142-143
Acute abdomen, 374-383
Acute cortical necrosis, 331
Acute disseminated intravascular coagulation, 465-466
Acute hepatitis, 74-75
Acute lung injury
  causes and management of, 284-291
  time course of, 309-310

Acute mesenteric ischemia, 382
Acute pancreatitis, 364-365
Acute phase of lung injury
  causes and management of, 287, 288
  time course of, 309-310
Acute renal failure
  diagnosis and treatment of, 331-339
  pancreatitis and, 371
  surgical patient and, 80-85
Acute subdural hematoma, 195
Acute tubular necrosis
  causes of, 333-334
  definition of, 331
  differentiating from renal failure and, 333
  surgical patient and, 80
ACV; *see* Assist control ventilation
Acyclovir
  herpesviruses and, 432
  immunocompromised patient and, 498-500
  renal impairment and, 149
  serum concentration of, 153
Acylampicillins, immunocompromised patient and, 496
Adducted contracture, 143
Adductors, spinal cord injuries and, 205
Adenosine
  atrioventricular nodal reentry tachycardia and, 238
  dysrhythmias and, 233
Adenosine deaminase, nutritional support and, 25
Adenosine triphosphate, hyperlactatemia and, 31
Adjusted-dose heparin, 121
Administration route of nutritional support, 24
Adrenal hemorrhage, 398
Adrenal insufficiency, 397-399
Adrenalin; *see* Epinephrine
Adrenergic agonists, bronchospasm and, 294, 295
Adrenocortical response to surgical stress or trauma, 482